Atlas of Reconstructive Surgery: A Case-Based Approach

Atlas of Reconstructive Surgery: A Case-Based Approach

Lee L.Q. Pu, MD, PhD, FACS, FICS

Professor of Plastic Surgery
Division of Plastic Surgery
University of California, Davis
Sacramento, California, USA

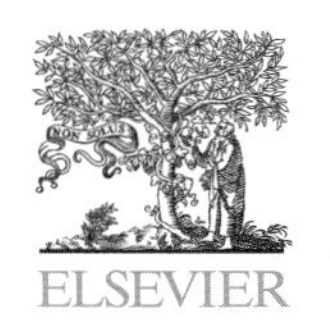
ELSEVIER

Elsevier
1600 John F. Kennedy Blvd.
Ste 1800
Philadelphia, PA 19103-2899

ATLAS OF RECONSTRUCTIVE SURGERY: A CASE-BASED APPROACH ISBN: 978-0-323-87553-0

ISBN: 978-0-323-87553-0

Content Strategist: Belinda Kuhn
Senior Content Development Specialist: Priyadarshini Pandey
Publishing Services Manager: Shereen Jameel
Project Manager: Nadhiya Sekar
Design Direction: Ryan Cook
Medical Illustrator: Sarah St. Claire

Printed in India
Last digit is the print number: 9 8 7 6 5 4 3 2 1

Dedications

To my wife, Yu-Shan (Emily), and my children, Felix, Dustin, and Adrian, whose love, sacrifices, understanding, and unselfish support have made editing and writing this book possible.

To my parents and my younger brother, who have supported me for all these years and have trusted me to pursue my dream to become an excellent plastic surgeon through more than a decade's effort.

To my professors and teachers who inspired me throughout my surgical education to set up a higher standard in my career and to work harder to achieve it.

To my worldwide friends and colleagues in plastic surgery who have made so many remarkable contributions to our specialty and have consistently encouraged me to do the same.

Lee L.Q. Pu, MD, PhD, FACS, FICS

Foreword

In an effort to share a senior surgeon's lifelong experience, Dr. Pu collected his cases from serving in academic institutions to provide a "grand rounds" flavor in managing complex problems in plastic surgery reconstructive practice. Although case reports are relegated to Level 5 evidence, they are still valuable because each case exemplifies plastic surgery principles to deduce a complex problem into manageable forms. The articulate approach in this textbook shares the journey through the lens of a senior surgeon whose vast reconstructive experience is distilled and promoted to the next generation. In most philosophies, a master conducts seminars whereby he or she shares one's life experience for the disciples. Using the similar teaching method, Dr. Pu strives to mentor others in his unique approach to solving complex defects for the vestige of the last general surgeon that defines our specialty. In this era of super specialization in which each plastic surgeon assumes an anatomic territory to master, it's equally important for our trainees to be well equipped to deal with multitude of problems throughout the body, which makes Plastic Surgery such an enticing profession in fluidity of creativity.

I congratulate Dr. Pu for this most arduous endeavor to share generously his vast experience to the world. I look forward to receiving this book so that I can learn from his remarkable voyage in our cherished field of Plastic Surgery.

Kevin C. Chung, MD, MS
Charles D. G. de Nancrede Professor of Surgery
Chief of Hand Surgery, Michigan Medicine
Professor, Plastic and Orthopaedic Surgery
Assistant Dean for Faculty Affairs
Associate Director of Global REACH
University of Michigan
Ann Arbor, Michigan
USA
Editor-in-Chief
Plastic and Reconstructive Surgery

Acknowledgments

I wish to express my gratitude to Belinda Kuhn and her entire publishing team from Elsevier, Inc. I am especially grateful that Elsevier, a world-renowned medical publisher, agreed to publish my personal Atlas in Reconstructive Plastic Surgery. Belinda is an incredible woman who can deliver unparalleled service in medical publishing. Under her leadership, this book project started with the table of contents, completing each chapter, editing and re-editing, until it has been well done. It has been my great pleasure and privilege to work with Belinda and her publishing team. They have ensured the best possible quality of each chapter and this Atlas could not be successful without the effort and hard work by such an amazing team.

I have been very fortunate to hold a full-time academic position at the University of Kentucky, in Lexington, Kentucky (2000—2007) and University of California Davis, in Sacramento, California (2007—present). These two renowned institutions have superb faculty, resident, nursing, and support staff. Many of my former and current faculty associates have created an intellectually stimulating environment for me to write and edit such an atlas in plastic surgery. Many of my former and current faculty colleagues have helped cover my patients while I was concentrating on writing the chapters or attending meetings. I would like to thank my previous administrative assistant, Mrs. Delia Luna, for her tireless administrative support in preparation of manuscripts for the atlas and the photographer from the department, Mr. Manny Dial, for his valuable help with many intraoperative photos for the atlas. I would also like to express my special appreciation to Sarah St. Claire, RN, MS, a certified medical illustrator, for her expertise creating the many schematic drawings used in the atlas.

Finally, I wish to express my heartfelt gratitude to my wife, Yu-Shan (Emily), who has supported me for all these years during my academic career and has kept everything in order at home so that I can concentrate on my work for this project in the late evenings and weekends, to my sons, Felix, Dustin, and Adrian, who have taught me the joy of life outside of work, and my younger brother, Lijun (Leo), who has always encouraged me to take on a difficult task. I also wish to express my gratitude and respect to my former professors and training program directors, Dr. Zhong-Gao Wang, Dr. James F. Symes, Dr. Marvin A. McMillan, and Dr. Thomas J. Krizek. With their inspiration, I have been able to write successfully this atlas. I also wish to express my gratitude to my worldwide friends and colleagues in plastic surgery who have encouraged and supported me during this book project.

Lee L.Q. Pu, MD, PhD, FACS, FICS

Contents

Section 1: Head and Neck

Section 2: Shoulder and Upper Extremity

Section 3: Chest, Abdomen, and Back

Section 4: Pelvis, Groin, Sacrum, Buttock, Perineum and Genitals

Section 5: Lower Extremity

SECTION 1

Head and Neck

1

Scalp Reconstruction

CASE 1

Clinical Presentation

An 85-year-old White male with recurrent squamous cell carcinoma of his central scalp underwent additional surgical excision of the scalp including deep margin by the surgical oncology service. Once the peripheral and deep margin assessments by intraoperative frozen sections confirmed cancer was not present, the patient had a 10 × 7 cm full-thickness scalp defect with exposed skull. In the central part of the defect, a portion of the outer table of the skull was also removed (Fig. 1.1).

Operative Plan and Special Considerations

After assessing his available scalp donor sites including the quality of his remaining scalp tissue and possible blood supply for the design of a large scalp rotation flap, it was decided that the flap could be designed based on the left occipital vessels.

Operative Procedures

The patient was placed in a prone position. The left occipital vessels were easily identified using a pencil Doppler and were used as the pedicle of a large posteriorly based scalp rotation flap (Fig. 1.2). The flap design was marked and all the proposed scalp incisions were infiltrated with 1% lidocaine with 1:100,000 epinephrine.

The procedure to free the periosteum from the subgaleal space was started within the scalp defect. The large scalp rotation flap was then elevated after incision of the scalp with knife and electrocautery. Elevation in the subgaleal space and an adequate rotation of flap to the defect were accomplished. During dissection, the contralateral side of the occipital vessel was divided in order to have more freedom of rotation. The flap was inset into the defect and secured temporarily with skin staples. The scalp flap donor site was covered with a meshed split-thickness skin graft harvested from the right lateral thigh (Fig. 1.3). A 10 flat JP was inserted under the flap and the closure was performed in two layers. The deep dermal layer was approximated with several interrupted 3-0 Monocryl sutures and the skin was approximated with staples (Fig. 1.4). The "dog ear" in the proximal flap was trimmed away from the flap and also approximated with skin staples (Fig. 1.5). The pedicle vessels were easily identified with a pencil Doppler at the end of procedure. The skin graft site was covered with Xeroform, bacitracin ointment, fluffs, and a VAC sponge, which was secured with multiple skin staples.

Follow-Up Results

The patient did well postoperatively without complications related to the flap reconstruction. He was discharged from the hospital on postoperative day 5. The drain was removed during the first week after discharge. His scalp flap reconstruction and skin graft sites healed uneventfully (Figs. 1.6—1.8).

Final Outcome

The patient's scalp flap reconstruction and skin graft sites healed well. He returned to his normal life and activities and no local recurrence was found during a 1-year follow-up.

Pearls for Success

The design of a large scalp rotation flap should be based on a vascular pedicle that would provide a more consistent and reliable blood supply to the flap. Depending on the location of the scalp defect, such a design can be based on the location of any vessels that provide blood supply to the normal scalp. The pedicle vessels can be easily identified by a pencil Doppler. Scoring the galea under the flap may expand the flap tissue and make the flap inset easier and its closure less difficult. The excess tissue in the proximal aspect of the flap can be excised on the nonflap site and by doing so, the "dog ear" can be safely excised primarily without compromising the blood supply to the flap.

CASE 2

Clinical Presentation

A 65-year-old White female had a scalp melanoma and underwent wide local excision of her occipitoparietal scalp lesion with a 1.5 cm margin after sentinel lymph node biopsy by the surgical oncology service (Fig. 1.9). She had a 3.5 × 3.5 cm scalp defect down to the periosteum (Fig. 1.10). The plastic surgery service was asked to perform a scalp reconstruction to repair the scalp defect.

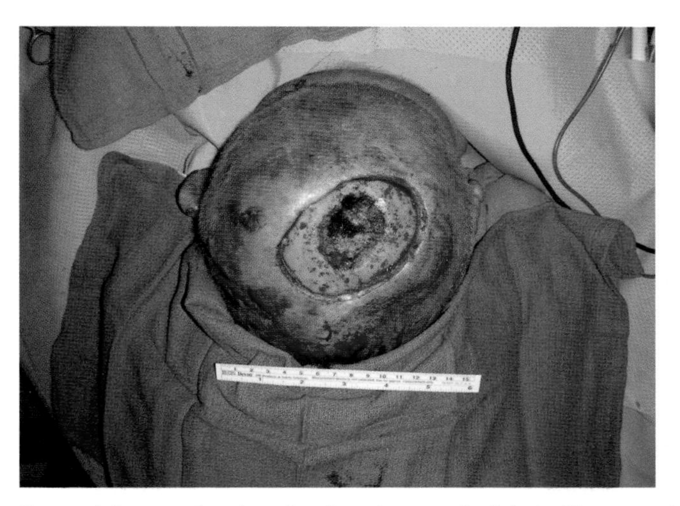

• **Fig. 1.1** Intraoperative view showing a large scalp defect with exposed skull after excision by the surgical oncology service.

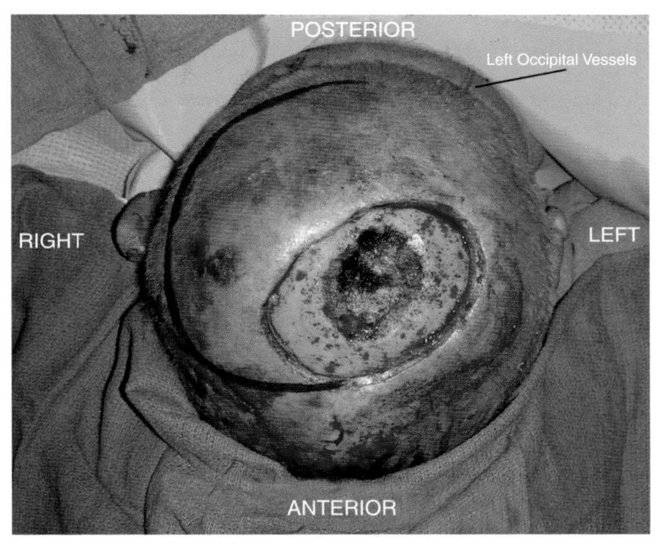

• **Fig. 1.2** Intraoperative view showing the design of a large posterior scalp rotation flap based on the left occipital vessels.

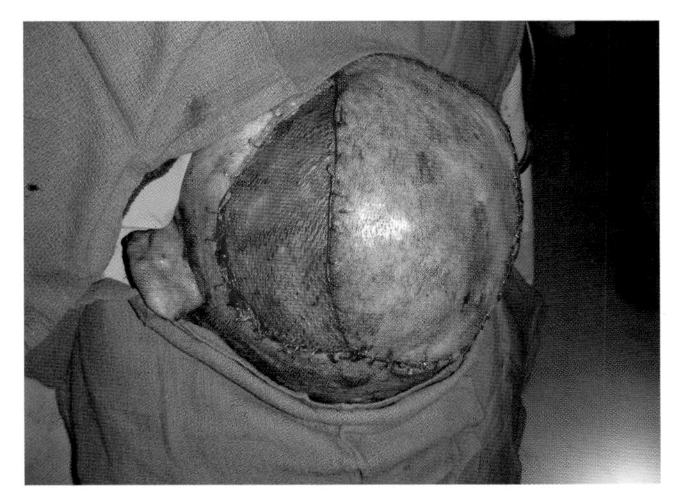

• **Fig. 1.3** Intraoperative view showing the completion of the large scalp rotation flap closure and skin grafted flap donor site.

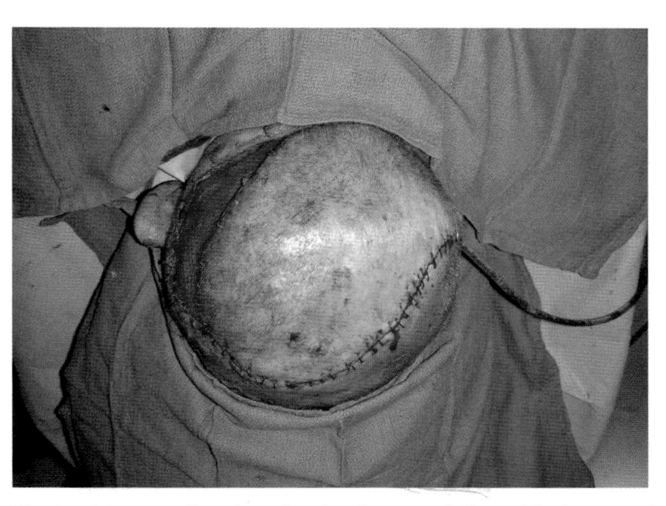

• **Fig. 1.4** Intraoperative view showing the completion of the large scalp rotation flap closure with a proper inset of the entire flap.

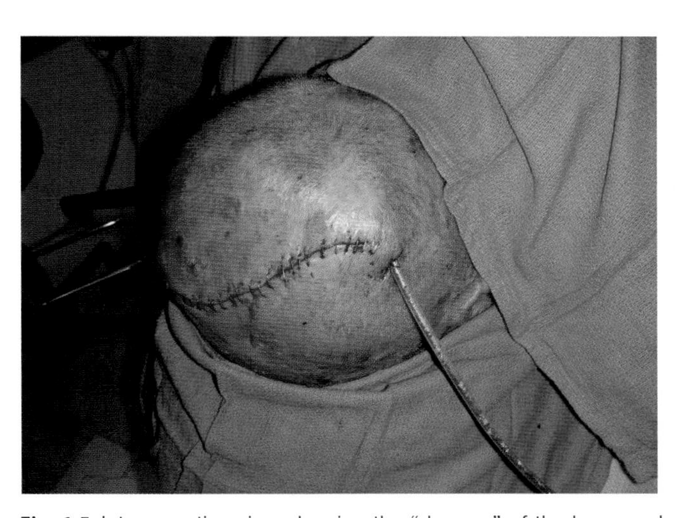

• **Fig. 1.5** Intraoperative view showing the "dog ear" of the large scalp rotation flap was reduced and closed toward nonflap site scalp as a one-stage procedure.

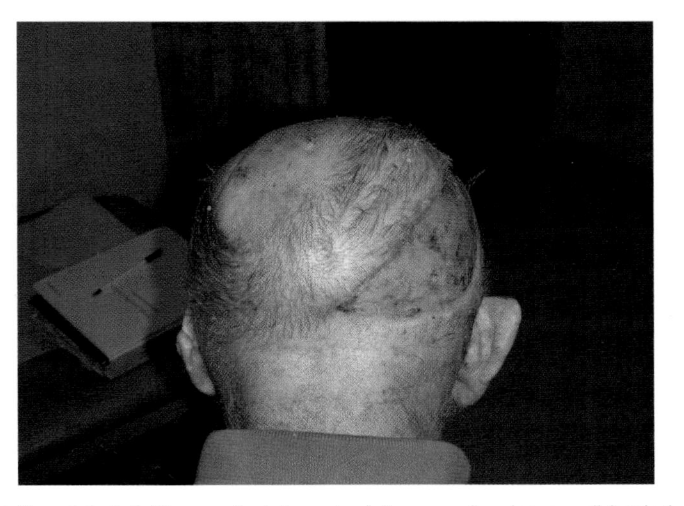

• **Figs. 1.6–1.8** The result at 4 weeks follow-up showing a well-healed scalp flap and skin graft sites.

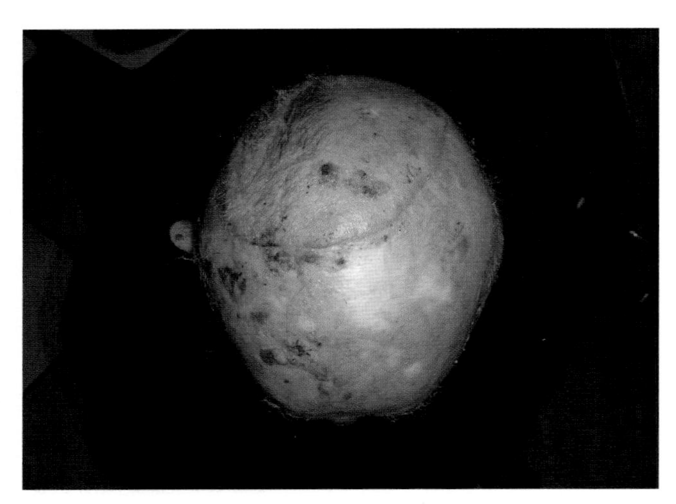

• **Figs. 1.6–1.8 cont'd**

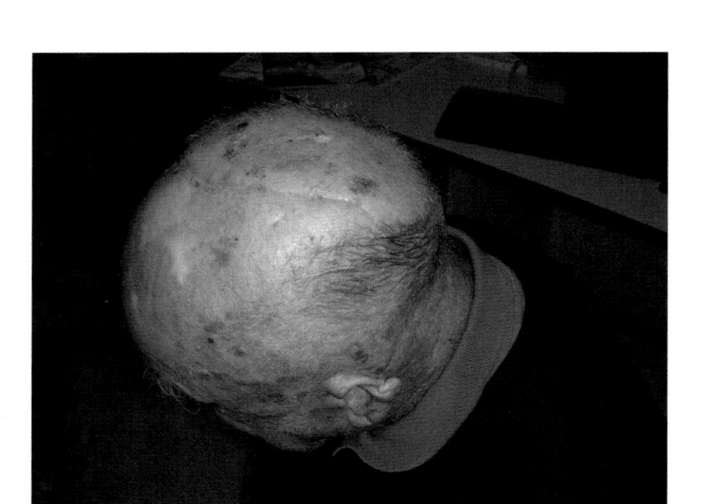

• **Figs. 1.6–1.8 cont'd**

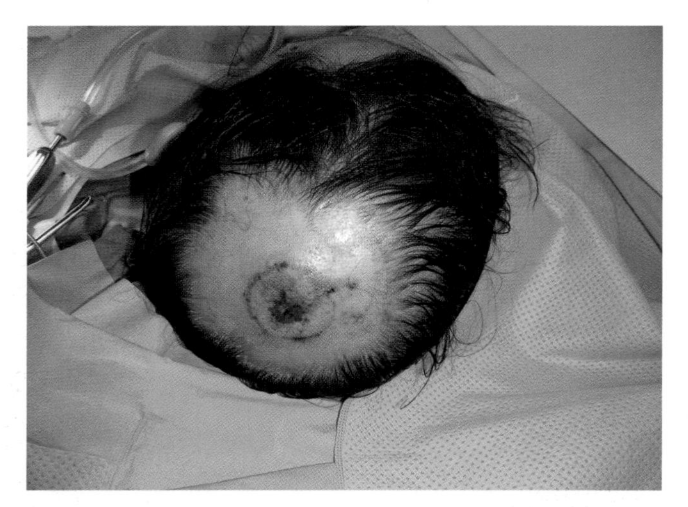

• **Fig. 1.9** Intraoperative view showing a large scalp melanoma after blue dye injection for sentinel lymph node biopsy by the surgical oncology service.

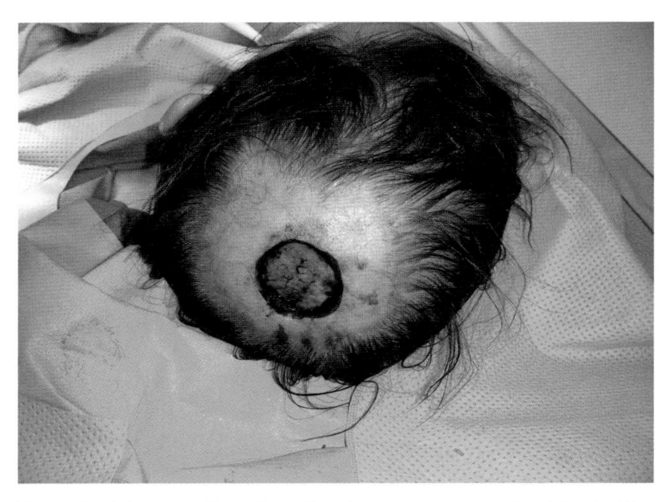

• **Fig. 1.10** Intraoperative view showing a sizable scalp defect after a wide local excision by the surgical oncology service.

Operative Plan and Special Considerations

Based on the size and shape of the scalp defect, bilateral rotation and advancement flaps (Yin-Yang flaps) were designed for this patient because the size of the defect was moderate and the shape of the defect was circular. In this way, her scalp defect could be closed primarily and no skin graft was needed. In addition, alopecia of the scalp after such a reconstruction could be avoided.

Operative Procedures

The bilateral scalp rotation and advancement (Yin-Yang) flaps were designed and marked (Fig. 1.11). Each flap was designed large enough to close this circular defect without changing hair-line style. All proposed incisions were infiltrated with 1% lido-caine with 1:100,000 epinephrine. The subgaleal dissection was

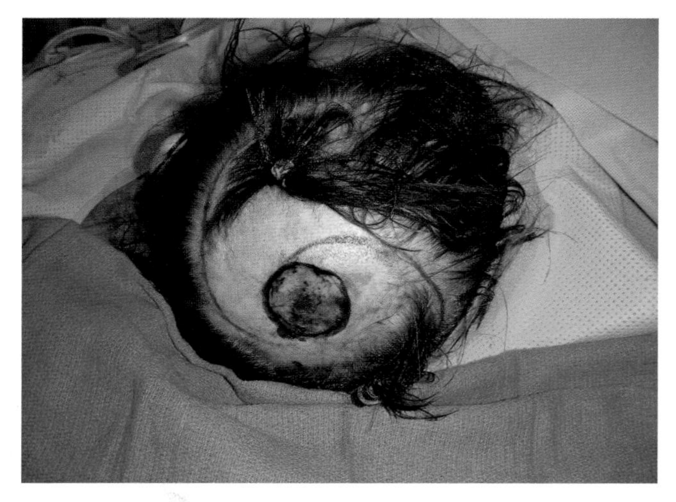

• **Fig. 1.11** Intraoperative view showing the design of bilateral rotation and advancement scalp flaps (Yin-Yang flaps).

then performed first inside the defect to raise more than half of the flap on each side. After that the incision was performed to raise the designed scalp flap on each side. Each flap was raised in half of the circular fashion so that it could be rotated and advanced into the defect and approximated in the midline of the circular defect. The extensive undermining was performed from the nonflap side scalp in order to close each flap's donor site. The scoring under the galea was done so that a relatively tension-free closure could be achieved. Excess scalp tissue of each flap was trimmed and the donor site was closed with several interrupted skin staples. A 7-mm JP drain was inserted under both flaps and a final scalp closure was completed in two layers with interrupted 3-0 PDS sutures for deep closure and the rest of the incision with multiple skin staples or interrupted 3-0 Prolene sutures (Fig. 1.12).

Follow-Up Results

The patient did well postoperatively without any complications related to the flap reconstruction. She was discharged from the hospital on postoperative day 2. The drain was removed during the first week follow-up visit. Her scalp flap sites healed well (Figs. 1.13 and 1.14).

Final Outcome

The scalp flap sites healed well. The patient returned to her normal activities and no local recurrence was identified during follow-up.

Pearls for Success

Each Yin-Yang flap should be designed as a rotation/advancement flap that can cover half of the circular defect. The subgaleal dissection is performed first within the defect on each side to facilitate scalp flap dissection. Scoring the galea under each flap is helpful for a closure with less tension. Extensive undermining of nonflap scalp should be performed to allow primary closure of each flap's donor site.

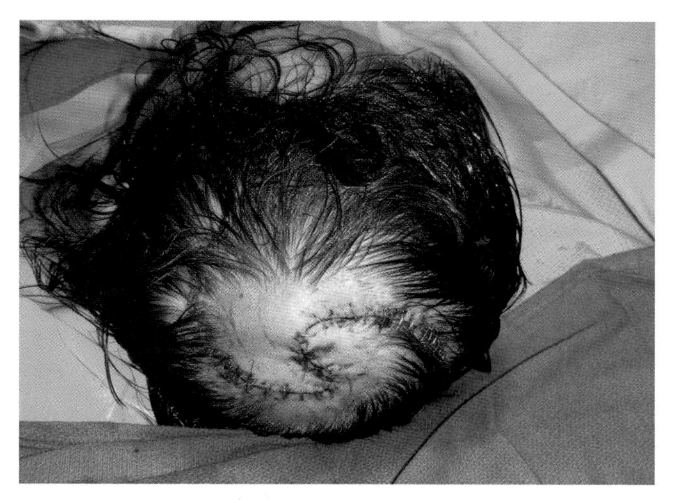

• **Fig. 1.12** Intraoperative view showing the closure of bilateral rotation and advancement scalp flaps (Yin-Yang flaps).

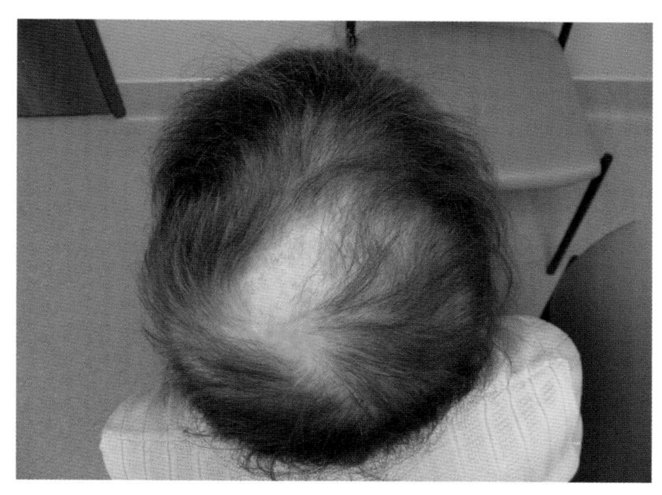

• **Figs. 1.13 and 1.14** The result at 4-month follow-up showing well-healed bilateral rotation and advancement scalp flap sites.

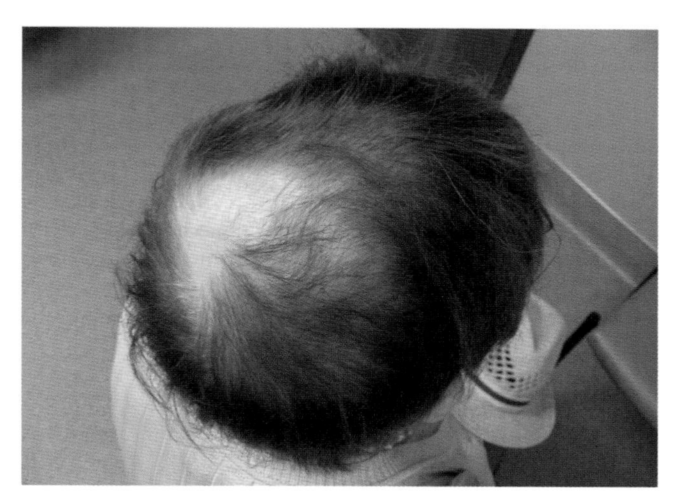

• **Figs. 1.13 and 1.14 cont'd**

CASE 3

Clinical Presentation

A 69-year-old White male with recurrent squamous cell cancer of his scalp had previous radiation and additional resection. The patient had developed a scalp wound with exposed skull. Several local reconstructive procedures were unsuccessfully attempted including Integra placement and local scalp rotation flap. He had a small scalp wound with exposed skull and had returned to his workplace in another state. One day ago, the patient was admitted to the neurosurgical service with subdural empyema. He was urgently taken to the operating room by our neurosurgeon for urgent debridement of the infected and necrotic skull and drainage of subdural empyema (Fig. 1.15). The plastic surgery service was asked to perform an emergency scalp reconstruction after neurosurgical procedures in the same setting.

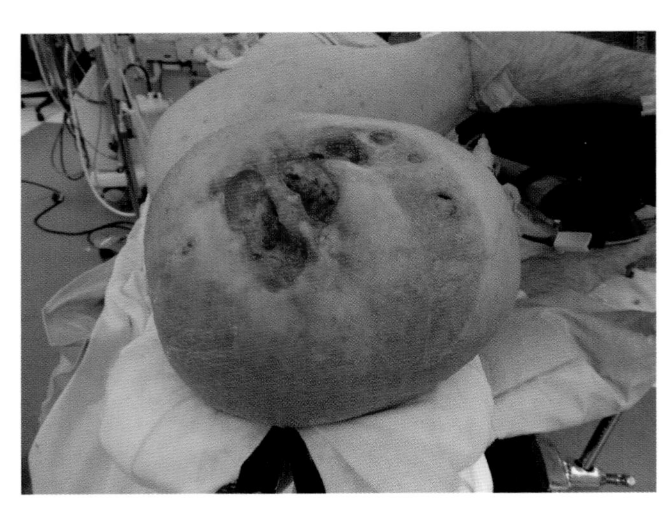

• **Fig. 1.15** Intraoperative view showing "infected" scalp wound and underlying skull.

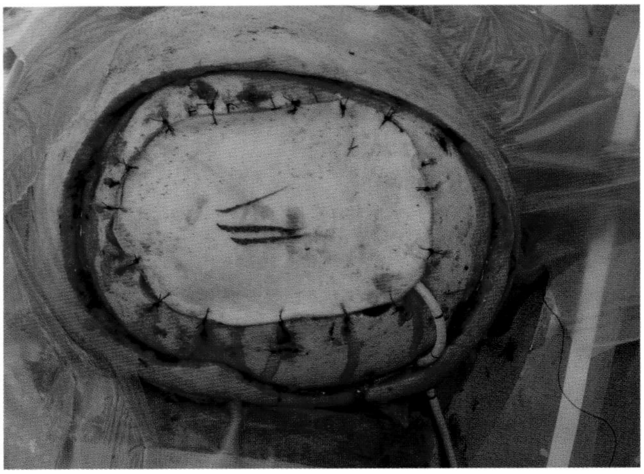

Operative Plan and Special Considerations

Because of the size of potential scalp defect after craniotomy by the neurosurgeon and clear clinical evidence of subdural infection as well as an emergency scalp reconstruction, a free latissimus dorsi muscle flap was selected for his scalp reconstruction. The latissimus flap is reliable and large enough to cover a large scalp wound. In addition, it has a long pedicle that can reach even facial vessels for microvascular anastomoses. A biological mesh, acellular dermal matrix (Strattice) was selected because of its biological nature and some rigidity.

Operative Procedures

After all neurosurgical procedures were completed, the scalp wound measured 18 × 15 cm and the skull defect measured 11 × 7 cm (Fig. 1.16). The skull defect was repaired first with Strattice. A large piece of Strattice was trimmed to 11 × 7 cm and with dermal side up, it was laid on the dural repair and secured with multiple 3-0 PDS sutures (Fig. 1.17).

Based on duplex scan finding, the superior temporal artery and vein were dissected next. A 5-cm preauricular incision was made through the skin, the subcutaneous tissue, and the SMAS layer down to the superficial temporal vessels (Fig. 1.18). Under loupe magnification, adequate length of both artery and vein were dissected free.

With an oblique incision, the latissimus dorsi muscle was first exposed (Fig. 1.19). Once the lateral border of the muscle was identified, the dissection was done to elevate the muscle off the chest wall. The muscle's attachment to the posterior iliac crest was divided under direct vision. The muscle was then elevated from its lateral, inferior, and also medial borders. The pedicle dissection was performed toward the axilla. The muscle attachment to the humerus was divided. With proper traction, the thoracodorsal nerve was dissected and divided, and the thoracodorsal artery and vein were dissected free and then divided with hemoclips from the

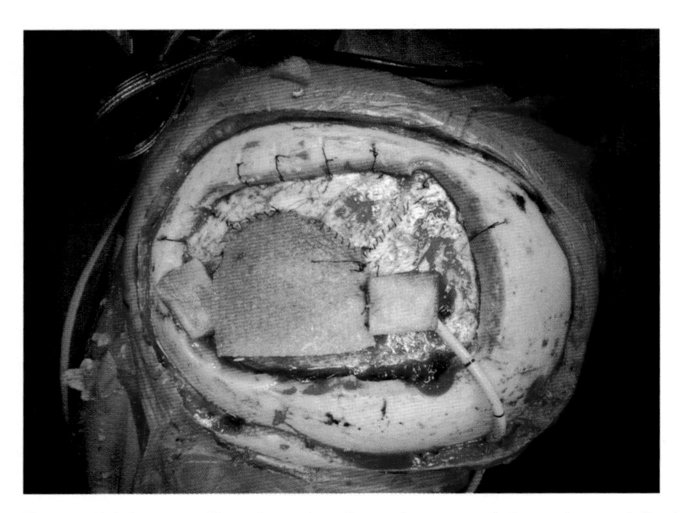

• **Fig. 1.16** Intraoperative view showing a large craniotomy bony defect associated with a large scalp defect after debridement and drainage of the subdural empyema by the neurosurgery service. The dura was also repaired by the same service.

• **Fig. 1.17** Intraoperative view showing the closure of the craniotomy skull defect with acellular dermal matrix mesh.

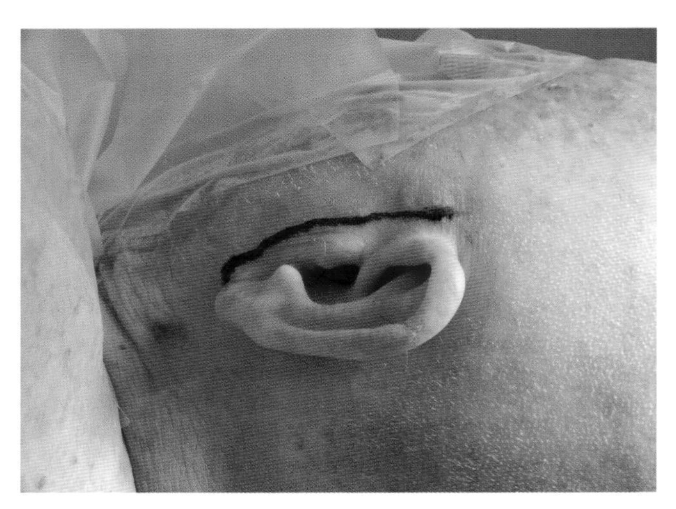

• **Fig. 1.18** Intraoperative view showing the design of a preauricular skin incision for exposure of the superficial temporal vessels for microvascular anastomoses.

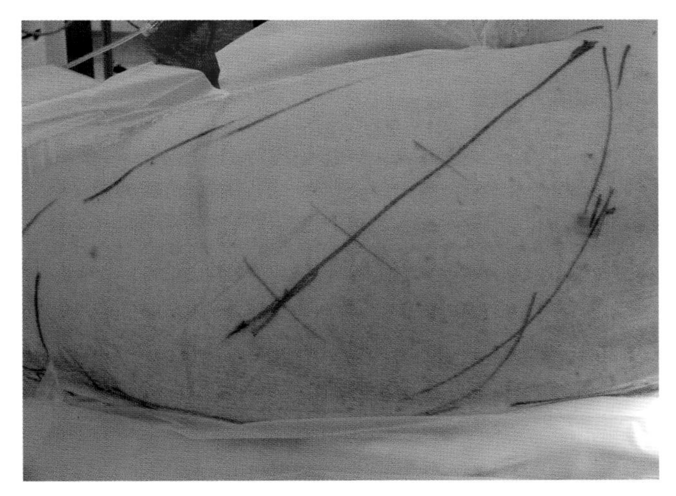

• **Fig. 1.19** Intraoperative view showing the design of the incision for the free latissimus dorsi muscle harvest.

subscapular vessels. The surgical dissection of a free latissimus dorsi flap was completed (Fig. 1.20).

The thoracodorsal artery and vein of the flap was prepared under loupe magnification. The pedicle vessels were flushed with heparinized saline solution. The muscle flap was temporarily inset into the scalp defect and a tunnel was made between the left preauricular area and scalp wound. Both pedicle vessels were then tunneled under the scalp and placed near the superficial temporal vessels.

Under a microscope, the superficial temporal vessels and the pedicle vessels were prepared further. The superficial temporal artery and vein were divided with hemoclips at the level of the tragus. The arterial microanastomosis was performed in an end-to-end fashion with interrupted 8-0 nylon sutures. For the venous microanastomosis, a 3-mm coupler device was used for an end-to-end anastomosis. Once all clamps were released, the muscle flap appeared to be well perfused with no sign of venous congestion. A Cook Doppler probe was placed on the pedicle artery distal to the arterial anastomosis.

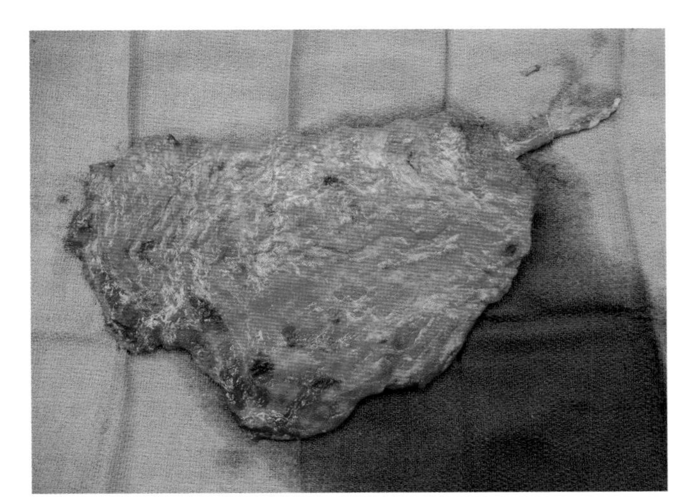

• **Fig. 1.20** Intraoperative view showing completion of the harvested free latissimus dorsi muscle flap.

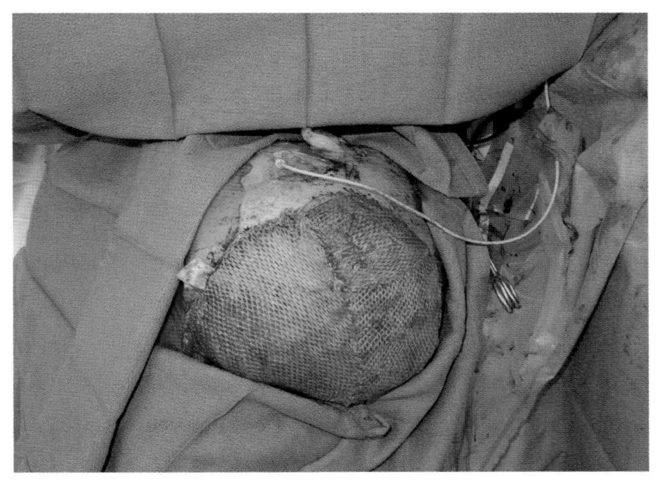

• **Fig. 1.21** Intraoperative view showing completion of a free skin-grafted latissimus dorsi muscle flap scalp reconstruction.

The preauricular incision was loosely approximated with several skin staples. The left latissimus dorsi muscle flap donor site was closed in two layers after placement of two drains.

The final inset of the latissimus dorsi muscle flap was performed after excess flap tissue had been excised. The flap was inset into the scalp defect with 3-0 Monocryl sutures in a half-buried horizontal mattress fashion. A Penrose drain was also inserted under the flap. A meshed split-thick skin graft was placed over the muscle flap (Fig. 1.21).

Management of Complications

The patient did well postoperatively and there were no flap-related complications. He was discharged home on postoperative day 7. Both the scalp reconstruction site and the flap donor site healed nicely. Unfortunately, he developed recurrent subdural empyema 5 months later (Fig. 1.22). He was urgently taken to the operating room by the neurosurgery service (Fig. 1.23). The well-healed latissimus muscle flap was reelevated by the plastic surgery

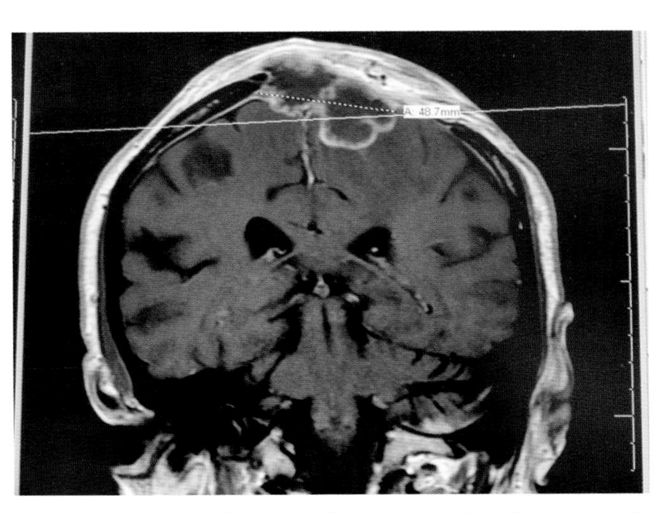

• **Fig. 1.22** A preoperative magnetic resonance imaging examination showing recurrent subdural empyema.

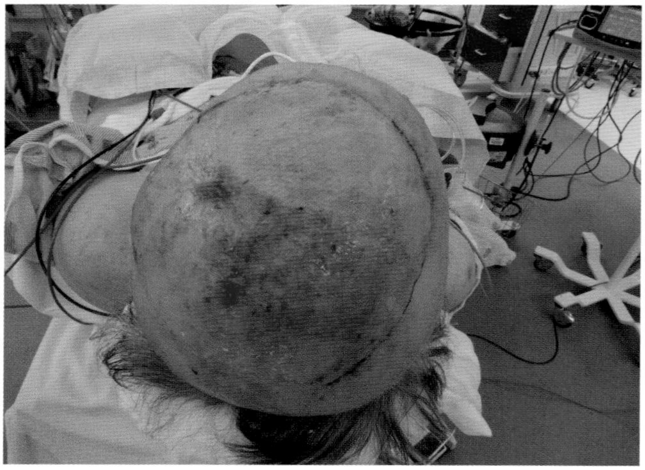

• **Fig. 1.23** Intraoperative view showing the design of elevation for well-healed free latissimus dorsi muscle flap.

service and the subdural empyema was debrided and drained after removal of previously placed Strattice (Fig. 1.24). The latissimus dorsi muscle flap was reinset with multiple half-buried horizontal mattress sutures (Fig. 1.25).

Follow-Up Results

The patient did well again postoperatively without any complications related to the free latissimus dorsi muscle flap reconstruction. He was discharged from the hospital on postoperative day 5. The drain was removed during a follow-up visit. His scalp flap reconstruction site again healed well (Fig. 1.26).

Final Outcome

The free latissimus dorsi muscle flap site healed well. The patient has resumed his normal activities and is followed by the neurosurgery service.

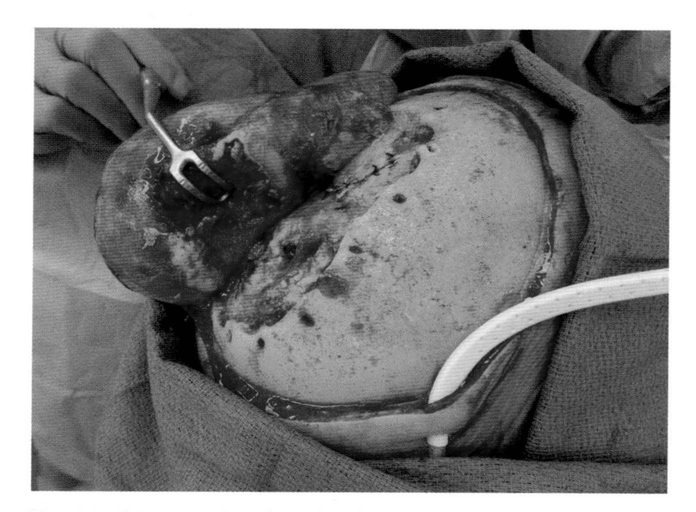

• **Fig. 1.24** Intraoperative view showing the completion of debridement and drainage of subdural empyema during reoperation.

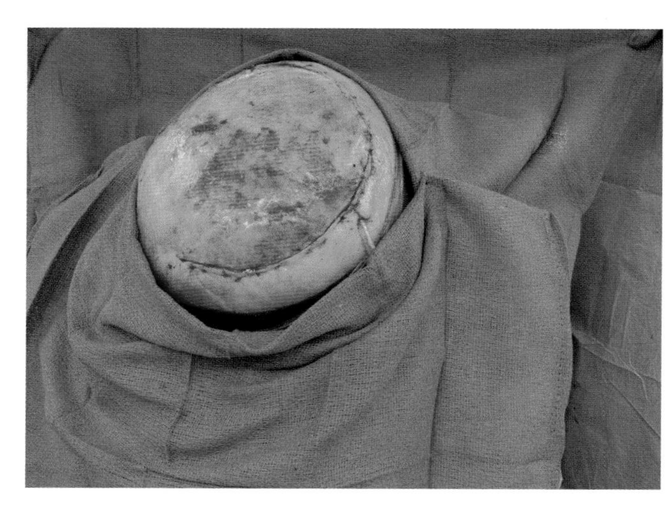

• **Fig. 1.25** Intraoperative view showing the completion of the second inset for the free latissimus dorsi muscle flap.

Pearls for Success

A free latissimus dorsi muscle is a large and reliable flap to reconstruct a large scalp defect. It has a long pedicle and can be harvested relatively fast in case an emergency free flap surgery is required. It should still be considered the flap of choice for scalp reconstruction when there is infection. Preoperative evaluation of the superficial temporal artery and vein with duplex scan should be performed if possible so that a better recipient vessel with adequate size of both artery and vein can be selected for relatively easier microvascular anastomoses. A near total flap reelevation could be safely performed with attention to the location of the pedicle vessels.

CASE 4

Clinical Presentation

An 86-year-old White male had scalp squamous cell cancer and had previously undergone excision and radiation to the area. He

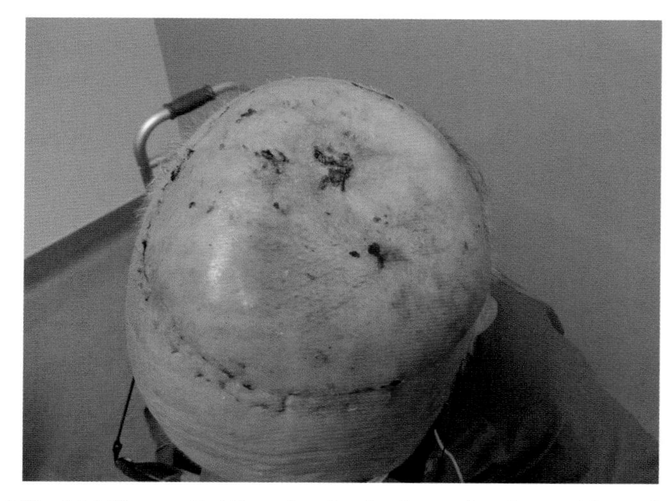

• **Fig. 1.26** The result at 3 weeks after the flap reelevation and 6 months after initial flap scalp reconstruction showing a well-healed free flap site.

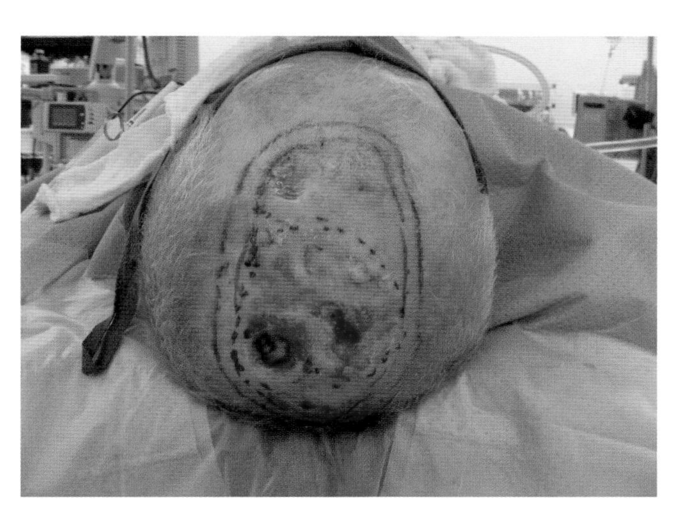

• **Fig. 1.27** Intraoperative view showing the extent of extensive scalp squamous cell cancer and ulcerated wounds with exposed skull. The *dotted line* indicating the outline of the scalp resection and the *solid line* indicating additional peripheral margins.

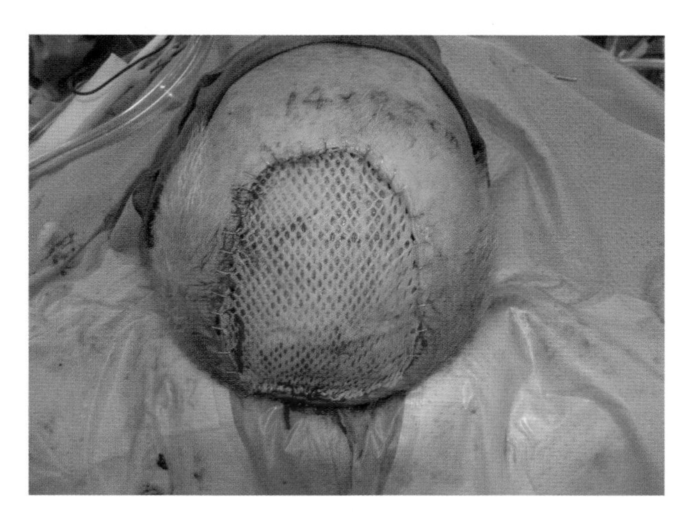

• **Fig. 1.29** Intraoperative view showing temporary coverage with an allo skin graft for the scalp defect while waiting for results from the permanent sections.

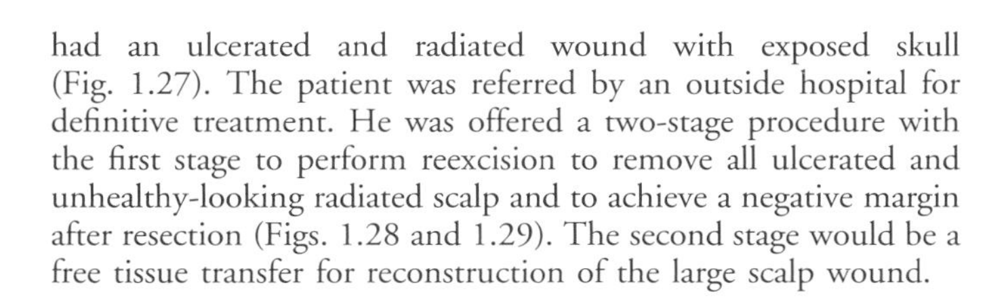

had an ulcerated and radiated wound with exposed skull (Fig. 1.27). The patient was referred by an outside hospital for definitive treatment. He was offered a two-stage procedure with the first stage to perform reexcision to remove all ulcerated and unhealthy-looking radiated scalp and to achieve a negative margin after resection (Figs. 1.28 and 1.29). The second stage would be a free tissue transfer for reconstruction of the large scalp wound.

Operative Plan and Special Considerations

Once a negative margin was confirmed by permanent section after reexcision of his ulcerated and radiated scalp wound, a free anterolateral thigh (ALT) perforator flap was offered to this patient to reconstruct the large scalp defect (15 × 12 cm) after definitive resection of scalp squamous cell cancer as well as radiated scalp tissue (Fig. 1.30). The superficial temporal vessels on both sides were evaluated by duplex scan to determine which side would be a better recipient site for microvascular anastomoses. In addition, perforators in each thigh's potential donor site were also mapped by duplex scan so that a preferred site for harvesting a free ALT perforator flap could be decided. A preoperative medical evaluation was also performed by the anesthesia preoperative clinic because of the patient's advanced age.

Operative Procedures

The left ALT perforator flap was selected based on the findings from preoperative duplex scan perforator mapping. The flap was designed based on a single large perforator with potential less extensive intramuscular dissection. A 27 × 11 cm skin paddle was designed and centered to this major perforator over the left ALT donor site (Fig. 1.31). The perforator was confirmed with a pencil Doppler. During elevation of the skin paddle, the fascia was incorporated as a fasciocutaneous flap. Several other less important

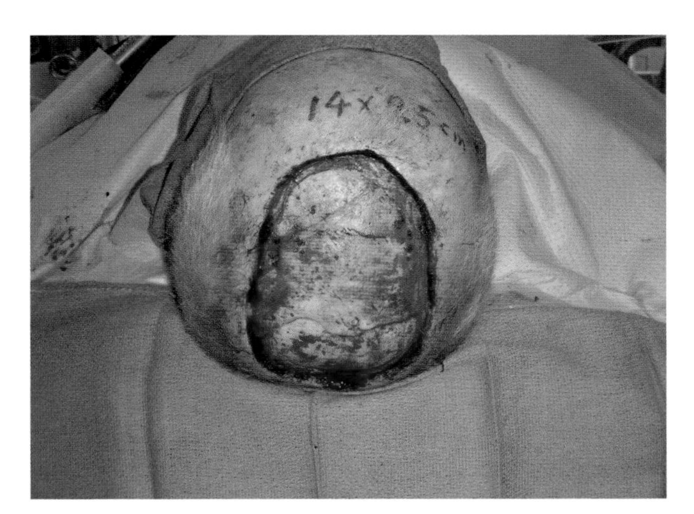

• **Fig. 1.28** Intraoperative view showing the extensive scalp defect after resection.

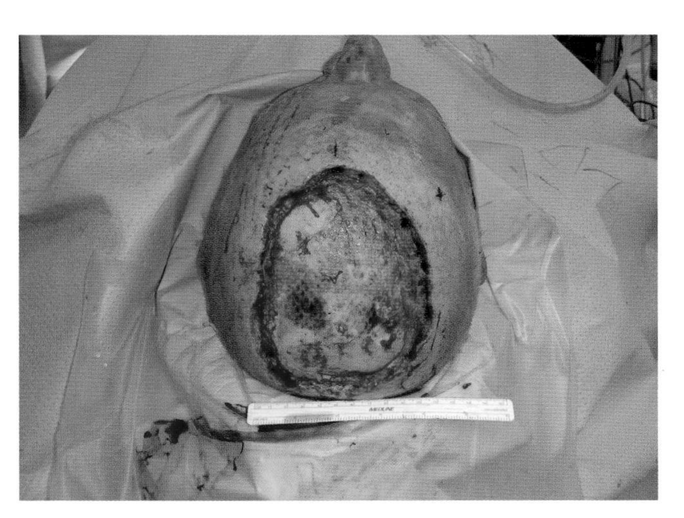

• **Fig. 1.30** Intraoperative view showing the extensive scalp defect after additional resection of the posterior scalp for a negative margin.

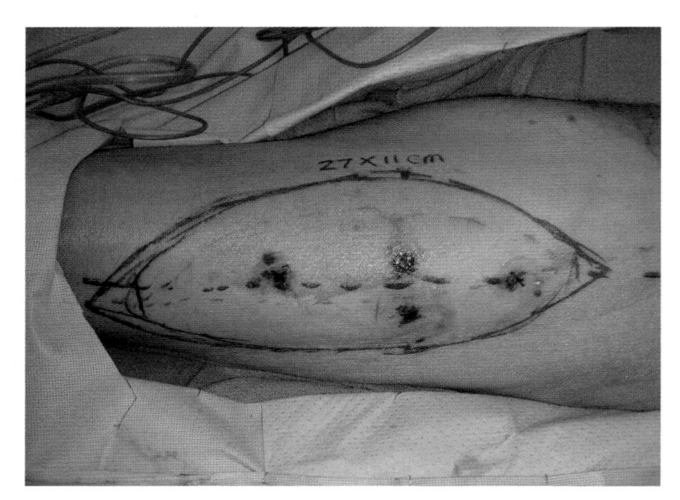

• **Fig. 1.31** Intraoperative view showing the design of a left anterolateral thigh perforator flap. Several perforators were identified during preoperative duplex scanning.

perforators were divided and only one major perforator, close to the septum between the rectus femoris and the vastus lateralis muscle, was followed and dissected free to the descending branch of the circumflex femoral vessels. During the pedicle dissection, the accompanied motor nerve was transected and was repaired with 8-0 nylon sutures. The pedicle dissection was done further to obtain more length of the pedicle so that it could reach the recipient vessels on the right side. The descending branch was divided as proximal as possible off the profunda vessels. One artery and two veins were divided with hemoclips and the flap dissection was completed (Fig. 1.32).

Based on the duplex scan's findings with the right superficial temporal vein being larger, a 5-cm right preauricular incision was made through the skin, subcutaneous tissue, and superficial fascia down to the superficial temporal vessels. Both the superficial temporal artery and vein were found to be adequate in size. The recipient vessel dissection was performed with loupe magnification and both the recipient artery and the vein were dissected free and ready for arterial and venous microanastomoses.

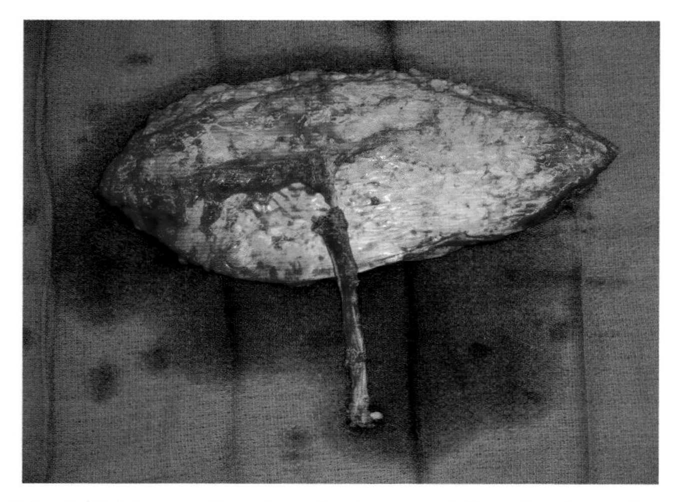

• **Fig. 1.32** Intraoperative view showing completion of a free anterolateral thigh perforator flap dissection.

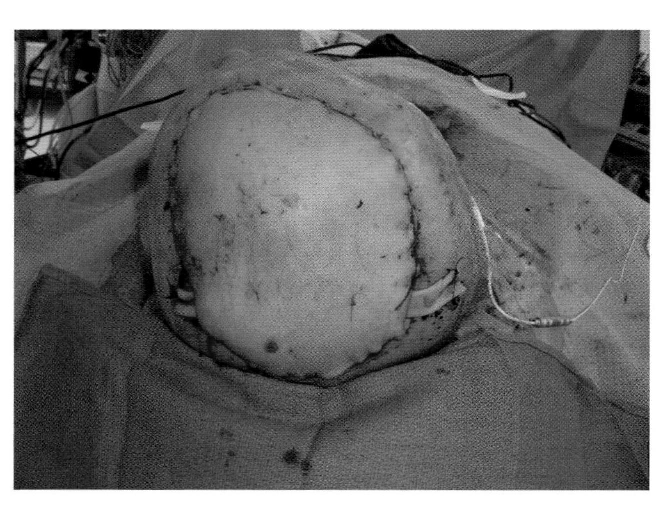

• **Fig. 1.33** Intraoperative view showing completion of a free anterolateral thigh perforator flap scalp reconstruction.

The pedicle of the flap was prepared under loupe magnification. With further proper dissection, one artery and two venae comitantes were identified. The artery was irrigated with heparinized saline solution. One smaller vena comitans was clipped with hemoclips. The flap was then placed into the scalp defect. A subcutaneous tunnel between the defect and the superficial temporal vessels was carefully made. A Penrose drain was used to pass the pedicle vessels through tunnel and proper orientation of the pedicle vessels was confirmed. Once the distal superficial artery and vein were divided, the arterial microanastomosis was performed in an end-to-end fashion with 8-0 nylon suture in an interrupted fashion under microscope. The venous microanastomosis was performed with a 2.5-mm Cook coupler device. Perfusion of the flap appeared to be good once all clamps were removed.

The final inset of the flap was performed with interrupted, half-buried horizontal mattress sutures after excess flap tissues were excised. A Penrose drain was placed under the flap. A Cook Doppler was connected with the machine to monitor venous outflow (Fig. 1.33). The left thigh flap donor site was closed in three layers after significant undermining.

Follow-Up Results

The patient did well postoperatively without any complications related to the free flap reconstruction. He was discharged from the hospital on postoperative day 7. The drain was removed before his discharge. The scalp flap reconstruction healed well (Fig. 1.34). Unfortunately, the flap site remained bulky after 1 year and a flap debulking procedure was done to improve his scalp contour (Fig. 1.35). The flap debulking procedure involved a liposuction to the flap followed by direct excision of the flap's excess skin from one side (Figs. 1.36 and 1.37). The flap contour was improved after debulking procedures (Fig. 1.38).

Final Outcome

The scalp reconstruction site healed well after the debulking procedures and the final contour has improved significantly (Fig. 1.39). The patient has resumed his normal life and no recurrent cancer has been found during follow-up.

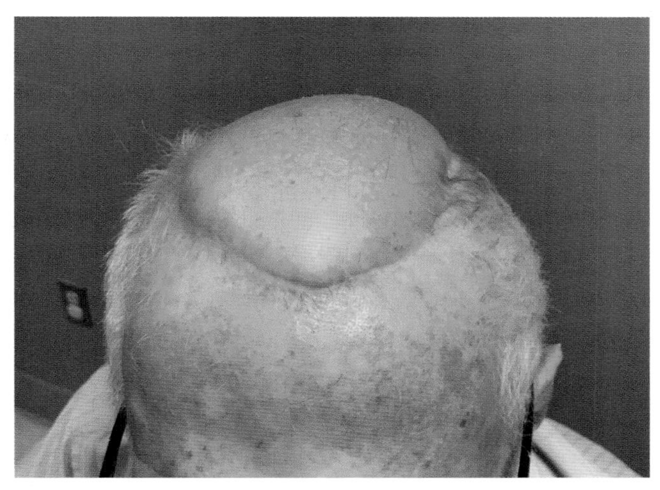

• **Fig. 1.34** The result at 11-month-follow-up. The bulk flap contour is shown.

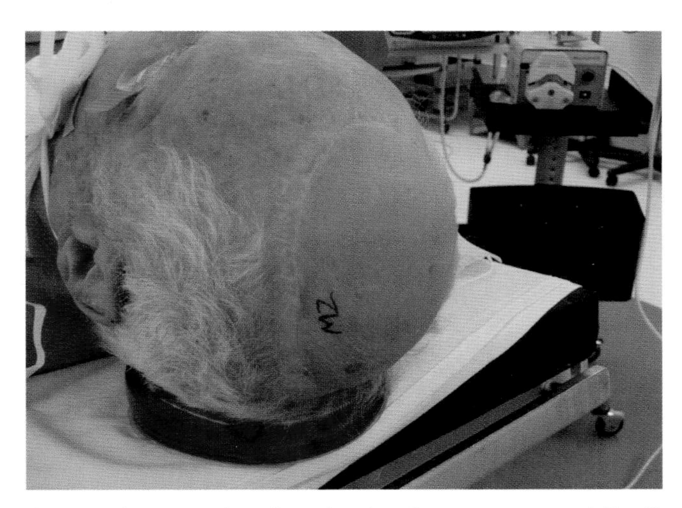

• **Fig. 1.35** Intraoperative view showing the appearance of the flap before its debulking procedure.

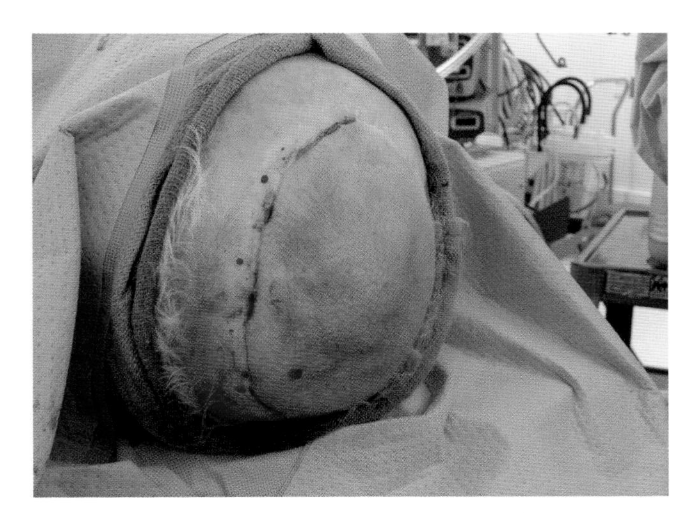

• **Fig. 1.36** Intraoperative view showing completion of liposuction to the flap. The bulkiness of the flap was reduced.

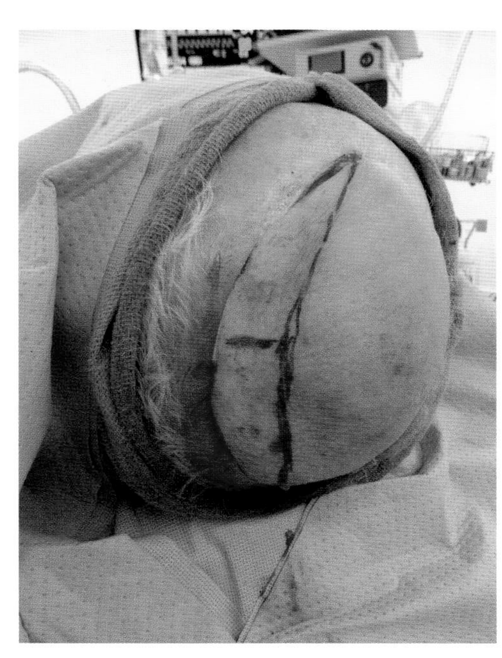

• **Fig. 1.37** Intraoperative view showing the amount of excess skin in the flap that would need to be excised.

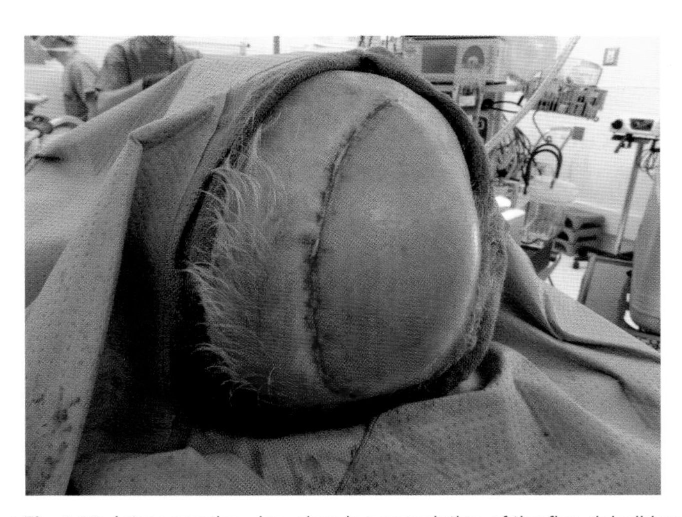

• **Fig. 1.38** Intraoperative view showing completion of the flap debulking procedure. The contour of the flap was significantly improved.

Pearls for Success

A free ALT perforator flap can be a good option for reconstruction of a large scalp defect. It has a long pedicle and can be harvested as a fasciocutaneous flap based on a single perforator for scalp reconstruction. However, its flap dissection can be time consuming. The tunneling of the pedicle should be performed very carefully and attention should be made to avoid avulsion injury of the perforator and to ensure the proper orientation of the pedicle.

Preoperative evaluation of the superficial temporal artery and vein with duplex scan should be performed so that a better recipient vessel with adequate size of both artery and vein can be selected and used for microvascular anastomoses. In addition, the perforator mapping with duplex scan can be helpful so that an

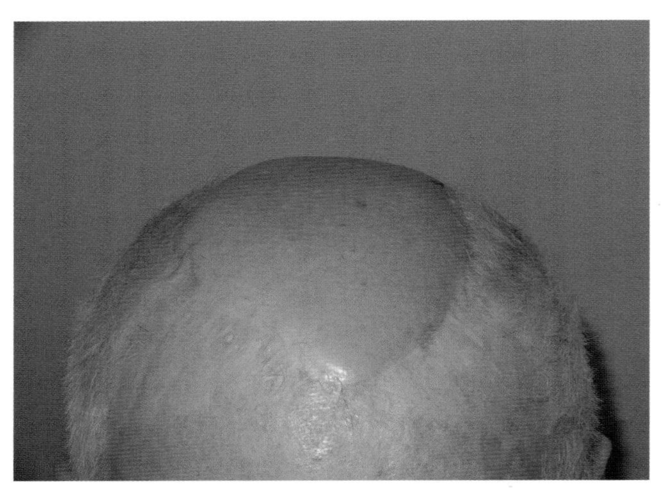

• **Fig. 1.39** The result at 2-month follow-up after the flap debulking procedure and 13 months after the flap scalp reconstruction showing a well-healed flap site with good contour.

easy side for perforator flap dissection can be selected. Unlike a free latissimus dorsi muscle flap, a free ALT perforator flap may remain bulky even after 1 year and a flap-debulking procedure can be performed to improve flap site contour.

CASE 5

Clinical Presentation

An 80-year-old White male with recurrent and advanced squamous cell carcinoma of the scalp underwent a wide local excision of scalp lesion by the surgical oncology service and craniotomy for resection of a full-thickness skull by the neurosurgery service. The dura was also repaired by the same service. The plastic surgery service was asked to perform a scalp reconstruction after the tumor resections (Fig. 1.40).

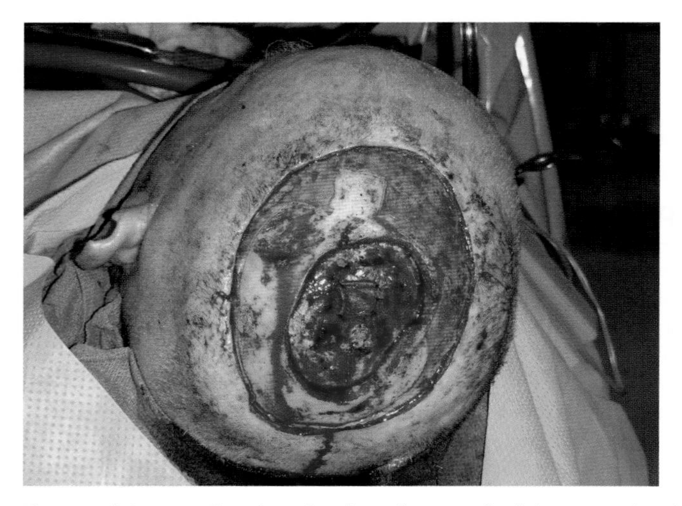

• **Fig. 1.40** Intraoperative view showing a large scalp defect associated with a skull defect after a wide local excision of recurrent and advanced squamous cell carcinoma in the scalp and craniotomy. The dura was repaired for the tear during such an extensive resection of the scalp cancer.

Operative Plan and Special Considerations

The scalp defect measured 12 × 10 cm and the full-thickness skull defect measured 7 × 5 cm. There was no obvious leak of cerebrospinal fluid in the dura repair site. Because of the size of the scalp defect, a free ALT perforator flap was offered to this patient. This patient was relatively thin and the contour after ALT flap reconstruction could be quite good. In addition, his skull defect should be reconstructed with a titanium mesh, as commonly done in cranioplasty.

Operative Procedures

Prior to the procedure, both ALT flap donor sites were mapped with a duplex scan. The left side had larger perforators with less intramuscular course and was selected for the ALT flap donor site. The left superficial temporal vessels were also mapped with a duplex scan. Both superficial temporal artery and vein were a good size and either side could be selected as recipient vessels. A 22 × 10 cm left ALT perforator flap was marked and the skin paddle with fascia was elevated (Fig. 1.41). One good perforator was identified and dissected free after a 5-cm intramuscular dissection. Another good perforator was also identified and dissected free after a 2-cm intermuscular dissection. The descending branch of the lateral circumflex femoral vessels was identified and dissected free to the profunda vessels. The pedicle was divided off the profunda. The flap was then prepared under loupe magnification. The flap was then ready for microvascular anastomosis (Fig. 1.42).

A left preauricular incision was made for exposure of the superficial temporal vessels. Both the superficial temporal artery and vein were dissected free and were also found to be a good size. The superior temporal vessels were ready for microvascular anastomosis.

The flap was temporarily inset into the scalp defect. The pedicle of the flap was carefully tunneled through the subgaleal space to the preauricular area without any twisting or tension. Both microvascular anastomoses were performed under a microscope. The arterial anastomosis was performed in an end-to-end fashion with interrupted 8-0 nylon sutures. The venous anastomosis was performed with a 2.5-mm coupler device (Fig. 1.43).

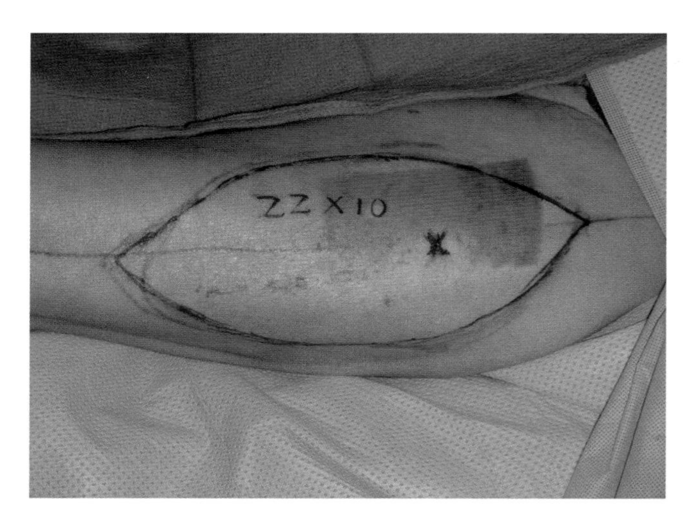

• **Fig. 1.41** Intraoperative view showing the design of the left free anterolateral thigh perforator flap. One large perforator was identified by preoperative duplex scan.

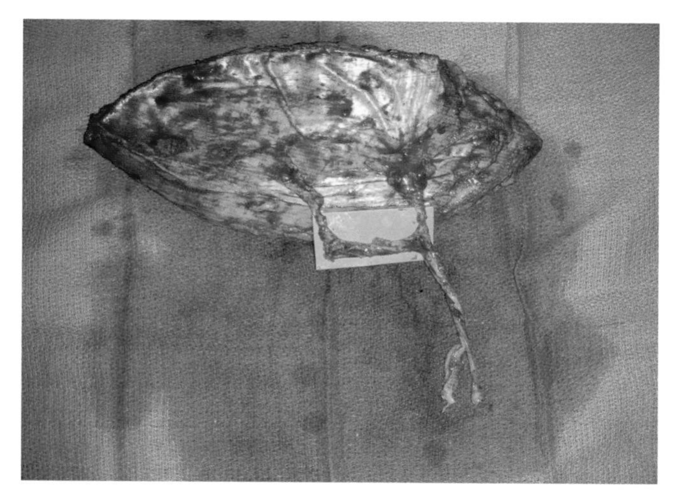

• **Fig. 1.42** Intraoperative view showing completion of the free anterolateral thigh perforator flap dissection based on two large perforators.

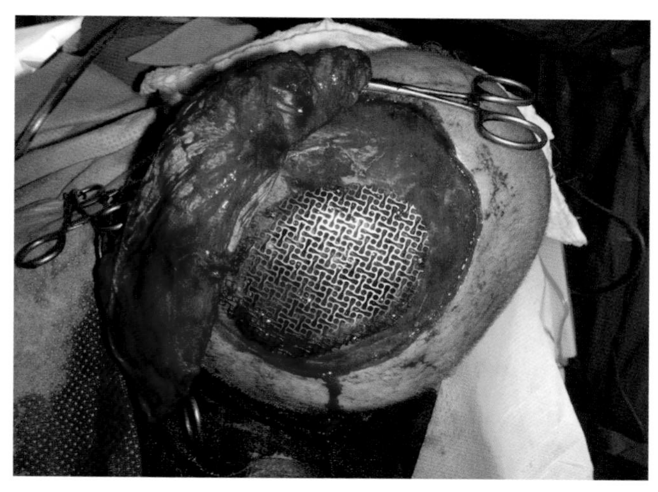

• **Fig. 1.44** Intraoperative view showing completion of a cranioplasty with a titanium mesh before the flap inset.

Once all clamps were removed, the flap appeared to be well perfused with a good Doppler signal.

The cranioplasty was performed with a slightly larger than 5 × 7 cm titanium mesh. The mesh was contoured and placed over the scalp defect and secured with multiple, self-tapping screws (Fig. 1.44).

The flap inset was then performed and flap excess was trimmed. A 10 flat JP was inserted under the flap and the entire flap inset was completed with several interrupted sutures in half-buried horizontal mattress fashion (Fig. 1.45). A preauricular incision was closed with skin staples. The left anterolateral donor site was closed in two layers after repair of the divided muscles.

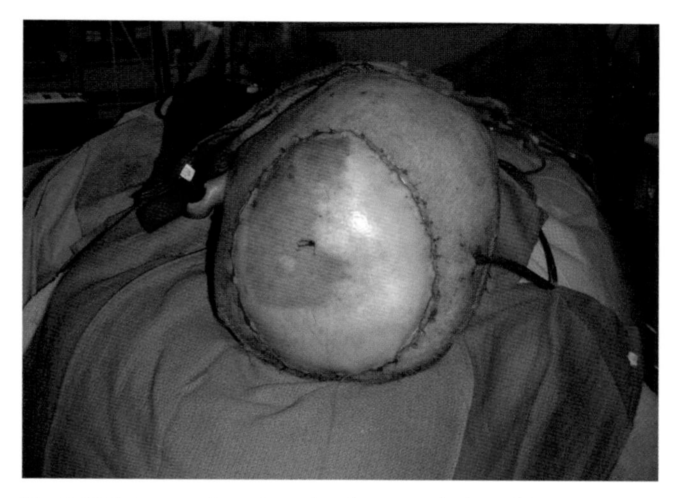

• **Fig. 1.45** Intraoperative view showing completion of the free anterolateral thigh perforator flap inset for scalp reconstruction.

Management of Complications

This patient had a well-healed scalp reconstruction during an early follow-up (Fig. 1.46). Unfortunately, he developed an extrusion of the titanium mesh in the periphery of the flap 4 months later, which was managed with removal of the mesh and replacement with a Medpor mesh (Figs. 1.47–1.50). He subsequently

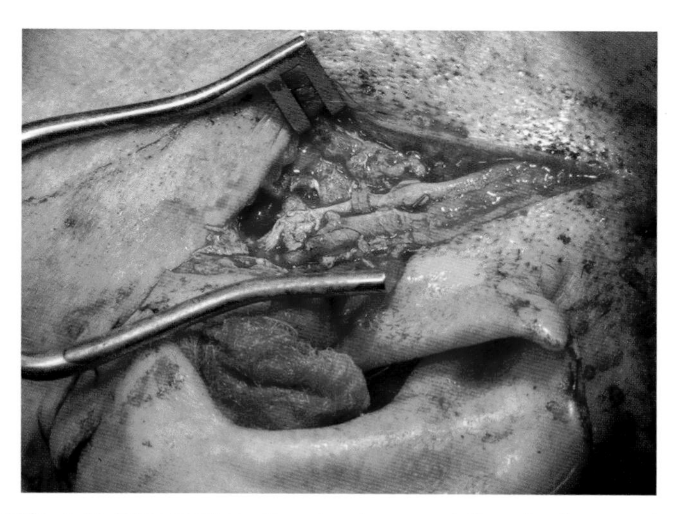

• **Fig. 1.43** Intraoperative view showing completion of microvascular anastomoses to the superficial temporal vessels.

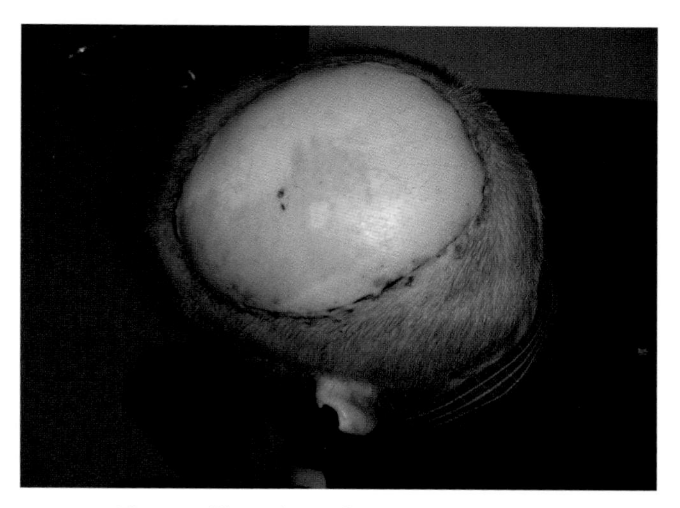

• **Fig. 1.46** The early result at 2.5-week follow-up.

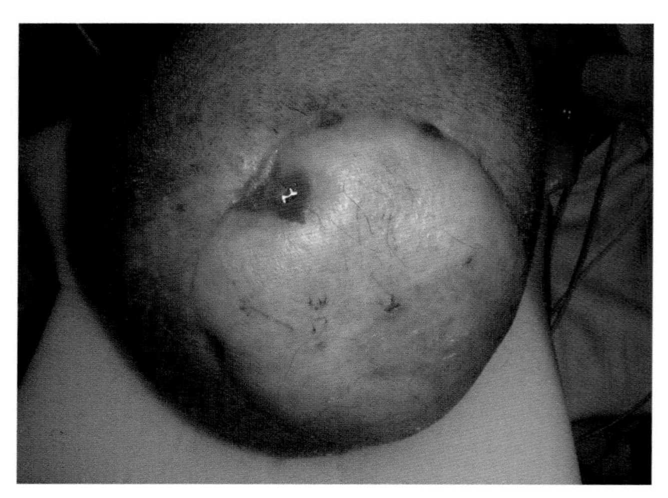

• **Fig. 1.47** Intraoperative view showing extrusion of titanium mesh used for cranioplasty.

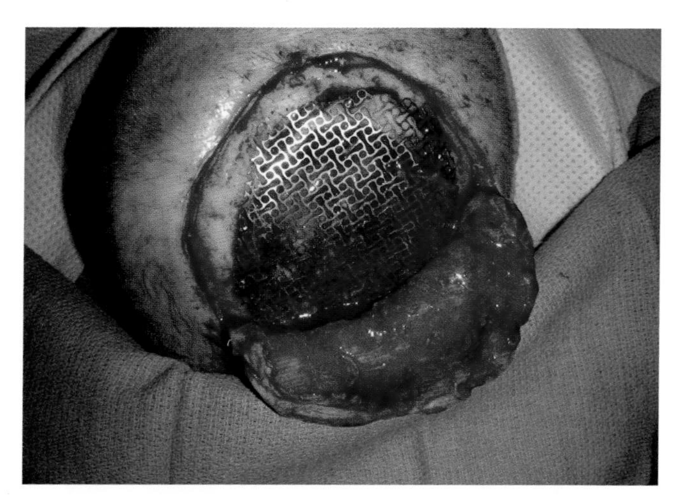

• **Fig. 1.48** Intraoperative view showing complete elevation of the anterolateral thigh flap to explore titanium mesh.

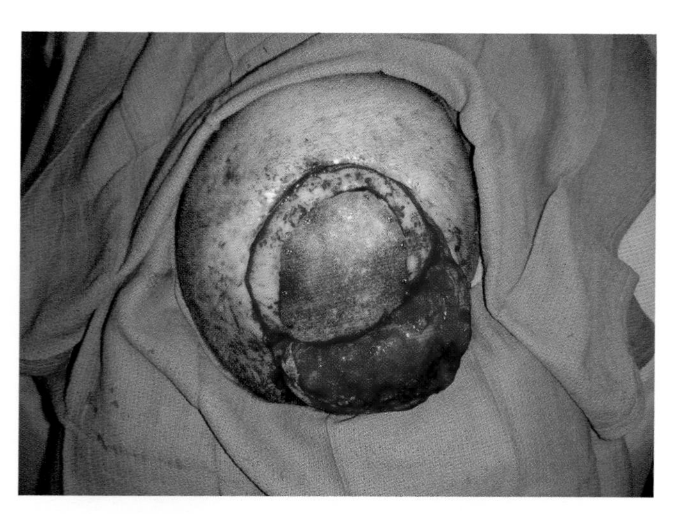

• **Fig. 1.49** Intraoperative view showing replacement of titanium mesh with Medpor mesh.

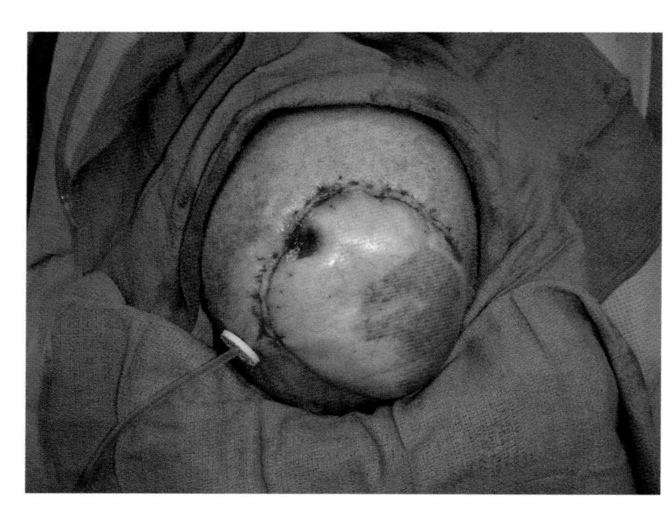

• **Fig. 1.50** Intraoperative view showing completion of the flap reinset after placement of Medpor mesh for cranioplasty.

developed multiple extrusions of the Medpor mesh in the periphery of the flap, which was managed with debridement and an adjacent local scalp rotation flap for coverage (Figs. 1.51–1.53). He later developed extrusions of the mesh in the center of the flap (Fig. 1.54).

Follow-Up Results

Because of multiple mesh extrusions, even with the Medpor mesh, the decision was made to remove the mesh and to debride unhealthy flap and scalp tissues (Figs. 1.55 and 1.56). A free latissimus dorsi muscle flap with a skin graft was performed for the scalp reconstruction (Figs. 1.57 and 1.58). The pedicle vessels were anastomosed to the right superficial temporal vessels. The procedure went well and the scalp reconstruction site again healed well (Fig. 1.59).

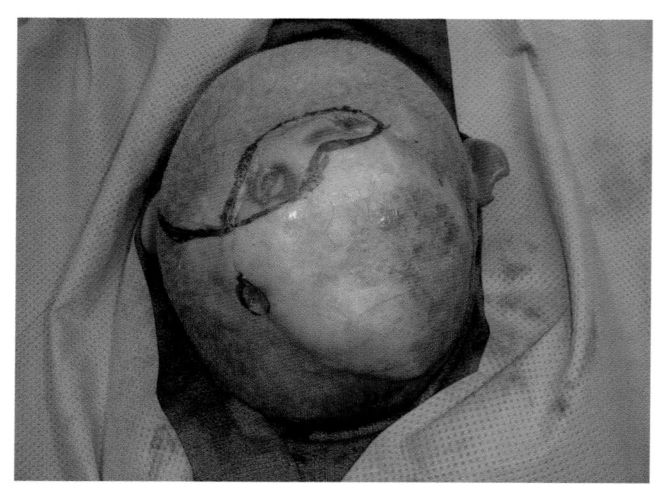

• **Fig. 1.51** Intraoperative view showing extrusion of Medpor mesh used for cranioplasty.

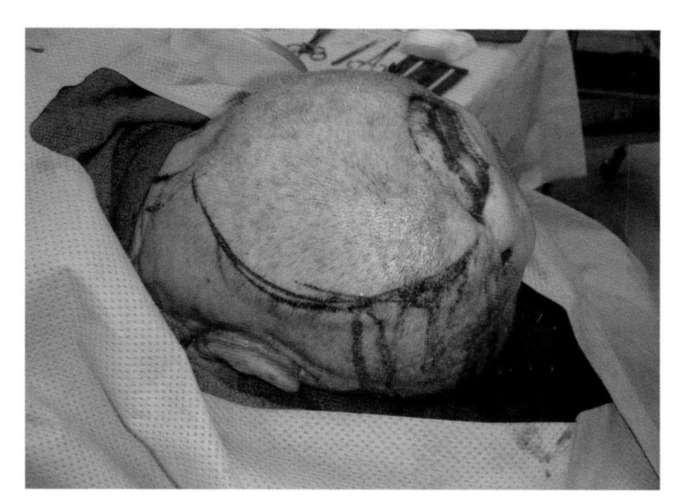

• **Fig. 1.52** Intraoperative view showing completion of the flap debridement and the design of a large posterior scalp rotation flap based on the occipital vessels for the coverage of the defect.

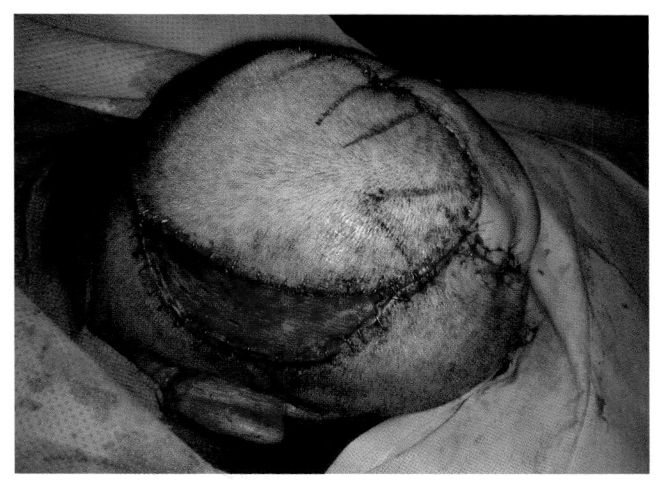

• **Fig. 1.53** Intraoperative view showing completion of the posterior scalp rotation flap for the defect closure and a skin graft for the closure of the flap donor site.

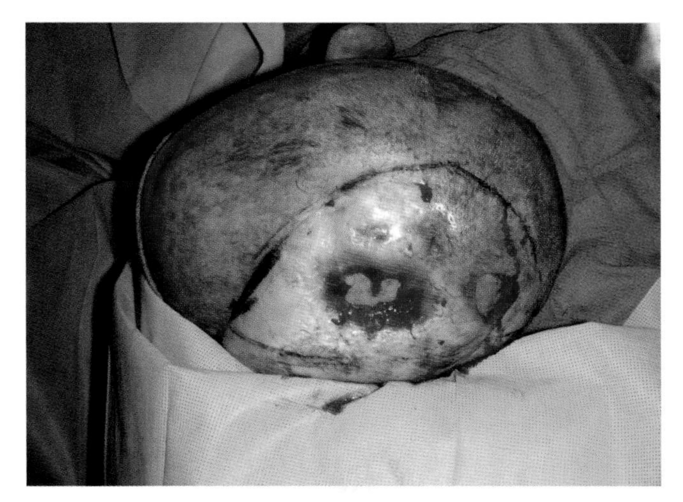

• **Fig. 1.54** Intraoperative view showing extrusion of Medpor mesh used for cranioplasty.

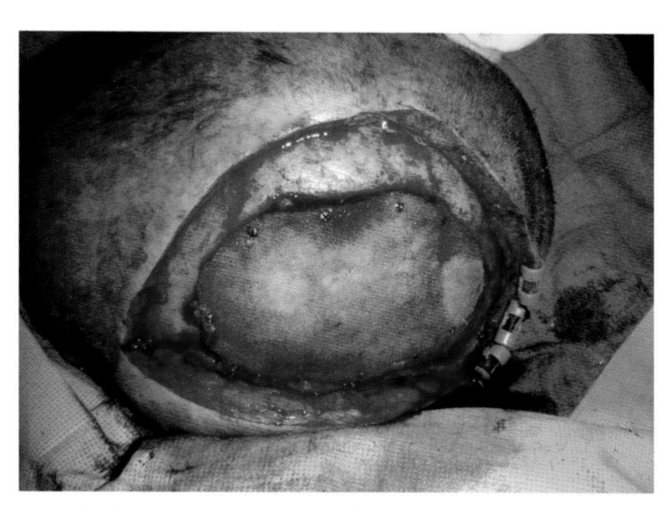

• **Fig. 1.55** Intraoperative view showing exposed Medpor mesh after debridement of the flap tissue.

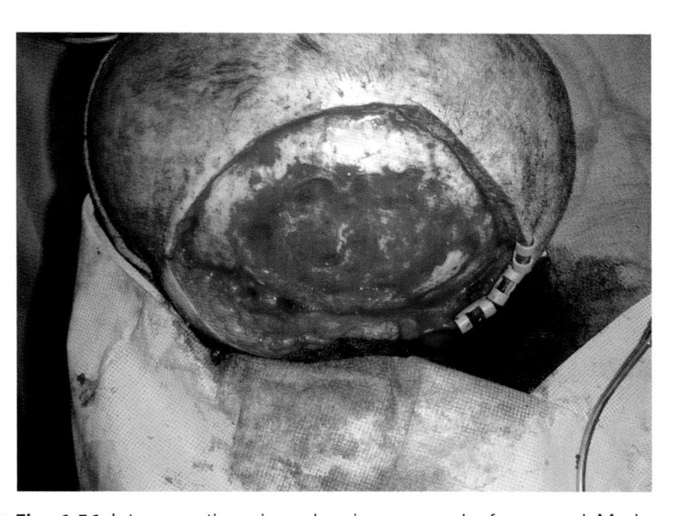

• **Fig. 1.56** Intraoperative view showing removal of exposed Medpor mesh.

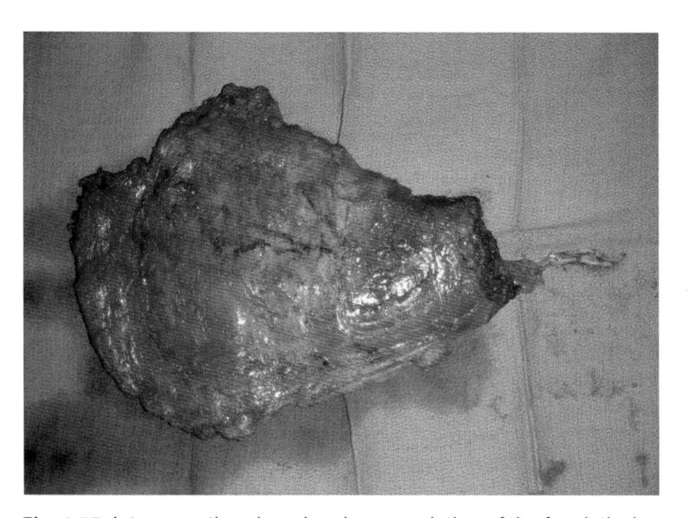

• **Fig. 1.57** Intraoperative view showing completion of the free latissimus dorsi muscle flap dissection.

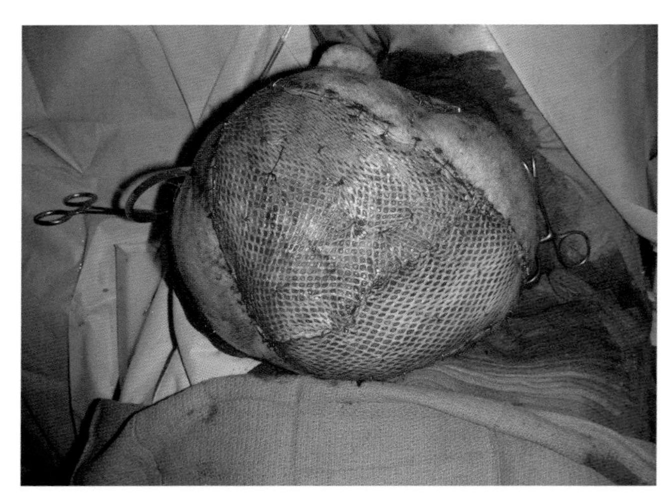

• **Fig. 1.58** Intraoperative view showing completion of the skin-grafted free latissimus dorsi muscle inset.

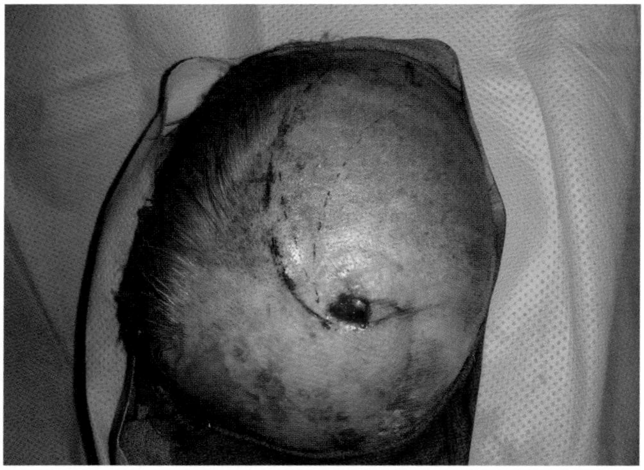

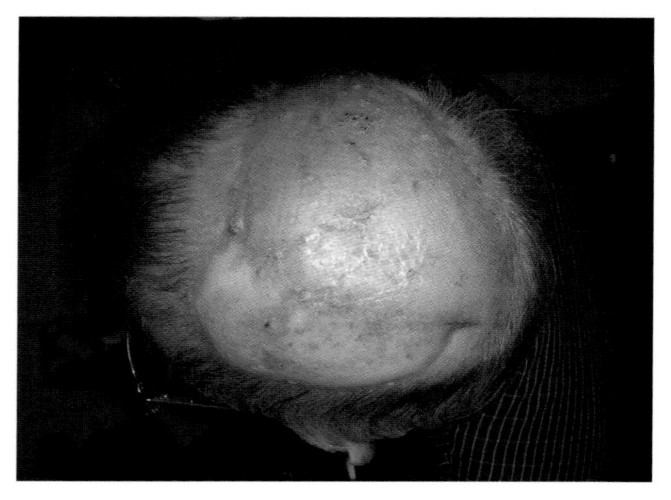

• **Fig. 1.59** The result at 3-month follow-up after the free latissimus dorsi muscle flap for scalp reconstruction.

Final Outcome

The patient's second scalp reconstruction site healed well. About 6 months later, he developed a small open wound at the junction of the new flap and remaining scalp (Fig. 1.60). This was reconstructed with an adjacent local scalp rotation flap (Fig. 1.61). Unfortunately, a small portion of the wound closure was reopened and this was reconstructed again with the same scalp rotation flap after wound debridement (Figs. 1.62 and 1.63). This patient finally had a stable and healed scalp wound and has returned to his normal life (Fig. 1.64). He had a total of six operations including two free tissue transfers over 16 months.

Pearls for Success

A free ALT flap can be an excellent choice for scalp reconstruction in a relatively thin patient. However, the flap tissue may not be durable enough long-term and extrusion of the mesh through the flap can occur. Removal of the exposed mesh may have to be done and a second free flap, such as a free latissimus dorsi muscle, can

• **Fig. 1.60** Intraoperative view showing a small wound dehiscence between the free latissimus muscle flap and the posterior scalp and the design of a posterior scalp rotation flap for wound coverage.

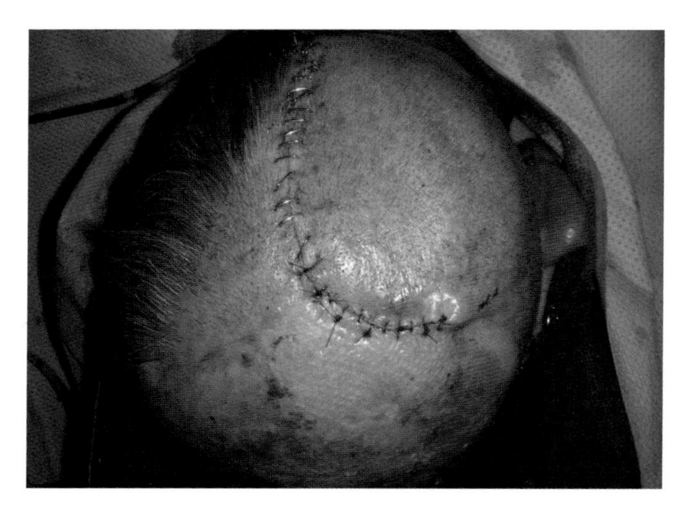

• **Fig. 1.61** Intraoperative view showing a successful wound closure with the posterior scalp rotation flap

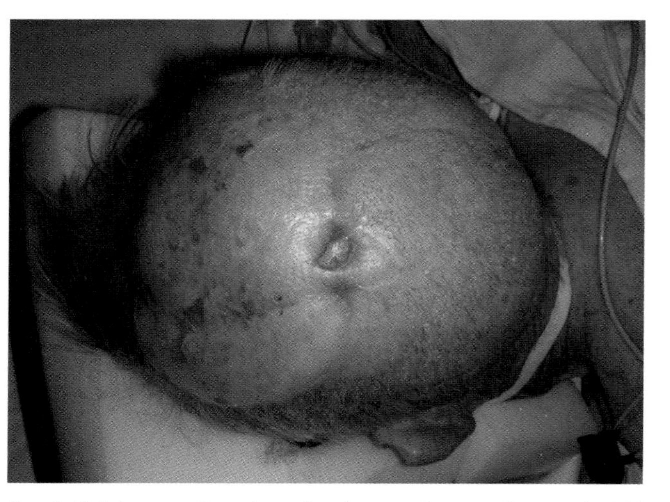

• **Fig. 1.62** Intraoperative view showing another small wound dehiscence between the free latissimus muscle flap and the posterior scalp.

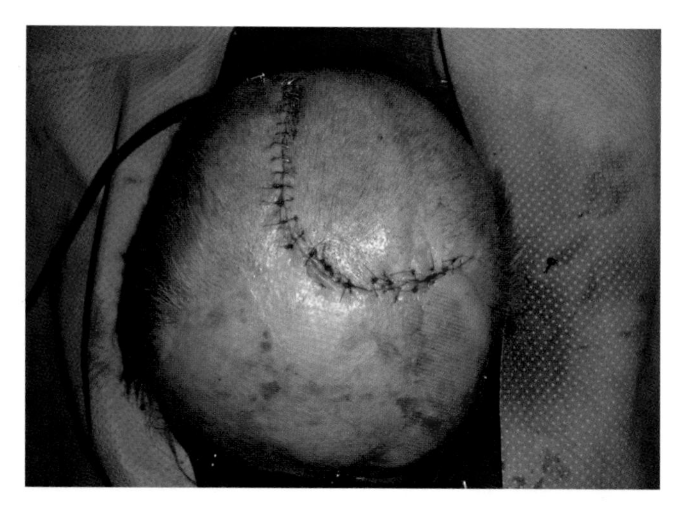

• **Fig. 1.63** Intraoperative view showing a readvancement of the previous posterior scalp rotation flap for the wound coverage.

be performed to provide more durable soft-tissue reconstruction. A wound dehiscence of the flap may occur and an adjacent local scalp rotation flap can be designed for wound closure. The complexity of a large scalp reconstruction in older bald male patients should be fully recognized.

CASE 6

Clinical Presentation

A 20-year-old previously healthy White female developed coccidioidomycosis meningitis and encephalitis with subsequent hydrocephalus. Over the course of her treatment, she developed complications such as pulmonary embolus, hematoma, and cranial osteomyelitis and became quadriplegic, requiring a tracheostomy and a gastrojejunostomy feeding tube. She had a cranioplasty for the skull defect secondary to decompression of elected intracranial pressure. Over 3 years, she underwent numerous revisions to her cranioplasty and ventriculoperitoneal shunt as a result of infection, persistent ventriculomegaly, and syringomyelia. The persistent soft tissue infections ultimately left her with several areas of threatened scalp over alloplastic cranioplasty material. A local scalp rotation flap was performed 6 months ago. Unfortunately, the patient developed two new areas of wound breakdown measuring 1 cm^2 each with exposed titanium mesh (Fig. 1.65).

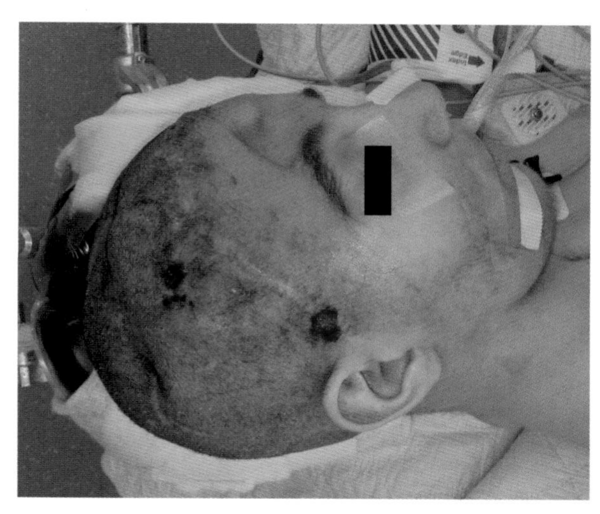

• **Fig. 1.65** Intraoperative view showing two small open wounds from the cranioplasty site.

Operative Plan and Special Considerations

There was a large area of questionable scalp over her right head and forehead (Fig. 1.66). There was concern for communication with the subdural space, so the decision was made to proceed with a muscle-based flap, because this would provide the best protection against contamination of the hardware in addition to the ability to resorb cerebrospinal fluid should a leak occur. A free latissimus dorsi myocutaneous flap was offered to this patient

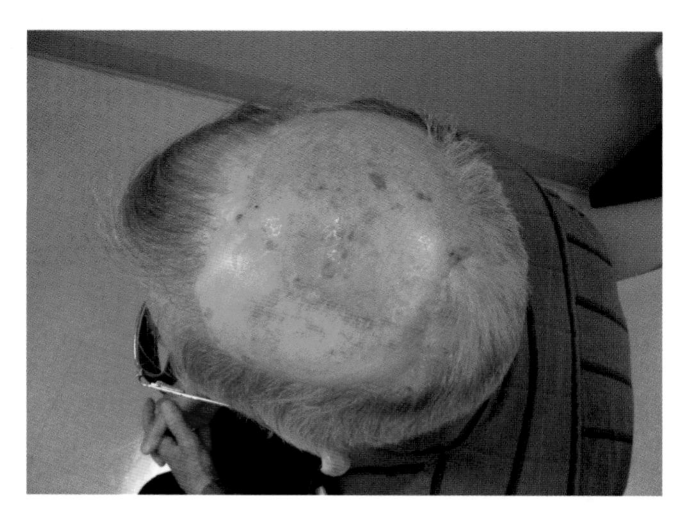

• **Fig. 1.64** The result at 3 months after the free latissimus dorsi muscle flap transfer and 16 months after the free anterolateral thigh perforator flap transfer showing a durable soft tissue coverage of the scalp.

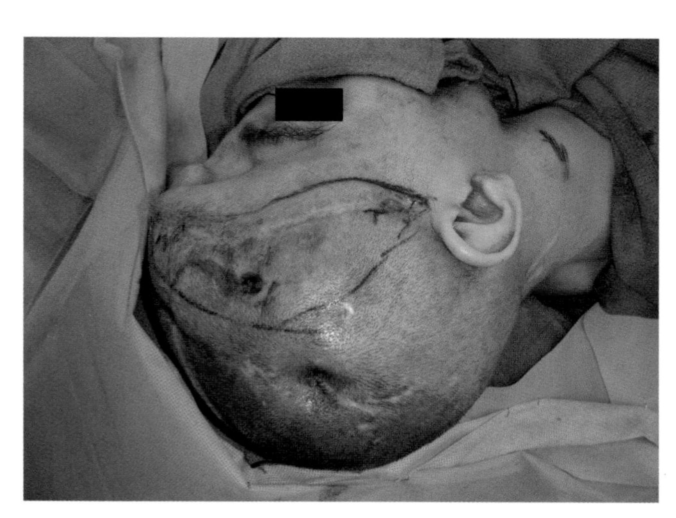

• **Fig. 1.66** Intraoperative view showing an outline of the compromised scalp that would need to be excised.

for the reasons previously mentioned as well as the size of the potential scalp defect after debridement. According to her neurosurgeon, she would require a free tissue transfer to her scalp as a lifesaving procedure, even though the procedure itself could be complex and difficult because of her comorbidities. In addition, because right superficial temporal vessels were transected during previous right frontal craniotomy, the right facial artery and vein were selected as recipient vessels for the free flap transfer.

Operative Procedures

The procedure started by exploring right facial artery and vein. Only the facial artery was visualized with a duplex scan. However, the facial vein was not visualized. Therefore, the recipient vessels were exposed first.

The facial artery was identified and appeared to be a good size. However, the facial vein appeared to be quite small. Fortunately, a large but deeper vein was found after further deep neck dissection. The vein appeared to be a good size and could be used as a recipient vein for microvascular anastomosis.

The area of the pending necrotic scalp over her right forehead and the middle head, measuring 15.5 × 6.0 cm, was resected. Based on the measurement of where the recipient vessels would be, a 14 × 8 cm skin paddle of the right latissimus dorsi muscle was marked over her right back in oblique fashion. In this way, some dog ear was also incorporated with the skin paddle.

The skin paddle of the latissimus dorsi muscle flap was incised to the muscle (Fig. 1.67). The dissection was performed both medially and laterally to free up the entire border of the muscle. Once the muscle's insertion to the posterior iliac spine was divided, the latissimus dorsi muscle along with its skin paddle was elevated.

The pedicle dissection was then performed toward the axilla. Once the serratus branch was divided, the thoracodorsal vessel was identified and dissected free toward the axilla. The proximal attachment of the muscle to the humerus was divided under direct visualization and the pedicel dissection was performed further toward the axillary vessels. The thoracodorsal nerve was divided first and the vascular pedicle was then divided off the axillary vessels. The pedicle artery and vein of the flap was then prepped under the loupe magnification. Both artery and vein were further prepped and ready for microvascular anastomosis (Fig. 1.68).

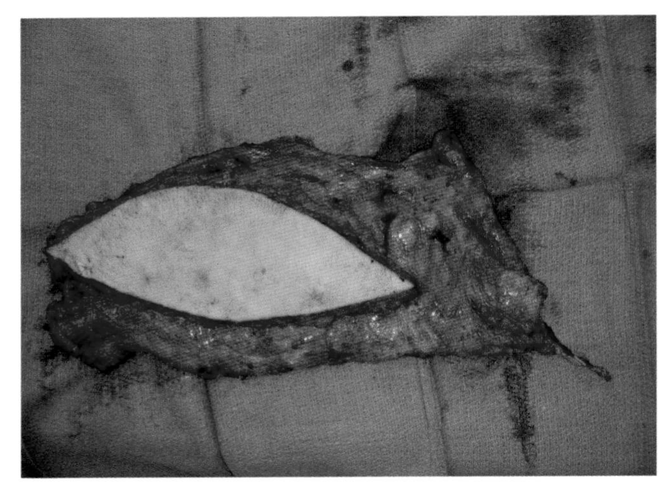

• **Fig. 1.68** Intraoperative view showing completion of the right free large latissimus dorsi myocutaneous flap dissection.

The flap was temporarily inset into the right forehead and middle head. The pedicle vessels were tunneled through the auricular skin to the neck. The arterial microanastomosis was performed in an end-to-end fashion with interrupted 8-0 nylon sutures. The venous microanastomosis was performed with a 3.0 coupler device also in an end-to-end fashion.

Debridement of the pending necrotic scalp was then performed. The flap inset was performed after the muscle-only portion of the flap was placed under the adjacent healthy-looking scalp. This skin paddle of the flap was approximated with adjacent scalp in two layers (Fig. 1.69). The neck incision was approximated with skin staples. The right back donor site was closed in two layers after drain placements.

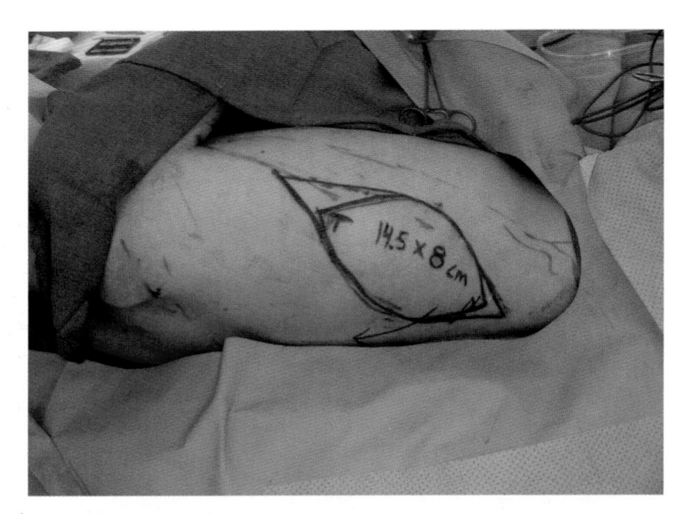

• **Fig. 1.67** Intraoperative view showing the design of the right free large latissimus dorsi myocutaneous flap.

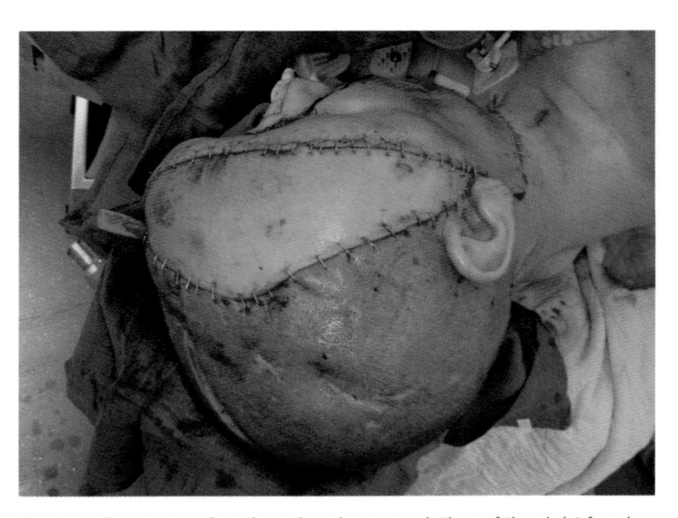

• **Fig. 1.69** Intraoperative view showing completion of the right free large latissimus dorsi myocutaneous flap for scalp reconstruction.

At the end of the procedure the flap appeared to be well perfused with good capillary refill and a strong Doppler signal in the skin paddle.

Management of Complications

For the first 2 days after a successful free latissimus dorsi myocutaneous flap for the scalp reconstruction, the patient unfortunately had several episodes of hypotension during the immediate postoperative period and had most likely partial thrombosis of the arterial anastomosis. She was urgently taken back to the operating room for reexploration and revision of microvascular anastomosis (Fig. 1.70).

The arterial anastomosis was reopened. There was a fresh blood clot to both sides of the anastomosis. Careful embolectomy was performed manually with microdilator and once the blood clot was removed, both sides of the vessel were irrigated thoroughly with heparinized saline. Tissue plasminogen activator (2 mg in 5 cc) was perfused to the arterial pedicle of the flap. Arterial anastomosis was then performed again in an end-to-end fashion and there was a good arterial flow to the flap (Fig. 1.71). A needle prick produced bleeding and there was a good Doppler signal within the skin paddle of the flap. The flap was successfully salvaged (Fig. 1.72).

Follow-Up Results

The patient unfortunately developed a hematoma under the flap (Fig. 1.73), but it was successfully evacuated (Fig. 1.74). However, her overall medical condition was deteriorating, and she eventually lost the flap (Fig. 1.75). As a salvage procedure for scalp reconstruction, two large scalp rotation flaps were performed to cover the scalp defect (Fig. 1.76). Unfortunately, she developed a partial flap necrosis from one scalp flap, which left an open wound. Because of her multiple medical conditions and persistent hypotension, the patient would not tolerate a second free tissue transfer for her definitive scalp reconstruction (Fig. 1.77). The patient was transferred to the medicine service for medical management and optimized care and was eventually discharged home for continued medical care.

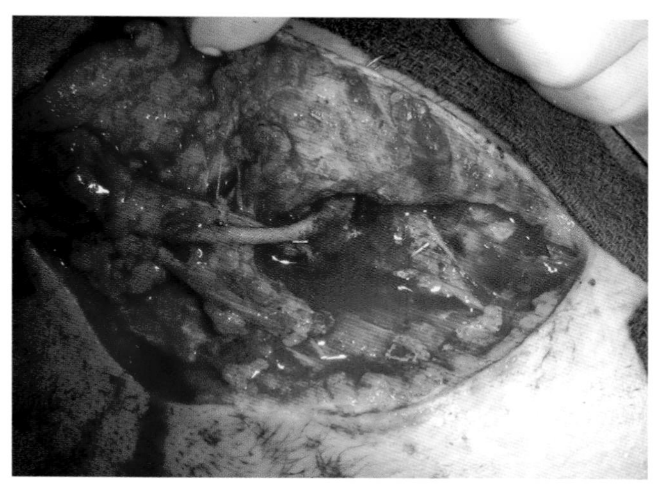

• **Fig. 1.71** Intraoperative view showing the patent arterial microvascular anastomosis after revision.

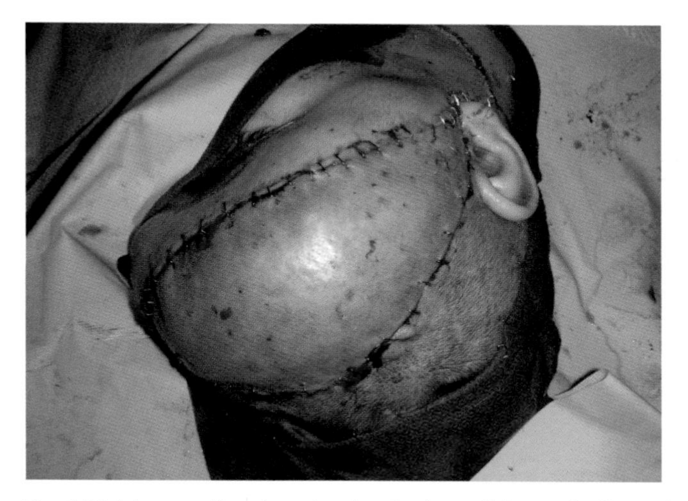

• **Fig. 1.72** Intraoperative view showing the immediate result after revision of the thrombosed arterial microvascular anastomosis.

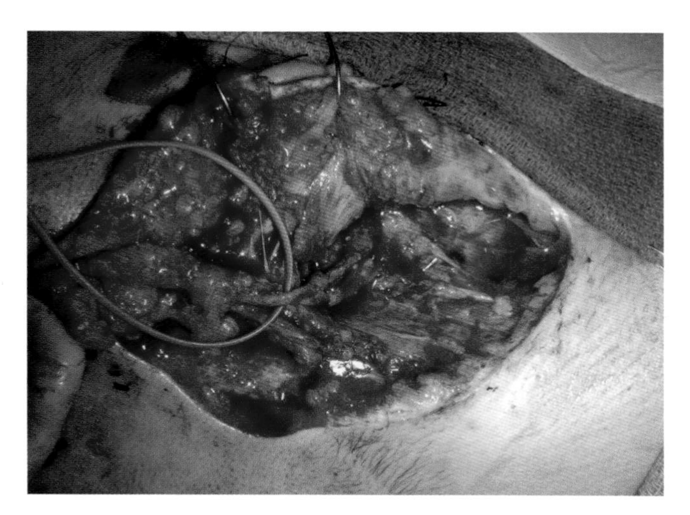

• **Fig. 1.70** Intraoperative view showing thrombosed arterial microvascular anastomosis during exploration.

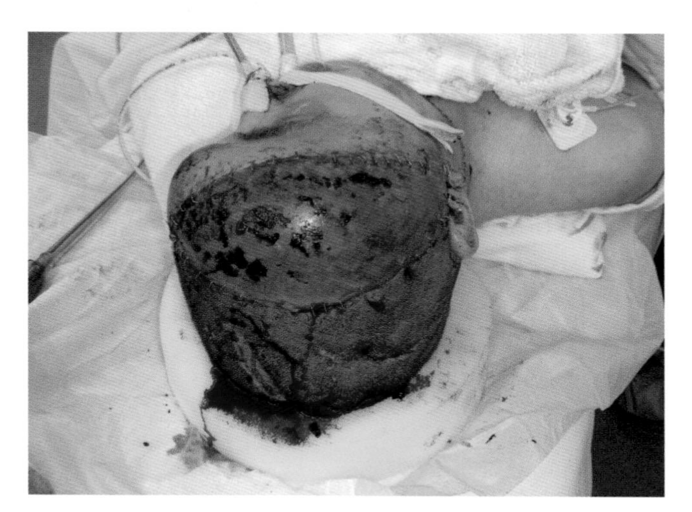

• **Fig. 1.73** Intraoperative view showing hematoma under the free latissimus dorsi muscle flap.

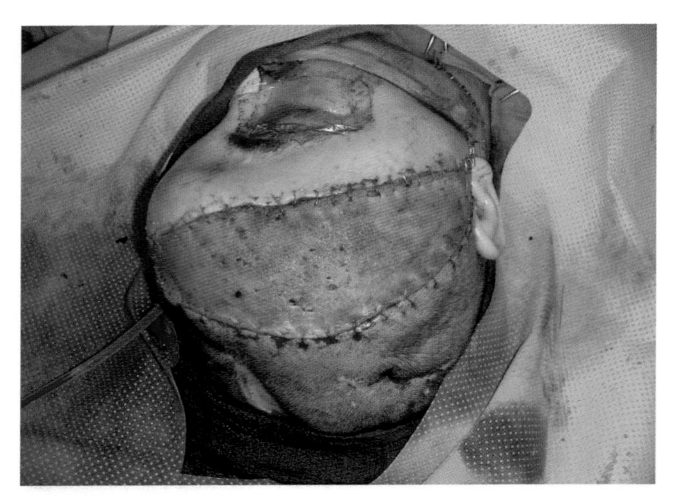

• **Fig. 1.74** Intraoperative view showing the viable flap after evacuation of the hematoma under the free latissimus dorsi muscle flap.

Final Outcome

After nearly 5 months of medical management, the patient was medically stable and optimized for definitive scalp reconstruction (Fig. 1.78). It was felt that the previous free flap failure was in large part caused by postoperative hypotension secondary to a long procedure and decreased bodily reserve. Given the numerous attempts for soft tissue coverage and salvage as well as the potential difficulty of exploring her facial vessels again as recipient vessels, the decision was made to proceed to a two-stage free flap reconstruction using the contralateral latissimus dorsi muscle. In light of the patient's prolonged and difficult postoperative course after her initial free tissue transfer, she was optimized for her cardiac status, nutritional status, and overall medical condition with the assistance of intensive care specialists.

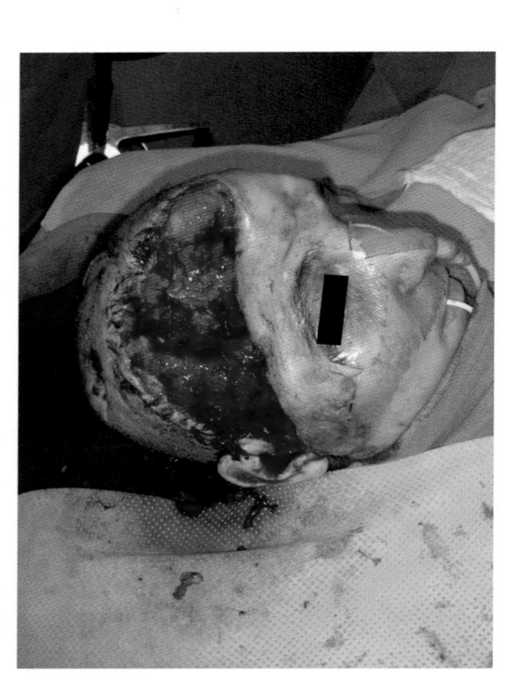

• **Fig. 1.75** Intraoperative view showing a large forehead scalp defect following debridement of the necrotic free latissimus dorsi flap.

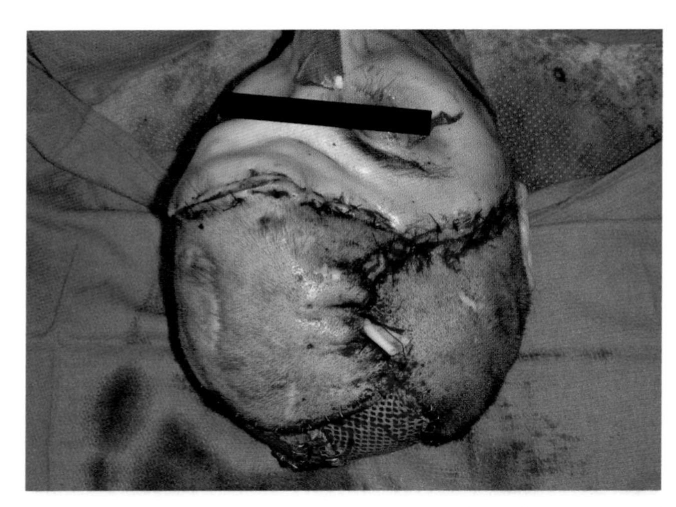

• **Fig. 1.76** Intraoperative view showing completion of two large adjacent scalp rotation flaps for closure of the large forehead scalp wound.

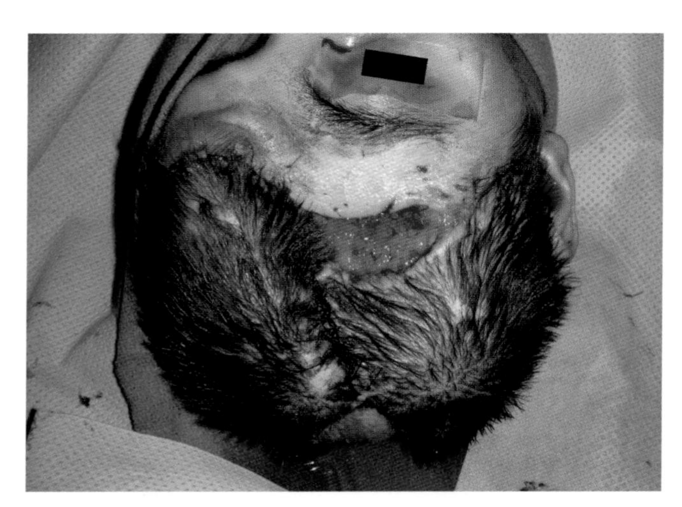

• **Fig. 1.77** Small portion of one scalp rotation flap became necrotic resulting in a forehead scalp defect. The wound had been left for granulation over the dura.

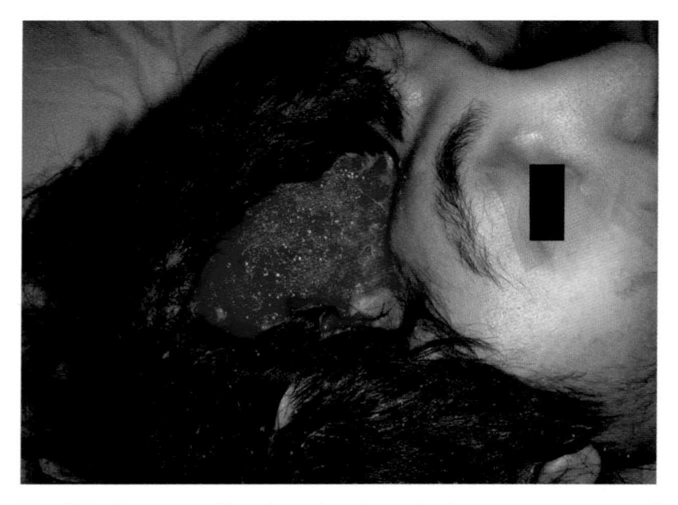

• **Fig. 1.78** A preoperative view showing a forehead scalp wound with good granulation at its base.

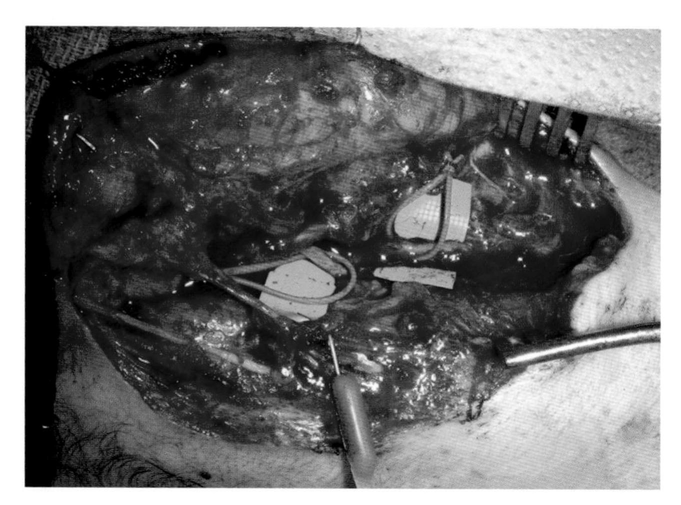

• **Fig. 1.79** Intraoperative view showing completion of both arterial and venous recipient vessel dissections in the neck. The procedure was performed under general anesthesia and took about 2 hours. Both recipient vessels were ready after the first-stage operation.

The first-stage procedure involved a right-sided neck exploration to identify suitable recipient vessels from the scarred area. A suitable vein was identified as a branch from the jugular vein to the face. The recipient artery was identified as the superior thyroid artery (Fig. 1.79). The first stage of the procedure allowed us to limit prolonged exposure to general anesthesia with the added benefit of shortening the operative time of the second-stage definitive free tissue transfer and also served as a test drive to see whether the patient could tolerate general anesthesia. The patient tolerated the first procedure of 2 hours well. Three days later, she underwent the left latissimus myocutaneous flap harvest and microsurgical free tissue reconstruction (Figs. 1.80 and 1.81). Her free tissue transfer went well this time and the entire procedure was significantly shortened to less than 4 hours because the recipient vessels were prepared before and ready for microvascular anastomoses (Figs. 1.82 and 1.83). Her postoperative course was also without any major issues. She was successfully discharged on postoperative day 7. Postdischarge follow-up showed a well-healed scalp wound after the second free tissue transfer (Fig. 1.84).

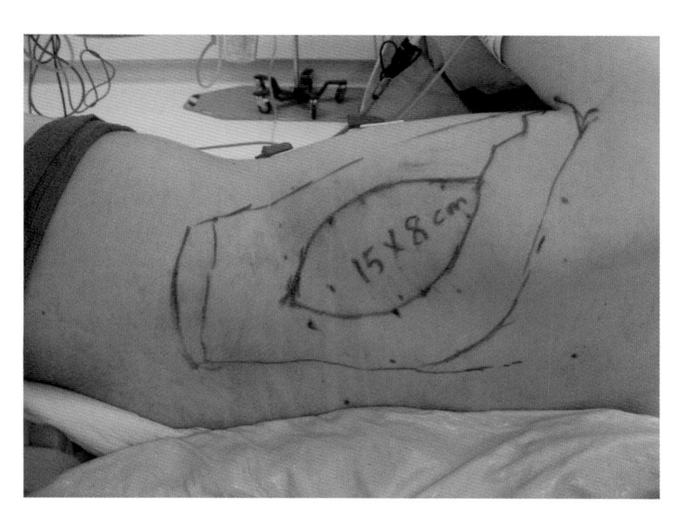

• **Fig. 1.80** Intraoperative view showing the design of the left free large latissimus dorsi myocutaneous flap.

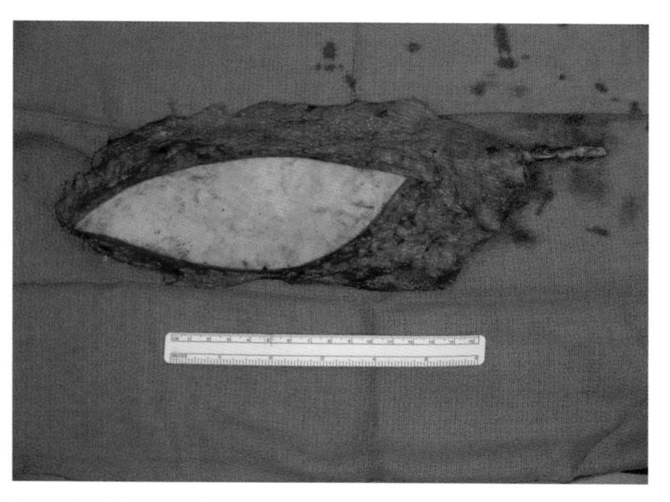

• **Fig. 1.81** Intraoperative view showing completion of the left free large latissimus dorsi myocutaneous flap dissection during the second-stage operation.

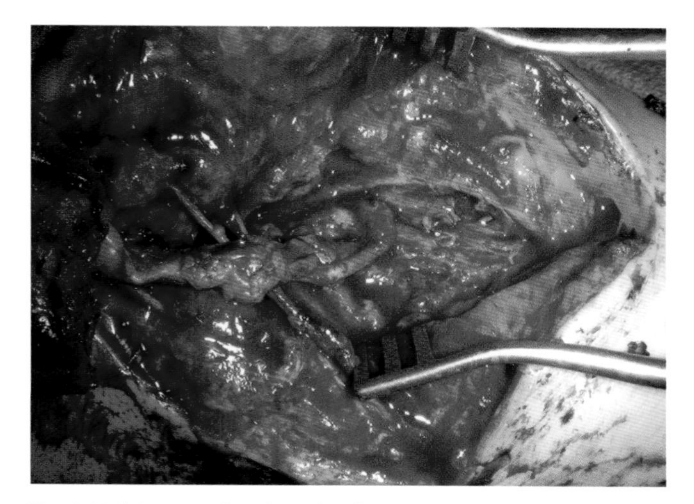

• **Fig. 1.82** Intraoperative view showing completion of both arterial and venous microvascular anastomoses in the neck during the second-stage operation.

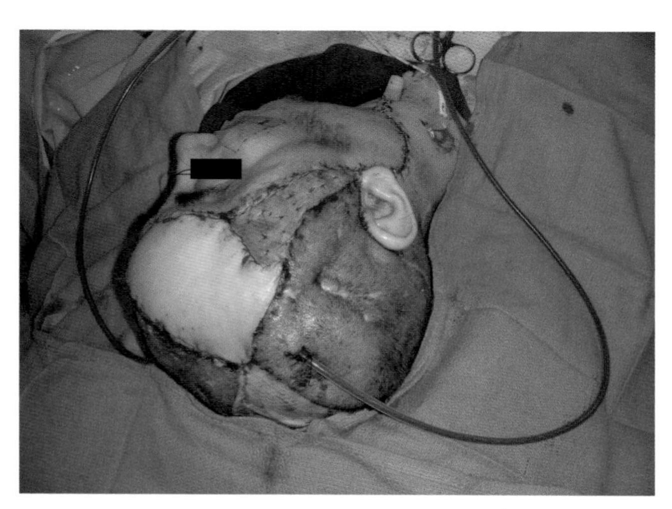

• **Fig. 1.83** Intraoperative view showing completion of the right free large latissimus dorsi myocutaneous flap for scalp reconstruction during the second-stage operation. The procedure took about 4 hours.

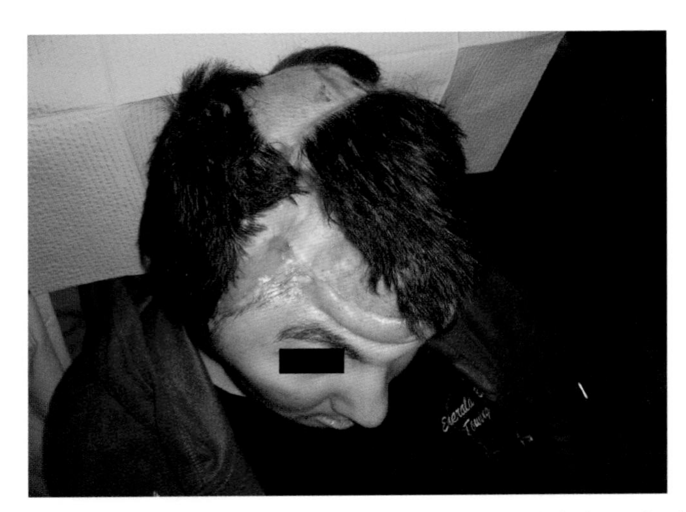

• **Fig. 1.84** The result at 2 months after her second free latissimus dorsi myocutaneous flap transfer and 11 months after her first free latissimus dorsi myocutaneous flap transfer showing a reliable soft tissue coverage to her scalp wound.

Pearls for Success

The case presented illustrates the surgical stratagem of staged free tissue transfer in light of known suboptimal patient and surgical conditions. In this specific scenario, proceeding with a second free flap without addressing the obvious risk factors would be imprudent and unadvisable. The key surgical plan in addressing this complex patient is that of staging the free flap into distinct phases in order to ensure the ultimate success of our reconstruction. If there is concern regarding whether the patient can tolerate a prolonged free tissue transfer or if the primary flap was not successful, the same procedure should not be repeated without careful consideration of how to improve the intraoperative approach.

In this case, we had to limit the exposure to prolonged general anesthesia and mitigate the risk of surgical stressors to the patient. Thus, we utilized the first-stage procedure in order to shorten the anesthetic exposure, but most importantly to precondition the patient and determine her tolerance to another anesthetic before proceeding with the definitive second free flap because the cause of the first free flap failure was perioperative hypotension. This second-stage procedure was again shorter than her initial latissimus dorsi free flap because of the staged approach and the patient tolerated the second stage better without any episodes of hypotension or respiratory distress.

Recommended Readings

Afifi A, Djohan RS, Hammert W, et al. Lessons learned reconstructing complex scalp defects using free flaps and a cranioplasty in one stage. *J Craniofac Surg*. 2010;21:1205–1209.

Amin A, Rifaat M, Civantos F, et al. Free anterolateral thigh flap for reconstruction of major craniofacial defects. *J Reconstr Microsurg*. 2006;22:97–104.

Dorfman D, Pu LL. The value of color duplex imaging for planning and performing a free anterolateral thigh perforator flap. *Ann Plast Surg*. 2014;72:S6–S8.

Hansen SL, Foster RD, Dosanjh AS, et al. Superficial temporal artery and vein as recipient vessels for facial and scalp microsurgical reconstruction. *Plast Reconstr Surg*. 2007;120:1879–1884.

Iblher N, Ziegler MC, Penna V, et al. An algorithm for oncologic scalp reconstruction. *Plast Reconstr Surg*. 2010;126:450–459.

Leedy JE, Janis JE, Rohrich RJ. Reconstruction of acquired scalp defects: an algorithmic approach. *Plast Reconstr Surg*. 2005;116:54e–72e.

Mehrara BJ, Disa JJ, Pusic A. Scalp reconstruction. *J Surg Oncol*. 2006;94:504–508.

Simunovic FS, Eisenhardt SU, Penna V, Thiele JR, Start GB, Bannasch H. Microsurgical reconstruction of oncological scalp defects in the elderly. *J Plast Recontr Aesthetic Surg*. 2016;69:912–919.

Song P, Jaiswal R, Pu LL. The second free tissue transfer after the first free flap loss for a complex scalp reconstruction: our strategy to success with a staged appraoch. *J Craniofac Surg*. 2022;33:e109–e111.

Sosin M, Schultz BD, De La Cruz C, et al. Microsurgical scalp reconstruction in the elderly: a systematic review and pooled analysis of the current data. *Plast Reconstr Surg*. 2015;135:856–866.

Uzum H, Bitik O, Ersoy US, Bilginer B, Aksu AE. Comparison of musculocutaneous and fasciocutaneous free flaps for the reconstruction of the extensive composite scalp and cranium defects. *J Craniofac Surg*. 2018;29:1947–1951.

2 Upper Facial Reconstruction

Clinical Presentation

A 52-year-old White male had a "large" melanoma in the right temporal area (Fig. 2.1) and underwent a wide local excision of the temporal melanoma with a 2-cm margin and sentinel lymph node biopsy in the face and neck by the surgical oncology service. He had a 4.5 × 4.5 cm skin defect down to the superficial temporal fascia involving the upper face, temporal area, and cheek (Fig. 2.2). The plastic surgery service was asked to close this large skin defect after the wide local excision and sentinel lymph node biopsy.

Operative Plan and Special Considerations

Based on the size and location of the skin defect and the existing incision for sentinel lymph node biopsy in the face and neck, and skin laxity in his neck, a large cervicofacial flap was designed for this patient. The procedure itself would be similar to a classic skin-only face lift performed by plastic surgeons for facial rejuvenation. In this procedure, the excess lower face and neck skin could be dissected free and used to reconstruct the large skin defect in the upper face and temporal area. Therefore, the defect could be closed primarily and no skin graft would be needed.

Operative Procedures

The cervicofacial skin rotation and advancement flap was designed based on the existing incision on the same side of the face and neck. The extent of the skin flap dissection was marked (Fig. 2.3). Its dissection should be extensive enough for the defect to be closed without very much tension. All proposed skin dissection areas were then infiltrated with 1% lidocaine with 1:100,000 epinephrine. The skin flap dissection was performed first from inside the defect and then followed to the existing face and neck incisions. Face lift scissors can be used to facilitate skin flap elevation. The extent of the cervicofacial flap dissect for this patient was similar to a unilateral face lift surgery, superomedially toward the orbicularis oculi muscle, medially to the nasolabial fold, inferiorly several centimeters below the mandibular boarder toward the midline. If necessary, cervical skin dissection could be more extensive both medially and inferiorly. The entire cervicofacial flap was then rotated and advanced to the skin defect and excess skin of the flap was trimmed. All closure was performed in two layers including the preauricular and neck incisions as for a

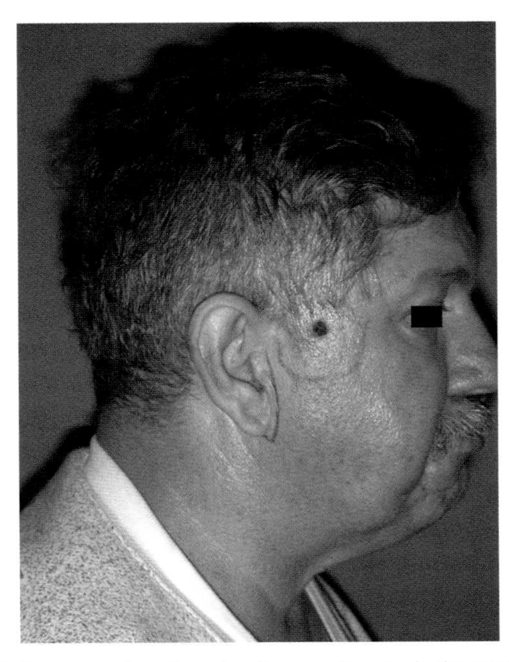

• **Fig. 2.1** A preoperative view showing a melanoma in the temporal and upper facial regions and an outline of potential margin for the wide local excision.

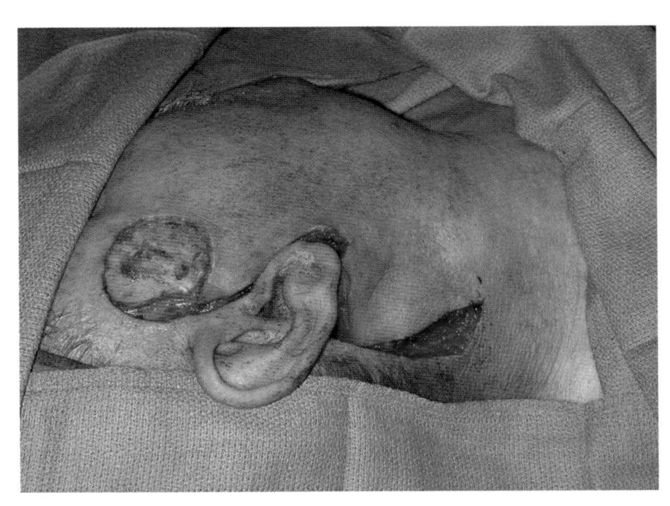

• **Fig. 2.2** An intraoperative view showing a large skin defect involving the temporal, upper facial regions and cheek as well as incisions for cervical lymph node dissection in the face and neck.

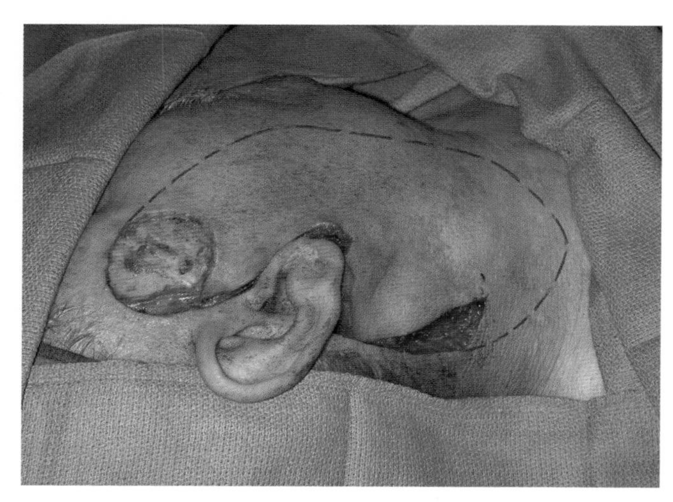

• **Fig. 2.3** An intraoperative view showing the extent of a cervicofacial skin flap dissection.

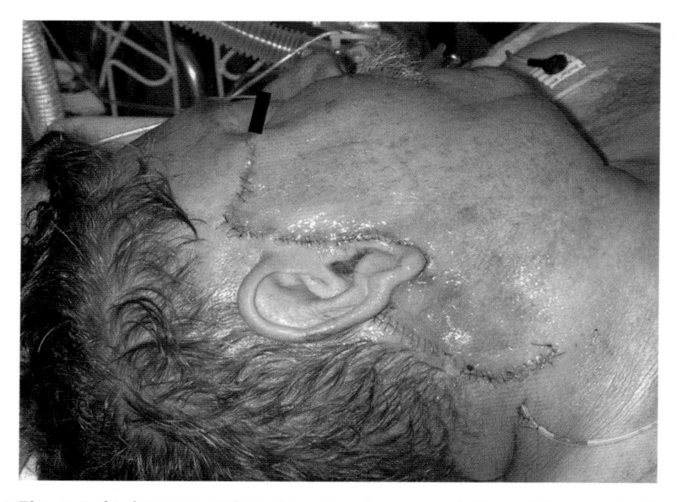

• **Fig. 2.4** An intraoperative view showing completion of the cervicofacial skin flap for closure of the defect.

standard face lift incision closure. A 7-mm JP drain was inserted under the flap (Fig. 2.4).

Follow-Up Results

The patient did well postoperatively without any complications related to his cervicofacial flap reconstruction. He was observed overnight in the hospital and discharged home next day. The drain was removed during the first week follow-up visit. The flap site and his preauricular and neck incisions all healed well (Fig. 2.5).

Final Outcome

His cervicofacial reconstruction site healed well without any problems. He has a reasonably good facial symmetry and nicely

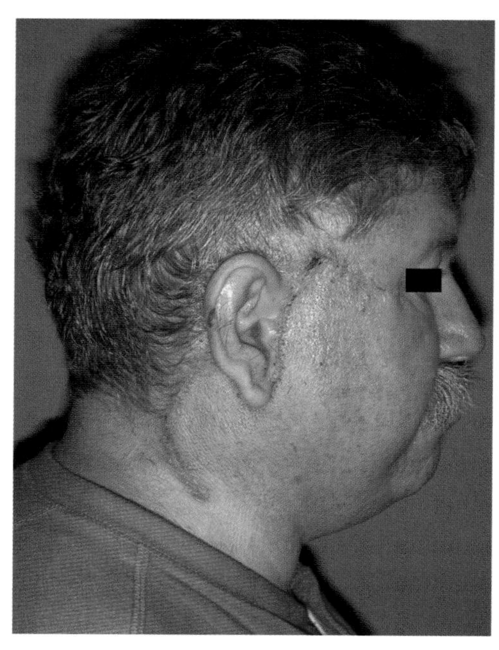

• **Fig. 2.5** Result at a 4-week follow-up showing well-healed flap site with minimal contour deformity and scarring.

faded scars. He returned to his normal life and has been followed by our surgical oncology service for routine melanoma follow-up.

Pearls for Success

Accurate preoperative evaluation is important to assess the amount of excess lower face and neck skin the patient has, especially for elderly patients. Extensive skin flap dissection could be performed just like a face lift surgery, but more neck skin dissection may be needed to create a tension-free closure. Face lift scissors can be helpful for performing such a skin flap dissection. The superficial musculoaponeurotic system fascia plication or even elevation may facilitate the skin defect closure or allow reduced neck skin dissection for the closure.

Recommended Readings

Austen Jr WG, Parrett BM, Taghinia A, Wolfort SE, Upton J. The subcutaneous cervicofacial flap revisited. *Ann Plast Surg*. 2009;62: 149–153.

D'Arpa S, Cordova A, Pirrello R, Zabbia G, Kalbermatten D, Moschella F. The face lift SMAS plication flap for reconstruction of large temporofrontal defects: reconstructive surgery meets cosmetic surgery. *Plast Reconstr Surg*. 2011;127:2068–2075.

Huang AT, Tarasidis G, Yelverton JC, Burke A. Novel advancement flap for reconstruction of massive forehead and temple soft-tissue defects. *Laryngoscopy*. 2012;122:1679–1904.

Sakellariou A, Salama A. The use of cervicofacial flap in maxillofacial reconstruction. *Oral Maxillofacial Surg Clin N Am*. 2014;26: 389–400.

3 Middle Facial Reconstruction

CASE 1

Clinical Presentation

A 51-year-old White male had a basal cell cancer over his left medial cheek and nasal sidewall. Mohs surgery was performed by our dermatological surgeon and the skin resection margins were all negative. The patient had a 6 × 2.5 cm skin defect involving the medial cheek and nasal sidewall near the medial canthus (Fig. 3.1). The plastic surgery service was asked to close this complex skin defect after a definitive cancer resection. The patient was also a heavy smoker and was unable to stop smoking prior to surgery.

Operative Plan and Special Considerations

Based on an analysis of the defect involving the medial cheek and nasal sidewall, the medial cheek advancement could be designed to cover the cheek defect and a portion of the nasal sidewall defect and a full thickness skin graft could also be used to cover the rest of the defect in the nasal sidewall.

Operative Procedures

The medial cheek advancement flap was designed superiorly parallel to the lower eyelid and medial to the nasolabial fold (Fig. 3.2). The flap area was infiltrated with 1% lidocaine with 1:100,000 epinephrine.

The flap was elevated under direct vision at the subcutaneous tissue plane and the area of the skin flap elevation measured 15 × 10 cm (Fig. 3.3). With a scissor dissection, the medial cheek skin flap was elevated and advanced to cover the entire medial cheek defect along with some of the inferior portion of the nasal sidewall (Fig. 3.4). Several tacking sutures were used with 4-0 nylon suture to hold the skin flap and facilitate closure of the defect. On the nasal side wall, the skin flap was also approximated to the nasal sidewall skin with 4-0 nylon sutures in half-buried horizontal mattress fashion. Some excess skin was excised for better donor site closure. The medial inferior portion of the flap was sutured to the nasal labial fold skin with 4-0 nylon sutures in simple interrupted fashion. The lower eyelid incision closure was done in the deeper dermal layer with 5-0 Monocryl sutures in a simple interrupted fashion, followed by the 5-0 nylon sutures for skin closure in a simple running fashion.

The excess portion of the distal flap was excised. This portion of the skin, which measured 2 × 1 cm, was defatted and placed over the left nasal side wall defect and secured with multiple 5-0 chromic sutures (Fig. 3.5). The skin graft was sutured to the wound bed and then secured with a tie-over dressing for skin graft immobilization.

Follow-Up Results

The patient did well postoperatively without any complications related to the medial cheek advancement flap. He was observed overnight in the hospital and discharged home the next day. His tie-over dressing was removed at postoperative day 5. The flap and skin graft sites both healed well. There was no entropion over his left lower eyelid (Figs. 3.6A–C).

Final Outcome

The medial cheek advancement flap to the medial cheek defect and full thickness skin graft to the nasal sidewall defect healed well without any issues. The patient has had a reasonably good cosmetic outcome and minimal scarring (Fig. 3.7A and B). He returned to normal life and has been followed by our demonologist for routine skin cancer follow-up.

Pearls for Success

The medial cheek advancement flap can be elevated to cover a medial cheek and even a portion of the nasal sidewall defects if the patient has some skin laxity in the cheek. The flap is elevated at the subcutaneous tissue plane above the fascia of the superficial musculoaponeurotic system. Superiorly it is parallel to the lower eyelid and medially it follows the nasolabial fold. Attention should be paid not to traumatize the orbicularis oculi muscle. Preoperative evaluation of the lower eyelid position may be helpful to predict whether the patient would need a lateral canthopexy. In a smoker, the distal portion of the flap may not be reliable. For this case, it was converted to a full thickness skin graft. With proper immobilization postoperatively, the full thickness skin graft can heal well and provide even better contour of the nasal sidewall for reconstruction.

CASE 2

Clinical Presentation

A 19-year-old White female sustained comminuted fractures of her maxilla secondary to a motor vehicle accident. She was

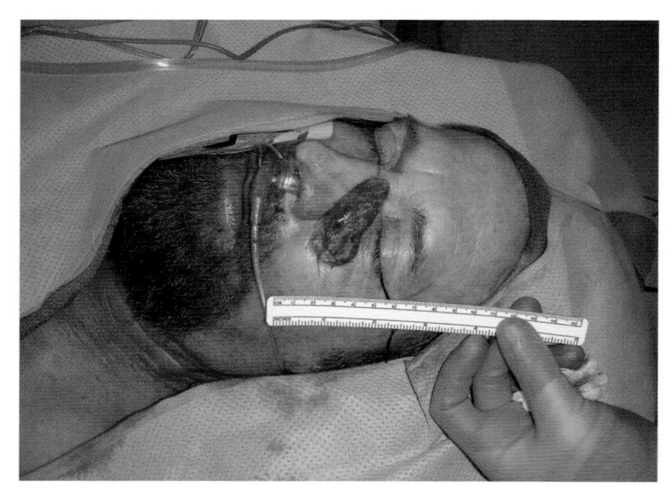

• **Fig. 3.1** Intraoperative view showing a large skin defect involving the medial cheek and nasal side wall after mons surgical resection with all negative margins.

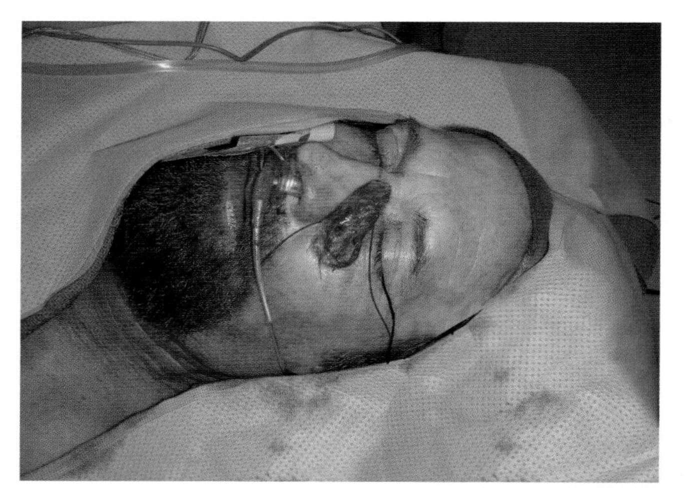

• **Fig. 3.2** Intraoperative view showing the design of a medial cheek advancement flap with marking of all proposed skin incisions.

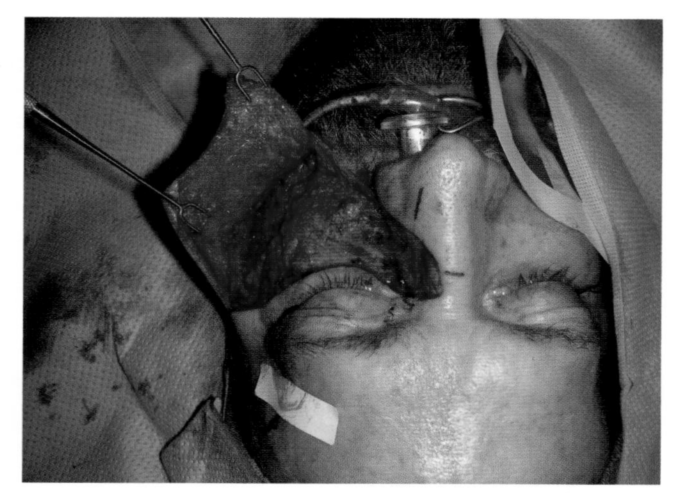

• **Fig. 3.3** Intraoperative view showing the extent of skin elevation for the medial cheek advancement flap.

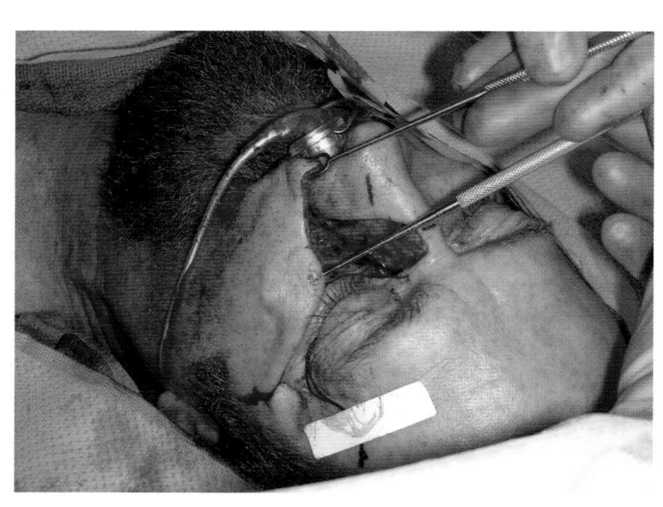

• **Fig. 3.4** Intraoperative view showing the amount of rotation and advancement from the medial cheek advancement flap for coverage of this large skin defect.

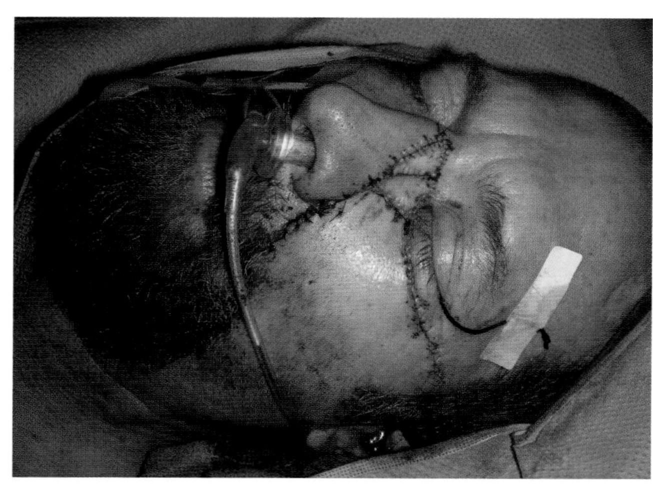

• **Fig. 3.5** Intraoperative view showing completion after the medial cheek advancement flap reconstruction and full thickness skin graft.

managed by an outside hospital initially for the soft tissue injury and acute trauma conditions and was transferred to our plastic surgery service for definite reconstruction of her middle facial bony defect. On examination, she had a significant midfacial collapse (Fig. 3.8). Intraoral examination showed poor quality and scarred gum tissue over the old fracture site. Her facial bone CT scan showed a significant bony defect in the central portion of the maxilla and a missing small bony portion of the nasal dorsum (Fig. 3.9).

Operative Plan and Special Considerations

This patient was also evaluated by our oral surgery service. A dental model was made for her and it showed the exact 8-cm bony defect of the maxilla and the amount of vascularized bone graft needed for such a reconstruction (Figs. 3.10 and 3.11). Because of the need for maxillary bony reconstruction and the poor quality of her intraoral soft tissue, a free fibula osteocutaneous flap

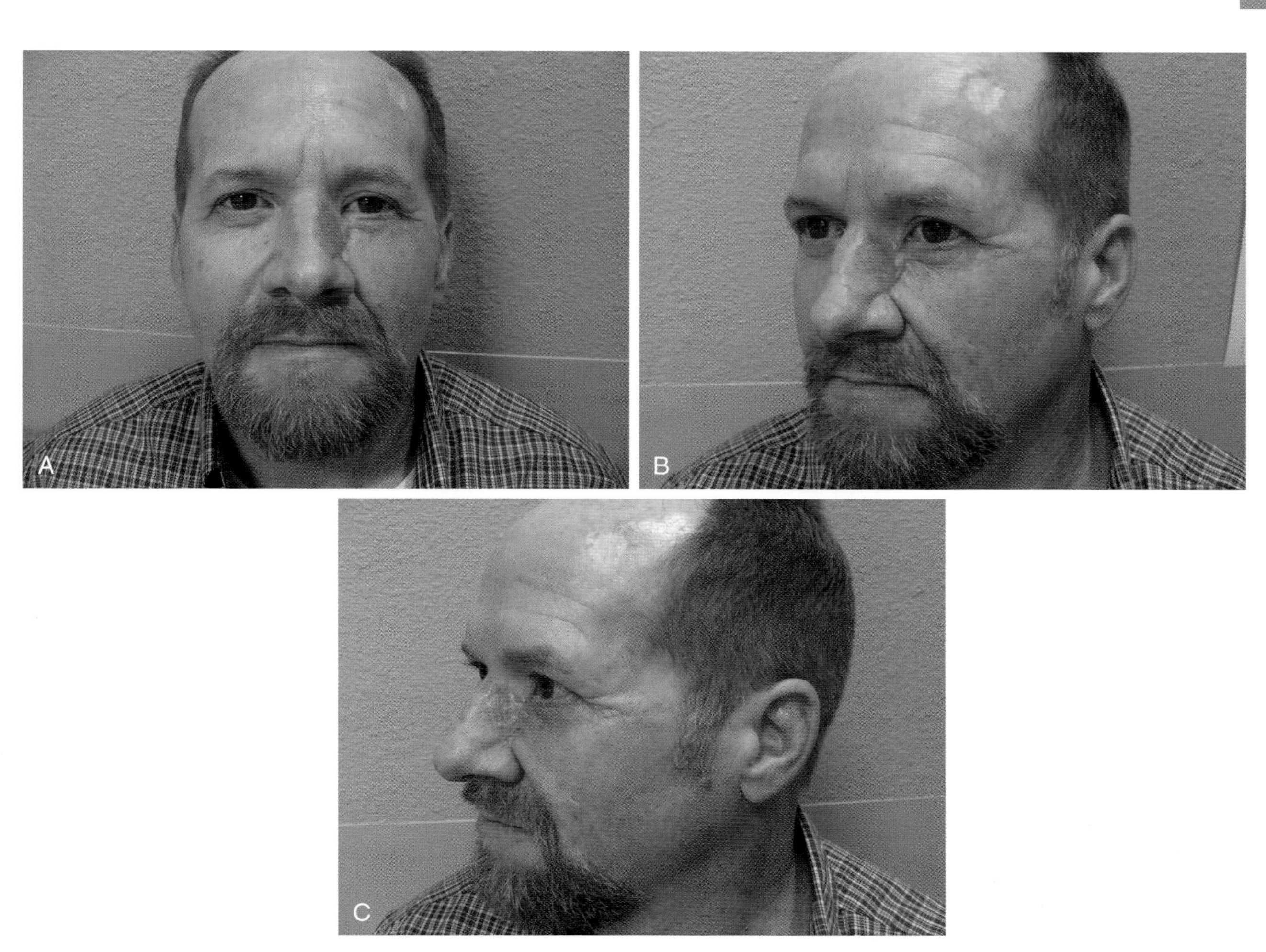

• **Fig. 3.6** (A–C) The result at 1-month follow-up. The patient's lower eyelid position is normal.

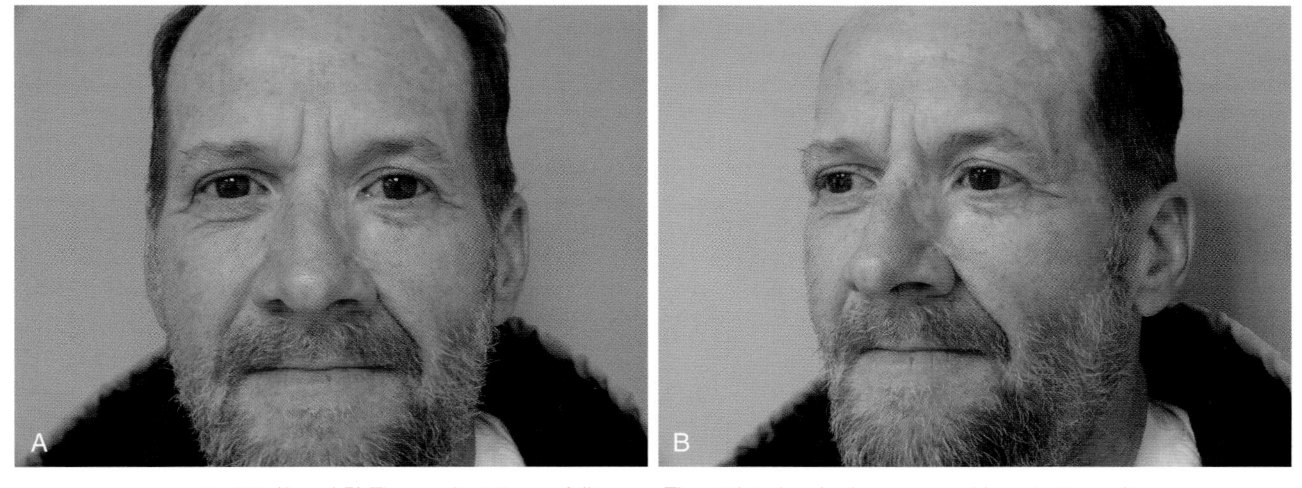

• **Fig. 3.7** (A and B) The result at 5-year follow-up. The patient has had a very good long-term result with nearly normal-looking face.

reconstruction was offered to this patient. Because the dental model had been made, the bony reconstruction could be performed simultaneously for potentially improved occlusion and future osteointegrated dental implants. A preoperative angiogram was performed to confirm a normal vascular structure of both legs.

Operative Procedures

The procedure was started by two teams simultaneously. Her old maxillary fracture site was explored by the oral surgery service. Her scarred gum tissue was removed and the residual maxillary fracture

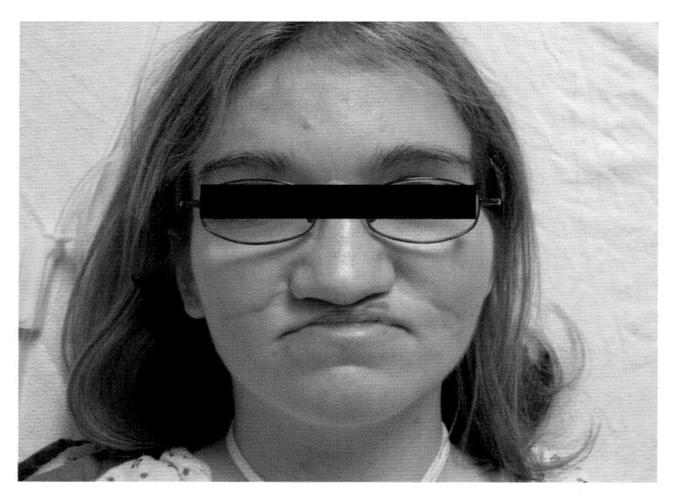

• **Fig. 3.8** A preoperative view showing a significant midface collapse and under-projection of her nose.

sites were explored. All of the mini bony fragments were removed. Her maxilla bony defect was confirmed as 8 cm after a direct measurement.

The left free fibula osteocutaneous flap was harvested by the plastic surgery service. A 12 × 4 cm of the skin paddle was designed (Fig. 3.12). Under tourniquet control, the skin paddle was incised through the fascia. The subfascial dissection was performed toward the posterior intermuscular septum (Fig. 3.13). Two septocutaneous perforators were identified in the septum. Attention was made to avoid direct or indirect injury to those perforators. The dissection was made to release the muscle attachment to the fibula from the soleus muscle. Once the peroneal vessels close to the fibula were identified, the distal osteotomy was performed at a level of about 6 cm proximal to the lateral malleolus. By further dissection of the hallucis longus muscle's attachment, the peroneal vessels and the fibula were dissected free. The proximal osteotomy was then performed and a 10-cm segment of the fibula was obtained. A longitudinal skin incision was extended further toward the fibular head. Following more dissection around the pedicle, the peroneal vessels were

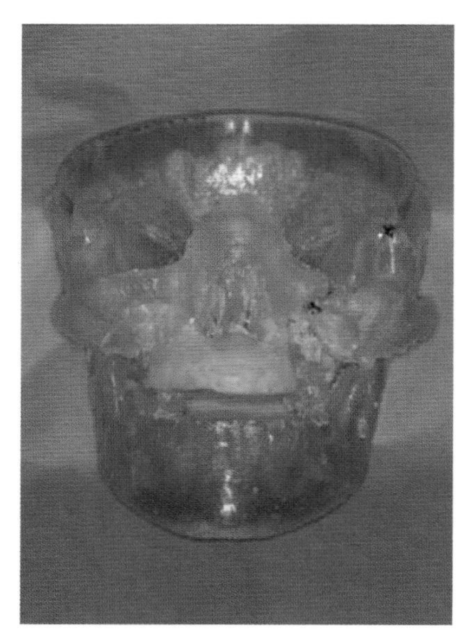

• **Fig. 3.10** Anterior view of preoperative 3-D model showing the exact amount of missed maxilla in this patient.

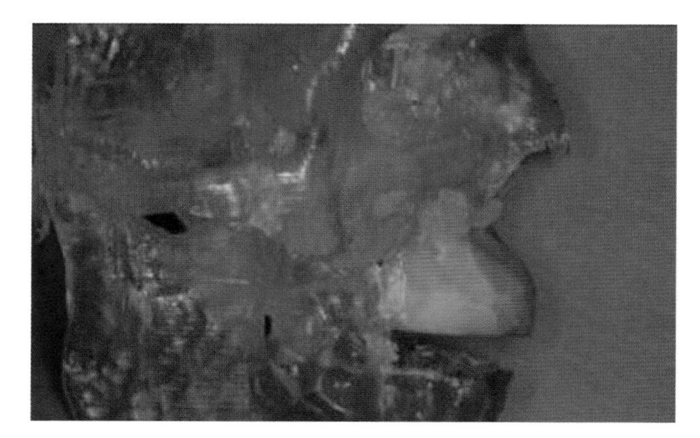

• **Fig. 3.11** Lateral view of preoperative 3-D model showing the exact amount of missed maxilla in this patient.

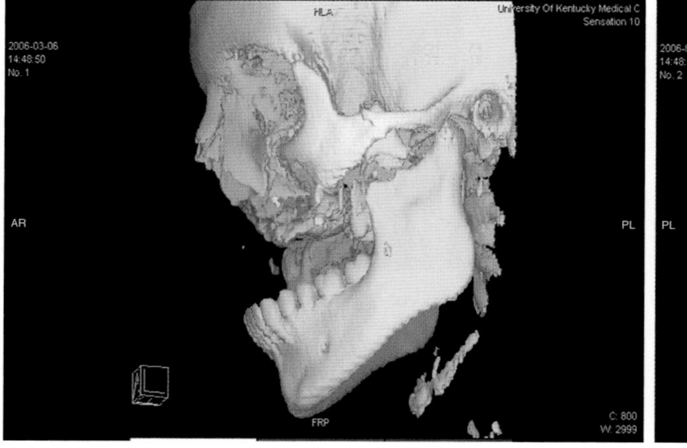

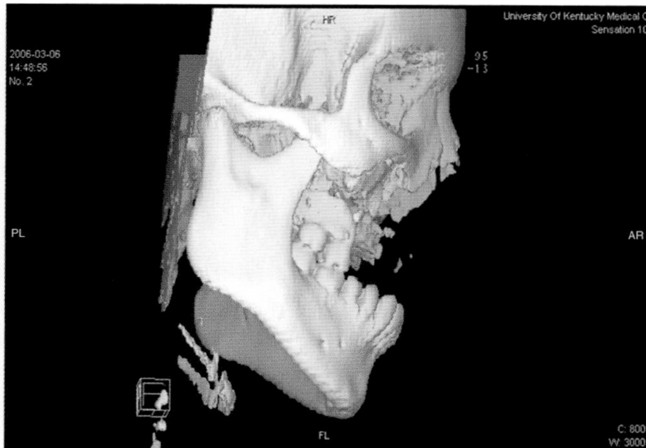

• **Fig. 3.9** Preoperative facial CT scans showing significant portion of the maxilla missing as a result of previous trauma.

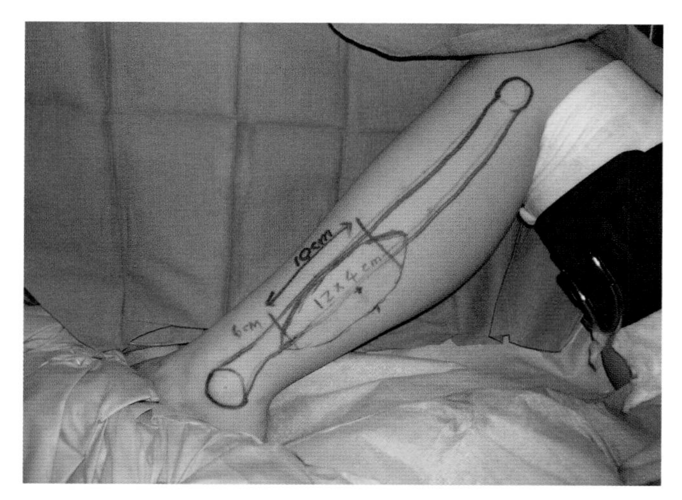

• **Fig. 3.12** Intraoperative view showing the design of the fibula osteocutaneous flap. A 12 × 4 cm skin paddle was designed and a perforator within the skin paddle was identified by Doppler scan.

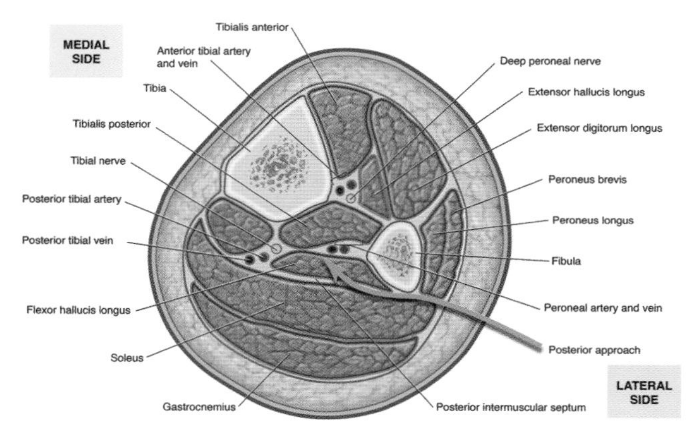

• **Fig. 3.13** A schematic diagram showing the posterior approach used for fibula osteocutaneous flap dissection.

dissected free toward its bifurcation with the posterior tibial vessels. Once the bifurcation was visualized, the pedicle was divided and the flap's dissection was completed (Fig. 3.14). With the guide of the dental model, two osteotomies were performed on the nonperiosteum attachment side (Fig. 3.15).

The harvested fibular osteocutaneous flap was then inset into the maxillary defect and secured with multiple 1.0 miniplates. Two osteotomy sites were secured with miniplates based on the contour of the bone. During the flap dissection, the excess portion of the fibula was removed and used as a free bone graft for the nasal dorsal augmentation that was secured with a screw via an open approach.

With a 5-cm submandibular incision, the right facial artery and the vein were explored. The facial artery appeared to be a good size, but the facial vein appeared to be small.

By tunneling through the cheek, both the pedicle artery and the vein were brought into the submandibular area. They were prepared under loupe magnification. Both end-to-end microvascular anastomoses were performed under a microscope. The vein

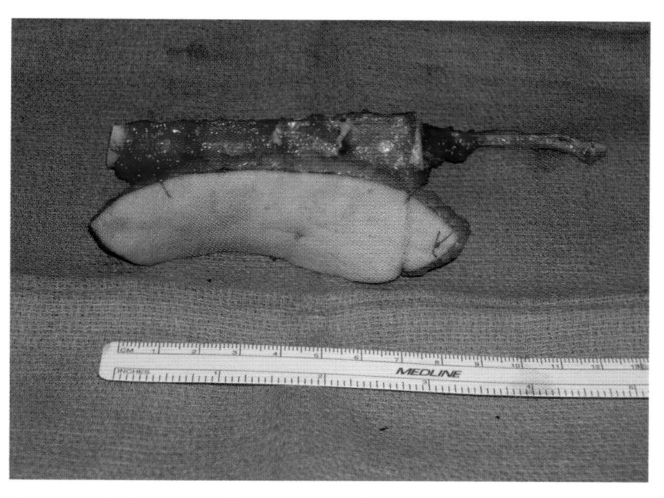

• **Fig. 3.14** An intraoperative view showing completion of the free fibular osteocutaneous flap.

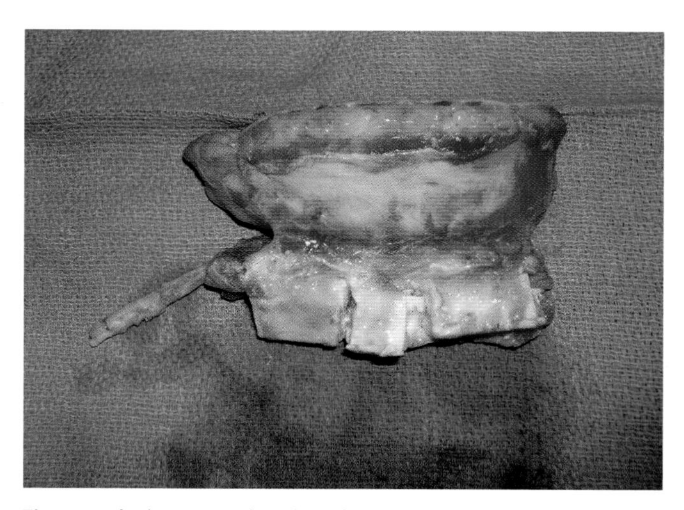

• **Fig. 3.15** An intraoperative view showing two osteotomies performed for the free fibular osteocutaneous flap.

was anastomosed first with 2.5-mm coupler device without any problems but there was a slight mismatch. With a double-armed Acland clamp, the arterial anastomosis was performed with an 8-0 nylon in a simple interrupted fashion. The total ischemia time was 2.5 hours.

Once both anastomoses were completed, the flap appeared to be well-perfused and with good Doppler signal sounds. The skin paddle of the flap was then inset into the upper intraoral cavity. Unfortunately, the skin paddle appeared to be too bulky, therefore it was removed. The fascial portion of the flap was sutured with several interrupted 3-0 Vicryl sutures in a half-buried horizontal mattress fashion to adjacent mucosa and the entire vascularized bone graft was well covered with the remaining fascia of the flap (Fig. 3.16).

The left leg fibular flap donor site was closed primarily in two layers after all muscles were approximated with several interrupted 2-0 Vicryl sutures. The submandibular skin incision was loosely closed with skin staples.

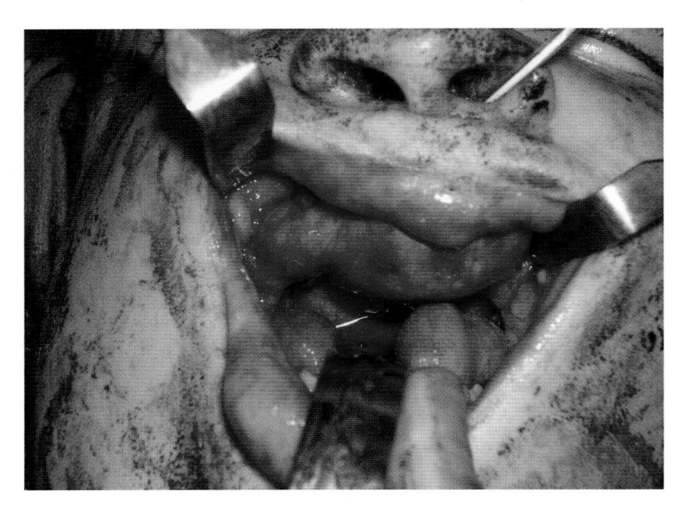

• **Fig. 3.16** An intraoperative view showing completion of the flap inset intraorally.

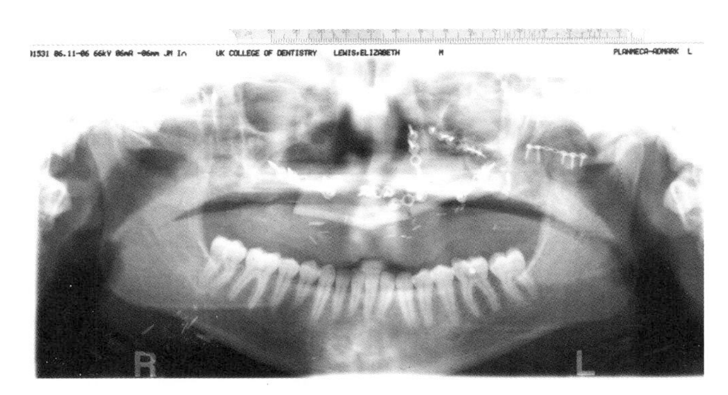

• **Fig. 3.17** Postoperative X-ray image showing the evidence of maxillary bony union at 6-week follow-up (anterior view).

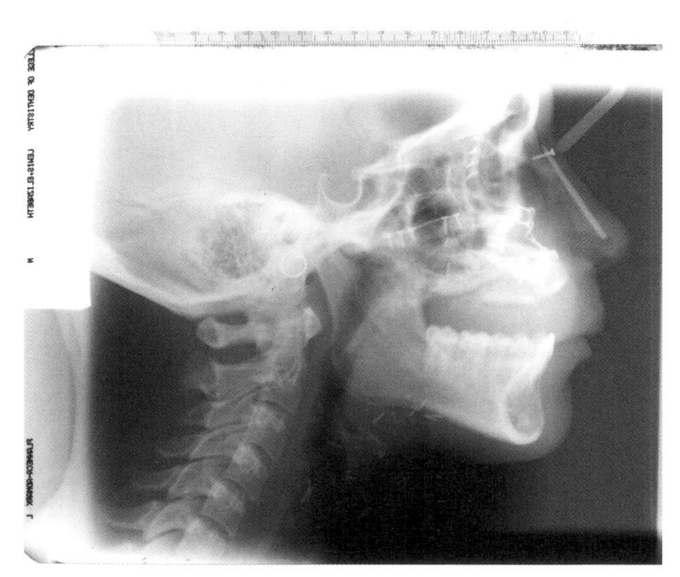

• **Fig. 3.18** Postoperative X-ray image showing the evidence of maxillary bony union at 6-week follow-up (lateral view).

Management of Complications

Postoperatively, venous congestion of the flap developed, probably because of the poor venous outflow. Therefore, the patient was brought back to the operating room at postoperative day 1 for revision of the venous anastomosis. A saphenous vein graft was harvested and a new and better recipient vein, the superior thyroid vein, was found. Each venous anastomosis of the vein graft was performed with a coupler device. Tissue plasminogen activator was used intraoperatively to resolve venous congestion within the flap.

Follow-Up Results

The patient did well after surgery and was discharged home at postoperative day 10. The intraoral flap site healed well and there was evidence of early bony healing of the fibular vascularized bone graft (Figs. 3.17 and 3.18). Her middle facial contour looks nearly normal. Her nasal dorsal projection is also improved (Figs. 3.19 and 3.20).

Final Outcome

The patient had complete bony union of the fibular vascularized bone graft site. Her intraoral flap site healed well (Fig. 3.21). She had a good cosmetic improvement of her middle facial contour and her nasal projection (Figs. 3.22–3.24). Her left leg flap donor site had no issues (Fig. 3.25). She was followed by the oral surgery service for future osteointegrated dental implants. She has returned to her normal life as a college student.

Pearls for Success

A 3-D dental model is very helpful in terms of preoperative planning. In this case, the size and contour of the fibular bone graft after osteotomy could be determined. Working with the oral surgery service ensures a better occlusion after the flap inset. In addition, the oral surgery service could predetermine the thickness of the fibular bone graft to ensure a better outcome for future

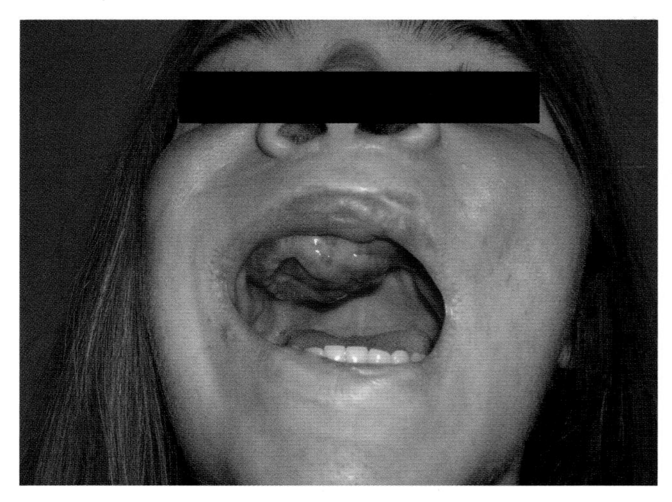

• **Fig. 3.19** The result at 3-month follow-up showing well-healed intraoral flap site.

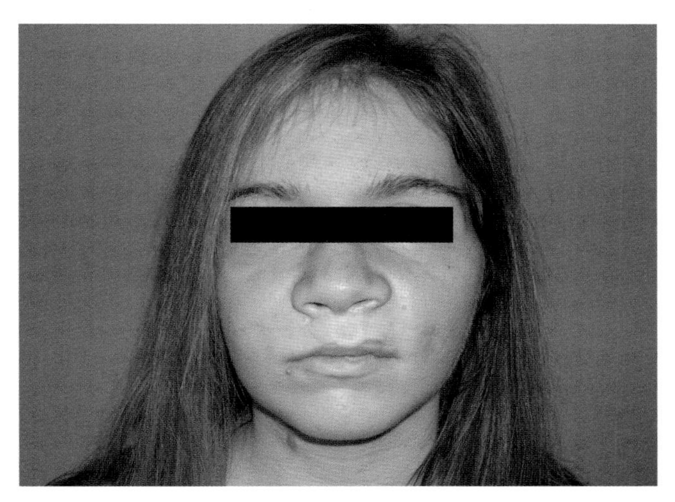

• **Fig. 3.20** The result at 3-month follow-up showing improved middle facial contour.

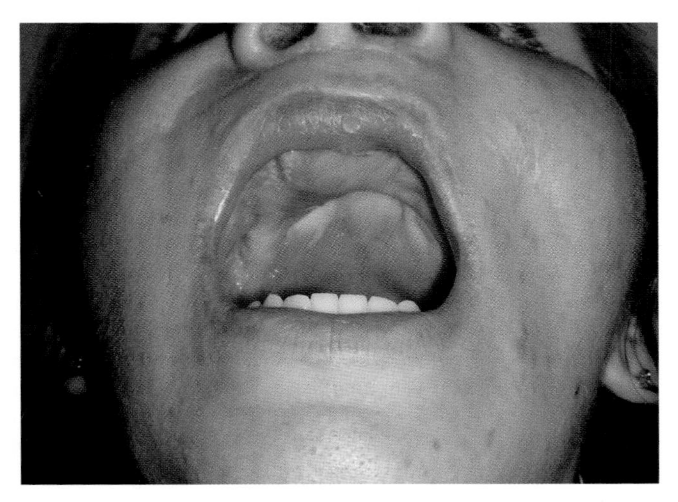

• **Fig. 3.21** The result at 7-month follow-up showing well-healed intraoral flap site.

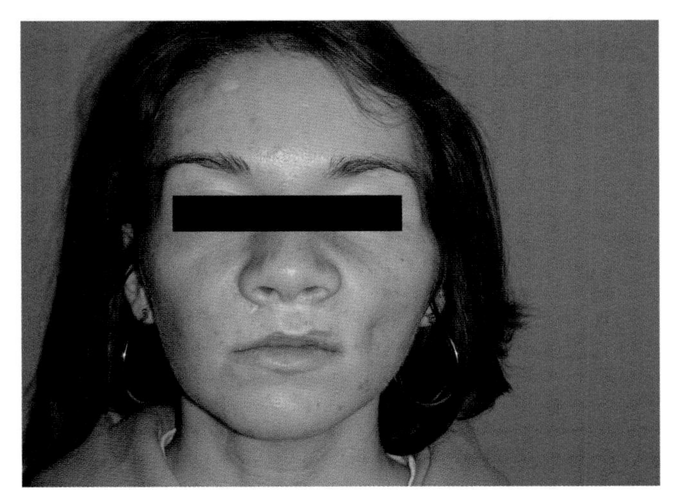

• **Fig. 3.22** 7-month follow-up showing improved middle facial contour (anterior view).

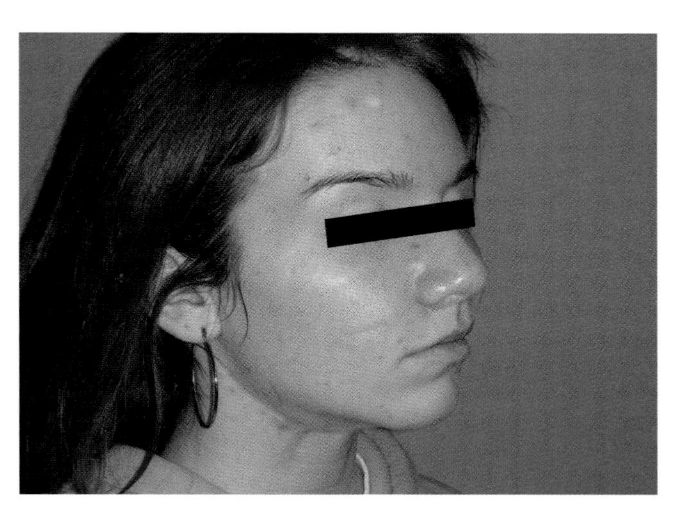

• **Fig. 3.23** 7-month follow-up showing improved middle facial coutour (right oblique view).

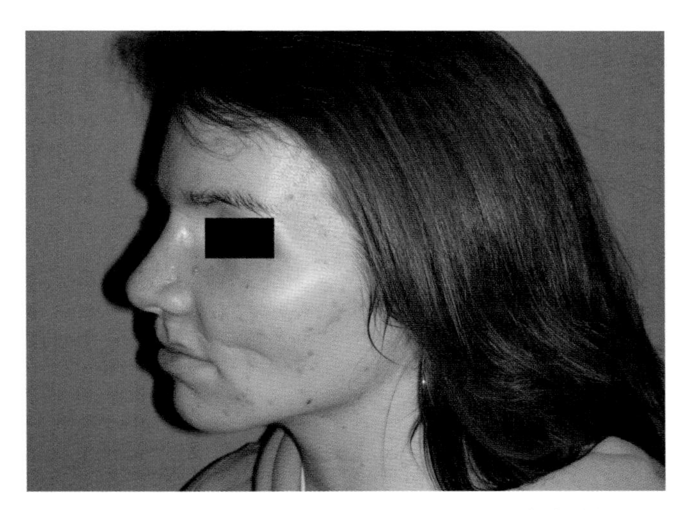

• **Fig. 3.24** 7-month follow-up showing improved middle facial contour (left oblique view).

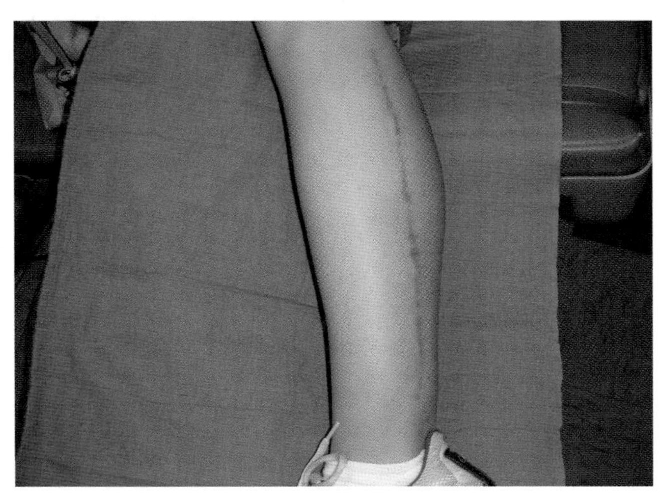

• **Fig. 3.25** The result at 7-month follow-up showing leg contour and scar after a free fibular osteocutaneous flap harvest.

osteointegrated dental implants. The narrow skin paddle could ensure a primary closure of the flap donor site for better cosmetic outcome. Intraoral soft tissue closure with the flap's fascial portion may be adequate after mucosalization. A better venous anastomosis with a vein graft to the good recipient vein should have been done initially to avoid potential venous outflow problem. However, this would be a surgeon's judgment call intraoperatively. Routine preoperative evaluation of the facial vessels as good recipient vessels can also be critical to the success of any free tissue transfer to the middle face.

CASE 3

Clinical Presentation

A 61-year-old White male with a history of squamous cell carcinoma (SCC) in the left temporal region, cheek, and ear had a recurrent SCC after previous excisions and radiation to the area. He had locally advanced SCC involving the left temporal bone and its adjacent soft tissue, including the left ear and cheek. He underwent radical resection including the temporal bone and ear by both otolaryngology and neurosurgery services for the local control and modified neck lymph node dissection. After these resections, there was a 14 × 11 cm soft tissue defect involving the temporal region, middle and lower face, and postauricular scalp with exposed underlying bones and the ear canal (Fig. 3.26).

Operative Plan and Special Considerations

For such a large soft tissue defect, a free vertical rectus abdominus musculocutaneous (VRAM) flap was selected for soft tissue coverage based on the preoperative evaluation of the abdominal wall. The flap itself is reliable and the flap dissection is relatively easy and quick. Although its pedicle may not be that long, the exposed facial artery and vein after the neck lymph node dissection would be adequate for an easy microvascular anastomosis (Fig. 3.27).

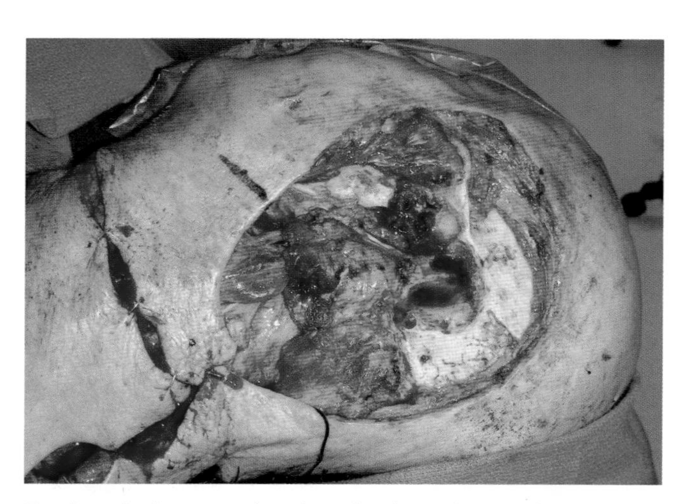

• **Fig. 3.26** An intraoperative view showing a large soft tissue defect involving the temporal region, middle and lower face, and postauricular scalp after resection with the exposed underlying bones and ear canal.

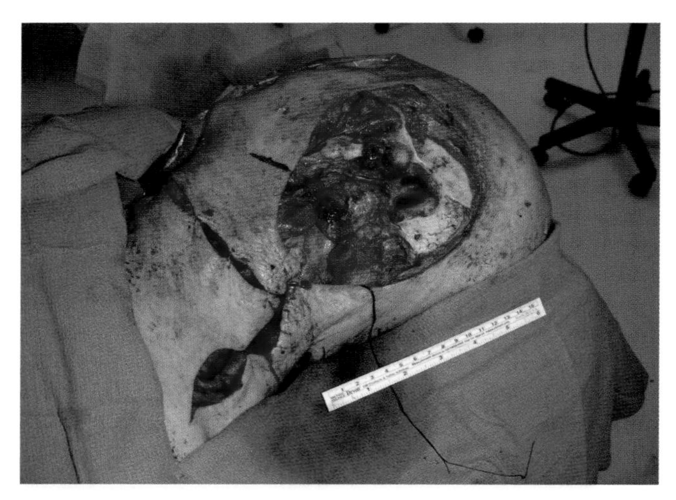

• **Fig. 3.27** An intraoperative view showing approximated neck wounds after the neck lymph node dissection with exposed facial artery and vein.

Operative Procedures

A free VRAM flap over the right rectus abdominus muscle was designed based on the skin laxity and a 14 × 11 cm skin paddle of the flap, oriented vertically, was marked (Fig. 3.28). Once the skin incision had been made to the anterior rectus sheath, the fascia was incised to the rectus muscle, and the rectus abdominis muscle was divided superiorly close to the costal margin. The flap was then elevated from the posterior rectus sheath after the superior epigastric vessels were divided with metal clips. The rectus abdominis muscle was then divided inferiorly and the free edge of the muscle was sown to the fascia with interrupted sutures to prevent sheer force between the muscle and fascia. Careful blunt dissection was performed to elevate the flap from superior to inferior, separating the posterior rectus sheath from the overlying muscle and vascular bundle. The inferior epigastric vessels were followed and dissected free toward their origin. The inferior deep

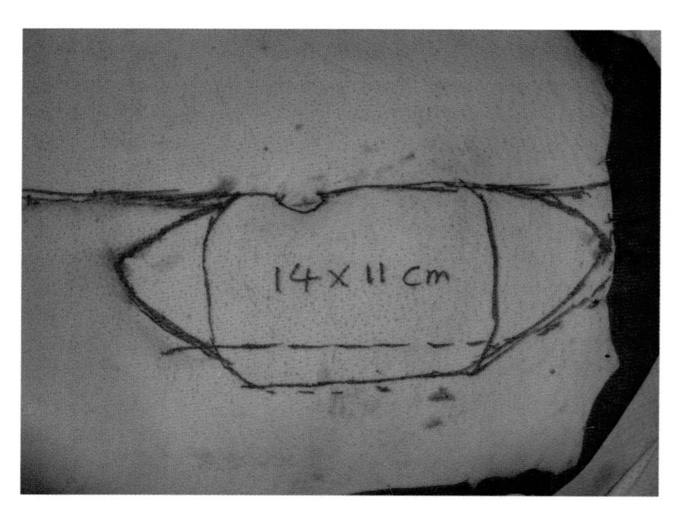

• **Fig. 3.28** Intraoperative view showing the design of the free vertical rectus abdominus musculocutaneous flap. The flap had a 14 × 11 cm skin paddle. In this case, less fascial resection was performed during the flap dissection.

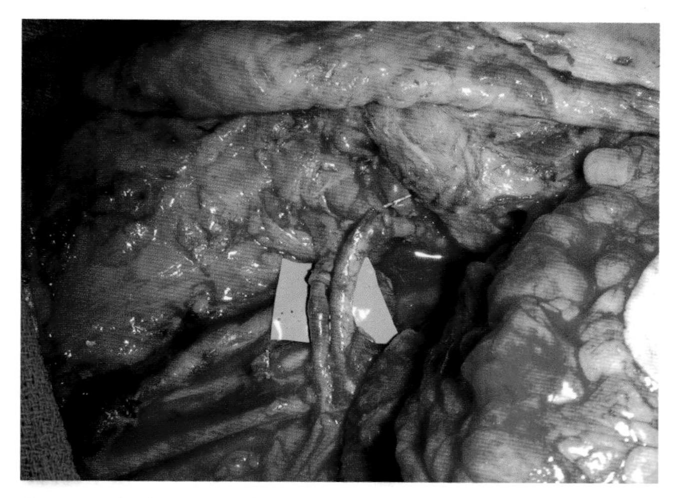

• **Fig. 3.29** An intraoperative view showing completion of both arterial and venous microvascular anastomoses to the facial artery and vein.

epigastric vessels were then divided at the level of the external iliac artery and vein.

The left facial vessels were found intact as well as the left internal jugular and external jugular veins. After further dissection, both facial artery and vein were found in good caliber and dissected proximally. Under a microscope, an end-to-end venous microvascular anastomosis was performed with a 3-mm venous coupler. The arterial microvascular anastomosis was also performed in an end-to-end fashion with interrupted 8-0 nylon sutures using a double-armed microclamp (Fig. 3.29).

The flap was then inset into the defect. Excess skin was trimmed around the periphery and the superior portion of the flap was debulked extensively to remove the excess subcutaneous fat. The flap was closed peripherally into the entire soft tissue defect including the abdominal wall fascia and Scarpa's fascia with interrupted sutures. A Penrose drain was placed near the anastomosis. Two other JP drains were brought out from under the flap into the scalp superiorly and over by the left neck wound inferiorly. The skin closure was performed with running 4-0 nylon (Fig. 3.30).

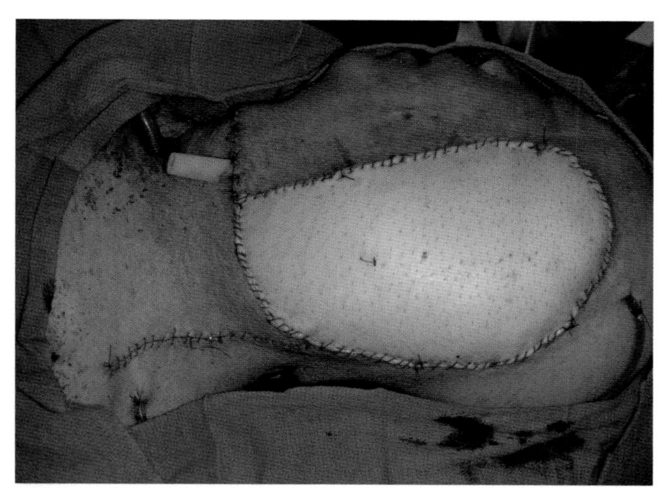

• **Fig. 3.30** An intraoperative view showing completion of the free vertical rectus abdominus musculocutaneous flap inset.

The abdominal flap donor site was closed in three layers: the anterior rectus sheath was approximated with a running 0 Prolene suture, the dermal layer with interrupted buried 3-0 Vicryl, and the skin with staples. A 15-Fr drain was placed in the subcutaneous tissue.

Management of Complications

At postoperative day 1, there was concern for an arterial inflow to the flap because it was slightly cooler and had very sluggish arterial bleeding. Although the Doppler signal in the flap was still present, it was felt that the signal was not as strong as immediate postoperatively. However, during the exploration, both arterial and venous anastomoses were found to be patent with no compromise for either the arterial inflow or the venous outflow of the flap.

Follow-Up Results

The patient did well postoperatively without any complications related to his free VRAM flap. His flap site had been healing well. He was discharged home at postoperative day 8. During follow-up, his flap site and abdominal donor site healed well (Fig. 3.31).

Final Outcome

His free VRAM flap reconstruction and abdominal donor site healed well without any issues. He remains cancer-free and underwent an upper eyelid procedure for his eyelid ptosis by a different service. He has returned to his normal life and has been followed by our otolaryngology service for routine cancer follow-up.

Pearls for Success

Although a free anterolateral thigh flap can be a good selection for the same reconstruction, a free VRAM can be harvested quickly and provide reliable soft tissue coverage as a "fast" free tissue transfer. Its flap dissection is relatively straightforward and its skin paddle is very reliable. Many refinements in the flap dissection have been focused on how to save more anterior rectus sheath as

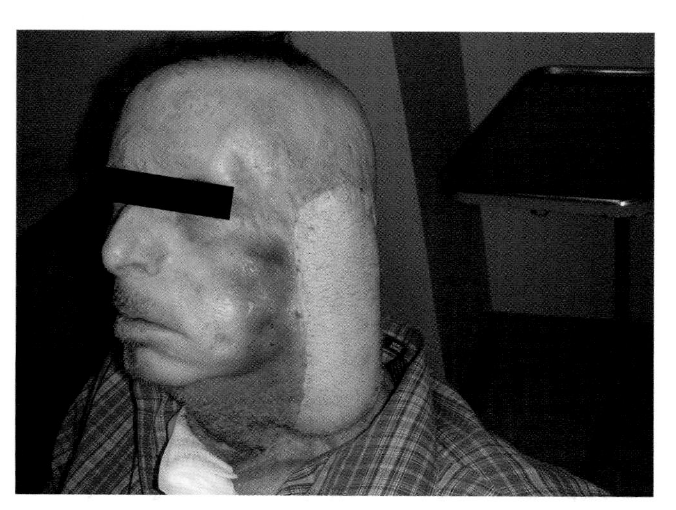

• **Fig. 3.31** The result at 1-month follow-up.

during a free transverse rectus abdominus myocutaneous flap dissection. However, the flap's pedicle length is relatively short and can only reach the facial vessels in the upper neck. Preoperative evaluation of the facial vessels can be critical to the success of a free VRAM flap transfer for a complex middle facial reconstruction.

Recommended Readings

Al Shetawi AH, Quimby A, Rui Fernandes R. The cervicofacial flap in cheek reconstruction: a guide for flap design. *J Oral Maxillofac Surg.* 2017;75:2708.e1–2708.e6.

Cordeiro PG, Santamaria E. A classification system and algorithm for reconstruction of maxillectomy and midfacial defects. *Plast Reconstr Surg.* 2000;105:2331–2346.

Largo RD, Garvey PB. Updates in head and neck reconstruction. *Plast Reconstr Surg.* 2018;141:e271–e285.

McCarthy CM, Cordeiro PG. Microvascular reconstruction of oncologic defects of the midface. *Plast Reconstr Surg.* 2010;126:1947–1959.

Patel NP, Matros E, Cordeiro PG. The use of the multi-island vertical rectus abdominis myocutaneous flap in head and neck reconstruction. *Ann Plast Surg.* 2012;69:403–407.

Runyan CM, Sharma V, Staffenberg DA, et al. Jaw in a day: state of the art in maxillary reconstruction. *J Craniofac Surg.* 2016;27:2601–2604.

Wei FC, Chen HC, Chuang C-C, et al. Fibular osteoseptocutaneous flap: anatomic study and clinical application. *Plast Reconstr Surg.* 1986;78:191–199.

Zhang WB, Wang Y, Liu XJ, et al. Reconstruction of maxillary defects with free fibula flap assisted by computer techniques. *J Craniomaxillofac Surg.* 2015;43:630–636.

4

Intraoral Reconstruction

CASE 1

Clinical Presentation

A 19-year-old White male with right alveolar squamous cell carcinoma (SCC) of the mandible underwent local surgical excision of the alveolar edge and the floor of the mouth and a marginal mandibulectomy via a lower lip split approach as well as a right modified neck lymph node dissection by the surgical oncology service (Fig. 4.1). Intraoperative frozen sections of the peripheral and deep margins were confirmed negative for SCC. Following resections, there was a 6.5 × 4.5 cm full-thickness intraoral mucosal defect with exposed alveolar bony bridge (Fig. 4.2).

Operative Plan and Special Considerations

After assessing the intraoral soft tissue defect including the alveolar defect of the mandible, a free radial forearm skin flap was selected for coverage of the floor of the mouth wound and the alveolar defect. The flap is reliable, versatile, and thin and could provide an excellent soft tissue coverage for such an intraoral defect with an easy inset and water-tight closure. In addition, the length of the flap's pedicle can reach any part of the neck recipient vessels.

Operative Procedures

A free radial forearm skin flap was designed on the nondominant side of the forearm after a negative Allen test. A 7.5 × 5.5 cm skin paddle of the flap, oriented longitudinally, was marked (Fig. 4.3). The skin incision was made through the fascia and subfascial dissection was performed for elevation of the skin paddle including the pedicle vessels that also contained the cephalic vein (Fig. 4.4). With a zig-zag incision, the dissection of the pedicle in the forearm was made between the flexor carpi radialis and brachioradialis muscles to the antecubital fossa. The radial artery and its venae comitantes as well as the cephalic vein were then divided with hemoclips.

The flap inset was done first to cover all intraoral soft tissue defect. A water-tight closure of the flap to the adjacent mucosa was performed with a 3-0 interrupted Vicryl suture in an interrupted half-buried horizontal mattress fashion. The pedicle of the flap was tunneled to the right neck where microvascular anastomoses were performed.

The right facial vessels were explored in the neck via the preexisting incisions for cancer resection and neck lymph node dissection. After further dissection, both the facial artery and vein were found to be a good size and dissected proximally for an adequate length. Under a microscope, an end-to-end venous microvascular anastomosis between the cephalic vein and the facial vein was performed with an 8-0 nylon sutures in an interrupted fashion using a double-armed microclamp. The arterial microvascular anastomosis was also performed in an end-to-end fashion with interrupted 8-0 nylon sutures. Additional intraoral closure was completed and the intraoral free radial forearm free flap reconstruction was completed (Fig. 4.5).

The lower lip and chin incisions were closed in two layers. The neck incision was also closed in two layers after a JP drain placement.

The forearm donor site skin incision was closed in two layers. A split-thickness skin graft was placed to the flap donor site, sutured to the adjacent normal skin edge, and secured with a tie-over dressing.

Management of Complications

The patient unfortunately developed a hematoma in the neck at postoperative day 2 and was brought back to the operating room for evacuation (Fig. 4.6). He had no recurrent hematoma after reoperation.

Follow-Up Results

The patient did well postoperatively without complications related to the free radial forearm flap reconstruction. He was discharged from the hospital on postoperative day 5. The drain was removed during the first week follow-up. His intraoral flap site as well as his lip and chin incisions healed well (Fig. 4.7). His left forearm flap donor site also healed well (Fig. 4.8).

Final Outcome

He looked nearly normal after the reconstruction for marginal mandibulectomy and local resection of his intraoral cancer (Fig. 4.9). He returned to his normal life and activities and was followed by the surgical oncology service for routine cancer follow-up.

Pearls for Success

Although other free skin flaps can be an option for the same reconstruction, a free radial forearm skin flap can be an excellent choice for an intraoral soft tissue coverage. The flap can be

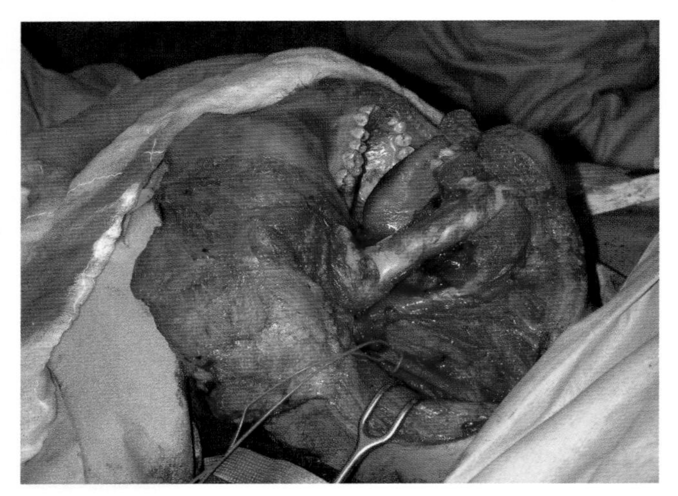

• **Fig. 4.1** Intraoperative view showing completion of the right marginal mandibulectomy, excision for the alveolar edge and floor of the mouth squamous cell carcinoma, and a modified neck lymph node dissection.

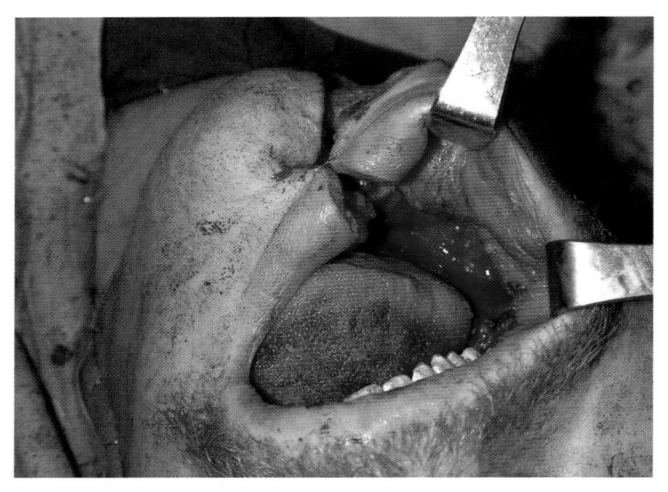

• **Fig. 4.2** Intraoperative view showing the intraoral soft tissue defect after excision for the alveolar edge and floor of the mouth squamous cell carcinoma.

harvested quickly and provide a thin and malleable soft tissue coverage as a "fast" free tissue transfer for an intraoral reconstruction. A water-tight intraoral flap closure should be done properly to prevent an orocutaneous fistula to the neck. The cephalic vein should be considered a dormant vein and selected for a single venous anastomosis. Many refinements in the radial forearm flap dissection have been focused on a suprafascial dissection of the skin paddle so that the flap donor sites can be closed with a split-thickness skin graft over the approximated fascial layer. In this way, the cosmetic appearance of the forearm donor site can be improved.

CASE 2

Clinical Presentation

A 61-year-old Black male with a SCC in the left floor of the mouth and the base of his tongue underwent surgical excision of the SCC including deep margin via a central lower lip splitting approach by the surgical oncology service. He also underwent a modified neck lymph node dissection during the same operation. Intraoperative frozen sections of the peripheral and deep margin were confirmed negative from SCC and following resections, there was a 6 × 2 cm soft tissue defect in the floor of his mouth and the base of his tongue (Fig. 4.10).

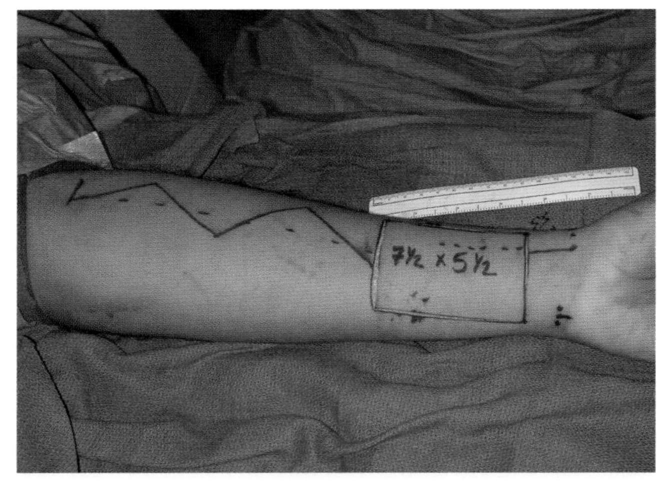

• **Fig. 4.3** Intraoperative view showing the design of a free radial forearm fasciocutaneous flap in the patient's left forearm.

Operative Plan and Special Considerations

After assessing the intraoral soft tissue defect and excess skin in the patient's left nasolabial fold, an inferiorly based nasolabial skin flap was selected for coverage of soft tissue defects in the floor of the mouth and at the base of the tongue. The flap receives blood supply from perforators of the angular artery, the terminal branch of the facial artery. It is thin and versatile and could provide a good soft tissue coverage of a small intraoral defect once it is tunneled through the cheek. The length of the flap is long enough and can easily reach the same side of the floor of the mouth and the base of the tongue defect. However, this is a two-stage procedure and the pedicle of the flap needs to be divided during the second stage.

Operative Procedures

The left inferiorly based nasolabial skin flap was marked and branches of the angular artery were mapped by a handheld Doppler. A 9 × 2.5 cm skin paddle of the flap was designed in an elliptical pattern (Fig. 4.11). After the skin incision was made down the muscle, the flap dissection was easily performed following this tissue plane (Fig. 4.12). The flap was elevated quickly but a relatively wide base of the flap was preserved (Fig. 4.13). The flap was then tunneled through the cheek into the oral cavity (Fig. 4.14). The flap was inserted into the defects of the floor of the mouth and the base of the tongue and a water-tight closure of the flap to the adjacent mucosa was performed with a 3-0 interrupted Vicryl suture in an interrupted half-buried horizontal mattress fashion (Fig. 4.15).

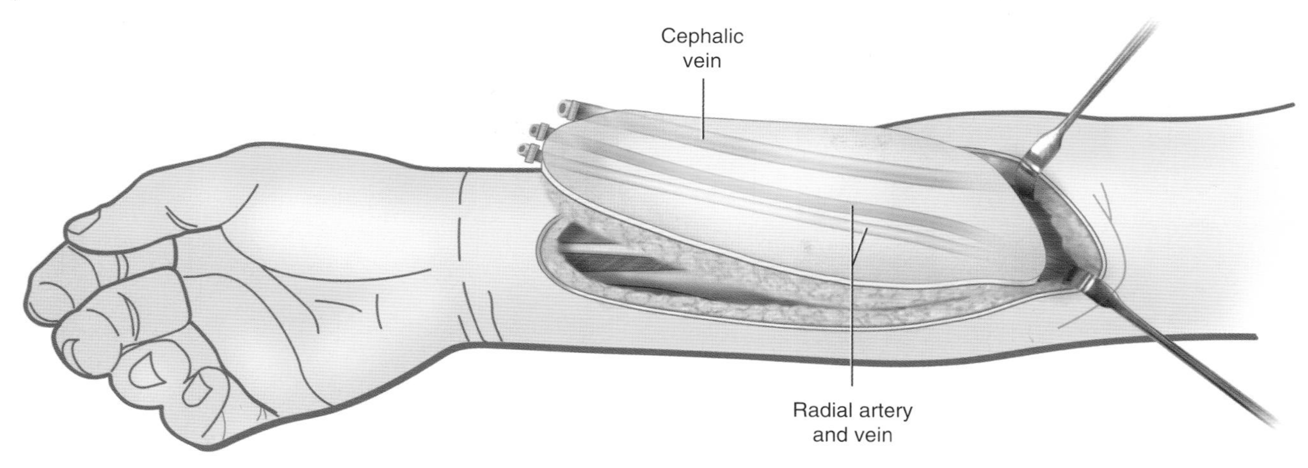

• **Fig. 4.4** A schematic diagram showing the vascular anatomy and dissection of a free radial forearm fasciocutaneous flap.

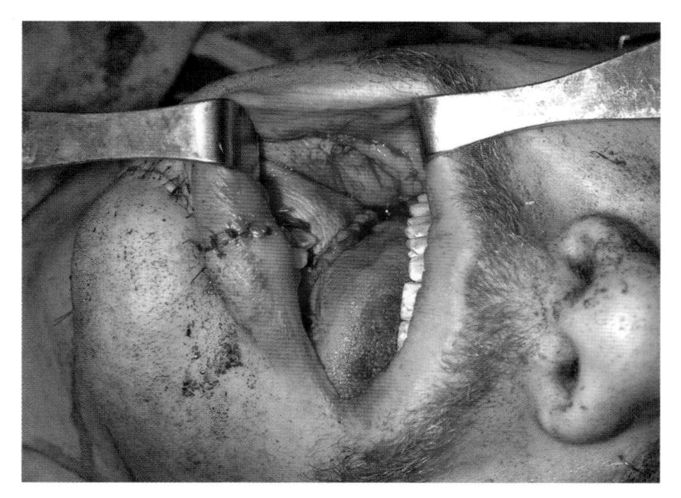

• **Fig. 4.5** Intraoperative view showing completion of the intraoral inset of the free radial forearm flap. A water-tight closure of the skin paddle was demonstrated.

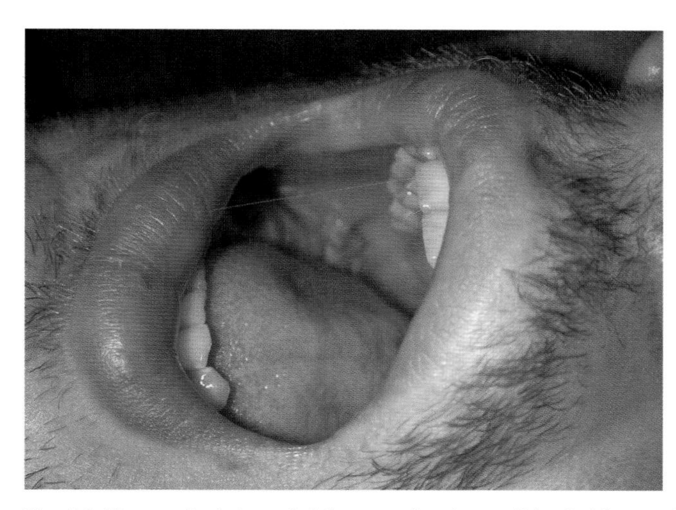

• **Fig. 4.7** The result at 4-week follow-up showing well-healed intraoral free radial forearm flap.

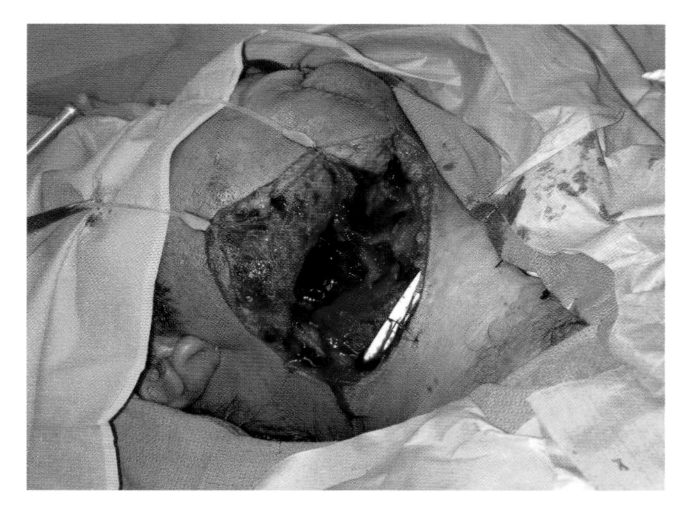

• **Fig. 4.6** Intraoperative view showing a hematoma in the right neck wound.

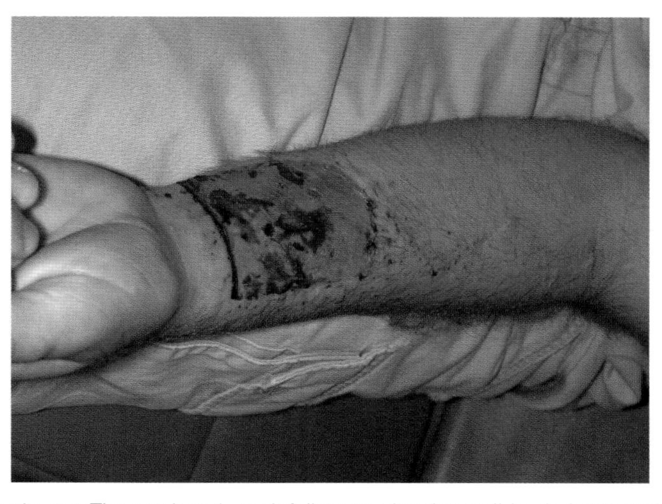

• **Fig. 4.8** The result at 4-week follow-up showing well-healed skin graft of the free radial forearm flap donor site.

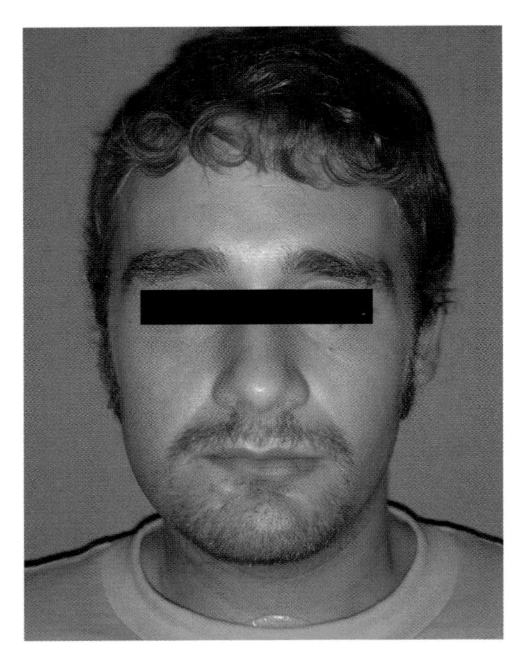

• **Fig. 4.9** The result at 6-month follow-up showing a nearly normal looking lower face with minimal scarring.

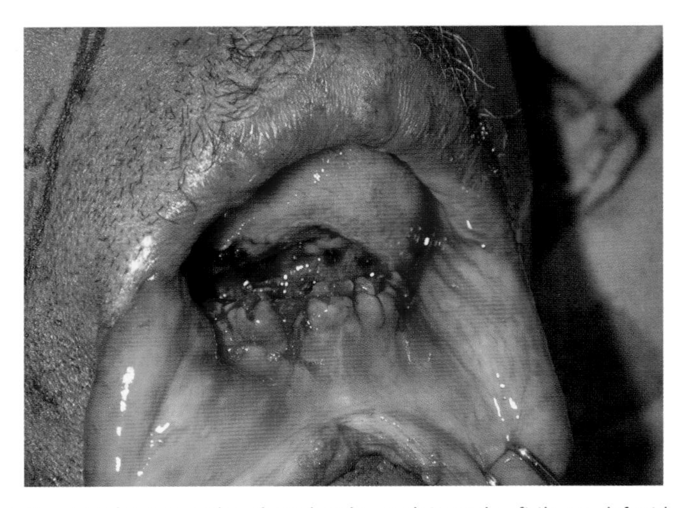

• **Fig. 4.10** Intraoperative view showing an intraoral soft tissue defect in the floor of the mouth and at base of the tongue after an excision of squamous cell carcinoma by the surgical oncology service.

The lower lip and chin incisions were closed in two layers. The neck incision was also closed in two layers after a JP drain placement. After the additional intraoral closure had been completed, the first-stage nasolabial flap intraoral reconstruction was completed (Fig. 4.16).

Four weeks later, the patient was brought back to the operating room for division of the flap pedicle as a second-stage procedure (Fig. 4.17). Once perfusion of the flap was judged adequate after the pedicle was temporarily occluded, the pedicle was then divided and the rest of the flap inset was repeated and closed to the adjacent mucosa accordingly (Fig. 4.18).

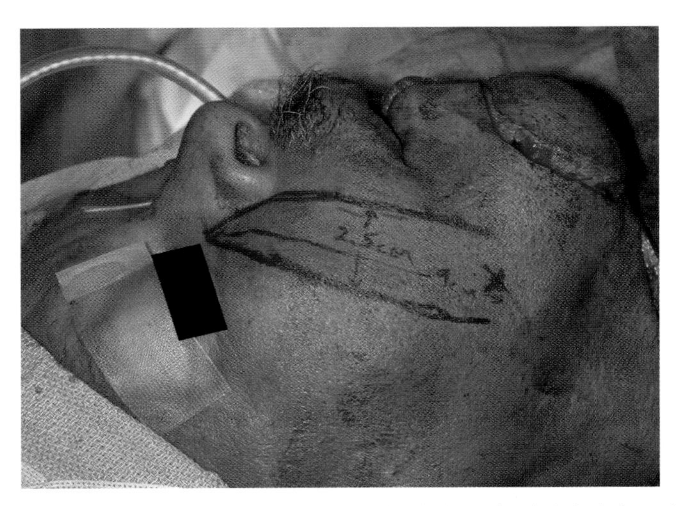

• **Fig. 4.11** Intraoperative view showing the design of an inferiorly based nasolabial flap, measured 9 × 2.5 cm. A large perforator at the base of the flap was marked.

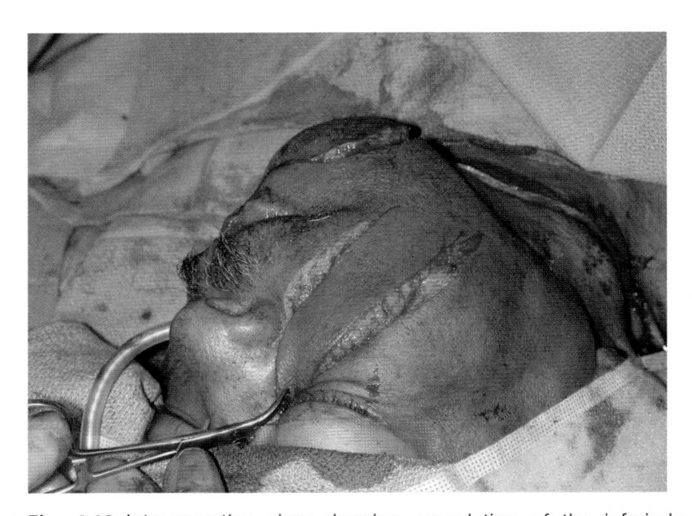

• **Fig. 4.12** Intraoperative view showing completion of the inferiorly based nasolabial flap elevation.

Follow-Up Results

The patient did well postoperatively after two-stage reconstructive procedures. His intraoral flap site healed uneventfully (Fig. 4.19) and his nasolabial flap donor site also healed well without problems (Fig. 4.20).

Final Outcome

The patient looked normal after the intraoral reconstructive procedures (Fig. 4.21). The nasolabial flap donor site healed well (Fig. 4.22). He returned to his normal life and activities and has been followed by the surgical oncology service for cancer follow-up. He also underwent laser hair removal over his intraoral flap.

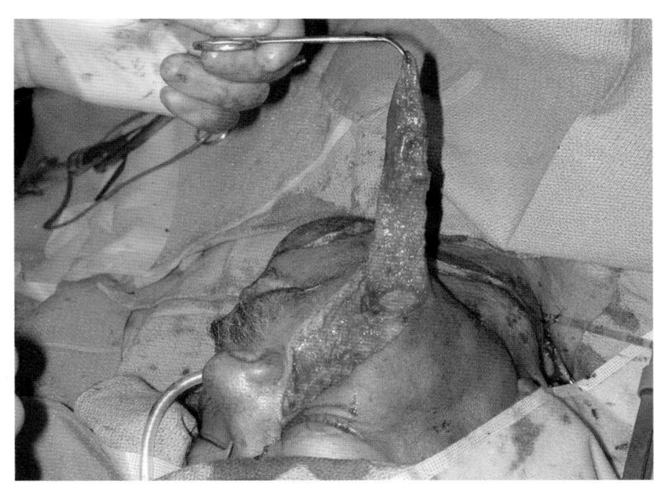

• **Fig. 4.13** Intraoperative view showing the base of the elevated inferiorly based nasolabial flap.

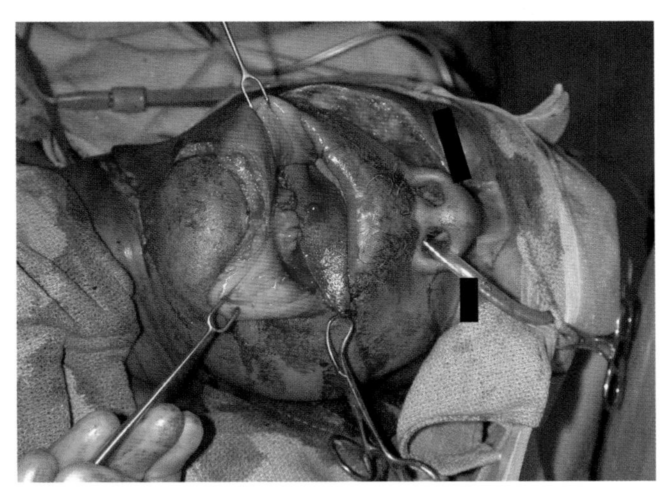

• **Fig. 4.14** Intraoperative view showing the tunneling of the inferiorly based nasolabial flap to the oral cavity.

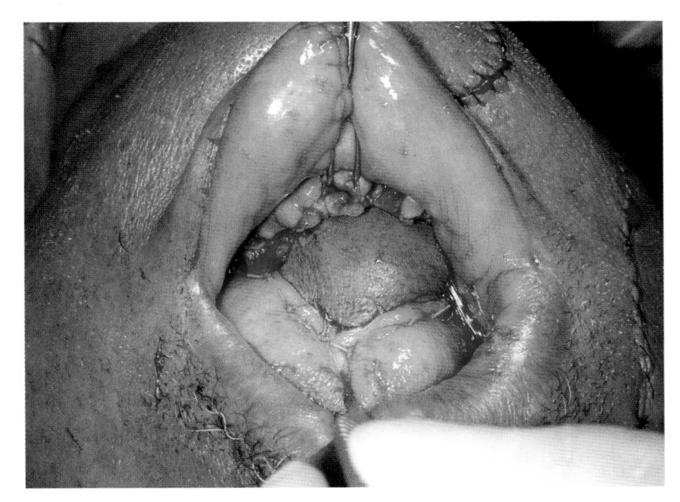

• **Fig. 4.15** Intraoperative view showing completion of the inferiorly based nasolabial flap inset intraorally.

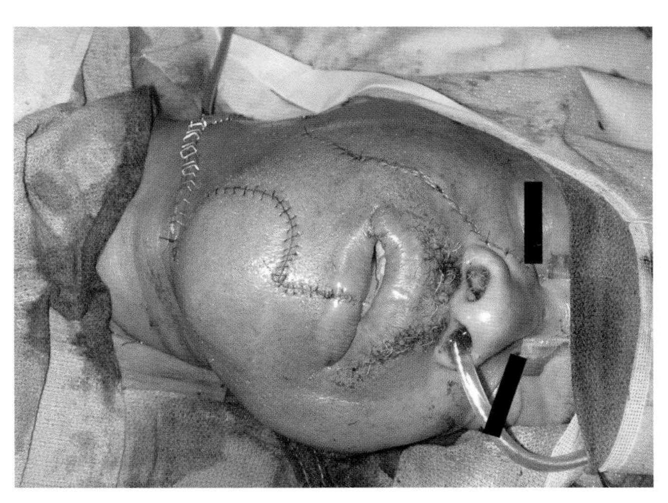

• **Fig. 4.16** Intraoperative view showing completion of the donor site closure for the inferiorly based nasolabial flap and the rest of incision's closure.

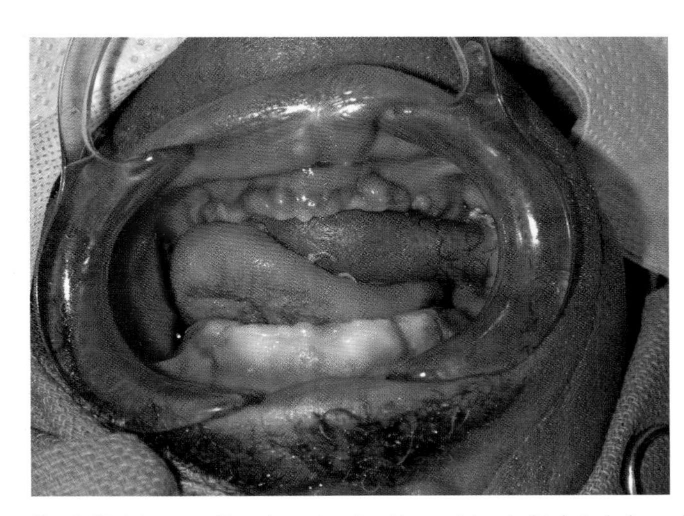

• **Fig. 4.17** Intraoperative view showing the well-healed inferiorly based nasolabial flap intraorally at 4 weeks before the division of the pedicle.

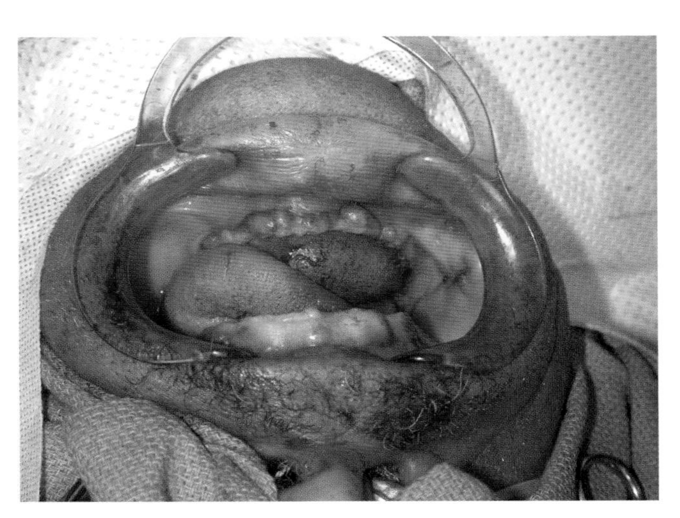

• **Fig. 4.18** Intraoperative view showing the viable inferiorly based nasolabial flap intraorally after the division of the pedicle.

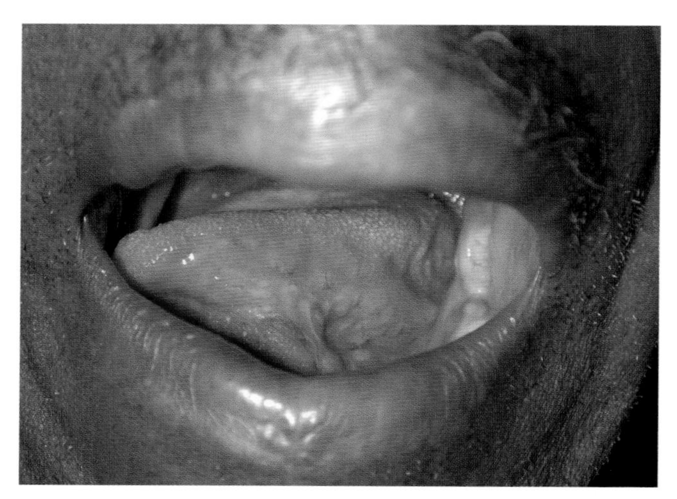

• **Fig. 4.19** The result at 4-week follow-up showing a well-healed intraoral inferiorly based nasolabial flap after the division of its pedicle.

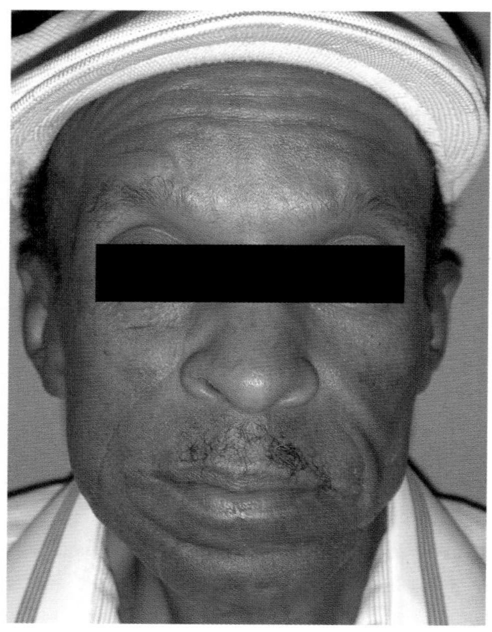

• **Fig. 4.20** The result at 4-week follow-up showing his nearly normal looking lower face following an inferiorly based nasolabial flap reconstruction after the division of its pedicle.

Pearls for Success

An inferiorly based nasolabial skin flap can be a good choice for coverage of a small intraoral defect in the floor of the mouth or at the base of the tongue. The flap can be harvested quickly and provide a malleable soft tissue coverage as a pedicle skin flap for intraoral reconstruction. A relatively wide base of the flap should be preserved based on the preoperative mapping of the pedicle vessels. A water-tight intraoral flap closure should be done to prevent an orocutaneous fistula to the neck. The width of the flap can be limited based on the skin laxity in the donor area. Two-stage procedures are necessary for a good intraoral reconstruction. Hairy flap can be a problem for certain male patients. The cosmesis of the flap donor site after healing can be quite good.

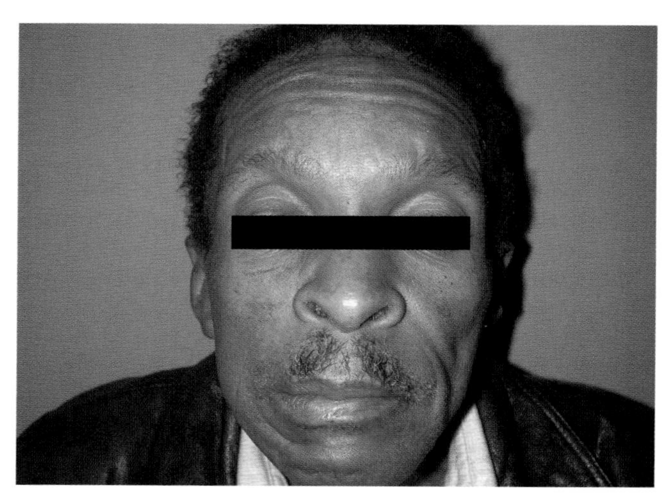

• **Fig. 4.21** The result at 7-month follow-up showing his nearly normal looking lower face with minimal scarring.

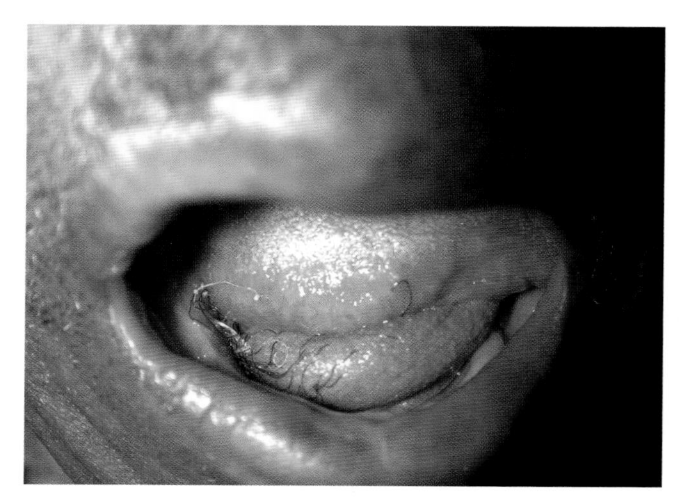

• **Fig. 4.22** The result at 7-month follow-up showing well-healed intraoral flap with some hair growth.

Recommended Readings

Chakrabarti S, Gupta DK, Gupta M, et al. Versatility and reliability of islanded pedicled nasolabial flap in head and neck cancer reconstruction. *Laryngoscope*. 2020;130:1967–1972.

Loreti A, Di Lella G, Vetrano S, Tedaldi M, Dell'Osso A, Poladas G. Thinned anterolateral thigh Cutaneous flap and radial fasciocutaneous forearm flap for reconstruction of oral defects: comparison of donor site morbidity. *J Oral Maxillofac Surg*. 2008;66:1093–1098.

Lutz BS, Wei FC, Chang SCN, Yang KH, Chen IH. Donor site morbidity after suprafascial elevation of the radial forearm flap: a prospective study in 95 cases consecutive cases. *Plast Reconstr Surg*. 1999;103:132–137.

Singh S, Singh RK, Pandey M. Nasolabial flap reconstruction in oral cancer. *World J Surg Onco*. 2012;10:227–232.

Smith GI, O'Brien CJ, Choy ET, Andruchow JL, Gao K. Clinical outcome and technical aspects of 263 radial forearm free flaps used in reconstruction of the oral cavity. *Br J Oral Maxillofac Surg*. 2005;43:199–204.

Wong CH, Lin JY, Wei FC. The bottom-up approach to the suprafascial harvest of the radial forearm flap. *Am J Surg*. 2008;196:e60–e64.

5

Lower Facial Reconstruction

Clinical Presentation

A 40-year-old White male had previously sustained a gunshot wound to his mandible and left mandibular bony reconstruction was unsuccessful. He had a significant deformity of his left lower face and desired a "good" mandibular reconstruction, not only to improve his lower face contour and deformity but also to have possible future reconstruction for osteointegrated dental implants (Figs. 5.1 and 5.2). A preoperative CT scan of his mandible was performed.

Operative Plan and Special Considerations

This patient was also evaluated by our oral surgery service. After a careful preoperative evaluation of the mandible including a dental model, a large, approximately 10-cm mandibular bony gap of the mandible was identified (Fig. 5.3). Because of the need for mandibular bony reconstruction, the future need for osteointegrated dental implant reconstructions and anticipated need for a skin coverage of the newly reconstructed mandible, a free fibula osteocutaneous flap reconstruction was offered to this patient. Because the dental model had already been made, a prebent 2.4-mm reconstruction plate was made preoperatively for secure occlusion and time saving in the operating room for plating the vascularized fibular bone graft. A preoperative angiogram was also performed to confirm a normal vascular anatomy of the left lower extremity.

Operative Procedures

The procedure was started by two teams simultaneously. His old mandibular fracture site was explored. All scarred soft tissue was removed and both mandibular fracture sites were dissected free (Fig. 5.4). Measurement of the left mandibular bony defect confirmed it to be 10 cm long. The previous submandibular incisions were reopened for a wide exposure.

The right facial artery and vein were explored and both recipient vessels appeared to be a good size.

The left free fibula osteocutaneous flap was harvested and a 13 × 4.5 cm skin paddle was created (Fig. 5.5). Under tourniquet control, the skin paddle was incised to the fascia. The subfascial dissection was performed toward the posterior intermuscular septum. Two septocutaneous perforators were identified within the septum and . Attention was given to avoid direct or indirect injury to them. The dissection was done to release the muscle attachment to the fibula from the soleus muscle. Once the peroneal vessels close to the fibula were identified, the distal osteotomy was performed at a level of about 6 cm proximal to the lateral malleolus. By further dissection of the hallucis longus muscle's attachment, the peroneal vessels and the fibula were dissected free. The proximal osteotomy was then performed and a 10-cm segment of the fibula was obtained. A longitudinal skin incision was extended toward the fibular head. After more dissection around the pedicle, the peroneal vessels were dissected free toward its bifurcation. Once the bifurcation was visible, the pedicle was divided and the flap's dissection was completed. With the guide of the dental model, only one osteotomy was performed on the nonperiosteum attachment side (Fig. 5.6).

A prebent reconstruction plate was placed over the mandibular bony gap and secured with multiple screws (Fig. 5.7). The free fibular osteocutaneous flap was inset into the mandibular bony defect and secured with multiple screws. Once a rigid fixation was completed, both microvascular anastomoses were performed. With loupe magnification, both pedicle and recipient vessels were prepared. All microvascular anastomoses were performed in an end-to-end fashion under a microscope. The vein was anastomosed with 2.5-mm coupler device without any problems. With a double-armed Acland clamp, the arterial anastomosis was performed with an 8-0 nylon in a simple interrupted fashion (Fig. 5.8). The total ischemia time was 2 hours.

Once both anastomoses were completed, the flap appeared to be well-perfused and with a good Doppler signal. The skin paddle of the flap was then inset into the left submandibular area to cover the portion of the reconstructed mandible (Fig. 5.9). The rest of the incisions were closed in two layers after a Penrose drain placement and a JP drain insertion under the left neck (Fig. 5.10).

The left leg fibular flap donor site was closed primarily in two layers after all muscles were approximated with several interrupted 2-0 Vicryl sutures. Although the skin closure was tight, the direct approximation was eventually possible.

Management of Complications

Although the patient's free fibular flap reconstruction was completely successful, he unfortunately developed a significant muscle necrosis in the flap donor site (Fig. 5.11). He underwent surgical debridement of necrotic muscles and a large open wound with exposed distal fibula remained (Fig. 5.12). A free skin-grafted rectus abdominis muscle flap was performed 4 weeks later to cover this large open wound from the free fibular osteocutaneous flap donor site. The arterial microvascular anastomosis was performed in an end-to-side fashion to the posterior tibial artery. The venous microvascular anastomosis was performed in an end-to-end fashion

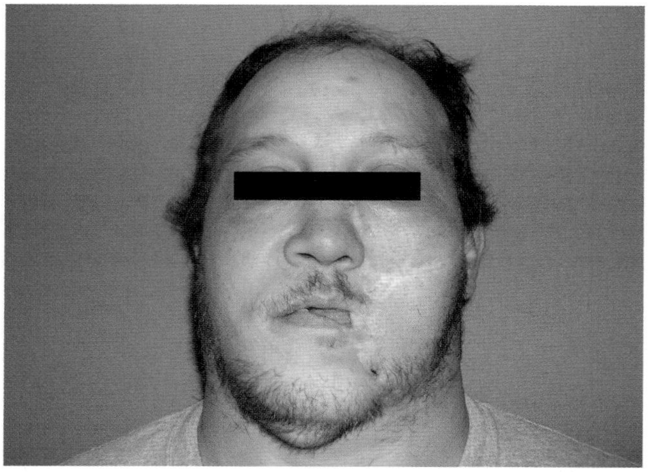

• **Fig. 5.1** A preoperative view showing a significant contour deformity of his left lower face with an incompetent lower lip.

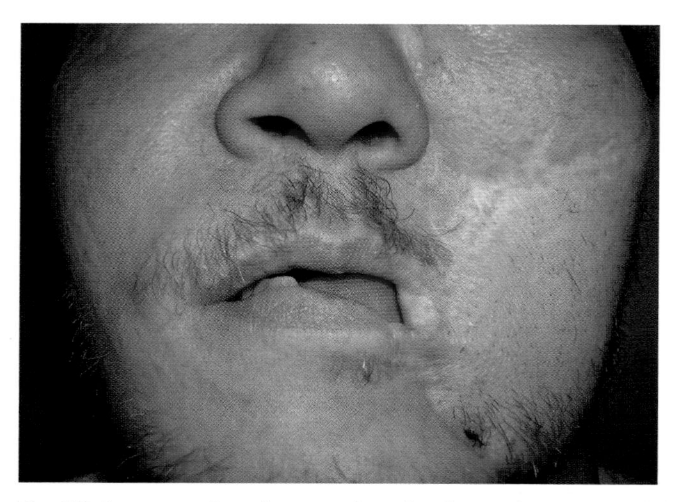

• **Fig. 5.2** A preoperative close-up view showing an incompetent left lower lip and missing most front teeth.

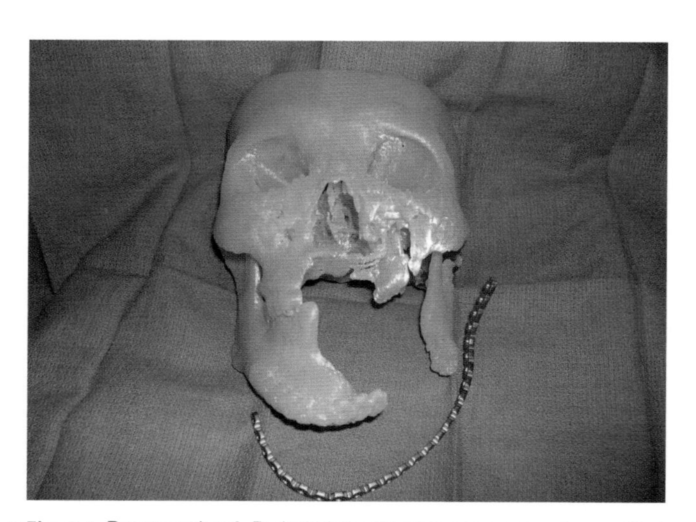

• **Fig. 5.3** Preoperative 3-D dental model showing an exact mandibular bony defect and a prebent reconstruction plate used for the reconstruction.

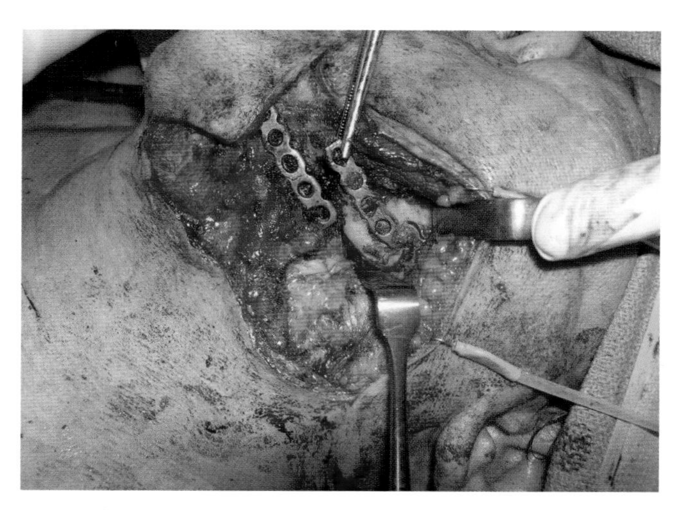

• **Fig. 5.4** Intraoperative view showing a fractured reconstructed plate used for previous mandibular reconstruction without vascularized bone graft. Two posterior septocutaneous perforators were identified and marked.

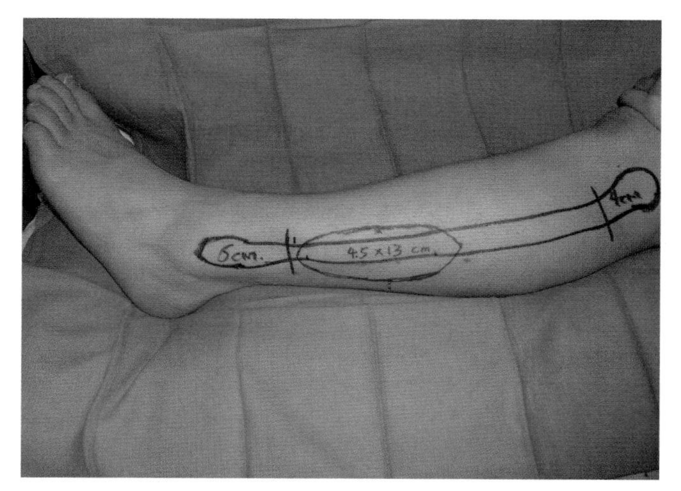

• **Fig. 5.5** Intraoperative view showing the design of a free fibular osteocutaneous flap.

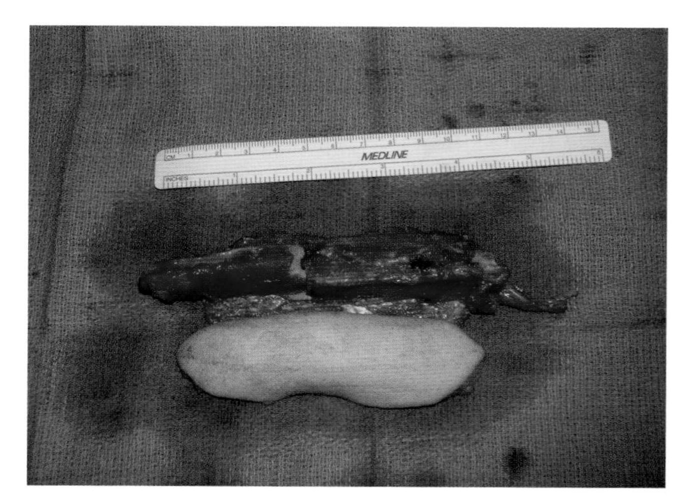

• **Fig. 5.6** Intraoperative view showing completion of a free fibular osteocutaneous flap dissection. Based on the 3-D dental model, only one osteotomy was performed.

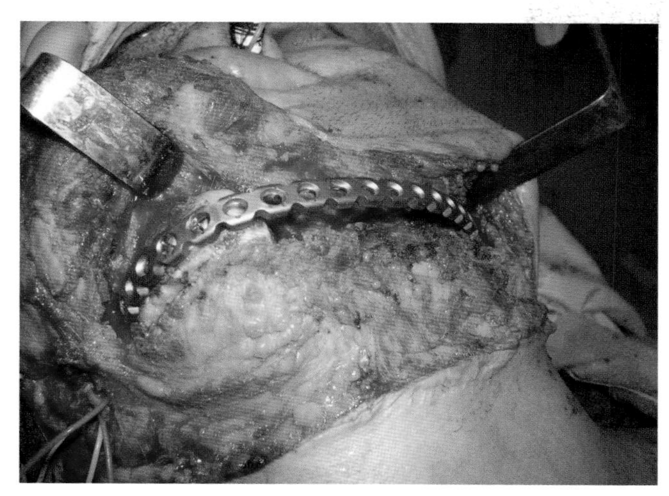

• **Fig. 5.7** Intraoperative view showing precise placement of the reconstruction plate.

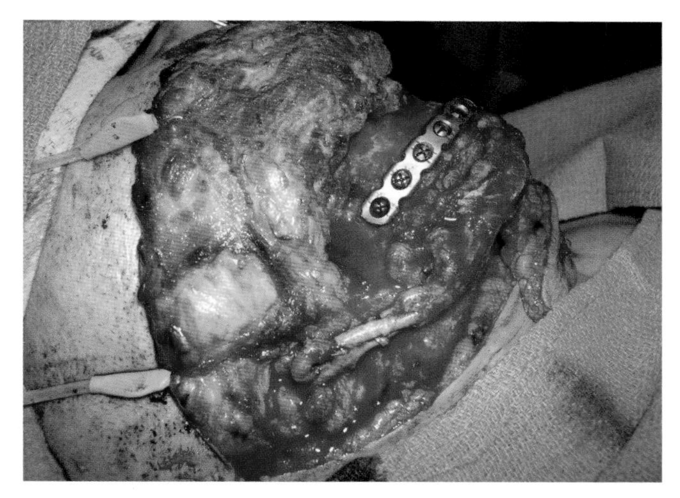

• **Fig. 5.8** Intraoperative right lateral view showing placement and fixation of the free fibular vascularized bone graft and completion of microvascular anastomoses.

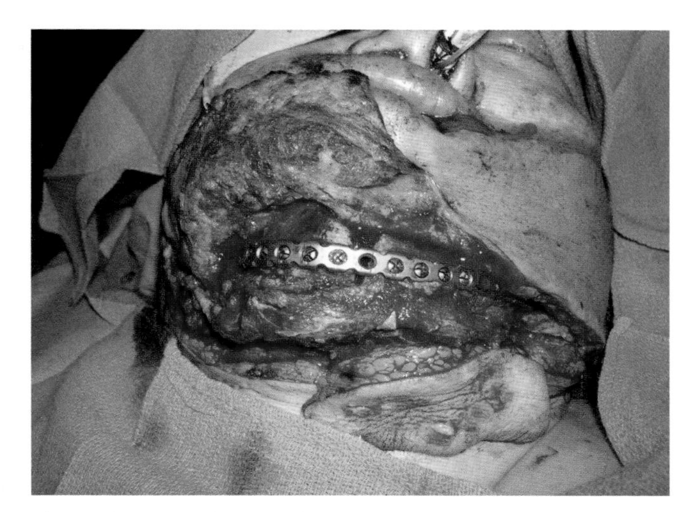

• **Fig. 5.9** Intraoperative view showing placement and fixation of the free fibular vascularized bone graft.

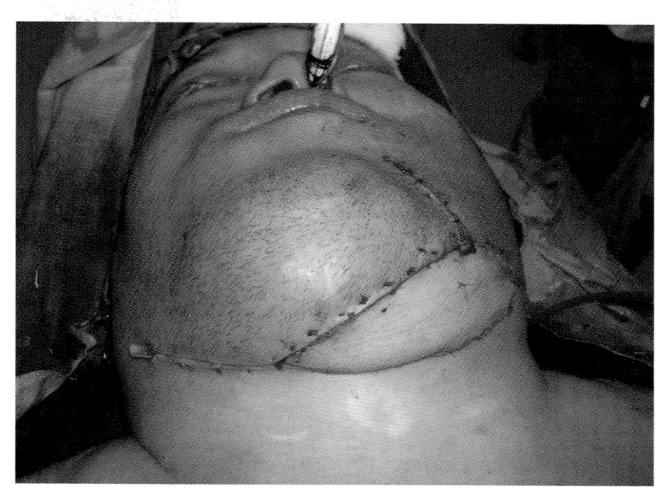

• **Fig. 5.10** Intraoperative view showing completion of the skin paddle inset of the free fibular osteocutaneous flap and closure of all incisions.

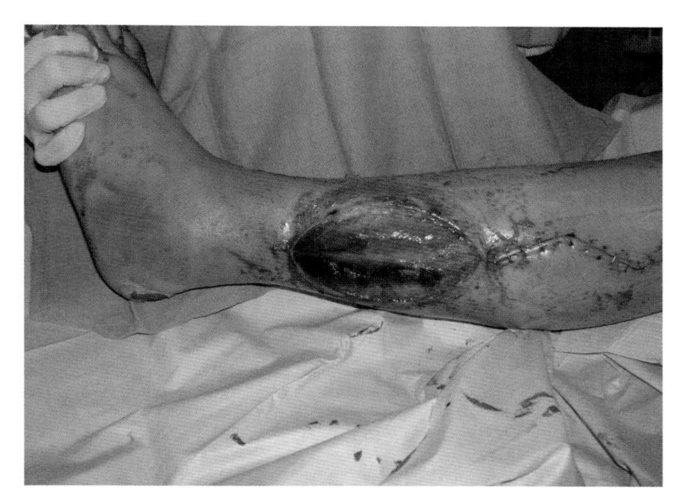

• **Fig. 5.11** Intraoperative view showing necrotic muscles in the free fibular osteocutaneous flap donor site after attempted direct wound closure.

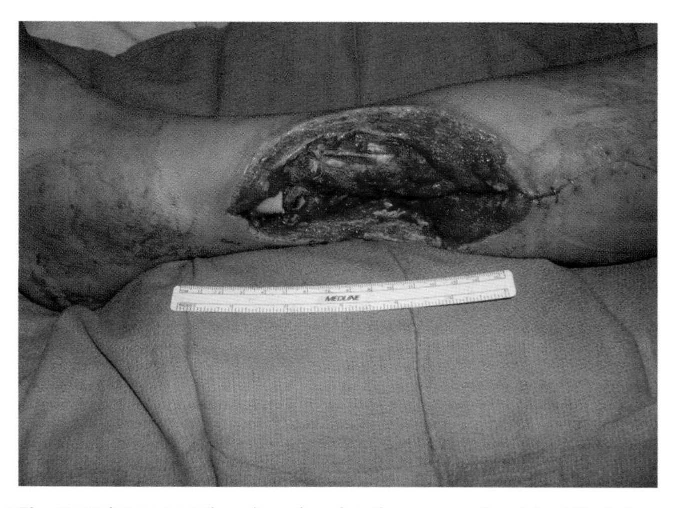

• **Fig. 5.12** Intraoperative view showing the exposed residual fibula bone and deep wound in the free fibular osteocutaneous flap donor site after surgical debridement.

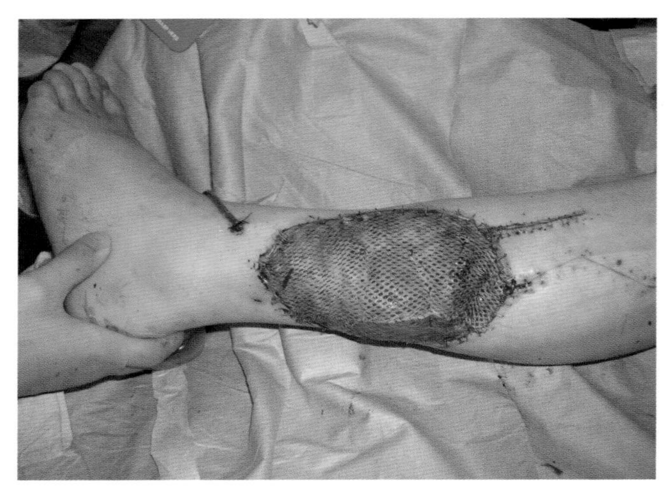

• **Fig. 5.13** Intraoperative view showing completion of a successful skin-grafted free rectus abdominis muscle flap for the wound coverage.

to the posterior tibial vein (Fig. 5.13). The patient did well after the operation and the large open wound in his left leg donor site healed.

Follow-Up Results

The patient did well after the operation with no complications related to the free fibular osteocutaneous flap for the mandibular reconstruction. The skin paddle of the flap healed well (Fig. 5.14). Early postoperative X-ray examination showed excellent alignment and early bony healing of the fibular vascularized bone graft (Fig. 5.15). The left leg donor site also healed after a successful free rectus abdominis muscle flap reconstruction for soft tissue coverage.

Final Outcome

The patient's left lower face contour improved after a successful one-stage free fibular osteocutaneous flap reconstruction for the mandibular reconstruction and soft tissue coverage in the left neck

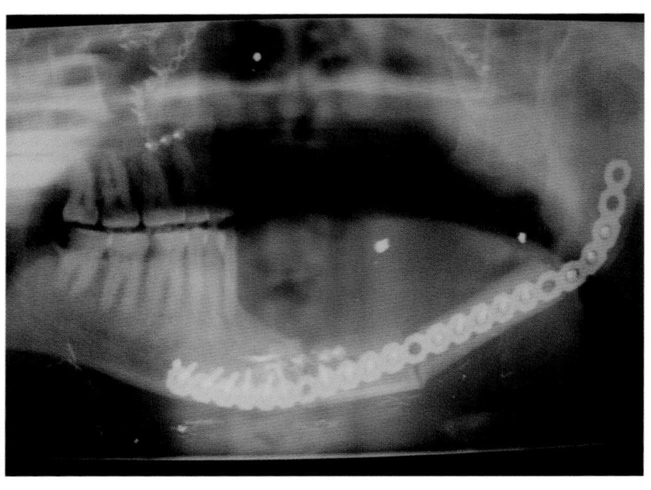

• **Fig. 5.15** Early X-ray examination at postoperative 6 weeks showing good alinement and fixation of the free fibular vascularized bone graft and early signs of bony healing.

(Fig. 5.16). He returned to his normal life and activities and was followed by the oral surgery service for osteointegrated dental implant surgery.

Pearls for Success

A 3-D dental model (or a virtual planning) can be very helpful for preoperative planning of mandibular reconstruction. It can guide the accurate measurement and harvest of a fibular vascularized bone graft and determine the number of osteotomies needed and the angle of each osteotomy. A reconstruction plate can be prebent to ensure optimal alignment and fixation of the fibular vascularized bone graft. Working with the oral surgery service could ensure a better occlusion after the flap inset for future placement of osteointegrated dental implants. In addition, the thickness of the fibular bone graft could be predetermined by the oral surgery service to ensure a better outcome for future osteointegrated dental implants. The narrow skin paddle (<5 cm) could ensure a primary

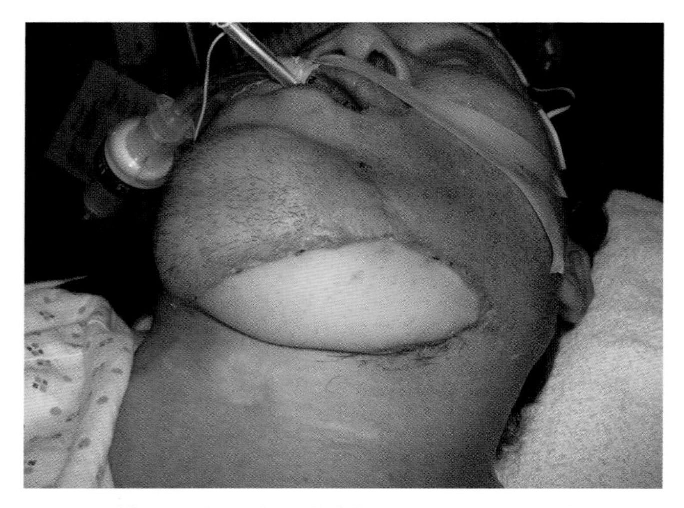

• **Fig. 5.14** The result at 4-week follow-up showing well-healed skin paddle of the free fibular osteocutaneous flap and the rest of the incisions.

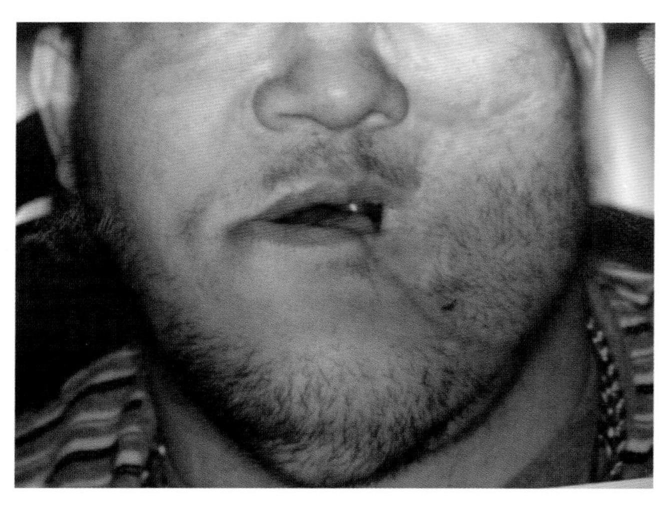

• **Fig. 5.16** The result at 9-week follow-up showing good contour of the left lower face and well-healed skin paddle of the free fibular osteocutaneous flap and the rest of the incisions.

closure of the flap donor site for better cosmetic outcome. However, a skin graft should be used initially for the leg donor site closure if attempted primary closure is under more than moderate amount of tension. Routine preoperative imaging evaluation for the facial vessels as good recipient vessels in the trauma patient can be critical to the success of any free tissue transfer to the face.

Recommended Readings

Hidalgo DA. Free flap mandibular reconstruction: a 10-year follow-up study. *Plast Reconstr Surg*. 2002;110:438–449.

Largo RD, Garvey PB. Updates in head and neck reconstruction. *Plast Reconstr Surg*. 2018;141:271e–285e.

Santamaria E, We FC, Chen HC. Fibular osteoseptocutaneous flap for reconstruction of osteoradionecrosis of the mandible. *Plast Reconstr Surg*. 1998;101:921–929.

Wallace CG, Chang YM, Tsai CY, Wei FC. Harnessing the potential of the free fibula osteoseptocutaneous flap in mandible reconstruction. *Plast Reconstr Surg*. 2010;125:305–314.

Wei FC, Celik N, Yang WG, Chen IH, Chang YM, Chen HC. Complications after reconstruction by plate and soft-tissue free flap in composite mandibular defects and secondary salvage reconstruction with osteocutaneous. *Flap Plast Reconstr Surg*. 2003;112:37–42.

6

Eyelid Reconstruction

Clinical Presentation

A 77-year-old White female sustained necrotizing fasciitis in her right periorbital area secondary to facial trauma. She was initially seen by an oculoplastic surgeon and urgently referred to the plastic surgery service for more definitive surgical management. On clinical examination, she had a periorbital soft tissue infection involving both upper and lower eyelids. She was urgently taken to the operating room for surgical debridement (Figs. 6.1 and 6.2). The debridement was performed to preserve as much of the eyelid tissue as possible. After the debridement, open wounds remained in the entire lower eyelid and lateral portion of the upper eyelid (Fig. 6.3).

Operative Plan and Special Considerations

After 4 weeks of proper local wound care, the upper and lower eyelid wounds were ready for definitive closure. Because the tissue at the base of the wounds was of good quality, the wounds could be closed with a full-thickness skin graft (Fig. 6.4). The supraclavicular area was an excellent donor site because a skin graft taken from that area ensures the best color match to the lower eyelid. In addition, a lateral canthopexy or canthoplasty may be needed for correction of ectropion if indicated.

Operative Procedures

The upper and lower eyelid wounds were further debrided. Tarsorrhaphy sutures were placed (Fig. 6.5). Once the size of the wounds was measured, a full-thickness skin graft with a proper size was harvested from the same side of the supraclavicular area by a direct excision. The skin graft was then defatted and placed on the upper and lower eyelid wounds and sutured in place with 5-0 chromic sutures in a simple running fashion. A xeroform gauze was placed over the skin graft site and a tie-over dressing was applied. The tarsorrhaphy sutures were left in place for a week. The skin graft donor site was closed in two layers after minimal undermining.

Follow-Up Results

The patient did well postoperatively without any complications related to the wounds and skin graft site. The tie-over dressing was removed 1 week postoperatively. Her wounds healed well with only a full-thick skin graft. Unfortunately, she developed ectropion of the lower eyelid over a period of 4 months (Fig. 6.6). This condition was corrected with a lateral canthopexy 6 months after her skin graft procedure. The canthopexy was performed by suturing the lateral tarsus to the periosteum of the lateral orbital rim at the level of the pupils with a double-armed 5-0 Mersilene suture (Ethicon, Somerville, USA).

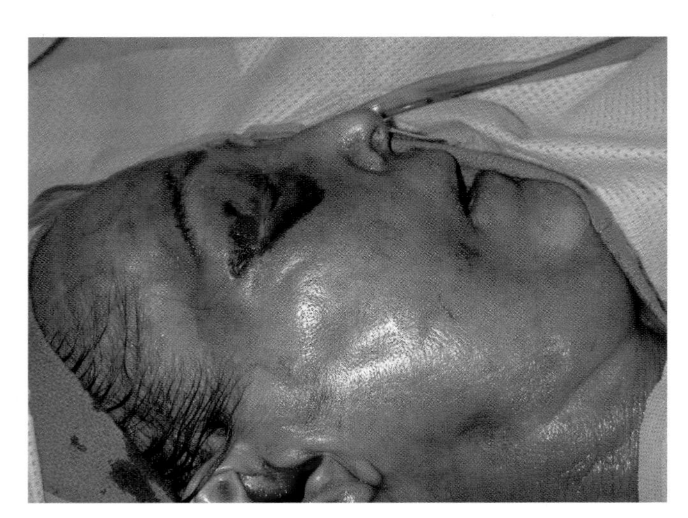

• **Fig. 6.1** An intraoperative view showing the extent of the right periorbital soft tissue infection involving both upper and lower eyelids.

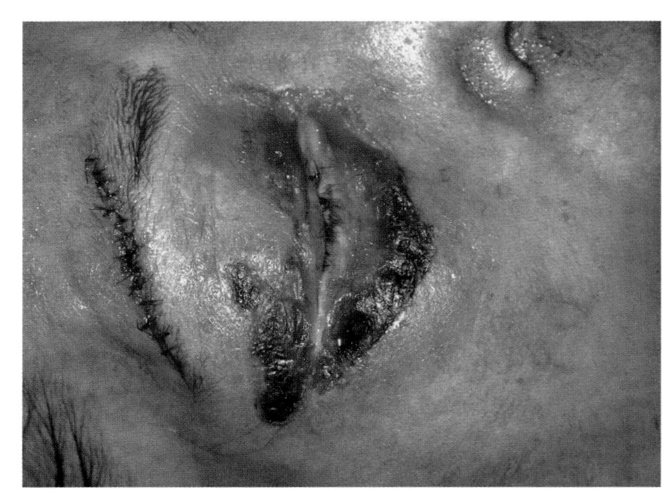

• **Fig. 6.2** An intraoperative close-up view showing the right periorbital soft tissue infection.

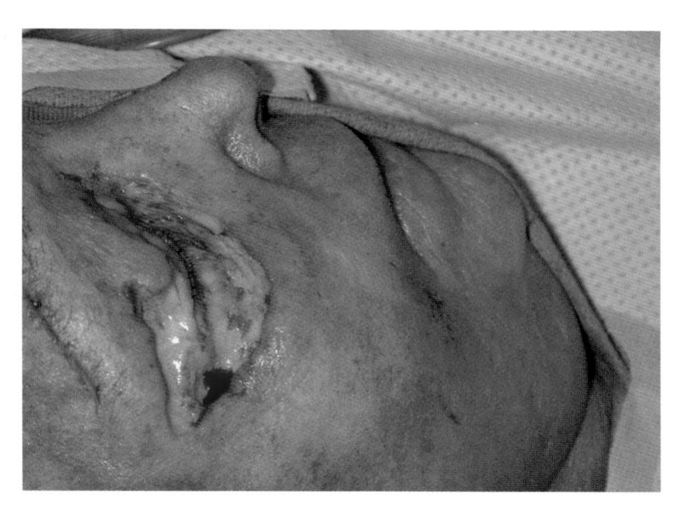

• **Fig. 6.3** An intraoperative view showing completion of adequate surgical debridement of both upper and lower eyelids.

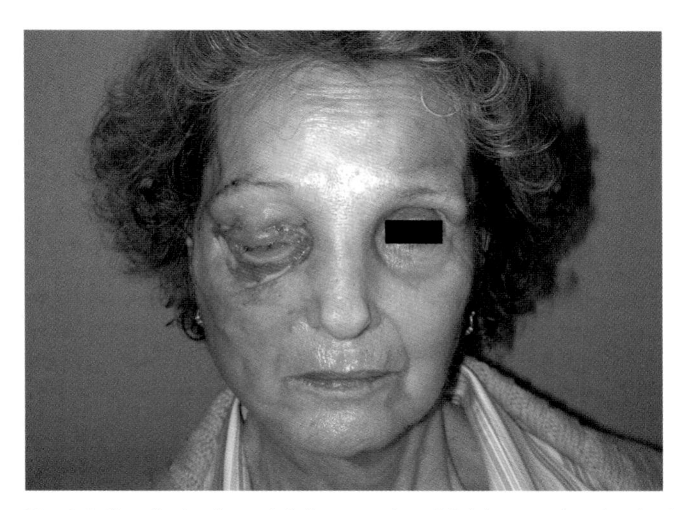

• **Fig. 6.4** Result at a 2-week follow-up after debridement showing both upper and lower eyelid wounds. At this point, the soft tissue infection was under control.

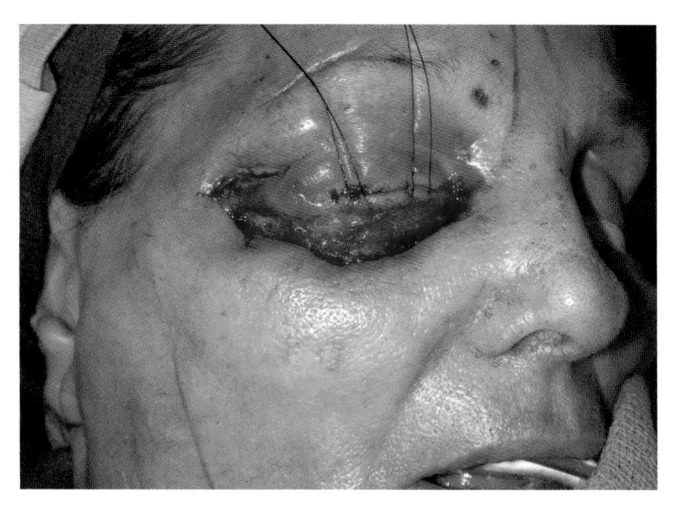

• **Fig. 6.5** An intraoperative view showing well-prepared wounds in both upper and lower eyelids after further careful debridement before a skin graft procedure.

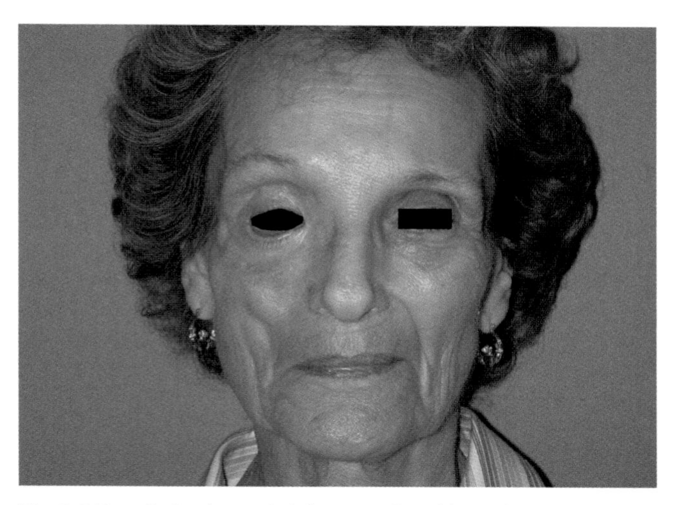

• **Fig. 6.6** Result at a 4-month follow-up after skin graft surgery showing well-healed upper and lower eyelid skin graft sites wounds. Unfortunately, the patient had developed ectropion of the lower eyelid.

Final Outcome

The skin graft site healed well without any issues and the ectropion was corrected after a lateral canthopexy (Fig. 6.7). The patient has had a reasonably good reconstructive outcome with minimal scaring. She returned to her normal life and has been followed by the plastic surgery service when needed.

Pearls for Success

Accurate preoperative evaluation to assess the amount of tissue loss after adequate debridement can be the first step to ensure the success of future reconstruction. After proper local wound care, a full-thick skin graft can be harvested for the eyelid wound coverage. Supraclavicular skin can be a good donor site for the best possible outcome because of its ideal thickness and color match. Ectropion may develop in an elderly patient and

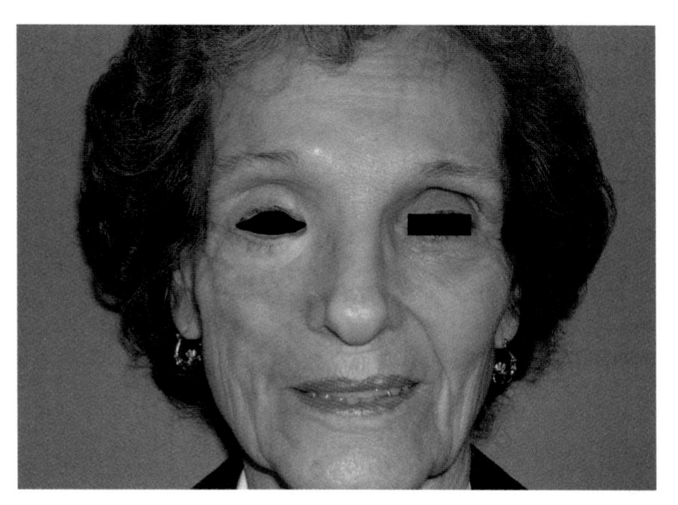

• **Fig. 6.7** Result at a 5-month follow-up after ectropion correction showing an improved lower eyelid position and nearly normal looking right upper and lower eyelids.

a lateral canthopexy or canthoplasty can be performed to correct such a condition successfully. Good reconstructive outcome can be expected after devastating periorbital soft tissue infection by using a simple full-thickness skin graft procedure with proper local wound care and adequate surgical debridement.

Recommended Readings

Alghoul MS, Bricker JT, Vaca EE, Purnell CA. Lower eyelid reconstruction: a new classification incorporating the vertical dimension. *Plast Reconstr Surg*. 2019;144:443–455.

Bortz JG, Al-Shweiki S. Free tarsal graft and free skin graft for lower eyelid reconstruction. *Ophthal Plast Recoconstr Surg*. 2020;36:605–609.

Custer P, Neimkin M. Lower eyelid reconstruction with combining sliding tarsal and rhomboid skin flaps. *Ophthal Plast Recoconstr Surg*. 2016;32:230–232.

Holds JB. Lower eyelid reconstruction. *Facial Plast Surg Clin N Am*. 2016;24:183–191.

Usla A. Use of a perforator/subcutaneous pedicled propeller flap for reconstruction of lower eyelid defects. *J Plast Reconstr Aesthetic Surg*. 2019;72:119–124.

Yordanov YP, Shef A. Lower eyelid reconstruction after ablation of skin malignancies: how far can we get in a single-stage procedure? *J Craniofacial Surg*. 2017;28:e477–e479.

7

Ear Reconstruction

CASE 1

Clinical Presentation

A 24-year-old Hispanic male sustained a human bite on his right ear. He had a partial ear amputation involving the helical rim and a small portion of antihelix as well as their overlying skin (Figs. 7.1 and 7.2). He was initially treated for the local wound and the open wound over his ear healed afterward (Fig. 7.3). Appropriate reconstruction for the composite tissue loss of his right ear was obviously desirable.

Operative Plan and Special Considerations

Based on the size and location of the ear composite tissue defect, a cartilage graft would be needed for the ear's frame reconstruction and a local skin flap would also be needed for coverage of the cartilage graft. A two-stage reconstruction was planned for this patient. During the first-stage reconstruction, the cartilage graft could be harvested from the contralateral ear and a local postauricular skin flap could be designed based on the postauricular skin as a random skin flap that would provide a skin coverage to the cartilage graft. During the second-stage reconstruction, the pedicle of the postauricular flap could be divided and a full-thickness skin graft from the supraclavicular region could be placed to close the postauricular donor site skin defect.

Operative Procedures

The first-stage reconstruction was performed under general anesthesia. The healed wound edge was reopened and refreshed with a knife. The size and shape of the cartilage defect was measured and a template was made. A contralateral ear cartilage graft was harvested from the concha via a posterior approach based on the template. Attention was paid to leave an adequate portion of the concha cartilage so that the shape of the contralateral concha could be maintained. The cartilage graft was then sutured in place with the remaining cartilage with interrupted 3-0 PDS sutures (Fig. 7.4). The postauricular skin flap was designed and marked (Fig. 7.5). Attention should be paid to make a wide enough skin flap to cover the cartilage graft and the flap itself should still receive adequate blood supply. The skin flap was inset and closed using interrupted 4-0 nylon sutures (Fig. 7.6).

Four weeks later, the second-stage reconstruction was performed (Fig. 7.7). Under general anesthesia, the skin pedicle at the base of the flap was clamped with a rubber band to assess whether the pedicle could be divided safely. After clamping for 5 minutes, the skin flap remained pink indicating that it could be divided without vascular compromise. The pedicle was then divided at the base of the flap and the postauricular open area of the flap was closed with interrupted 4-0 nylon sutures as much as possible. The rest of the open area was closed with a full-thickness skin graft harvested from the supraclavicular area and secured with a Xeroform tie-over dressing (Fig. 7.8).

Follow-Up Results

The patient did well postoperatively without any complications related to his two-stage composite partial ear reconstruction. Both the postauricular skin flap and the cartilage graft sites healed well. The supraclavicular skin graft site also healed well without any problems (Fig. 7.9).

Final Outcome

The two-stage partial ear reconstruction healed well with minimal scaring (Figs. 7.10–7.13). The shape of the reconstructed ear compared favorably with the contralateral normal ear. The patient has returned to his normal life and has been followed by the plastic surgery service as needed.

Pearls for Success

Two-stage partial ear reconstructions with an ear cartilage graft harvested from the contralateral ear and a postauricular skin flap for soft tissue coverage can be successfully used for reconstruction of a composite partial ear defect if the amount of missing cartilage can be replaced. The postauricular skin flap is a good local option to provide a reliable soft tissue coverage after reconstruction of the ear's cartilage framework. Unfortunately, the postauricular skin flap should be performed in stages and a good final outcome may be expected once the pedicle of the flap is divided. Attention should be paid to raise a relatively wide flap base during the initial flap design and to make sure the flap can be divided safely during the second-stage reconstruction. A minimum of 4 weeks should be left between the first- and second-stage reconstructions.

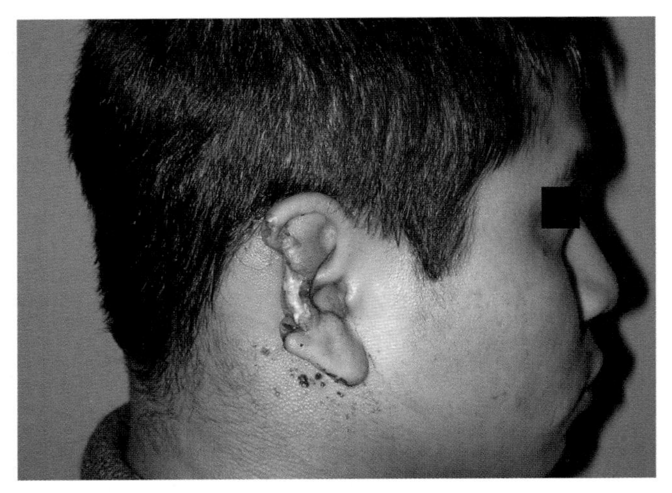

• **Fig. 7.1** A preoperative view showing a sizable partial composite defect of the right ear involving skin and cartilage of the helix, scapha, and antihelix.

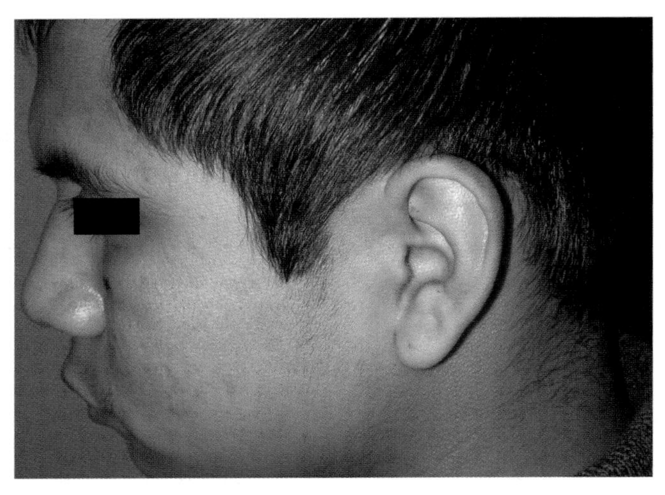

• **Fig. 7.2** A preoperative view showing the patient's normal left ear.

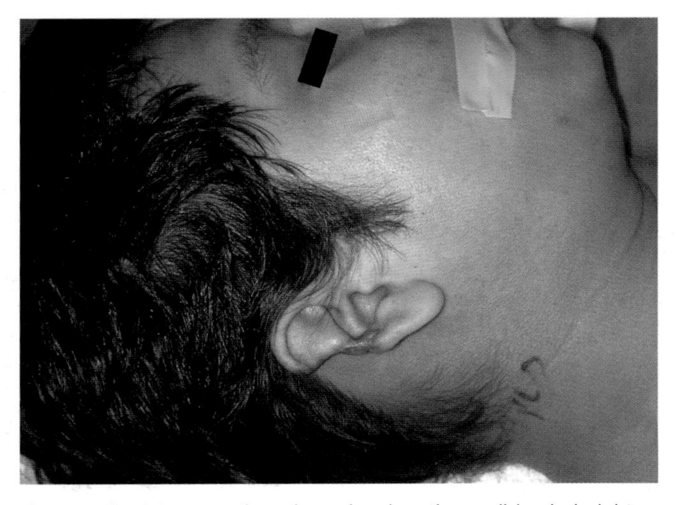

• **Fig. 7.3** An intraoperative view showing the well-healed right ear defect wound before reconstruction.

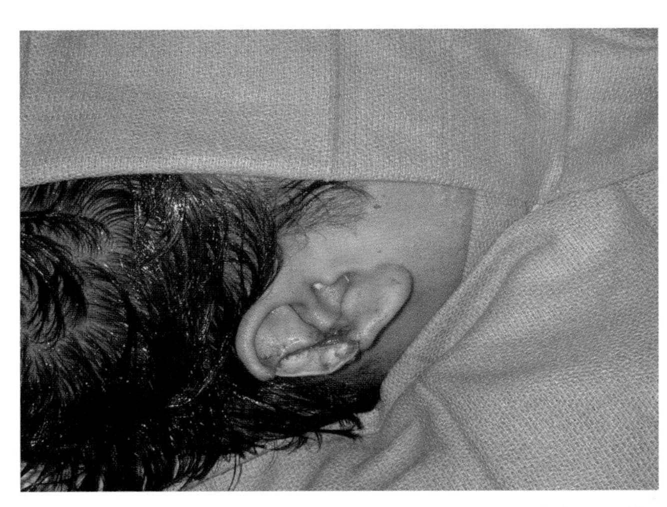

• **Fig. 7.4** An intraoperative view showing completion of the cartilage graft placement for structure reconstruction of the right ear defect.

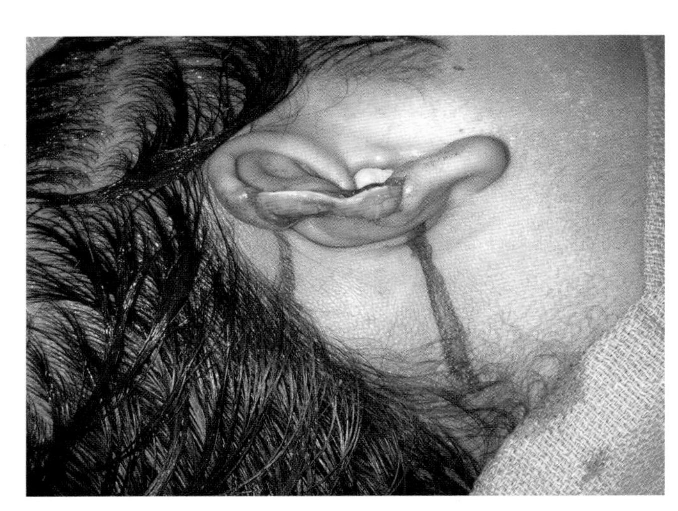

• **Fig. 7.5** An intraoperative view showing the design of the postauricular skin flap for skin coverage of the cartilage graft.

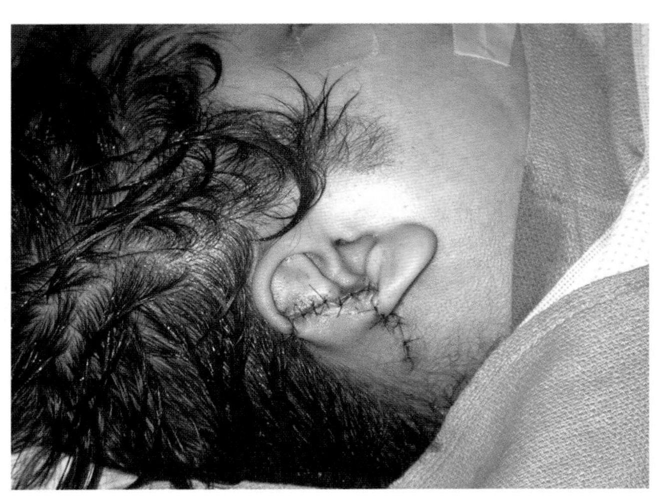

• **Fig. 7.6** An intraoperative view showing completion of the postauricular flap inset and the flap donor site closure.

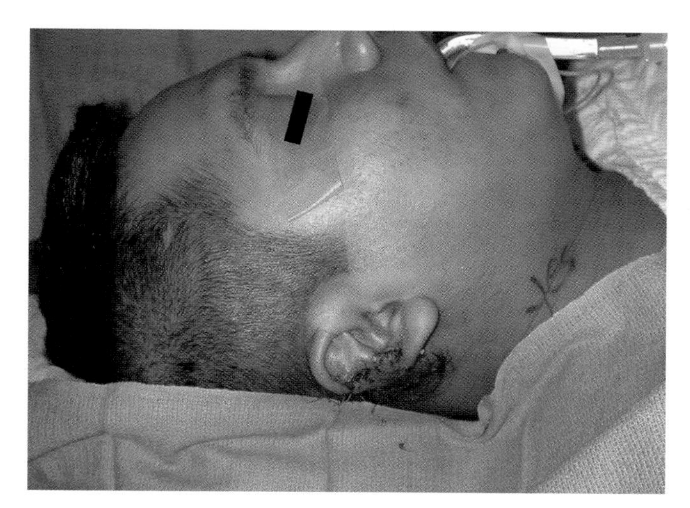

• **Fig. 7.7** An intraoperative view before the second-stage reconstruction showing well-healed postauricular skin flap site 3 weeks after the flap reconstruction just before the division of the flap's pedicle.

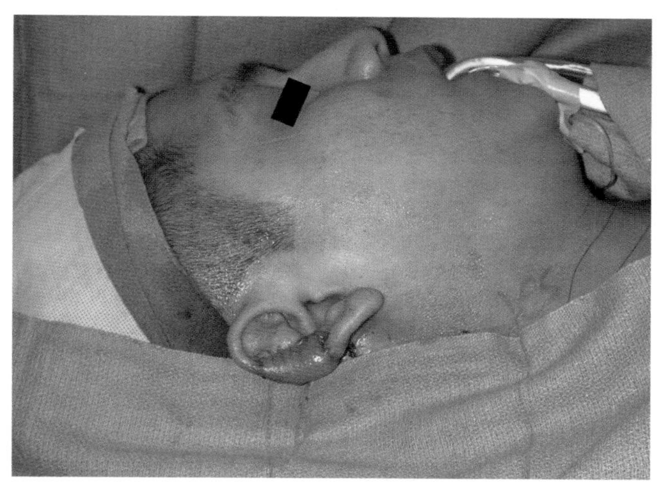

• **Fig. 7.8** An intraoperative view showing completion of the division of the postauricular flap's pedicle.

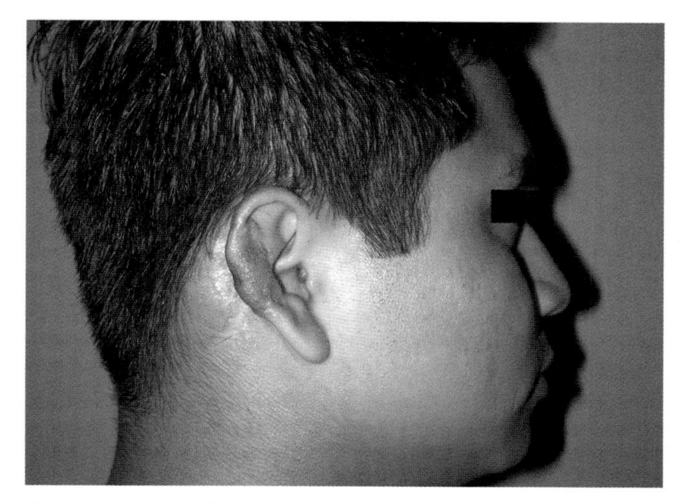

• **Fig. 7.9** Result at a 3-month follow-up showing well-healed composite reconstruction of the partial ear defect.

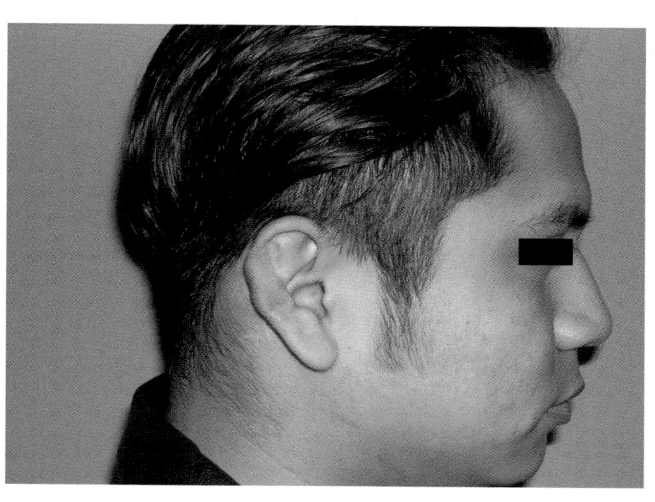

• **Fig. 7.10** Result at 7-month follow-up after the second-stage reconstruction showing nearly normal-looking reconstructed right ear.

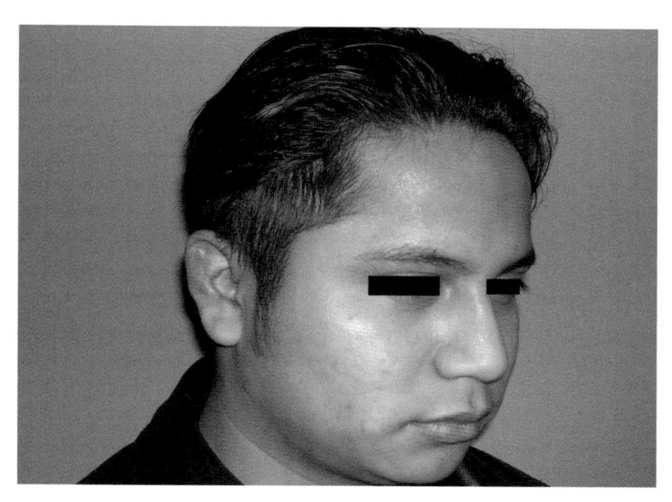

• **Fig. 7.11** Result of the reconstructed ear from right oblique view at 7-month follow-up after the second-stage surgery.

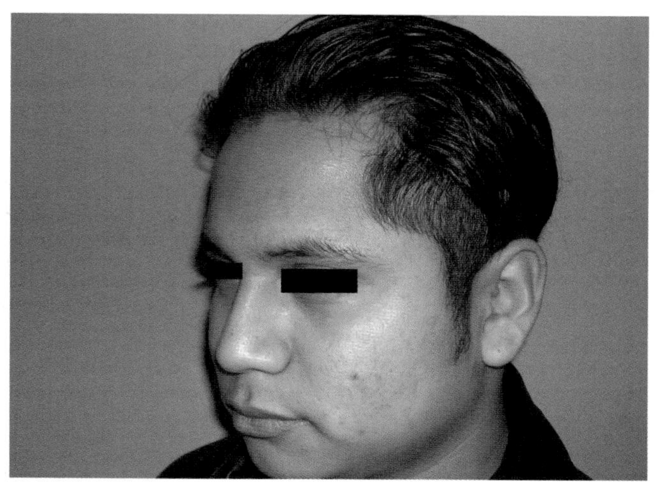

• **Fig. 7.12** View of the patient's normal ear for comparision.

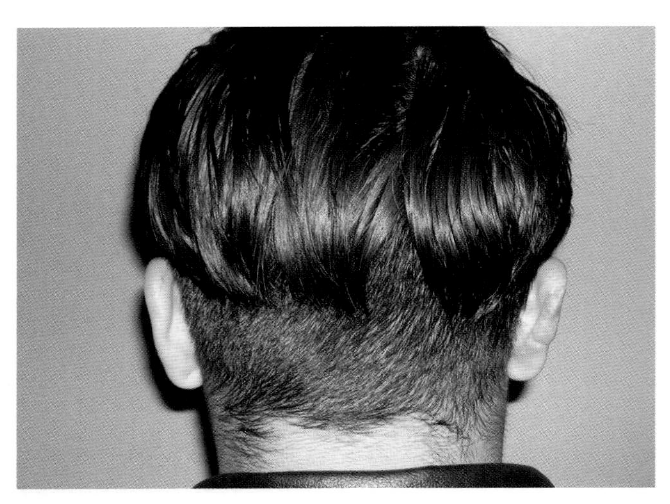

• **Fig. 7.13** Comparison of reconstructed ear with normal ear at 7-month follow-up is favorable.

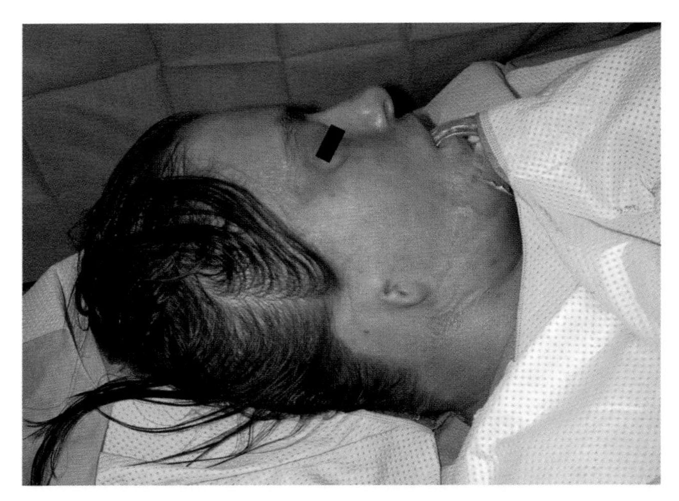

• **Fig. 7.14** A preoperative view before surgery showing a typical microtia of the right side. The patient only had a small amount of remaining cartilage and ear lobe.

CASE 2

Clinical Presentation

A 39-year-old White female had a congenital right microtia and presented to the plastic surgery service for a total ear reconstruction. On physical examination, she had a true total microtia with only remnants of the ear structures such as an earlobe and associate ear cartilages (Fig. 7.14).

Operative Plan and Special Considerations

Because of her age and the need for a total ear reconstruction, one-stage reconstruction with a Medpor implant and temporoparietal fascia flap was offered to this patient. The Medpor implant for total ear reconstruction has been recommended by others with a good long-term result. Such a reconstruction is especially indicated for adult patients because rib cartilage grafts may not be suitable for a total ear reconstruction. In addition, the framework of an ear made by a Medpor implant is readily available and significant time can be saved in the operating room. A pedicled temporoparietal fascia flap is an excellent choice for the soft tissue coverage of a Medpor implant because it is thin, large, and well vascularized. The flap will be covered by a sheet split-thickness skin graft for completion of one-stage reconstruction.

Operative Procedures

The temporoparietal fascia flap was designed and marked based on the Doppler mapping of the superficial temporal vessels. After the scalp incision was infiltrated with 1% lidocaine with 1:100,000 epinephrine, the incision was made down to the superficial temporal fascia. The extent of the scalp was elevated sharply with a knife in the subcutaneous plane to explore the entire temporoparietal fascia flap. The periphery of the flap was incised and the flap was then sharply elevated along the avascular subgaleal plane once the terminal branches of the superficial temporal vessels were divided with hemoclips. During the flap dissection, attention should be made to avoid injury to the pedicle vessels and the frontal branch of the facial nerve (Fig. 7.15).

Two-pieces of Medpor ear implant were sutured together with 3-0 clear nylon sutures (Fig. 7.16). Once the skin flap was elevated and the remnants of the ear cartilages were exposed, the ear framework made by Medpor implant was placed in the normal ear location over the mastoid fascia and secured with multiple clear 2-0 nylon sutures. The Medpor implant was inserted into the earlobe that had been created (Fig. 7.17). The temporoparietal fascia flap was inserted to cover the entire framework of the ear with multiple interrupted 3-0 Vicryl sutures.

The temporoparietal scalp incision was closed with skin staples after a drain placement. An unmeshed split-thickness skin graft was harvested from the patient's right lateral thigh with a dermatome. The skin graft was sutured to the temporoparietal fascia flap with multiple interrupted 5-0 chromic sutures. A suction tube was inserted under the skin graft and with suction, it was adherent to the underlying the temporoparietal fascia flap nicely (Fig. 7.18). The reconstructed ear was covered with a Xeroform gauze.

Follow-Up Results

The patient did well postoperatively without any complications related to the temporoparietal fascia flap and skin graft. She was observed in the hospital for 5 days and discharged home on postoperative day 6. The drain was removed during the second week follow-up visit. Her total ear reconstruction healed well during the first 8 months. Unfortunately, the Medpor implant developed an extrusion near the junction of the flap and earlobe tissues although the remaining earlobe tissues were without

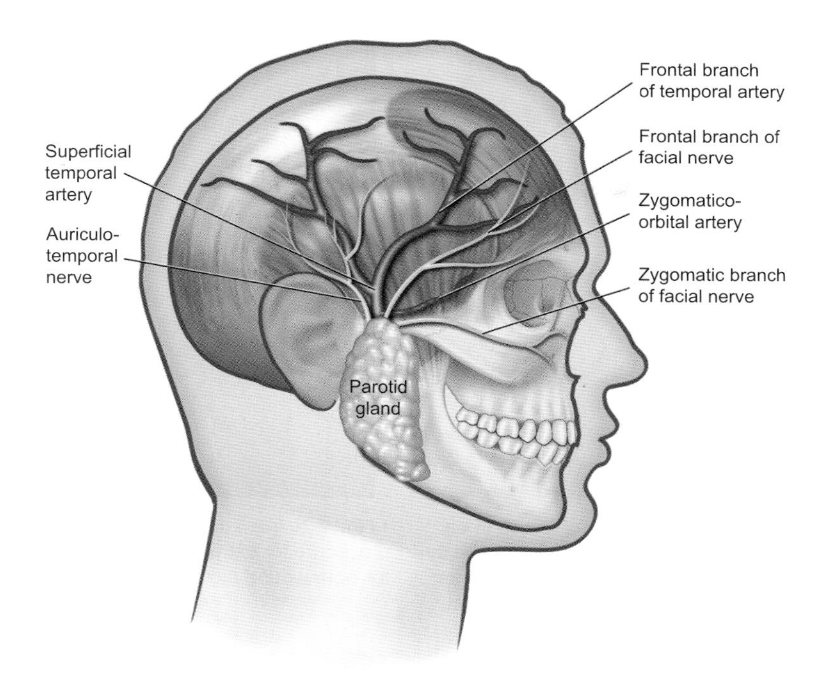

• **Fig. 7.15** A schematic diagram showing the extent of the temporoparietal fascia flap and its relevant anatomy.

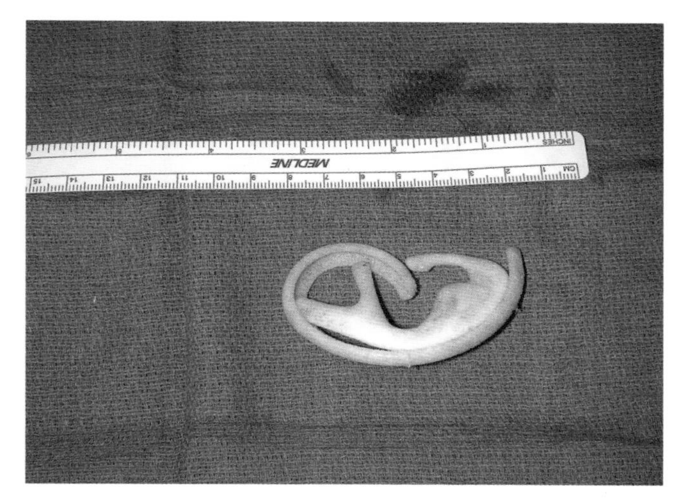

• **Fig. 7.16** An intraoperative view showing two pieces of Medpor ear framework that were sutured together.

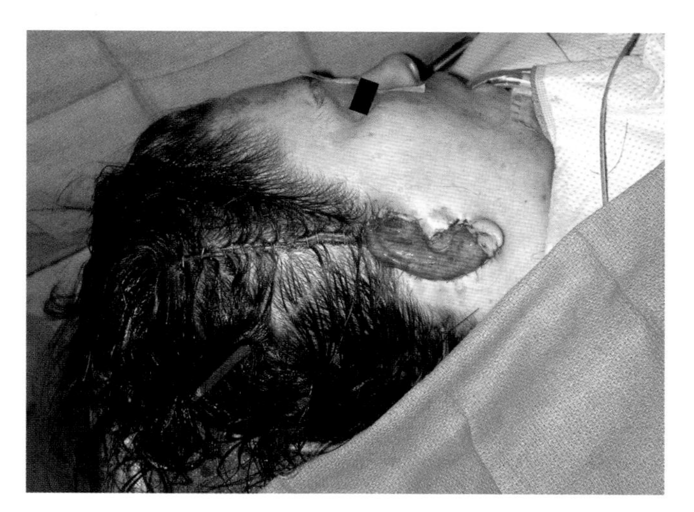

• **Fig. 7.17** An intraoperative view showing completion of placement for ear framework that was covered with a pedicled temporoparietal fascia flap. The remaining ear lobe was rotated inferiorly and incorporated into the ear framework. The temporoparietal flap donor site was closed with skin staples.

infection at 10 months postoperatively (Fig. 7.19). This was salvaged by debridement and adjacent skin flap for coverage (Fig. 7.20).

Final Outcome

The Medpor implant extrusion sites healed initially after the salvage procedure. Unfortunately, for an unknown reason, the patient developed implant extrusion again 6 months later but this time the Medpor implant was infected (Fig. 7.21). Her Medpor implant was removed during a subsequent procedure. The initial successful total ear reconstruction failed because of delayed implant extrusion for unknown reasons.

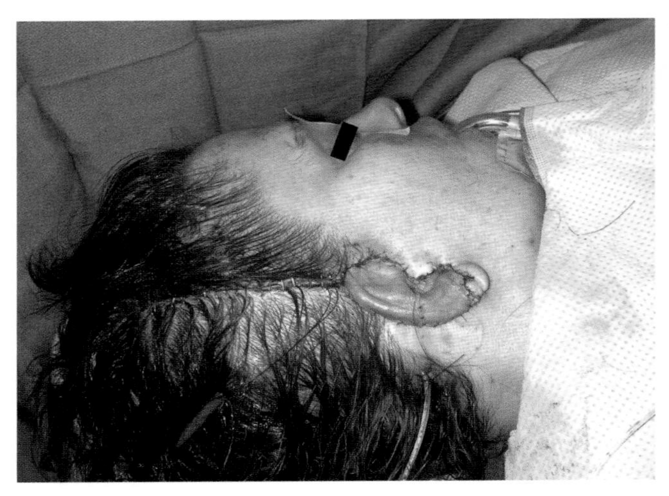

• **Fig. 7.18** An intraoperative view showing completion of the total ear reconstruction with the Medpor implant, a pedicled temporoparietal fascia flap, and a sheet split-thickness skin graft. A test tube drain was inserted under the flap so that the detailed structures of the reconstructed ear could be seen and maintained.

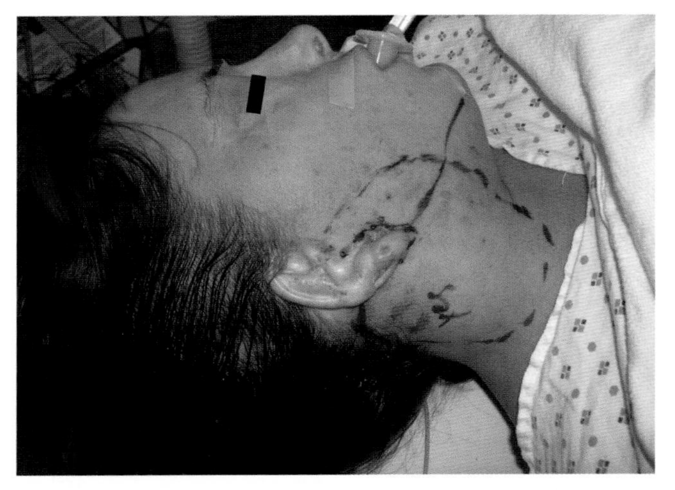

• **Fig. 7.19** A preoperative view at 10 months after total ear reconstruction before a salvage procedure showing two extruded areas of the Medpor implant in the reconstructed ear.

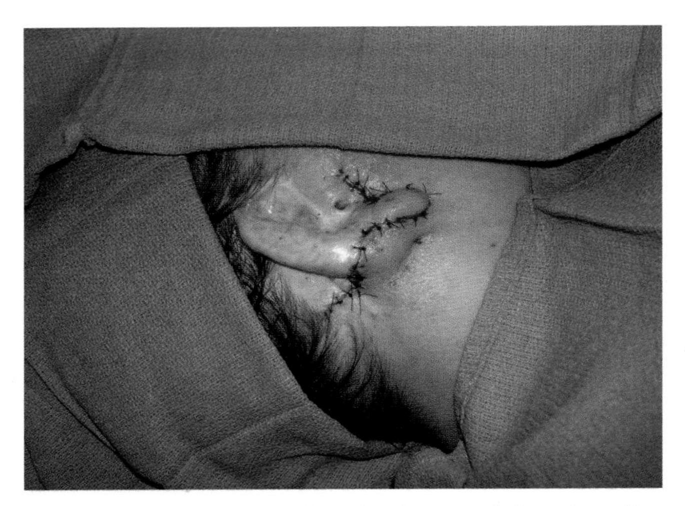

• **Fig. 7.20** An intraoperative view showing completion of a salvage procedure for extruded Medpor implant with local tissue rearrangement for both wound closures.

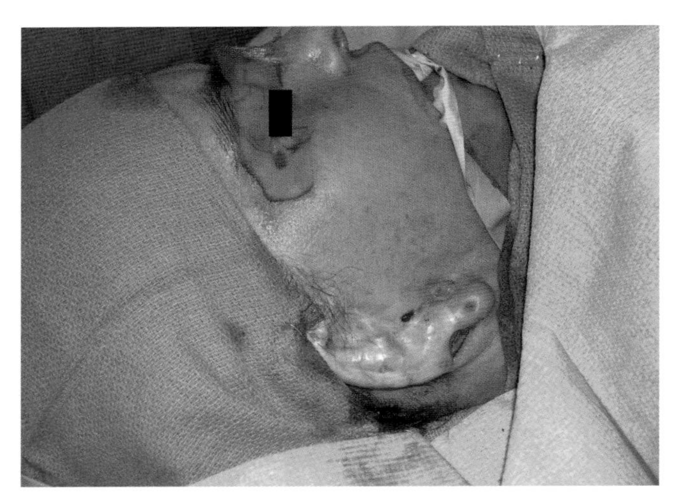

• **Fig. 7.21** An intraoperative view at 6 months after previous salvage procedure showing recurrent extrusion of the Medpor implant in the reconstructed ear.

Pearls for Success

A total ear reconstruction for microtia with a Medpor implant as a framework has been recommended by others as an effective solution for total ear reconstruction especially in adult patients. The commercially made Medpor implants are easily put together as a framework for a total ear reconstruction. Such an ear implant can then be covered by a pedicled temporoparietal fascia flap followed by a sheet split-thickness skin graft. The flap elevation is relatively straight forward as long as the pedicle of the flap, usually visible, is well protected during the procedure. A closed suction drain made from a test tube can be used effectively to promote better adhesion of the skin graft to the flap. Unfortunately, although there might be an initial success of the total ear reconstruction with the techniques described here, an implant extrusion may develop in the long-term as a result of the lack of protective sensation in the reconstructed ear. The implant extrusion is a known problem after this kind of total ear reconstruction and an effective option for surgical management may not always be sucessful. A Medpor implant is more resistant to infection compared with other implants because there can be good vascular ingrowth from the adjacent tissue to the implant. Therefore, the exposed Medpor implant can be washed out and reclosed with local tissue rearrangement. However, if there is clinically evidenced infection, it still needs to be removed just like any other implant.

Recommended Readings

Braun T, Gratza S, Becker S, Schwentner I, et al. Auricular reconstruction with porous polyethylene frameworks: outcome and patient benefit in 65 children and adults. *Plast Reconstr Surg*. 2010;126:1201–1212.

Gault D. Post traumatic ear reconstruction. *J Plast Reconstr Aesthetic Surg*. 2008;61:S5–S12.

Reinisch J, Hovell tot Westerflier, van C, Gould DJ, Tahiri YT. Secondary salvage of the unsatisfactory microtia reconstruction. *Plast Reconstr Surg*. 2020;145:1252–1261.

Reinisch J, Tahiri Y. Polyethylene ear reconstruction: a State-of-the-Art surgical journey. *Plast Reconstr Surg*. 2018;141:461–470.

Sanniec K, Harirah M, Thornton JF. Ear reconstruction after Mohs cancer excision: lessons learned from 327 consecutive cases. *Plast Reconstr Surg*. 2019;144:719–729.

Thorne CH, Wilkes G. Ear deformities, otoplasty, and ear reconstruction. *Plast Reconstr Surg*. 2012;129:701e–716e.

8 Nasal Reconstruction

Clinical Presentation

A 58-year-old White female sustained a dog bite to her nasal tip. Apparently, she lost a significant amount of nasal tip cartilage and also had a sizable nasal skin defect. After a period of local wound care, the nasal skin wound healed (Figs. 8.1 and 8.2). She desired appropriate reconstruction for the partial composite defect of her nose and was brought to the operating room for definitive but delayed nasal reconstruction about 4 weeks after her initial injury.

Operative Plan and Special Considerations

This patient required nasal frame reconstruction with cartilage grafts and distal nasal skin defect reconstruction with a paramedial forehead flap. All necessary cartilage grafts could be harvested from the ear and a paramedial forehead flap from either side of the forehead based on the supratrochlear vessels could be used to provide adequate nasal skin coverage. The paramedial forehead is a good option for a partial nasal skin coverage when the size of the nasal skin defect is greater than 2 × 2 cm. The nasal reconstruction was done in staged procedures because a better outcome can be accomplished through several flap debulking procedures after initial reconstruction. The flap debulking procedure may be more reliable and effective while the pedicle of the flap is still intact. No internal nasal lining was needed for this patient.

Operative Procedures

The first goal of the nasal reconstruction was to reopen healed nasal wounds and to recreate all composite defects of the nasal cartilages and nasal skin. Under general anesthesia, all scar tissue was excised and the wound was irrigated with normal saline solution (Fig. 8.3).

Contracture release surgery was performed for the nasal tip, alar septum, and columella. Under direct vision, the contracted wound was released with the scissors and the residual structures of the nasal skin and the cartilage-supporting structures were identified. The dissection was done to free the caudal septum, columella, nasal cartilage, and alar cartilage on each side. After these releases, it appeared that the patient would require extensive septal graft, the columellar strut, both right and left lower cartilage grafts for support and maintenance of the normal nasal shape (Fig. 8.4). The decision was made to harvest cartilage grafts from each ear.

A posterior approach was used to harvest ear cartilage grafts. The proposed incision was infiltrated with 1% lidocaine with 1:100,000 epinephrine. Once the skin incision was made, the skin dissection was done to free ear cartilage. With preservation of the rim of the cartilage in the concha, a 2 × 1 cm of the cartilage was harvested from each ear and placed in the normal saline solution.

Based on the template, a septal cartilage extension graft was placed first. This was done with a cartilage graft and sutured to the caudal portion of the septum with several interrupted 5-0 PDS sutures. The columellar strut graft was placed to the nasal spine and secured to the adjacent soft tissue with 5-0 PDS sutures. It was also secured to the caudal portion of the septum.

The right lower lateral cartilage graft was placed and sutured with several interrupted 5-0 PDS sutures. Both alar rim grafts were placed next to the columellar strut graft and secured with several interrupted 5-0 PDS sutures. At the end of procedure, the structure support of the nose was reestablished (Figs. 8.5 and 8.6).

The paramedian forehead flap was designed and marked based on the left supratrochlear vessel, identified and mapped with a Doppler. The flap was extended to the frontal hairline and the the size of the flap was about 3 × 2 cm. The width of the pedicle was 1.5 cm (Fig. 8.7). The flap dissection was done first to elevate the skin portion in the distal part and down to the midportion of the forehead and then converted to the subgaleal plane. The rest of the flap elevation was easily performed with more extended skin dissection in order to facilitate the flap inset. The distal portion of the flap was defatted primarily as long as its perfusion looked good. The flap was precisely inserted into the skin defect of the nose with several interrupted 5-0 nylon sutures. Each side of the soft triangle was reconstructed with the flap and the distal portion of the flap was also folded to cover the columellar graft. Two through-and-through sutures were placed to secure the closure of the distal part of the flap. The raw surface of the pedicle was covered with Xeroform.

The posterior ear donor site was closed in two layers. A bolster dressing was applied for compression to the ear cartilage graft donor side. The paramedian forehead flap donor site was approximated after significant undermining with 2-0 Prolene sutures in a simple interrupted fashion. The most distal part was left open (Fig. 8.8).

Eight weeks later under general anesthesia, the well-healed paramedian forehead flap was elevated from both nasal closure sides (Fig. 8.9). The distal portion of flap was completely elevated with the intact distal skin closure. Under direct vision, the debulking procedure was performed with scissors. The amount of tissue debulking was dependent on whether adequate perfusion in this part of the flap could be maintained. Once completed, each side of the elevated flap was then put back and approximated with several interrupted 5-0 Prolene sutures (Fig. 8.10). The raw surface of the pedicle was again covered with Xeroform.

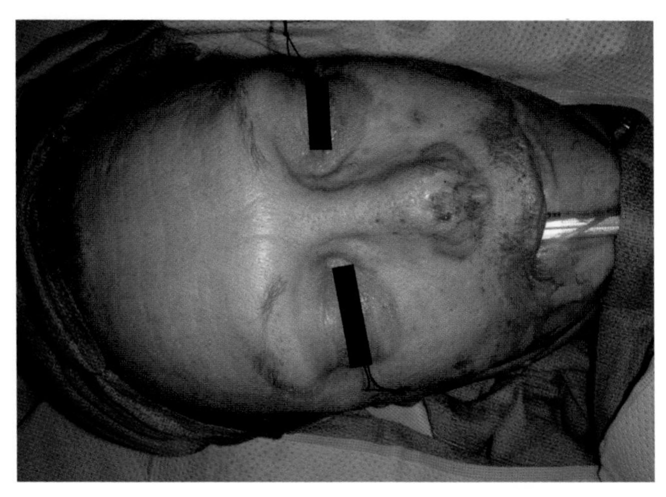

• **Fig. 8.1** Intraoperative view before the patient's first-stage nasal reconstruction showing well-healed composite nasal defects involving skin and underlying cartilage structures.

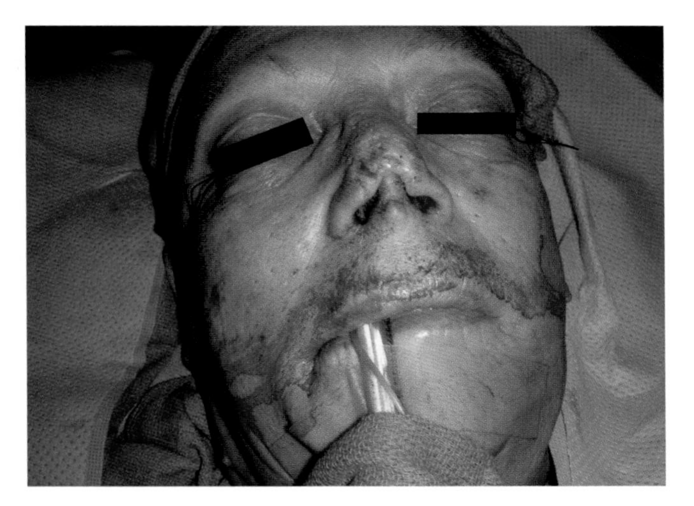

• **Fig. 8.2** Intraoperative basal view showing well-healed composite nasal defects involving skin and underlying cartilage structures.

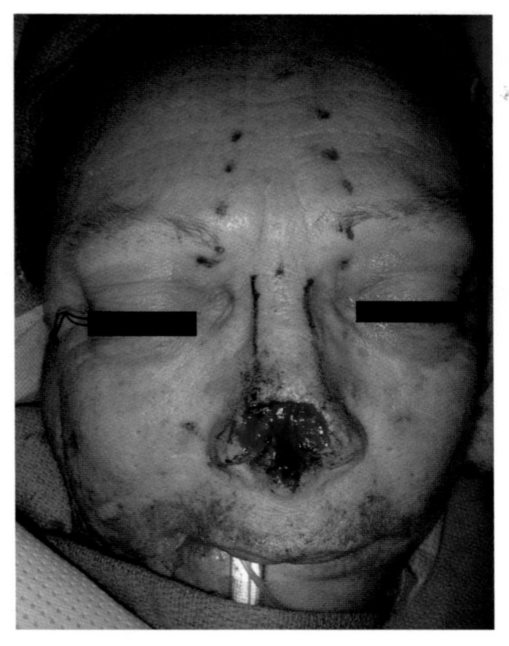

• **Fig. 8.3** Intraoperative view showing true composite nasal defects after scar excision and release.

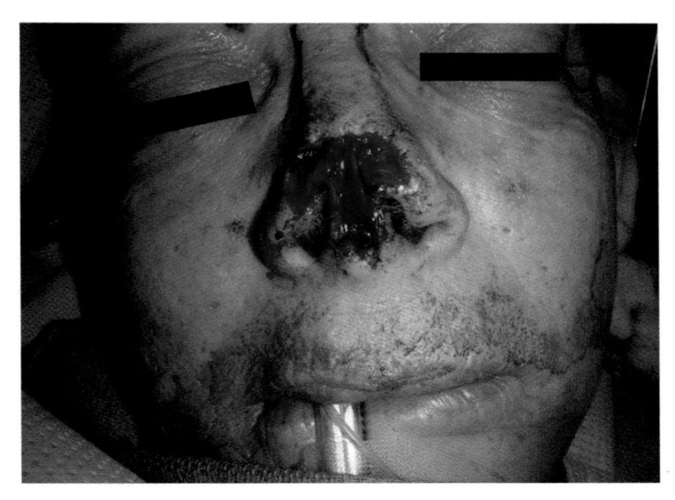

• **Fig. 8.4** Intraoperative close-up view showing residual cartilage structures of nasal tip, inferior lateral cartilage, and columella.

Eight weeks later and again under general anesthesia, the pedicle of the well-healed paramedian forehead was temporarily clamped with a Penrose (Fig. 8.11). Once the distal flap remained pink after 10 minutes, the pedicle could be safely divided. The division of the pedicle was performed with a 15 blade and there was good evidence of blood supply to the remaining flap (Fig. 8.12). It was further debulked proximally with scissors and a knife. The excess skin was then trimmed off and the closure was performed with a 4-0 Monocryl suture in a simple interrupted fashion, followed by the 5-0, fast-absorbing suture in a simple interrupted fashion. The left glabellar skin defect was closed with local tissue rearrangements. The medial half of the left eyebrow position was adjusted again with local tissue rearrangement (Fig. 8.13).

About another 8 weeks later and under general anesthesia, the well-healed flap was elevated superiorly with a knife and the defatting of the flap was again performed with both knife and scissors under direct vision. Care was taken to remove any excess tissue and not to injure the dermal plexus of the flap skin. The excess skin of the flap was also excised for better contour. The final closure was performed with 5-0 Prolene sutures in a simple interrupted fashion.

Follow-Up Results

This patient did well postoperatively after each surgery. There were no complications related to the paramedian forehead flap and cartilage grafts or to subsequent procedures including flap debulking and pedicle division. She had successful multistaged nasal reconstructions and the flap and cartilage grafts healed well.

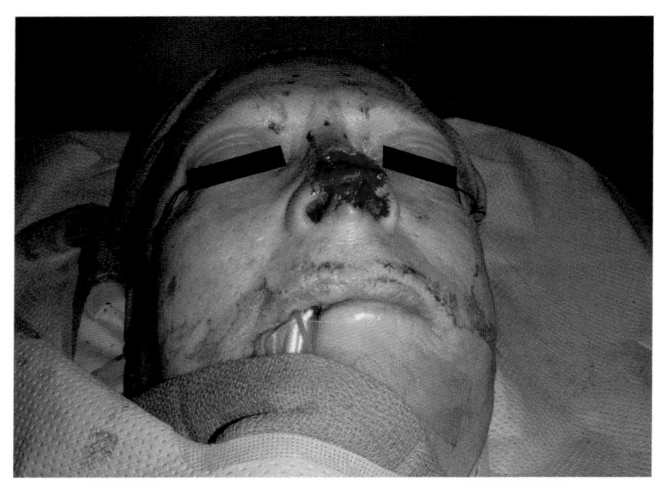

• **Fig. 8.5** Intraoperative view showing the completion of the cartilage graft placements to the septum, lateral cartilages, and columella.

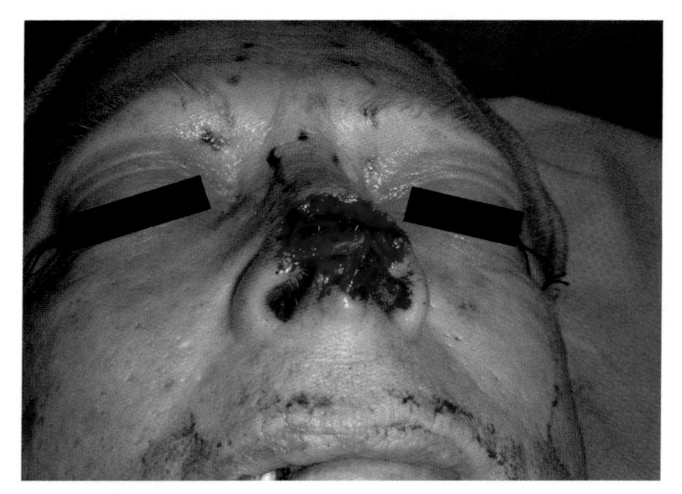

• **Fig. 8.6** Intraoperative close-up view showing the completion of the cartilage graft placements to the septum, lateral cartilages, and columella.

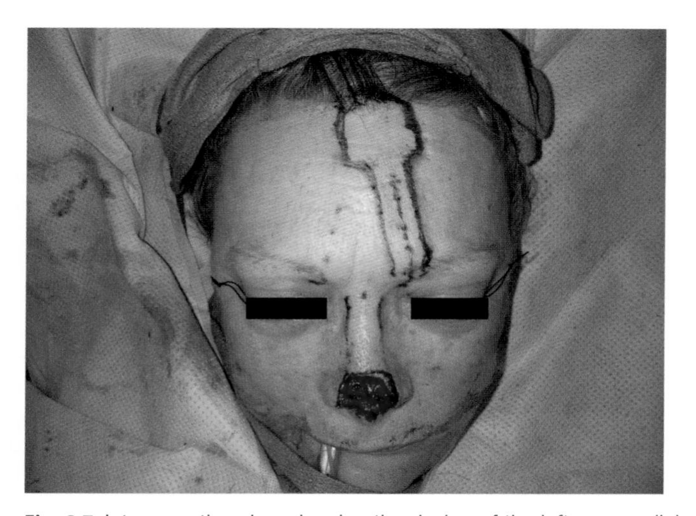

• **Fig. 8.7** Intraoperative view showing the design of the left paramedial forehead flap for nasal tip skin coverage after cartilage graft placements.

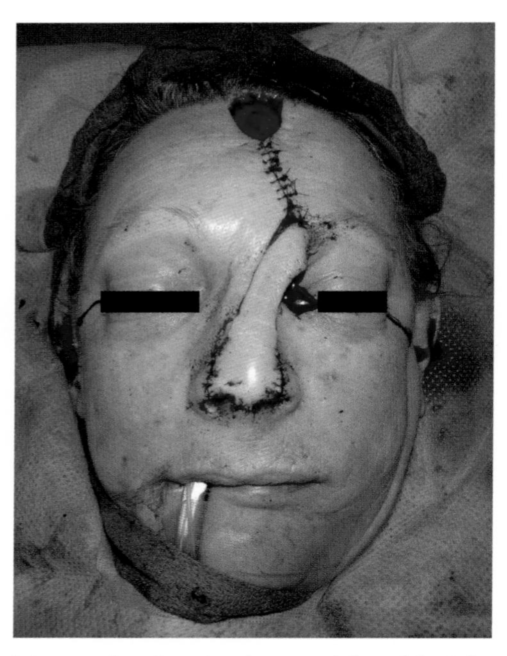

• **Fig. 8.8** Intraoperative view showing completion of the left paramedial forehead flap for nasal tip skin coverage and cartilage graft placements as the first-stage nasal reconstruction.

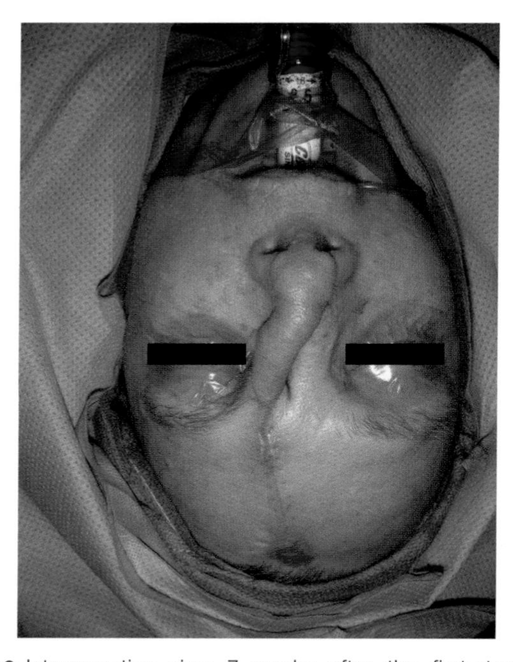

• **Fig. 8.9** Intraoperative view 7 weeks after the first-stage nasal reconstruction before the flap debulking procedure showing a well-healed paramedial forehead flap for nasal tip skin coverage.

Final Outcome

This patient has had a good partial nasal composite reconstruction with acceptable cosmetic outcome after a paramedian forehead flap with cartilage grafts. Although additional revisions could be performed to improve the cosmetic outcome, at this point the patient declines any additional procedures because she lives far

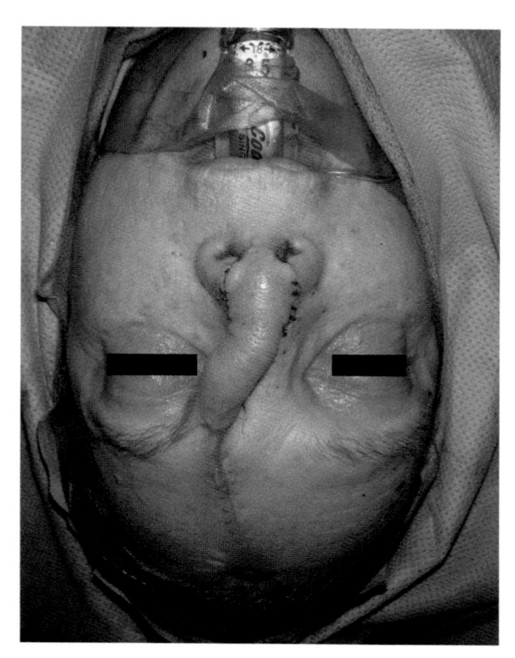

• **Fig. 8.10** Intraoperative view showing the immediate result after the debulking procedure of the paramedial forehead flap for nasal tip skin coverage.

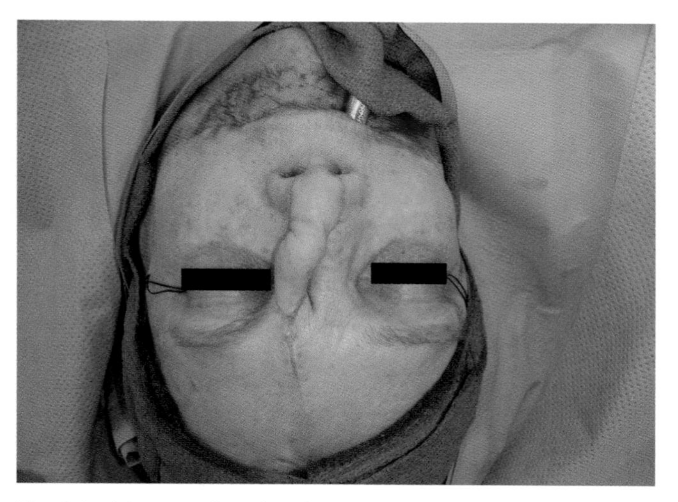

• **Fig. 8.11** Intraoperative view 8 weeks after the flap debulking procedure just before the division of the flap's pedicle showing a well-healed paramedial forehead flap for nasal tip skin coverage.

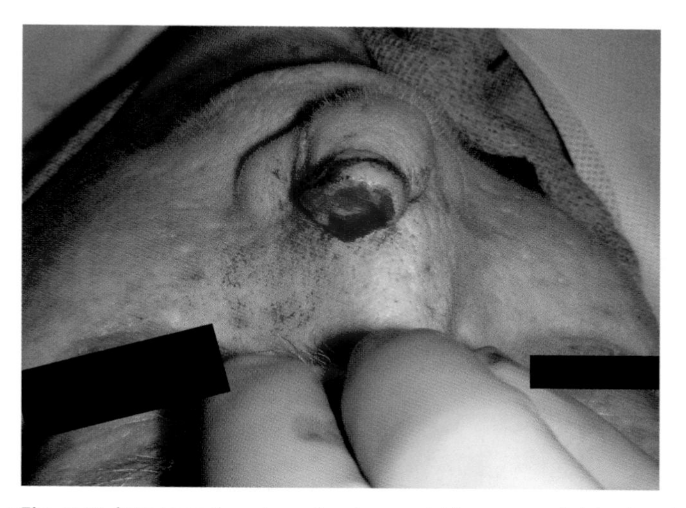

• **Fig. 8.12** Intraoperative view showing a viable paramedial forehead flap for nasal tip skin coverage after the division of the flap's pedicle.

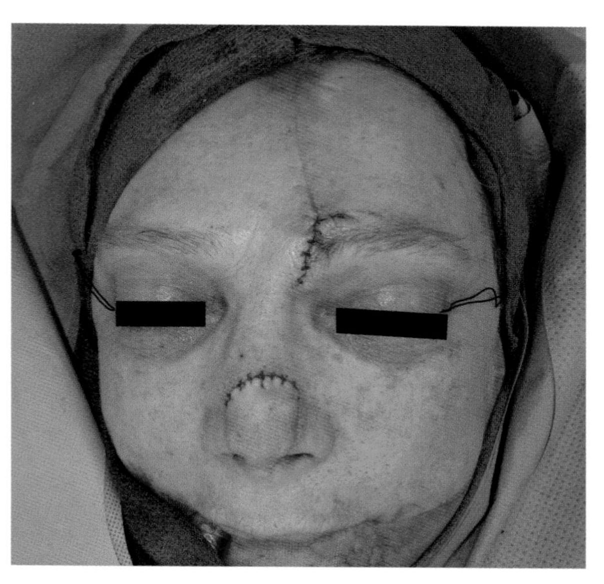

• **Fig. 8.13** Intraoperative view showing the immediate result after the division of the paramedial forehead flap's pedicle.

away from our hospital. She returned to her normal life and activities and has been followed by the plastic surgery service as needed.

Pearls for Success

Partial or total nasal reconstruction for a composite tissue defect remains challenging because such a reconstruction involves nasal framework reconstruction and nasal skin coverage. Cartilage grafts can be harvested from ears or ribs although ear cartilage grafts are more commonly harvested. A posterior approach behind the ear offers a good exposure and no visible scar. The amount of the cartilage grafts obtained from both ears is usually adequate for a partial nasal reconstruction as demonstrated in this case. A paramedian forehead flap is a classic option to provide soft tissue coverage for almost any size of nasal defect. In most patients, the pedicle can be easily mapped by a handheld Doppler and the width of the flap pedicle can be safely designed as narrow as 1 cm. The flap dissection is relatively straightforward and the tissue plane would be submuscular when its dissection is close to the pedicle vessels. Attention should be paid not to twist the pedicle while the flap is turned over to cover the nasal skin defect. When necessary, the flap dissection can be extended into the anterior hair line so that the flap can be folded to reconstruct nostrils and columella. In addition, the distal scalp defect can be left open and heal by secondary intention. The subsequent procedures such as pedicle division or flap debulking can be performed every 6 to 8 weeks until the contour of the reconstructed nose satisfies both the patient and the surgeon. The initial flap debulking can be performed while the pedicle of the flap is still intact. In this way, more excess tissues can be removed while adequate blood supply can be maintained. After pedicle division, one or more flap debulking procedures may be needed for additional thinning. In addition, dermal abrasion may be needed to improve the appearance at the junction between the flap and native nasal skin.

Recommended Readings

Cavadas PC, Torres A. Total reconstruction with prefabricated and prelaminated free flap. *Ann Plast Surg.* 2019;83:e35–e38.

Constantine FC, Lee MR, Sinno S, Thornton JF. Reconstruction of the nasal soft triangle subunit. *Plast Reconstr Surg.* 2013;131:1045–1050.

Menick FJ. A 10-year experience in nasal reconstruction with the three-stage forehead flap. *Plast Reconstr Surg.* 2002;109:1839–1855.

Menick FJ. Nasal reconstruction. *Plast Reconstr Surg.* 2010;125:138e–150e.

Torto FL, Redi U, Cigna E, et al. Nasal reconstruction with two stages versus three stages forehead fap: what is better for patients with high vascular risk? *J Craniofac Surg.* 2020;31:e57–e60.

Weng R, Li Q, Gu B, Liu K, Shen G, Xie F. Extended forehead skin expansion and single-stage nasal subunit plasty for nasal reconstruction. *Plast Reconstr Surg.* 2010;125:1119–1128.

9 Lip Reconstruction

CASE 1

Clinical Presentation

A 58-year-old White female had a 4 × 4 cm skin lesion of cancerous appearance above her central lower lip (Fig. 9.1). She underwent a local excision of the lower lip lesion with a 5-mm margin by the plastic surgery service (Fig. 9.2). All peripheral and deep margins were confirmed negative for basal cell carcinoma, a tissue diagnosis in the operating room, by intraoperative frozen sections. The defect over her central lower lip extended to the muscle but in the most area it was a full-thickness through-and-through defect (Fig. 9.3). A definitive lower lip reconstruction was planned for this patient by the same service.

Operative Plan and Special Considerations

Based on the location and size of the lower lip defect, which was about two-thirds of the entire lower lip, bilateral Karapandzic flaps were planned for this patient. The flap, performed bilaterally, would be ideal for the reconstruction of a large central lower lip defect. In this case, the excess lower face and cheek skin could be incorporated with each flap to facilitate both flaps' approximation in the midline so that the defect could be closed primarily without much tension.

Operative Procedures

Bilateral Karapandzic flaps were designed based on the existing skin crease in each side of the lower face and extended to the nasolabial fold (Fig. 9.4). All proposed skin incisions and dissection areas were infiltrated with 1% lidocaine with 1:100,000 epinephrine. The connected portion of the lower lip was excised, to facilitate the approximation of bilateral Karapandzic flap closure to the midline. Once the transverse skin incision had been made through the subcutaneous tissue to the orbicularis oris muscle, the muscle fibers were spread apart longitudinally to aid the flap's rotation and advancement to the midline. Care was taken to preserve the neurovascular pedicle of the flap on each side (Fig. 9.5). The skin incision was extended to the nasolabial fold and with additional muscle fiber spreading, both flaps could be approximated in the midline without tension. The midline closure was done in four layers from the mucosa, muscle, and subcutaneous tissue to the skin. The rest of the flap closure was done in two layers from the subcutaneous tissue to the skin. The back cut was extended to each side of the cheek to facilitate the flap's rotation and advancement. All skin closure was performed with 5-0 nylon suture in either interrupted or running fashion. The actual closure of the mucosa in the lower lip was done with 5-0 chromic sutures in an interrupted fashion (Fig. 9.6).

Follow-Up Results

The patient did well postoperatively without problems related to the bilateral Karapandzic flaps. She was observed overnight in the hospital but unfortunately developed sudden onset of chest pain and hypoxia. A prompt diagnosis of pulmonary embolism was made and she was fully anticoagulated. She remained asymptomatic and was discharged home at postoperative day 5 on oral anticoagulant. The lower lip flap reconstruction site healed well (Figs. 9.7A and B).

Final Outcome

The bilateral Karapandzic flap site healed well without any problems. The patient has a reasonably normal appearance and good function of her lower lip with minimal scarring (Fig. 9.8). The patient returned to normal life and has been followed by the plastic surgery service for routine skin cancer follow-up.

Pearls for Success

Bilateral Karapandzic flaps are an excellent reconstructive option for a large central lip defect. During the flap dissection, the orbicularis oris muscle should only be spread apart longitudinally and direct division of the muscle fibers should be avoided to preserve as much function of the muscle as possible. The neurovascular pedicle should be visualized and protected for maximum function of the lip after reconstruction. Skin back cut can be extended to the cheek to allow more rotation and advancement of each flap toward the midline closure. The ultimate reconstructive result can be excellent and a good lip function can be maintained.

CASE 2

Clinical Presentation

A 20-year-old White female had a 4 × 2 cm skin lesion of cancerous appearance over her central upper lip involving skin and mucosa (Fig. 9.9). She underwent a local excision of the upper lip lesion with a 5-mm margin by the plastic surgery service. All

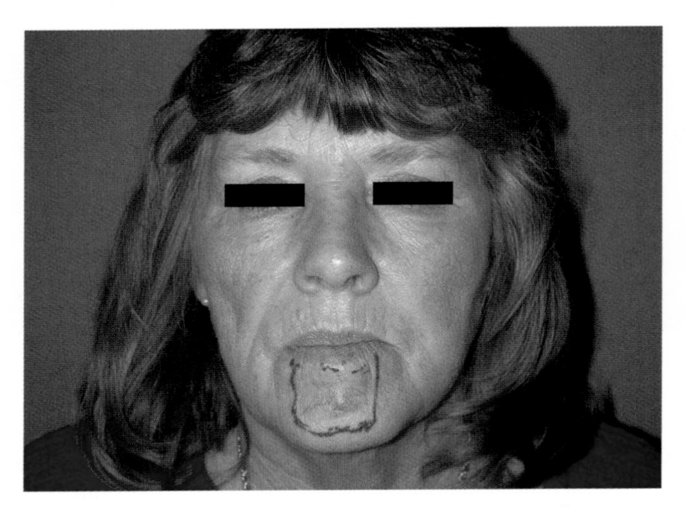

• **Fig. 9.1** A preoperative view showing a skin lesion of cancerous appearance in the central part of the patient's lower lip.

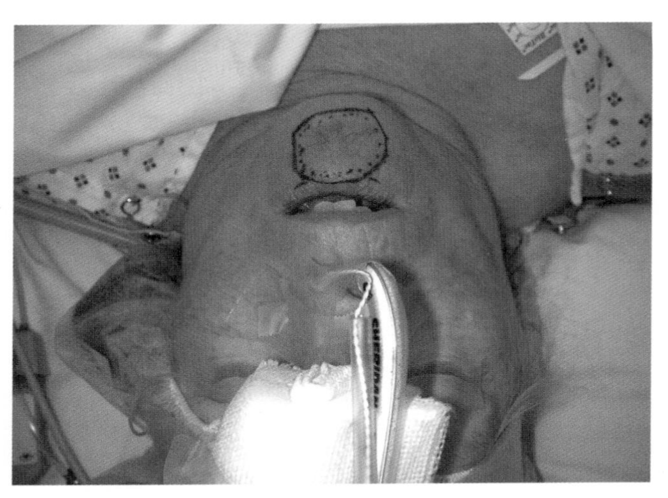

• **Fig. 9.2** An intraoperative view showing an outline of the skin lesion of cancerous appearance *(dotted line)* and an outline of the excision *(solid line)*.

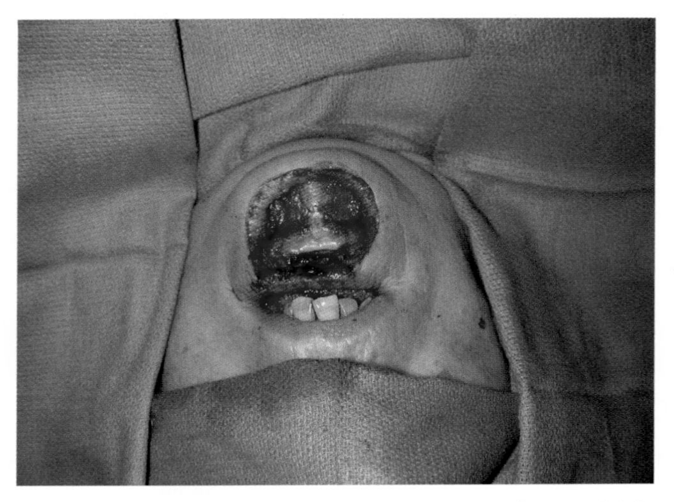

• **Fig. 9.3** An intraoperative view showing a large lower lip central defect after complete excision of the basal cell cancer lesion.

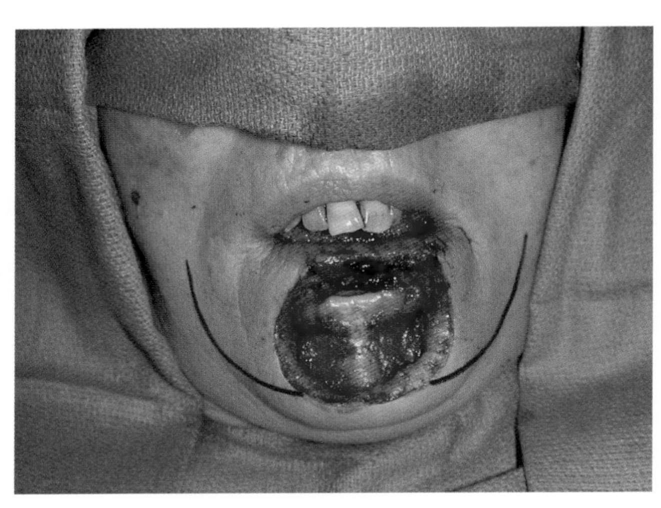

• **Fig. 9.4** An intraoperative view showing the design of bilateral Karapandzic flaps for closure of this large lower lip defect.

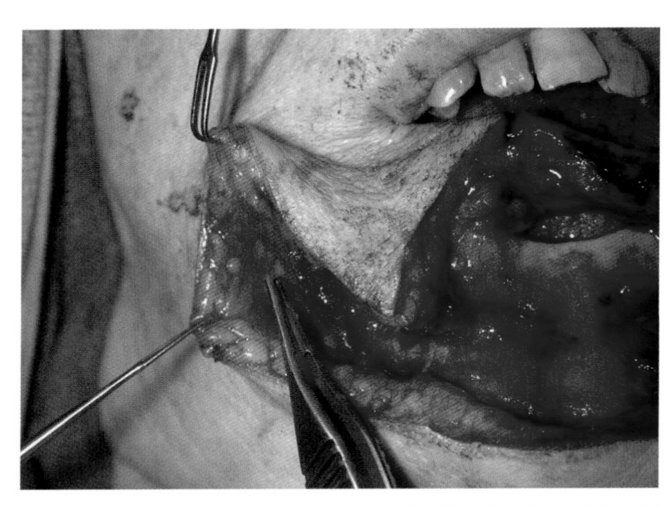

• **Fig. 9.5** An intraoperative view showing the flap elevation of the right Karapandzic flap. The orbicularis oris muscle was spread apart. The neurovascular pedicle of the flap, pointed by forceps, was identified.

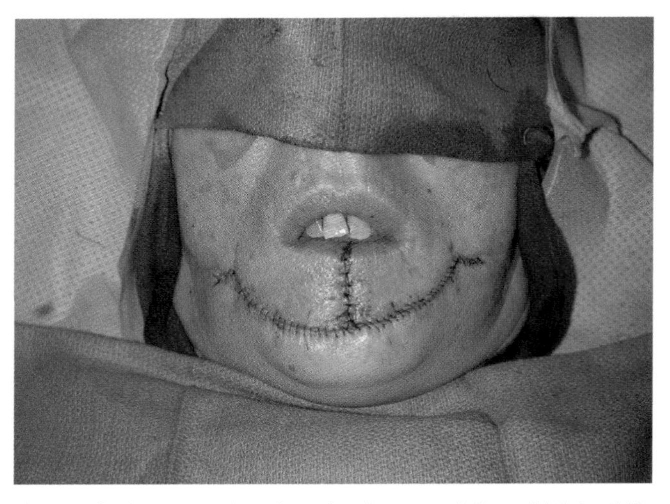

• **Fig. 9.6** An intraoperative view showing completion of bilateral Karapandzic flap reconstruction.

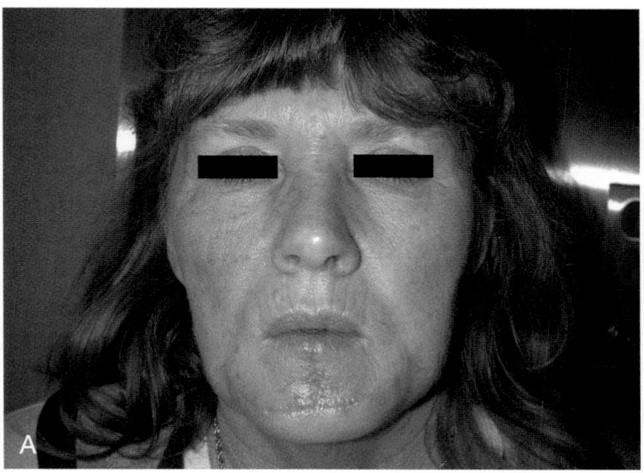

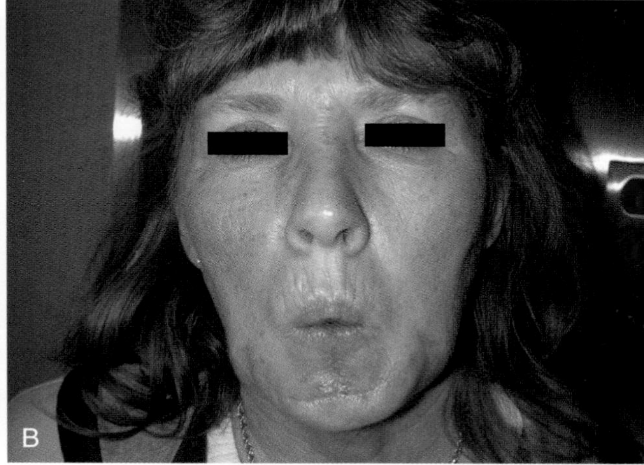

• **Fig. 9.7** Result at a 3-week follow-up showing (A) well-healed flap site with minimal contour deformity and scarring and (B) good function of the reconstructed lower lip.

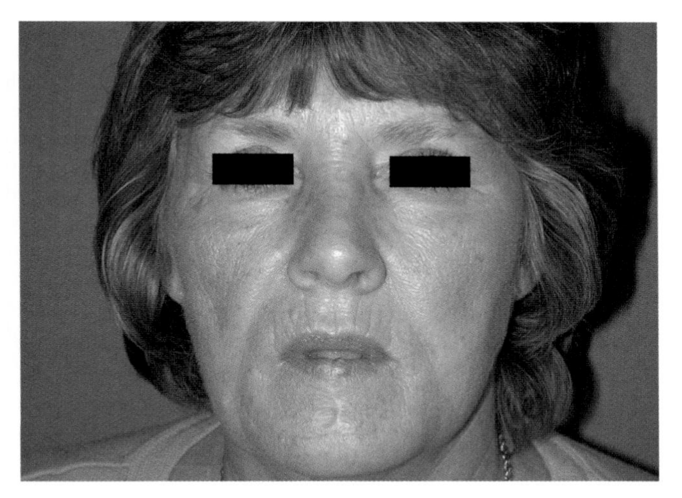

• **Fig. 9.8** Result at 8-month follow-up showing well-healed flap site with nearly normal looking lower lip and minimal scarring.

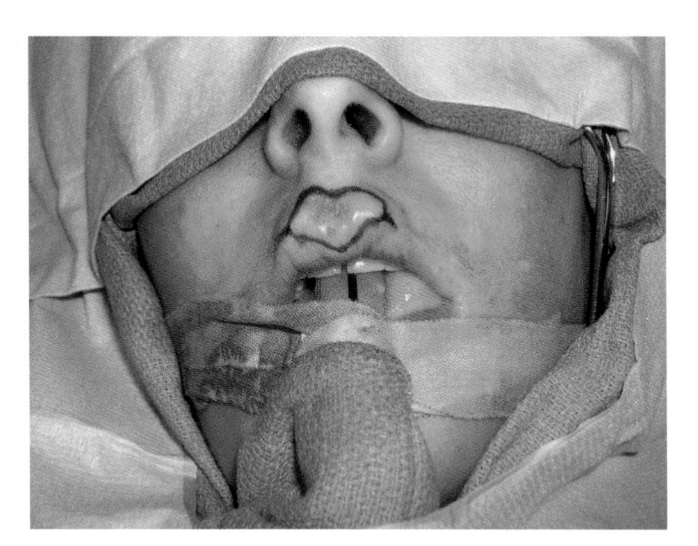

• **Fig. 9.9** A preoperative view showing an outlined squamous cell cancer of the central upper lip involving both skin and mucosa.

peripheral and deep margins were confirmed negative for squamous cell carcinoma by a tissue diagnosis in the operating room and by intraoperative frozen sections. The defect extended to the muscle. A definitive upper lip reconstruction was planned for this patient by the same service.

Operative Plan and Special Considerations

Based on the location and size of the central lip defect involving skin and mucosa, which was about half of the entire upper lip, two flaps were planned for this patient. V-to-Y mucosal advancement for reconstruction of the upper lip mucosal defect and bilateral upper lip skin advancement flaps for reconstruction of the upper lip skin defect. In this way, this complex upper lip defect can be reconstructed with like-to-like tissues and may potentially have a better reconstructive outcome.

Operative Procedures

Once both philtral columns were marked, bilateral upper lip skin advancements were designed and marked at the base of the nose with the ala on each side (Fig. 9.10). All proposed skin and mucosal incisions and dissection areas were infiltrated with 1% lidocaine with 1:100,000 epinephrine. Each side of the upper lip skin flap was elevated at the subcutaneous tissue plane and extended along the base of the nose superior to the junction between mucosa and inferior to the skin. The central part of the excess upper lip skin was excised and two upper lip skin advancement flaps were approximated in the midline and closed with two layers. The subcutaneous tissue was closed with 4-0 Monocryl sutures and the skin with 5-0 nylon sutures in an interrupted fashion. The V-to-Y mucosal advancement flap was elevated intraorally, advanced toward to the vermilion boarder, and closed in a V-to-Y fashion with 5-0 chronic suture in an interrupted fashion (Fig. 9.11).

Follow-Up Results

The patient did well postoperatively with no problems related to the bilateral upper lip skin advancement flaps and V-to-Y mucosal

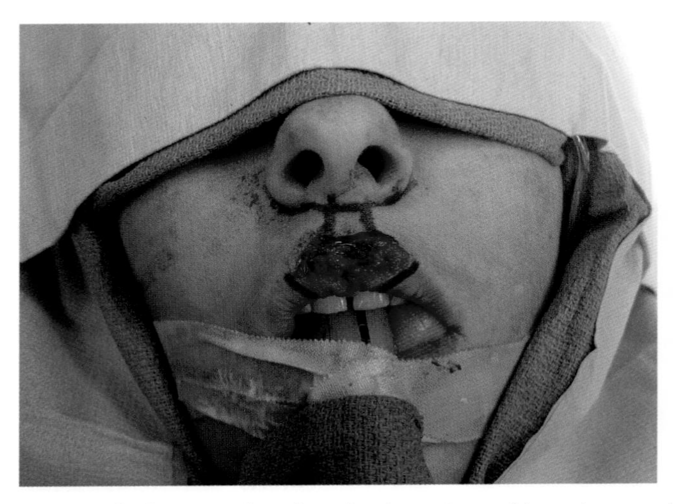

• **Fig. 9.10** An intraoperative view showing a large skin and mucosal defect of the central upper lip and a design for bilateral upper lip skin advancement flaps and V-to-Y mucosal advancement flap.

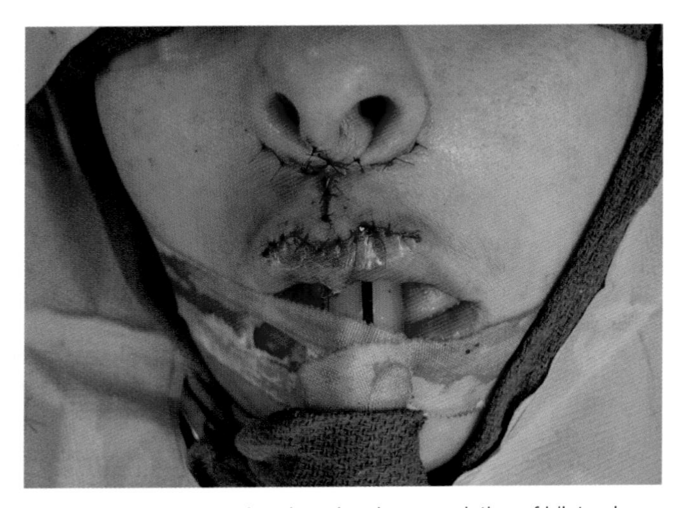

• **Fig. 9.11** An intraoperative view showing completion of bilateral upper lip skin advancement flaps and V-to-Y mucosal advancement flap.

advancement flap. She was observed overnight and was discharged next day from the hospital. The upper lip flap reconstruction site healed well.

Final Outcome

The reconstruction for her upper lip complex defect with bilateral upper lip skin advancement flaps and V-to-Y mucosa advancement flap healed well without problems. She has had a reasonably good outcome and normal function of the upper lip with minimal scarring (Fig. 9.12). The patient returned to normal life and has been followed by the plastic surgery service for routine skin cancer follow-up.

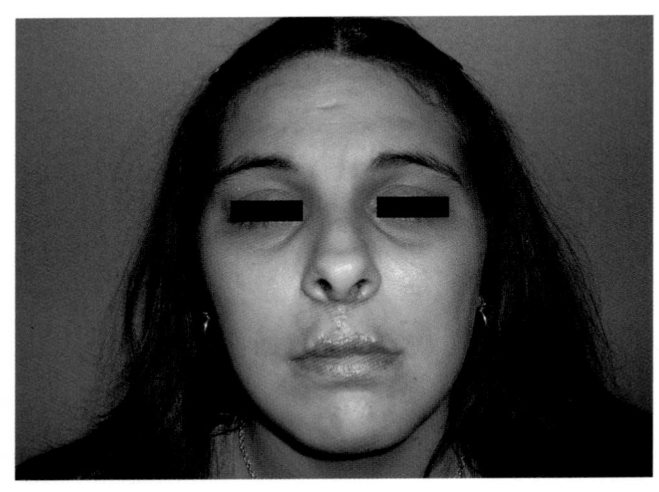

• **Fig. 9.12** Result at a 6-week follow-up showing well-healed flap site with minimal contour deformity and scarring.

Pearls for Success

For a complex upper lip defect involving skin and mucosa, each tissue component should be reconstructed with like-to-like tissue. In this case, bilateral upper lip skin flaps can be used to reconstruct the skin defect. With adequate dissection of each skin flap in the subcutaneous tissue plane, both flaps can be approximated in the midline of the upper lip. If needed, each skin flap can be advanced more by extending the skin incision following the alar base with more flap elevation. A V-to-Y mucosal flap can be used to reconstruct the mucosal defect. The width of the flap should be designed as the same length of the mucosal defect. The amount of the flap advancement is about 0.5 to 1 cm. Complete release in the distal part of "V" is important to ensure the flap's advancement.

Recommended Readings

Ethunandan M, Macpherson DW, Santhanam V. Karapandzic flap for reconstruction of lip defects. *J Oral Maxillofac Surg*. 2007;65:2512–2517.

Isik D, Garca MF, Durucu C, Goktas U, Atik B. Reconstruction of lower lip with myomucosal advancement flap. *Head Neck*. 2012:1562–1569.

Kim J, Lee Y, Choi H. A Rotational flap combined with a mucosal advancement flap for the lip reconstruction. *J Craniofac Surg*. 2019;30:e615–e617.

Madorsky S, Meltzer O. Myomucosal lip island flap for reconstruction of small to medium lower lip defects. *Facial Plast Surg Aesthet Med*. 2020;22:200–206.

Pantalena L, Bordeaux JS. Reconstruction of a multi-subunit defect on the lip, nose, and cheek. *Dermatol Surg*. 2017;43:293–296.

Salibian AA, Zide BM. Elegance in upper lip reconstruction. *Plast Reconstr Surg*. 2019;143:572–582.

10 Complex Facial Reconstruction After Trauma

CASE 1

Clinical Presentation

An 18-year-old man fell off a moving vehicle and was then struck by the same vehicle. He was intubated and was in critical condition. Initial injuries included an open skull fracture with exposed intracranial contents, scalp avulsion, left-sided facial avulsion, left superior and lateral orbital wall fractures, bilateral sphenoid sinus fractures, bilateral temporomandibular joint fractures with extension into the intraarticular space on the right, left mastoid fracture, and a cervical spine fracture. Once stabilized, the patient was immediately taken to the operating room by the trauma service for debridement of open wounds. He was found to have a soft-tissue defect measuring 10 × 14 cm of the left face and scalp with a missing zygomatic arch, avulsed left ear, and avulsed left facial nerve. Nine days later, a second facial wound debridement was performed by the plastic surgery service and careful planning for reconstruction was done in the operating room (Figs. 10.1 and 10.2).

Operative Plan and Special Considerations

Because of the size of this large facial wound and the missing zygomatic arch and portion of the zygoma, the initial definitive reconstruction would include a free anterolateral thigh (ALT) perforator flap for soft tissue coverage after adequate bony reconstruction for the left zygomatic arch and zygoma. Once the soft tissue wound healed, the patient would need several staged reconstructive and cosmetic procedures to improve the final outcome. Possible future procedures would include a flap debulking procedure, lateral canthopexy or canthoplasty to reposition the lower eyelid position, hairline reconstruction via scalp tissue expansion, scar revisions, and epidermal skin graft to improve the flap's colour match. The patient was informed about the expected outcomes with conventional and contemporary reconstructive and cosmetic procedures. Preoperatively, the left facial artery and vein were evaluated by duplex scan to determine whether they could be used as recipient vessels for microvascular anastomoses. In addition, perforators in each thigh were mapped by duplex scan so that a preferred site for harvesting a free ALT perforator flap could be decided. In addition, the patient's other trauma issues were properly managed or cleared by the trauma service for his initial definitive reconstruction.

Operative Procedures

Under general anesthesia, the entire open facial wound and exposed bones were debrided. After irrigation, the wound appeared to be clean and fresh and ready for definitive soft tissue reconstruction.

The midface bony reconstruction was performed first. The left zygoma including part of the zygomatic arch was reconstructed with a 7 × 2 cm Medpor implant. The Medpor implant was fashioned to replace the missing bony parts of the midface after being soaked with antibiotic solution. The Medpor implant was used to restore the lateral cheek and lateral orbital rim. This additional fixation was performed with a 1.5-mm plate and secured with multiple screws. A 2.4-mm titanium plate was contoured and placed to act as a zygomatic arch. It was secured with multiple screws (Fig. 10.3).

The left facial artery and vein were identified and explored next. The facial artery and the vein were dissected free and prepared under loupe magnification for microvascular anastomoses.

The left ALT perforator flap was harvested (Fig. 10.4). A 15 × 9 cm skin paddle was marked and a single perforator was identified and dissected out. The flap was dissected more superiorly, laterally, and inferiorly in order to have a bigger skin paddle. After about 3-cm intramuscular dissection, the junction of the perforator to the descending branch of the lateral circumflex vessels was identified. During the dissection, a motor nerve to the vastus lateralis muscle was preserved. The pedicle dissection was performed in a retrograde fashion and the most proximal dissection was performed toward the profunda. The pedicle was then divided with a hemoclip (Fig. 10.5).

The flap was prepared under loupe magnification. Both the artery and the vein were prepared with microscissors and flushed with the heparinized saline solution. The flap was temporarily placed on the left facial wound. A skin tunnel was made and the pedicle was placed through the tunnel.

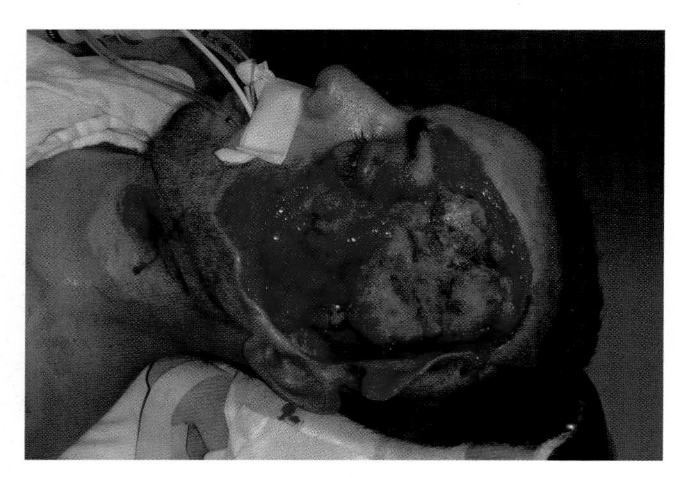

• **Fig. 10.1** Intraoperative view after initial debridement showing extensive soft tissue defect measuring 10 × 14 cm of the left face and scalp with missing left zygomatic arch, avulsed left ear, and avulsed left facial nerve. The left ear canal was stented with a plastic tube.

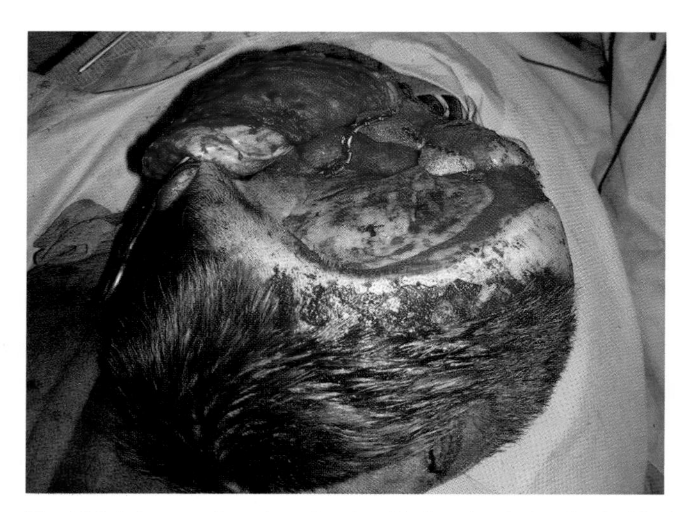

• **Fig. 10.3** Intraoperative view showing Medpor implants, fixed with titanium plates, for alloplastic bony reconstruction of the zygomatic body and lateral orbital rim. A 2.4-mm titanium plate was contoured to act as the reconstructed zygomatic arch.

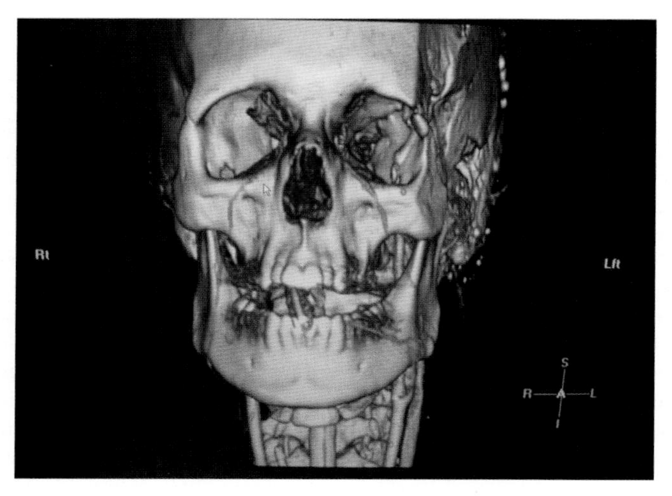

• **Fig. 10.2** The 3-D facial bone CT scan showing the extent of facial bone injury in the left face. The entire zygomatic arch, portion of the lateral orbital rim, and zygomatic body were missing.

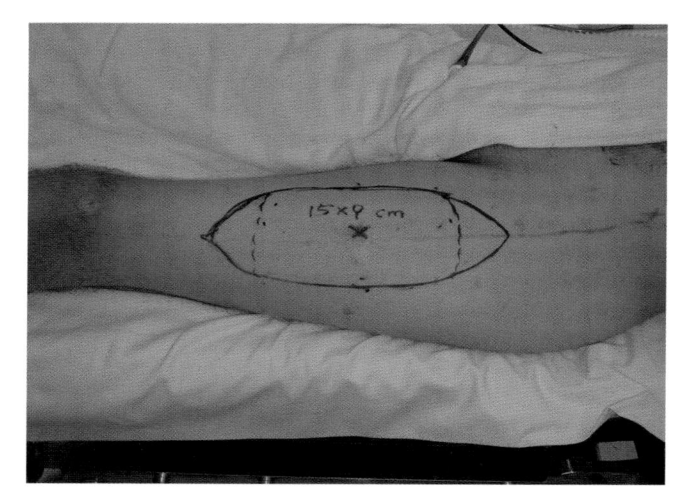

• **Fig. 10.4** Intraoperative view showing the design of the left free ALT perforator flap based on a single perforator.

The microvascular anastomosis was performed under microscope. Both facial artery and vein were divided with hemoclips. The arterial microvascular anastomosis was performed in an end-to-end fashion with 8-0 nylon suture. The venous microvascular anastomosis was performed with a 2.5-mm coupler in an end-to-end fashion. Once both arterial and venous anastomoses were completed, there was a good arterial and venous flow and the flap appeared to be well perfused.

A 3 × 0.5 cm full-thickness skin graft was harvested from the distal portion of the flap. The skin graft was defatted and approximated as a small tube with 5-0 chromic sutures. It was sutured to reconstruct the left ear canal and immobilized with a plastic tube.

The flap inset was inserted into the facial defect with multiple 3-0 Monocryl sutures in half-buried mattress fashion after placing a drain. Some of the skin closure was done with a staple. The left neck skin wound was simply approximated with skin staples (Fig. 10.6). The left thigh flap donor site was closed in two layers for deep dermal and skin closure.

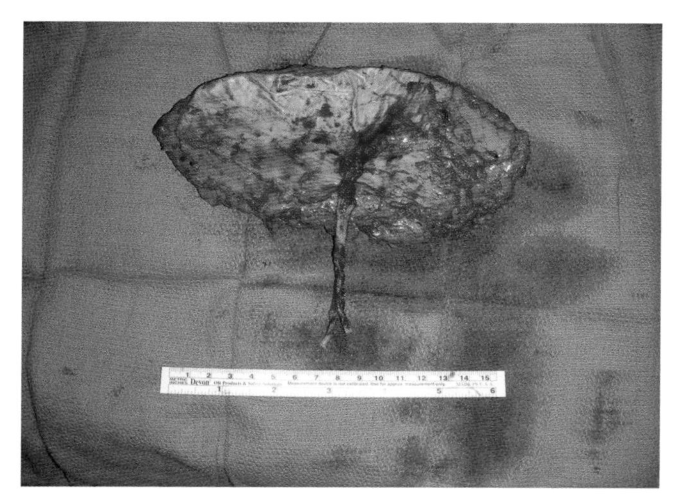

• **Fig. 10.5** Intraoperative view showing successful dissection of the free ALT perforator flap.

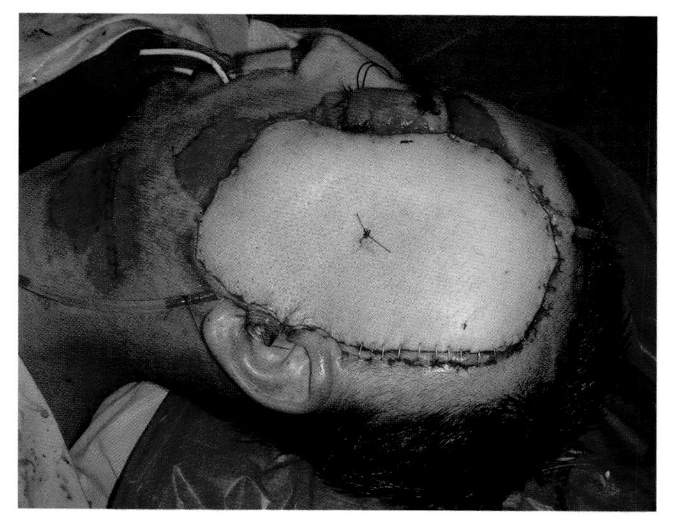

• **Fig. 10.6** Intraoperative view showing the immediate result after the free ALT perforator flap reconstruction for soft tissue coverage.

• **Fig. 10.7** Intraoperative view showing the immediate result after exploration of both arterial and venous microanastomoses. The flap remained well perfused.

Follow-Up Results

On postoperative day 1, moderate venous congestion of the ALT perforator flap was noted and duplex scan also demonstrated possible venous microvascular stenosis. The patient was taken emergently to the operating room for exploration. However, both arterial and venous pedicles appeared patent without twisting or kinking (Fig. 10.7). The flap was monitored through the rest of his hospitalization and remained viable. He was doing well and was discharged from the hospital on postoperative day 10.

The patient subsequently developed lower eyelid ectropion secondary to the lateral orbital scarring and the "pulling" force from the ALT flap (Figs. 10.8A and B). Five weeks after the initial reconstruction, he underwent release of the contracture, lateral canthoplasty, resuspension of the ALT flap, and full-thickness skin grafting to a resulting area of open wound (Figs. 10.9 and 10.10).

During subsequent office visits, the patient was noted to have developed hypertrophic scarring of his face and neck, in addition to persistent tearing and difficulty in fully closing his left eye (Fig. 10.11). He was treated with scar massaging and two rounds of Kenalog injections. There was bulkiness of the free flap and thinning of the left midface (Fig. 10.12). About 8 months after his initial revision surgery, he underwent repeated left lateral canthoplasty, debulking of the ALT flap, left midface suspension, and cheek augmentation using Medpor implant (Figs. 10.13 and 10.14).

The ectropion was corrected (Fig. 10.15) and the patient then underwent placement of a scalp tissue expander for hairline scalp reconstruction (Figs. 10.16 and 10.17). Over the next 3 months, he underwent fills to a final volume of 230 mL (Figs. 10.18 and 10.19). The expander was then removed and the resultant expanded temporoparietal scalp flap was advanced to reestablished the anterior temperal hairline scalp (Fig. 10.20).

Once the scalp hairline reconstruction had healed, an additional procedure was undertaken to improve the color mismatch between the ALT flap and the native face/scalp skin (Fig. 10.21). An epidermal skin graft was taken from the parietal scalp and sutured to the flap after de-epithelialization of a 14×8 cm region (Figs. 10.22–10.24). The resultant color match was noted to be

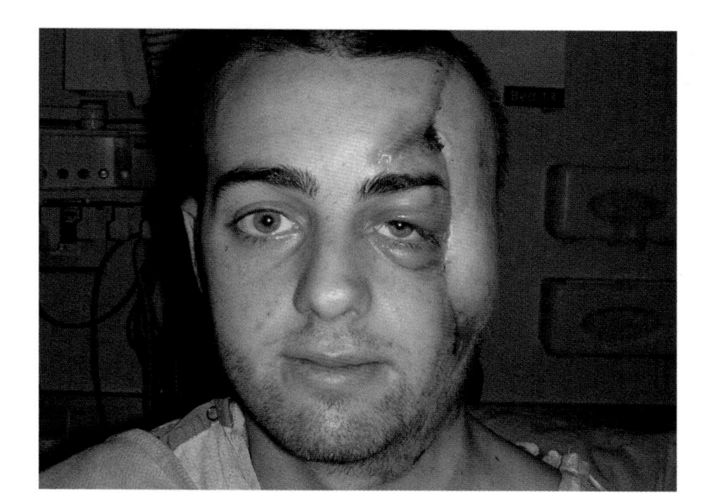

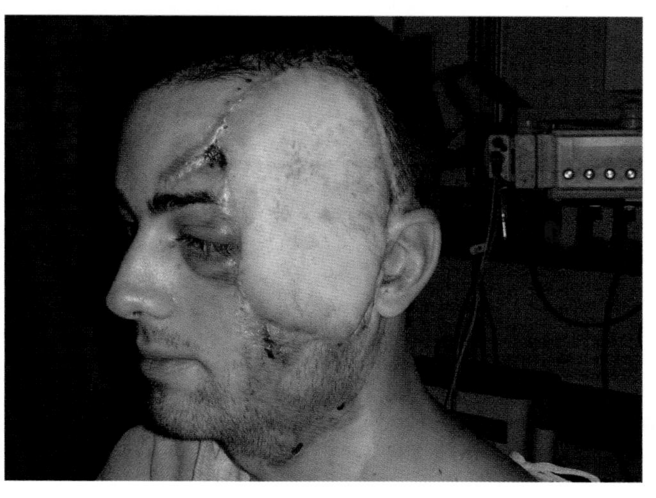

• **Fig. 10.8** (A) and (B), The result at 5-week follow-up after the initial free ALT perforator flap reconstruction and bony reconstruction with Medpor implants and titanium plates.

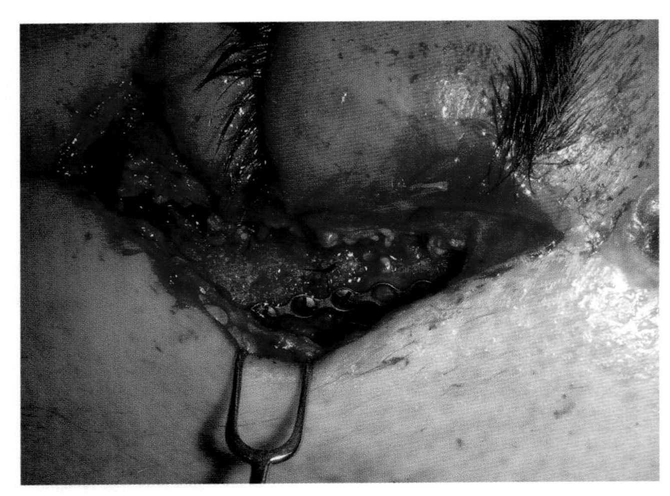

• **Fig. 10.9** Intraoperative view showing completion of the left lateral canthoplasty for reposition of the left lower eyelid.

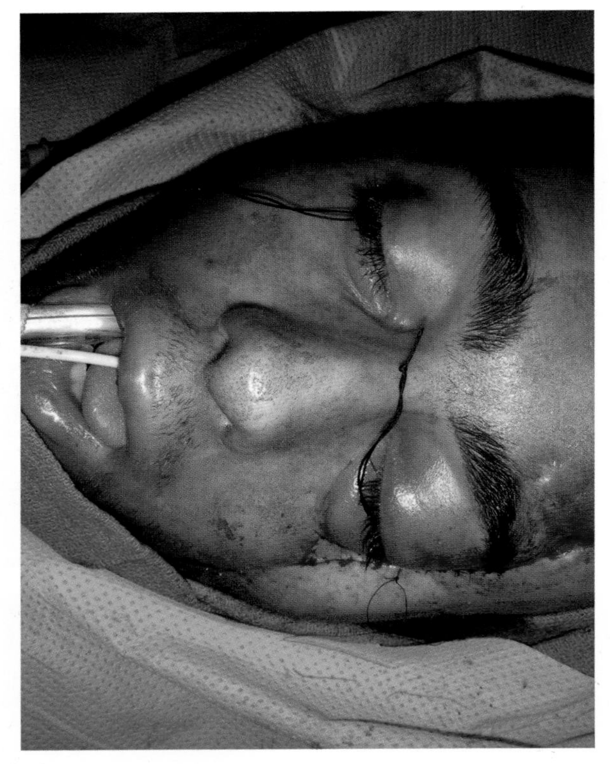

• **Fig. 10.10** Intraoperative view showing completion of the free ALT perforator flap's resuspension.

greatly improved and the graft had near complete take (Figs. 10.25 and 10.26).

Final Outcome

This patient underwent five reconstructive surgical procedures over a 2-year period. He had well-healed soft tissue reconstruction from his free ALT flap and stable bony reconstructions with Medpor implants and titanium reconstruction plates. At follow-up, the

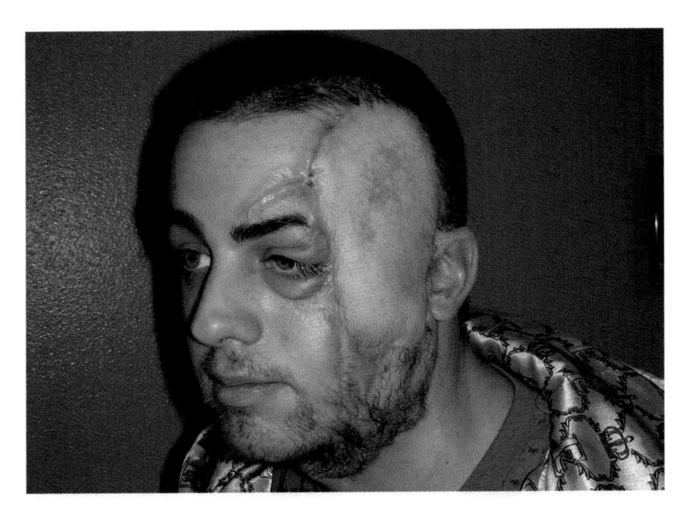

• **Fig. 10.11** The result at 9-week follow-up after the left lateral canthoplasty and the flap's resuspension showing persistent malposition and swelling of the left lower eyelid and facial hypertrophic scar.

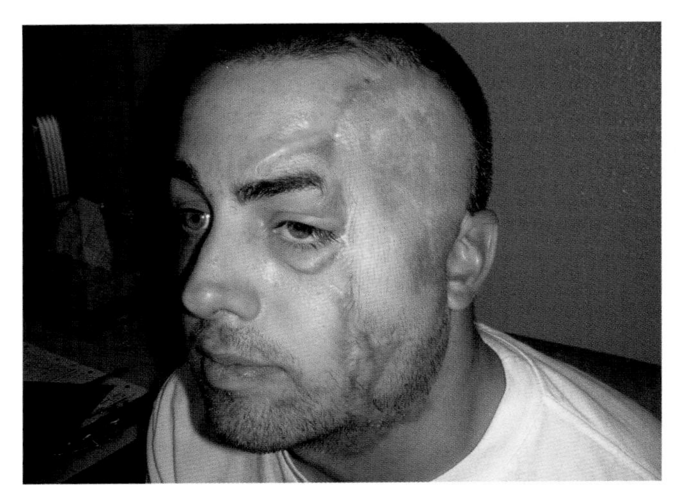

• **Fig. 10.12** The result at 8-month follow-up after the left lateral canthoplasty and the flap's resuspension also showing persistent malposition and swelling of the left lower eyelid and facial hypertrophic scar.

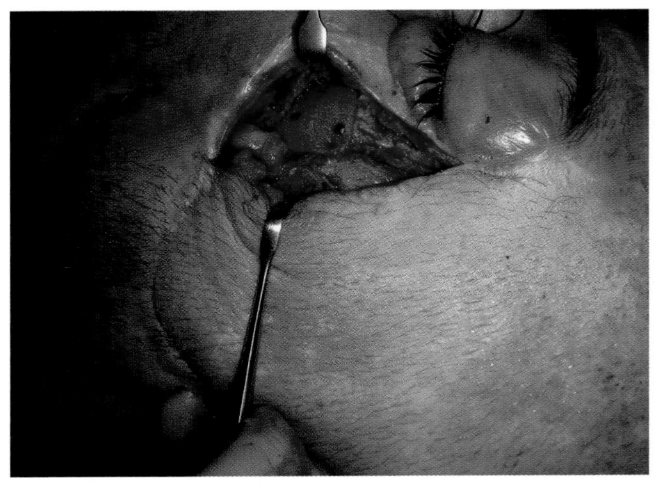

• **Fig. 10.13** Intraoperative view showing placement of a Medpor implant for the midfacial augmentation. In this way, the malposition of the patient's left lower eyelid might be improved.

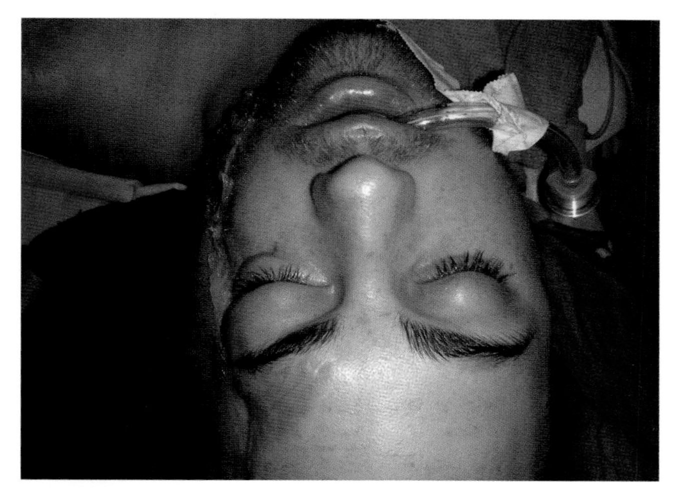

• **Fig. 10.14** Intraoperative view showing completion of the repeat left lateral canthoplasty, debulking of the ALT flap, left midface suspension, and cheek augmentation using Medpor implant.

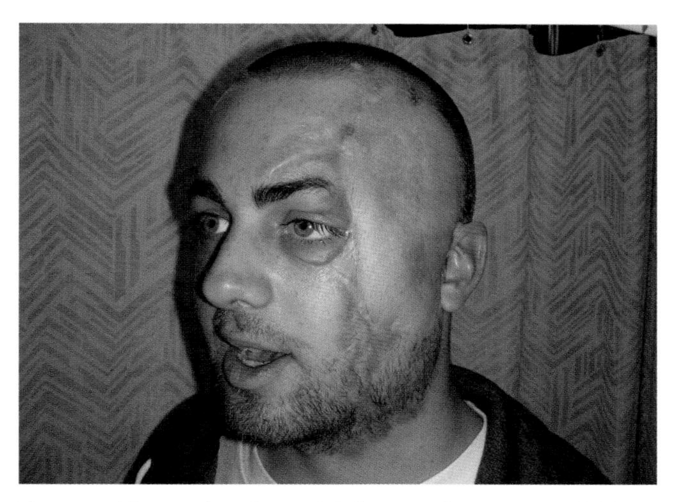

• **Fig. 10.15** The result at 4-month follow-up after the repeat left lateral canthoplasty, debulking of the ALT flap, left midface suspension, and cheek augmentation showing improved left eyelid position, swelling, and hypertrophic facial scar.

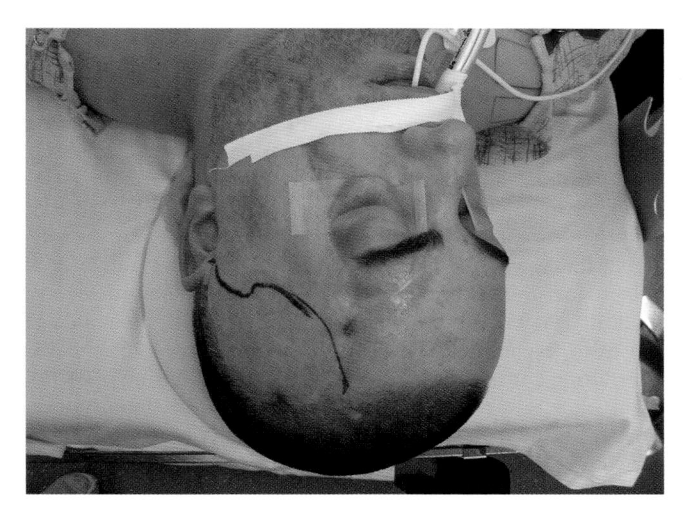

• **Fig. 10.16** Preoperative view showing the proposed hairline in the temporoparietal region.

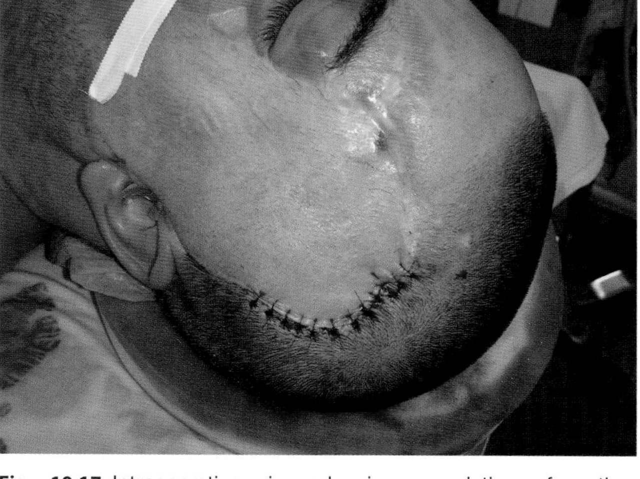

• **Fig. 10.17** Intraoperative view showing completion of a tissue expander placement.

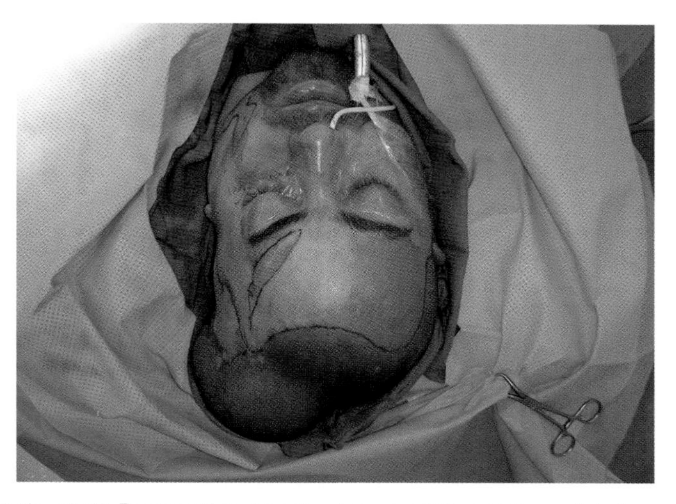

• **Fig. 10.18** Preoperative view showing completion of the scalp's tissue expansion in the temporoparietal region.

patient's only complaint was some edema in the lower eyelid area, which may represent persistent lymphedema, although at this point he did not want to undergo any other procedures and was satisfied with his cosmetic outcome after such extensive and complex injuries.

Although the skin color match of the ALT flap may continue improving, the persistent swelling in his lower eyelid region remains. He also has persistent scleral show and facial nerve paralysis on the injured side, but he has no major functional issues such as dry eye symptoms. At this point, the patient declines any further major reconstructive procedures such as facial nerve reconstruction. He has near normal-looking appearance and facial contour (Figs. 10.27 and 10.28). He has resumed his normal life and has been followed by the plastic surgery service as needed.

Pearls for Success

The complex facial trauma presented in this case poses a reconstructive challenge for plastic surgeons. Multiple contemporary reconstructive surgical techniques can be used to give the patient

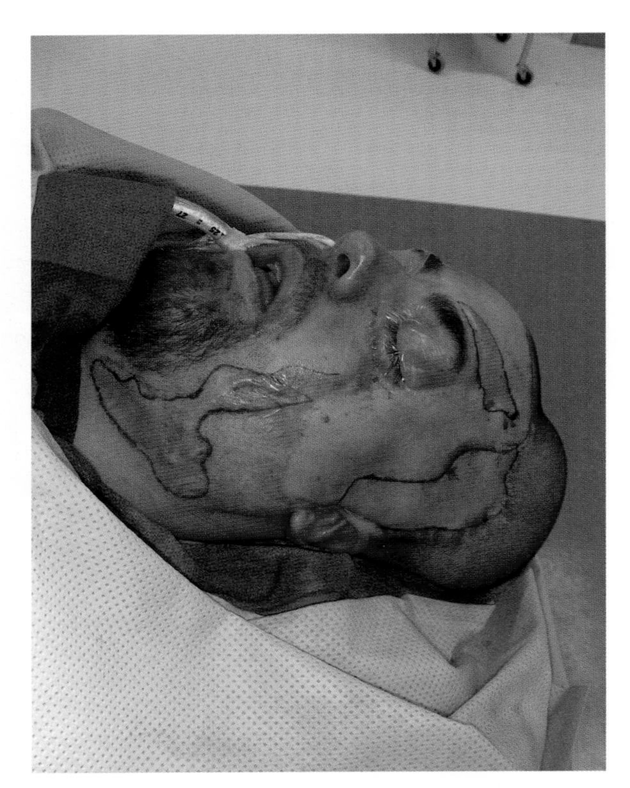

• **Fig. 10.19** Preoperative lateral view showing completion of the scalp's tissue expansion in the temporoparietal region.

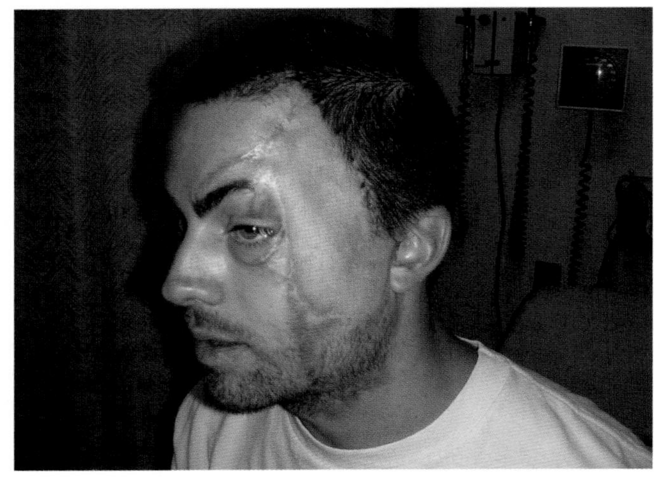

• **Fig. 10.20** The result at 3-week follow-up after the scalp's hairline reconstruction in the temporoparietal region.

an optimal outcome following extensive facial trauma. Medpor implants are composed of porous high-density polyethylene. When implanted in the face, they are stable and resistant to degradation. The advantages include ease of contouring and handling, resistance to infection, and incorporation into the host tissue via vascular ingrowth. Multiple recent studies, however, have shown similar functional outcomes when comparing Medpor implant reconstruction with bone graft, with the advantage of avoiding donor-site morbidity and shorter operating time.

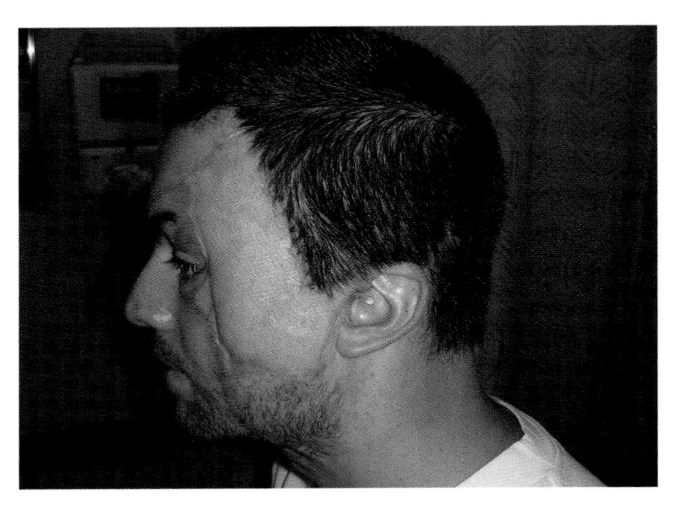

• **Fig. 10.21** The result at 3-week follow-up after the scalp's hairline reconstruction in the temporoparietal region.

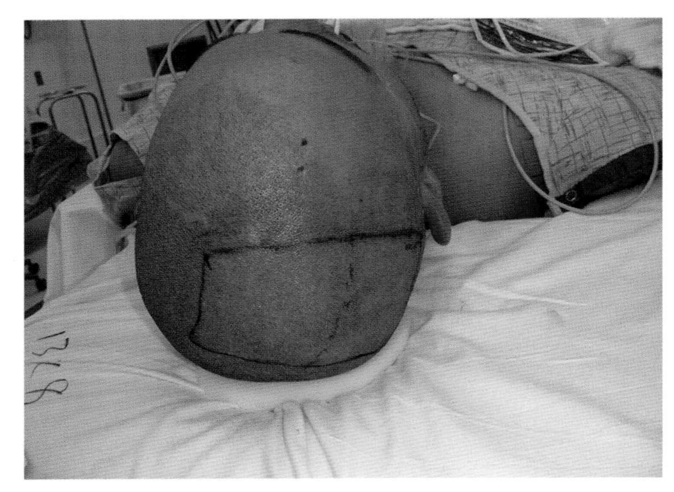

• **Fig. 10.22** Preoperative view showing the donor site of epidermal skin graft in the normal scalp.

The free ALT perforator flap has a large pedicle length, minimal donor-site morbidity, large and reliable skin paddle, customization of flap size to fulfill soft tissue reconstruction of the facial soft tissue defect. The flap is amenable to thinning, either at the initial operation or at a later stage. A tissue expander can be used for the reconstruction of hair-bearing scalp and epidermal grafting can be used to improve the color match after a facial fasciocutaneous flap reconstruction.

Numerous contemporary reconstructive techniques, including a free ALT perforator flap for soft tissue coverage and Medpor implant for initial midface reconstruction, followed by flap debulking, lateral canthoplasty, midface augmentation and lift, scalp tissue expansion for hairline reconstruction, and epidermal skin grafting for optimal skin color matching, can be used for a patient after severe facial trauma associated with significant soft tissue and bony loss. Good cosmetic and functional outcome can be achieved with our approach, but multiple staged reconstructions are often necessary to yield the best possible reconstructive outcome.

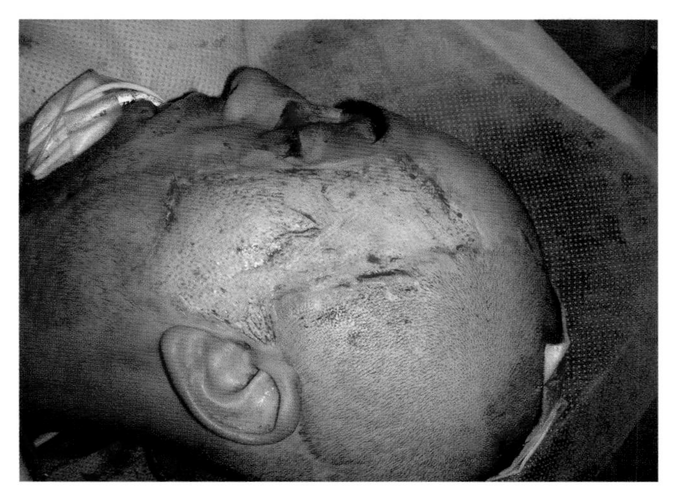

• **Fig. 10.23** Intraoperative view showing completion of the de-epithelized ALT flap.

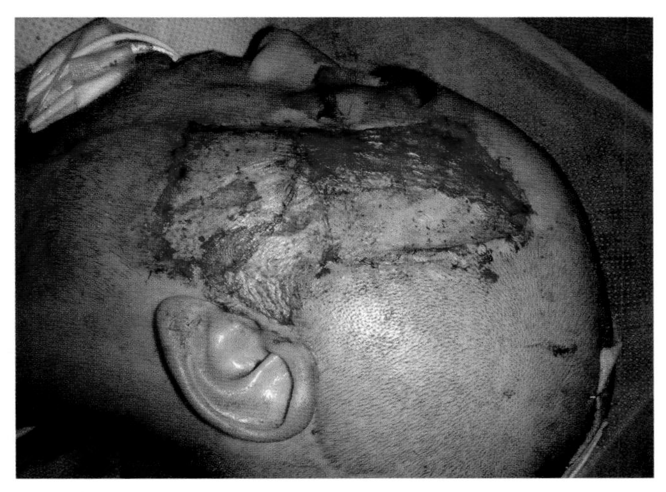

• **Fig. 10.24** Intraoperative view showing placement of epidermal skin grafts to the de-epithelized ALT flap.

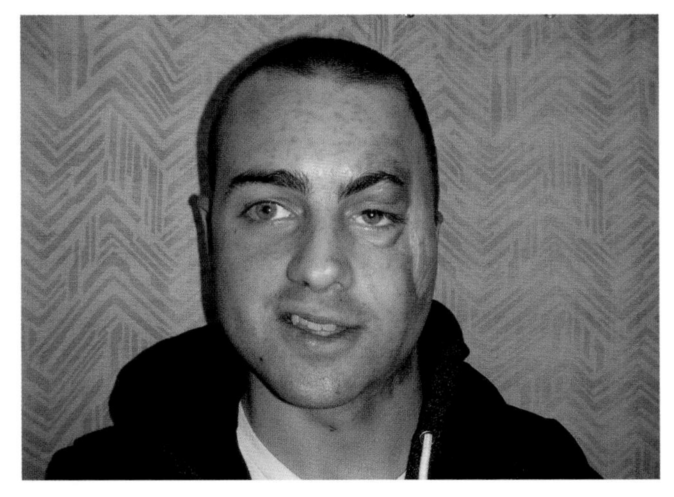

• **Fig. 10.25** The result at 6-month follow-up after placement of epidermal skin grafts to the de-epithelized ALT flap (anterior view).

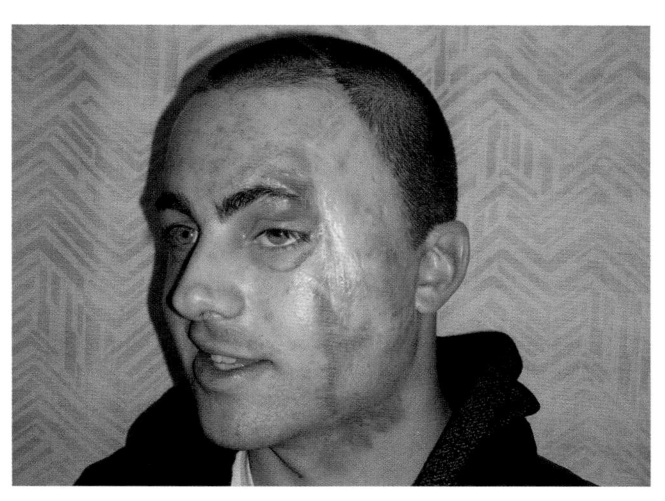

• **Fig. 10.26** The result at 6-month follow-up after placement of epidermal skin grafts to the de-epithelized ALT flap (oblique view). Good colour match was seen.

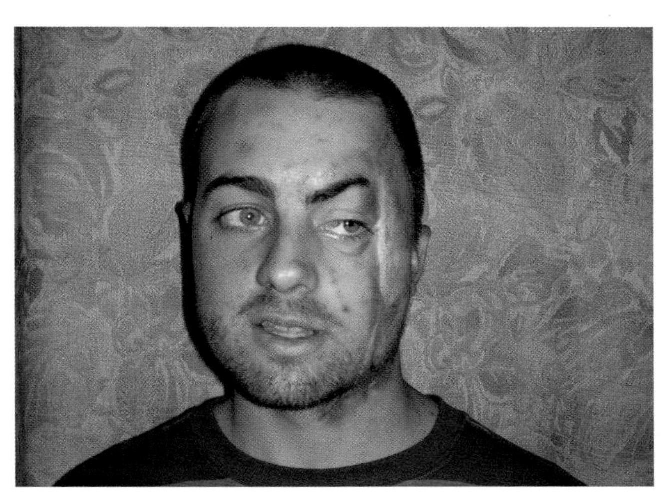

• **Fig. 10.27** The final result at 2-year follow-up after initial reconstruction showing good and acceptable reconstructive outcome (anterior view).

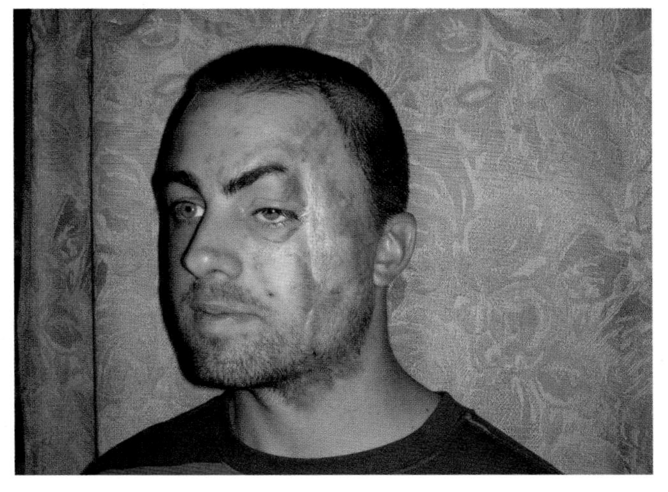

• **Fig. 10.28** The final result at 2-year follow-up after initial reconstruction showing good and acceptable reconstructive outcome (oblique view). No facial nerve reconstruction was performed for this patient.

CASE 2

Clinical Presentation

A 56-year-old White male sustained a self-inflicted gunshot wound to his left face. He had extensive left facial soft tissue wounds and comminuted fractures of the left zygoma and mandible. An on-call plastic surgeon carried out debridement of the facial soft tissue wounds, placement of multiple external fixators for the comminuted mandibular fractures, and repair of soft tissue wounds (Figs. 10.29 and 10.30). The patient's care was transferred to the author for more definitive reconstruction of facial soft tissue wounds including an intraoral soft tissue defect and bony fixations for comminuted fractures of the left zygoma and mandible.

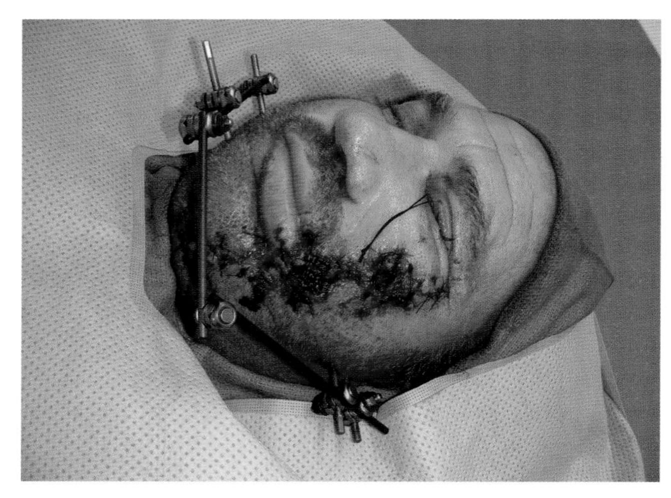

• **Fig. 10.30** Preoperative lateral view showing facial gunshot wounds after initial wound debridement and repair and placement of external fixators for temporary stabilization of comminuted mandibular fractures.

Operative Plan and Special Considerations

The first goal for this patient with extensive comminuted fractures of the zygoma and mandible would be to perform open reduction and internal fixation of those fractures with titanium plates after a wide exposure. This could be accomplished by reopening all previous facial repairs and extending incisions as needed. After good and adequate bony fixation of all facial fractures, the facial soft tissue wound could be reclosed more accurately. The intraoral soft tissue defect was less than 5 cm wide and could be closed with a pedicled supraclavicular island flap from the same side. The flap could be designed so that it would be tunneled into the mouth to cover the exposed reconstruction plate and mandibular fracture sites. The patient was informed of possible future procedures including a flap debulking procedure or osteointegrated dental implants and the expected outcomes with conventional reconstructive procedures.

Operative Procedures

This patient's definitive reconstruction was performed in two stages. During the first stage, under general anesthesia, all the facial fractures on the left side of the patient's face were exposed through the gunshot wounds. His comminuted zygomatic fractures were reduced and fixed with multiple titanium miniplates. The orbital floor fracture was repaired with an ultrathin Medpor implant (Fig. 10.31). His comminuted mandibular fracture was reduced and fixed with a large reconstruction plate and several small miniplates (Fig. 10.32). All external fixators were removed and facial soft tissue wounds were repaired. His nasal fractures were also reduced and splinted. A maxillomandibular fixation was placed. After the first-stage reconstruction, all the facial fractures were properly reduced and fixed. The patient's facial skeleton was restored (Fig. 10.33). In addition, all his facial soft tissue wounds were accurately repaired.

The second-stage procedure was performed 10 days later for intraoral soft tissue reconstruction. Under general anesthesia, the left supraclavicular artery island flap was designed based on the Doppler mapping. The pedicle was mapped with Doppler and a 23 × 5 cm flap was designed from the area above the clavicle to

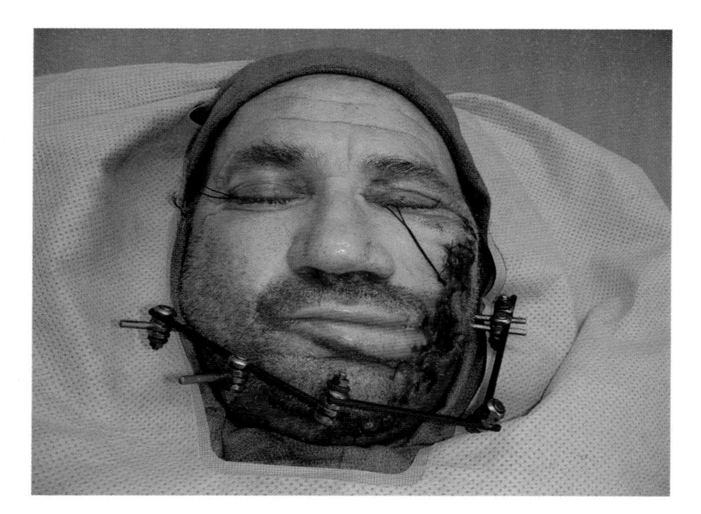

• **Fig. 10.29** Preoperative anterior view showing facial gunshot wounds after initial wound debridement and repair and placement of external fixators for temporary stabilization of comminuted mandibular fractures.

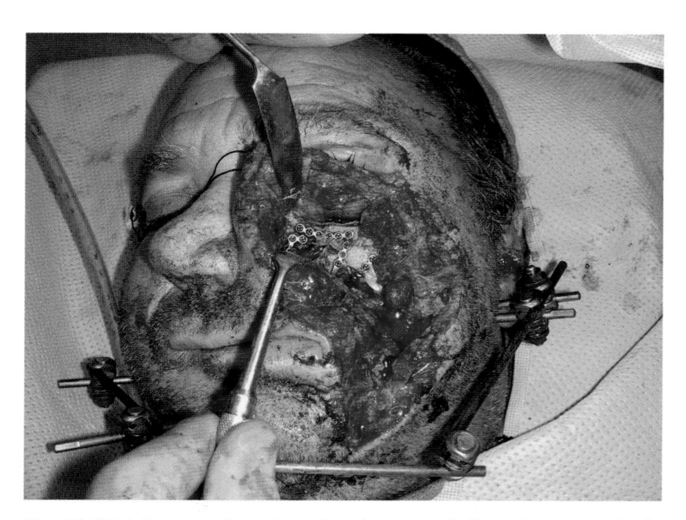

• **Fig. 10.31** Intraoperative view showing completion of open reduction and internal fixation for comminuted zygomatic fractures with multiple miniplates and placement of a Medpor implant for orbital floor fracture.

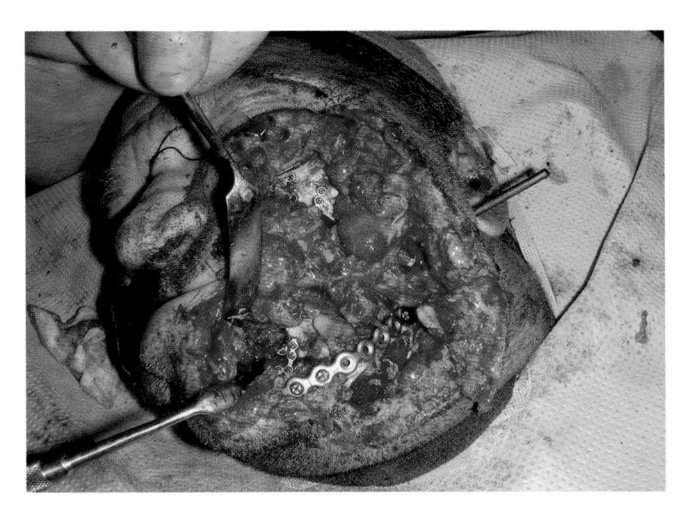

• **Fig. 10.32** Intraoperative view showing completion of open reduction and internal fixation for comminuted mandibular fractures with a large reconstruction plate and miniplates.

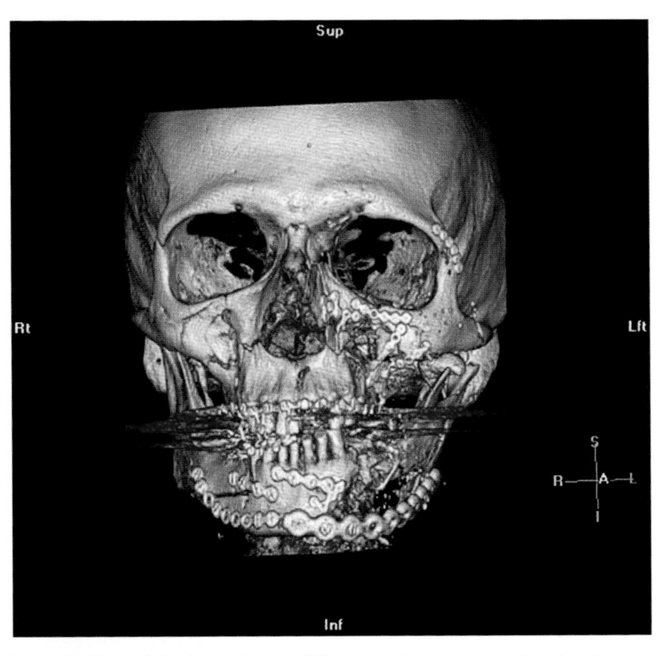

• **Fig. 10.33** A 3-D facial bone CT scan showing good reduction and fixation of comminuted zygomatic and mandibular fractures.

the midpoint of the deltoid. A triangular design was used to extend the tip of the flap more distally so that a dog-ear closure could be avoided (Fig. 10.34). The intraoral soft tissue defect measured 10 × 4 cm, therefore the width of the designed flap would cover the entire intraoral soft tissue wound.

The flap elevation was performed from more distally to the fascia under direct vision to proximal in a subfascial plane. After the flap's pedicle had been identified, additional dissection was performed to raise the flap, including the pedicle (Fig. 10.35). Additional dissection was done around the pedicle and some muscle attachments were divided. The distal skin was also incised so that the flap became an island flap (Fig. 10.36). The previous maxillomandibular fixation was released and a proxoimal portion

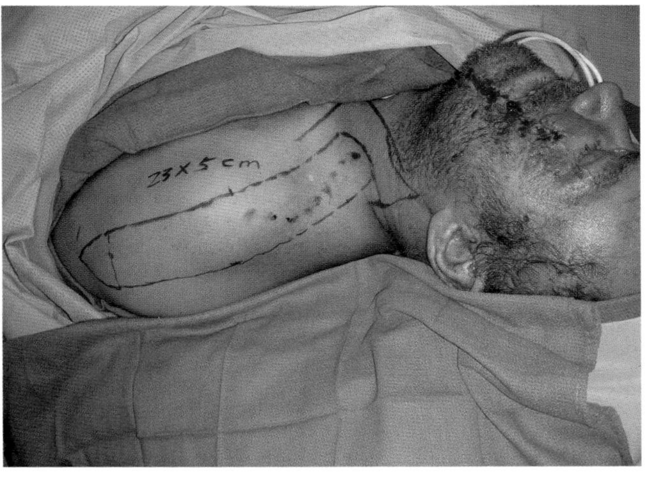

• **Fig. 10.34** Intraoperative view showing the design of the left supraclavicular artery island flap.

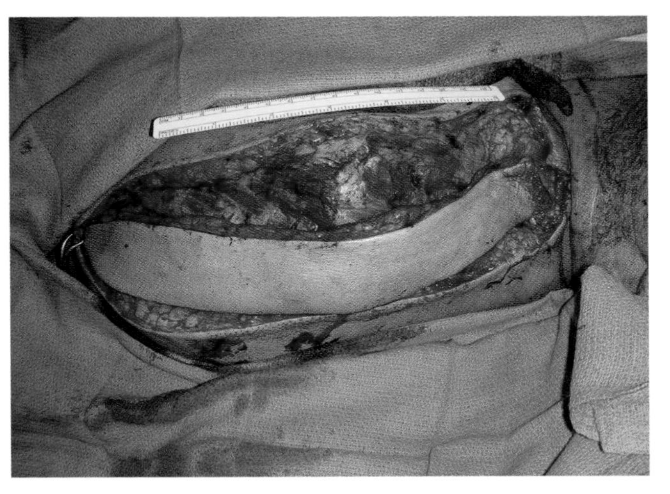

• **Fig. 10.35** Intraoperative view showing the extent of the left supraclavicular artery island flap dissection.

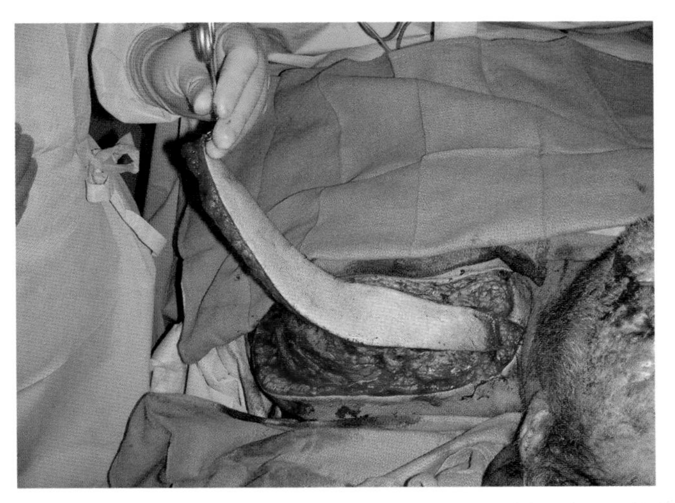

• **Fig. 10.36** Intraoperative view showing completion of the elevated left supraclavicular artery island flap.

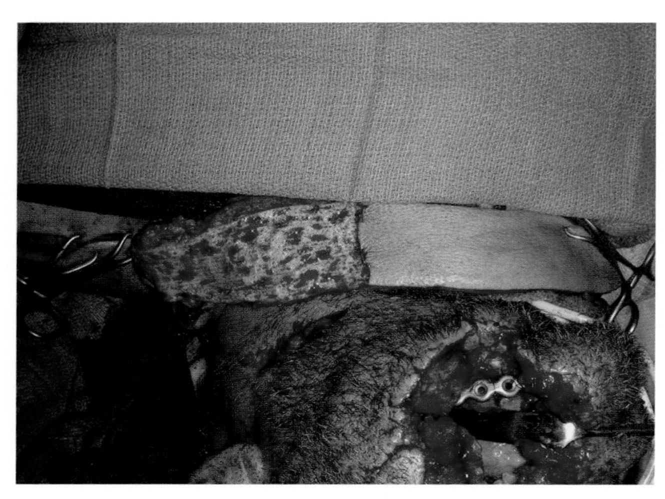

• **Fig. 10.37** Intraoperative view showing the de-epithelized portion of the left supraclavicular artery island flap that will be tunneled under the neck skin.

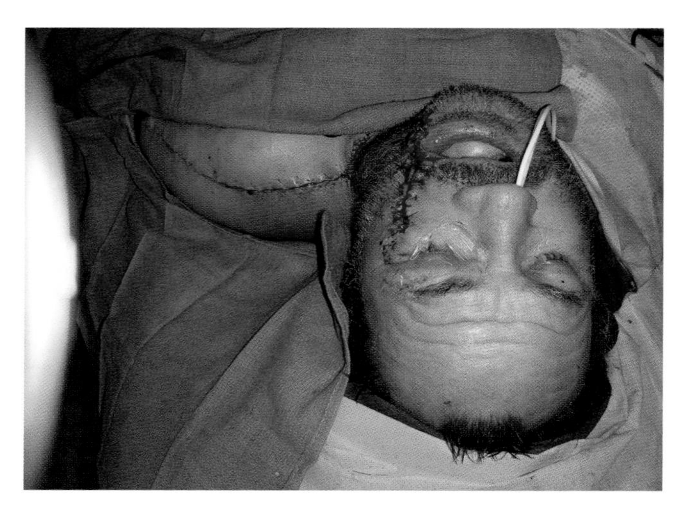

• **Fig. 10.39** Intraoperative view showing completion of the left supraclavicular artery island flap reconstruction after the donor site direct closure and facial wound repairs.

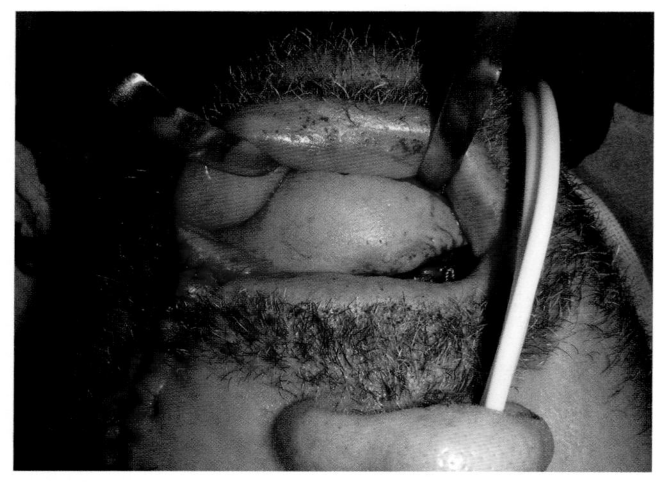

• **Fig. 10.38** Intraoperative view showing completion of the left supraclavicular artery island flap intraoral inset.

of the facial wound was reopened for better intraoral exposure. The tunneling of the neck was performed in a subcutaneous layer. The flap was then tunneled through and placed intraorally. The area of de-epithelialization of the flap was determined and completed (Fig. 10.37). The flap was then placed intraorally (Fig. 10.38). The flap's skin paddle was approximated to the adjacent intraoral tissue with 3-0 half-buried horizontal mattress sutures for watertight closure. All exposed reconstruction plates and mandibular fracture sites were completely covered with the flap. The left shoulder flap donor site was closed in two layers after significant undermining and the rest of the facial wound was reclosed in two layers (Fig. 10.39).

Follow-Up Results

The patient did well postoperatively without any complications related to the facial fracture repairs and intraoral supraclavicular flap reconstruction. He was discharged from the hospital 2 weeks following his initial injuries. His facial gunshot wounds, fractures, and intraoral flap reconstruction site healed well.

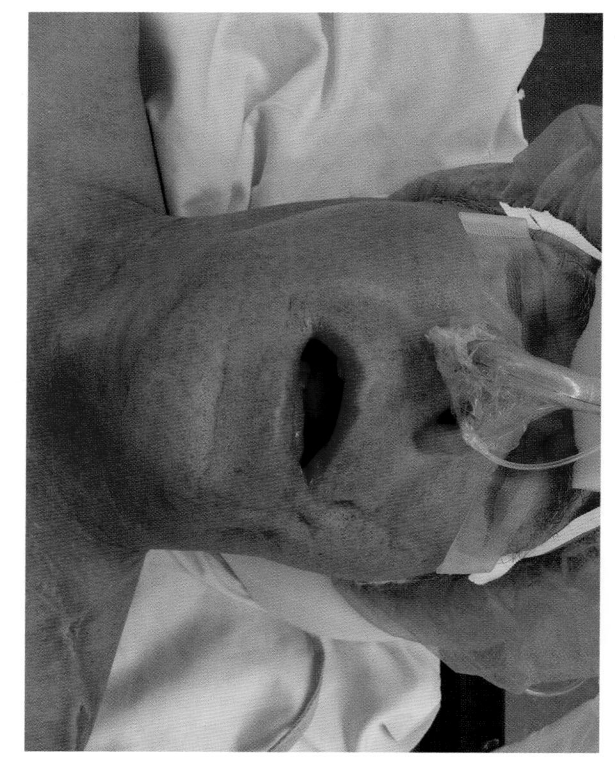

• **Fig. 10.40** Results at 5-month follow-up after multiple facial fracture repairs and the flap intraoral reconstruction.

Unfortunately, his intraoral flap site remained bulky after 5 months postoperatively and a flap debulking procedure was performed to reduce the size of his intraoral flap (Figs. 10.40 and 10.41). The flap debulking procedure involved a direct excision of the excess flap tissue (Figs. 10.42 and 10.43), which improved the flap contour (Figs. 10.44 and 10.45). The patient underwent additional debulking procedure via a direct excision of the excess flap tissue 2.5 years after the first debulking procedure for further contour improvement over the reconstructed plate and mandibular fracture sites intraorally (Figs. 10.46 and 10.47).

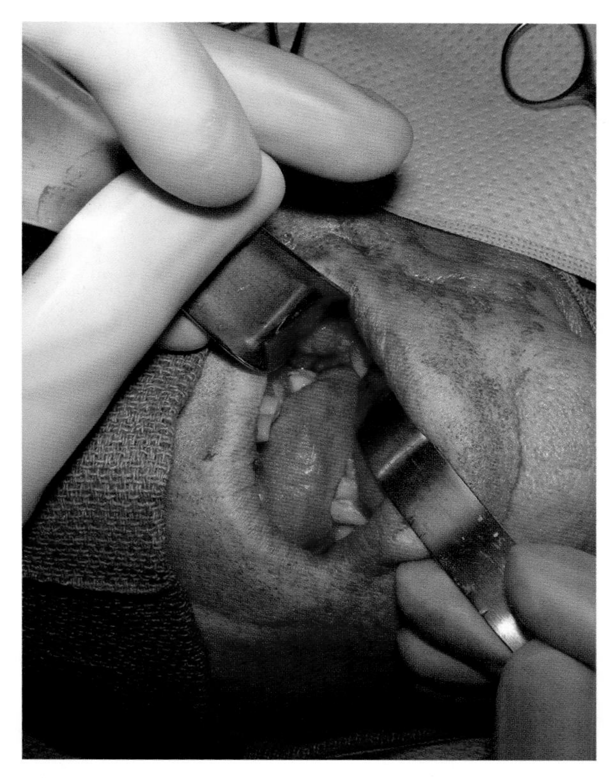

• **Fig. 10.41** Close up view showing the intraoral flap reconstruction at 5-month follow-up.

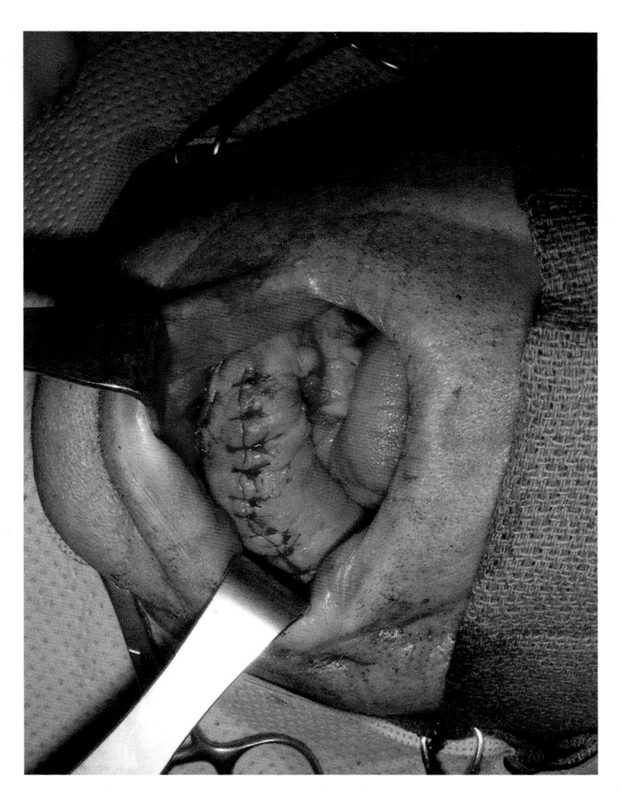

• **Fig. 10.42** Intraoperative view showing completion of the flap debulking of the left supraclavicular artery island flap reconstruction.

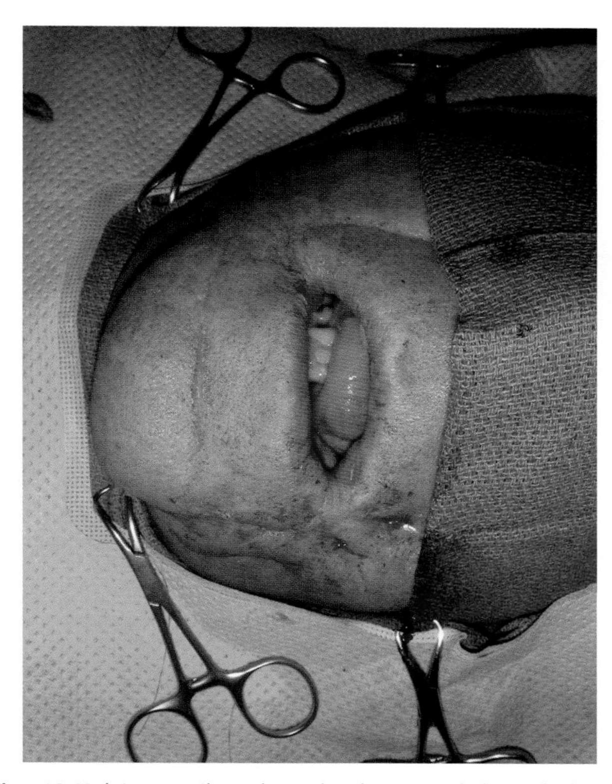

• **Fig. 10.43** Intraoperative view showing completion of the flap debulking of the left supraclavicular artery island flap reconstruction.

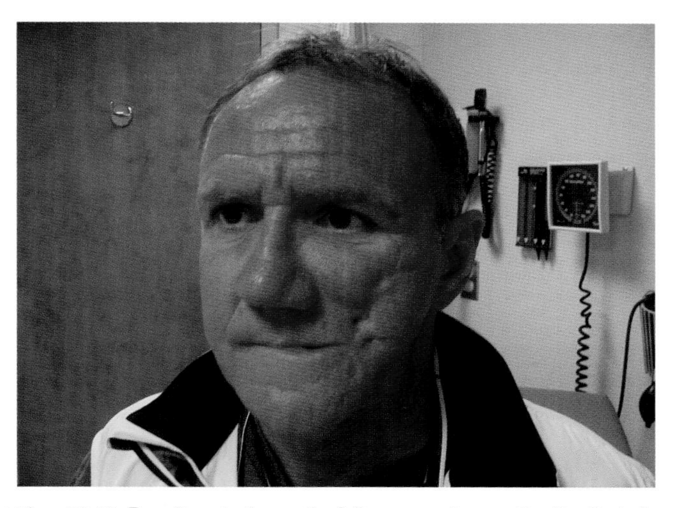

• **Fig. 10.44** Results at 4-month follow-up after patient's first flap debulking procedure of the left supraclavicular artery island flap reconstruction.

Final Outcome

The patient continued doing well. He had well-healed facial fracture sites and soft tissue wounds. Intraorally, he also had a well-healed supraclavicular flap over the mandible after two debulking procedures with an excellent contour. He has refused additional procedures such as fat grafting to improve the facial contour and osteointegrated dental implants (Figs. 10.48 and 10.49). He has returned to his normal life and has been followed as needed.

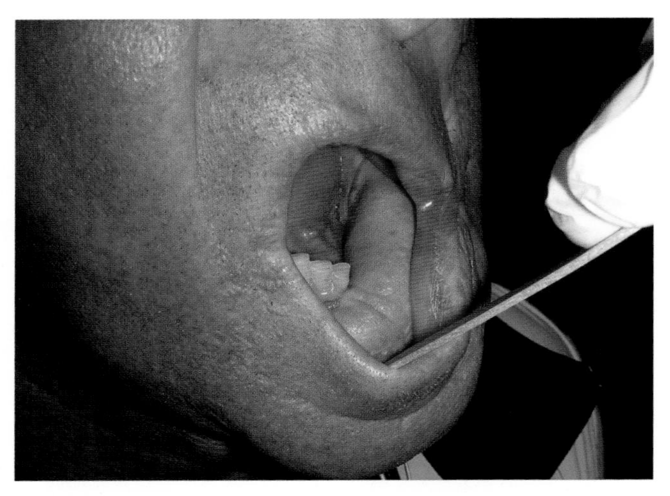

• **Fig. 10.45** Close up view at 4-month follow-up after first flap debulking procedure of the left supraclavicular artery island flap reconstruction site.

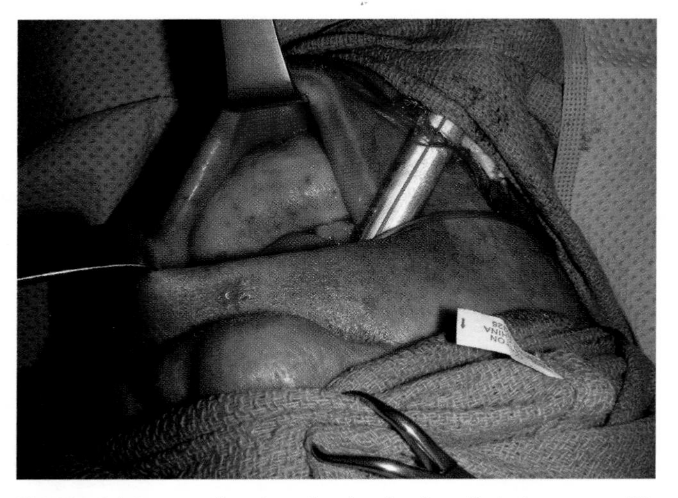

• **Fig. 10.46** Intraoperative view showing the flap site before second flap debulking procedure of the left supraclavicular artery island flap reconstruction.

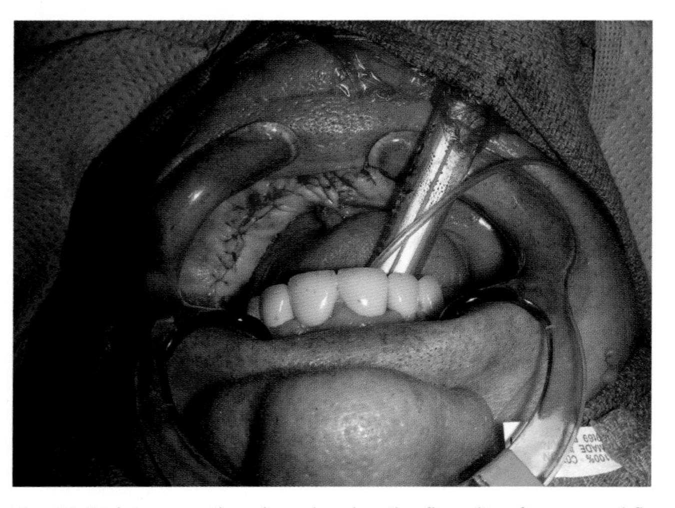

• **Fig. 10.47** Intraoperative view showing the flap site after second flap debulking procedure of the left supraclavicular artery island flap reconstruction.

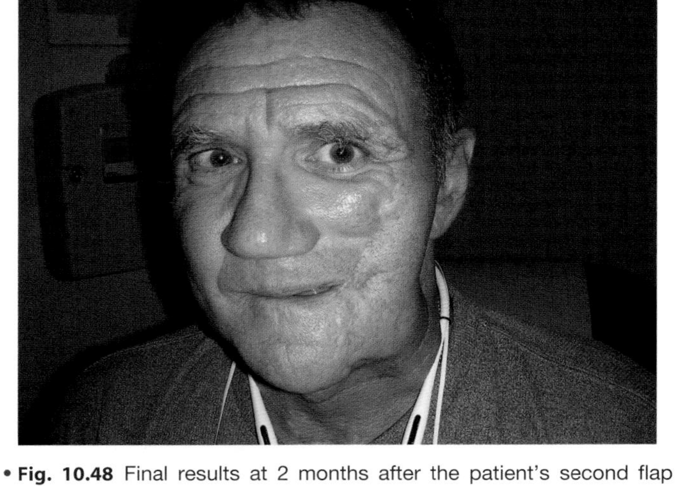

• **Fig. 10.48** Final results at 2 months after the patient's second flap debulking procedures and 2.5 years after his first flap debulking procedure. His face looks nearly normal.

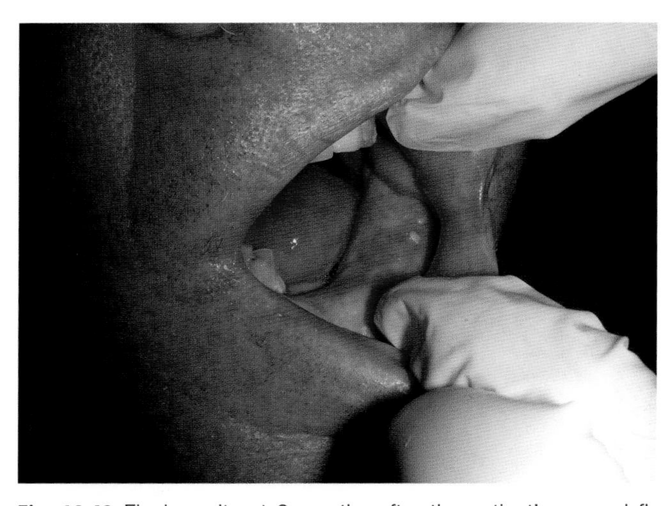

• **Fig. 10.49** Final results at 2 months after the patient's second flap debulking procedures and 2.5 years after his first flap debulking procedure with thin but adequate soft tissue coverage intraorally.

Pearls for Success

Complex facial trauma following gunshot wounds requires more extensive and complex repair and reconstruction. Comminuted facial fractures can be managed with multiple miniplates for reduction and fixation and a large reconstruction plate can be used for mandibular fracture. Wide exposure is often needed for better anatomic bony reduction and fixation. Soft tissue reconstruction is often required and a supraclavicular artery island flap can be an excellent choice for coverage of a relatively small intraoral wound. During the flap elevation, the pedicle of the flap should be identified and included in the flap dissection. For most patients, the flap can be extended into the deltoid area. A 5-cm donor site wound can be closed primarily after extensive undermining. When the flap is tunneled under the neck and facial skin into the oral cavity, care should be taken not to twist or compress the pedicle of the flap. If the flap remains bulky intraorally, flap debulk can be safely performed by direct excision of the excess flap tissue.

CASE 3

Clinical Presentation

A 24-year-old White male sustained a self-inflicted ballistic gunshot wound to his face. He was quickly transferred to our hospital, a level one trauma center in the area, for life support and definitive care. On initial examination, he apparently had significant composite injuries to his upper, middle, and lower face with extensive soft tissue wounds and multiple comminuted fractures (Figs. 10.50 and 10.51). The trauma service performed an emergency tracheotomy to secure his airway and the plastic surgery service then performed initial wound debridement, facial fracture stabilizations, and soft tissue repair. The trauma service also inserted a gastric feeding tube. The patient was stabilized after these urgent surgical procedures and supportive medical care.

His reconstructive surgical care was transferred to the author. Five days later, the patient was brought to the operating room for examination under general anesthesia. During this procedure, the detailed composite tissue defects were assessed and recorded. From the reconstructive surgery point of view, the composite tissue deficits included a significant soft tissue loss in the central portion of the mid and lower face, with a 7-cm maxillary defect and a 4-cm mandibular defect. He also lost anterior palate, right orbital rim, anterior nasal spine and septum, the entire ethmoid, and 50% of the right upper and lower lip soft tissues including right commissure (Figs. 10.52 and 10.53). Fortunately, his vision was intact on both sides. A 3-D model was made after his initial bony stabilization procedure to show his bony defects and the placement of multiple titanium plates and a reconstruction plate (Fig. 10.54).

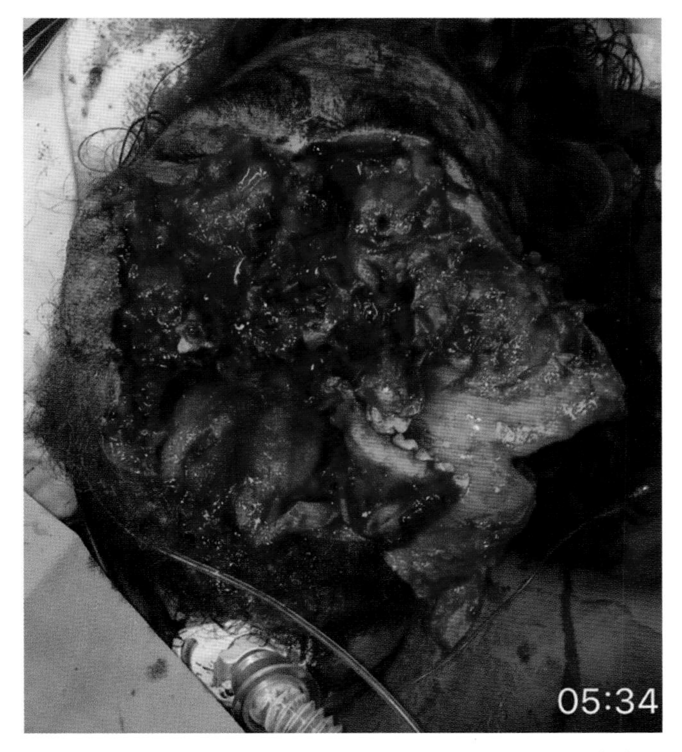

• **Fig. 10.50** Extensive composite facial tissue loss during initial presentation after self-inflicted gunshot wound.

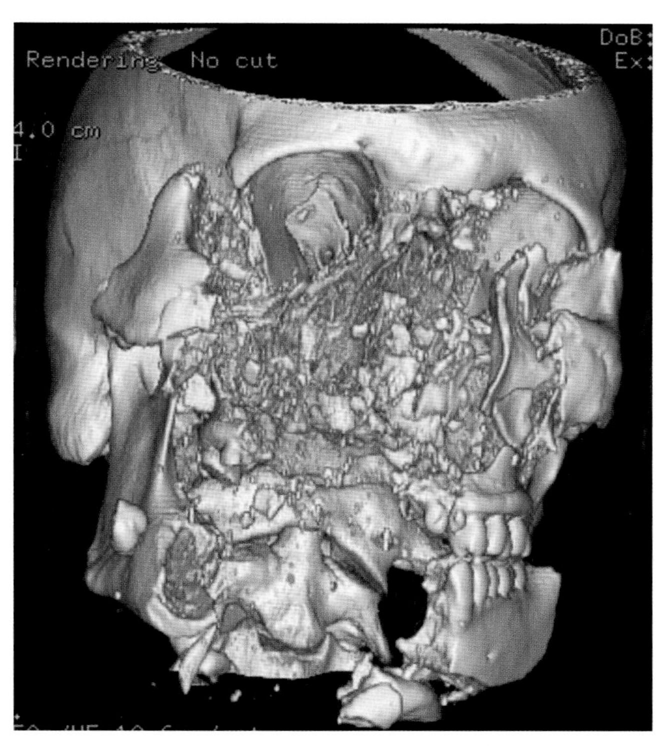

• **Fig. 10.51** Three-dimensional facial bone computed tomography scan image showing comminuted and multiple facial fractures during initial presentation after self-inflicted gunshot wound.

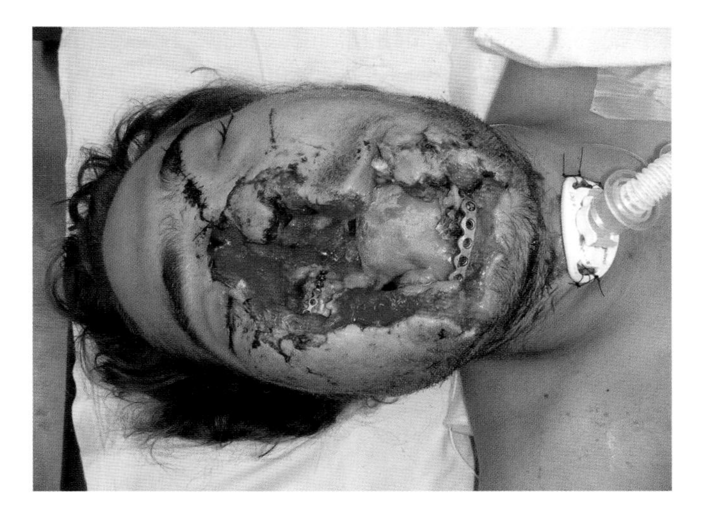

• **Fig. 10.52** Intraoperative view showing the extent of soft tissue defects and facial fractures and bony gaps after initial wound debridement and bony fixations with miniplates and reconstruction plates.

Operative Plan and Special Considerations

The complex and extensive soft tissue injuries and multiple comminuted fractures meant that this was considered an "irreparable" facial injury. This was particularly true because his central face had a significant ballistic injury with associated comminuted fractures of the nasal and palatal bones and ethmoid. The functional and aesthetic goals of reconstruction for this patient were beyond that which can be achieved with contemporary reconstructive techniques, typically requiring many procedures over

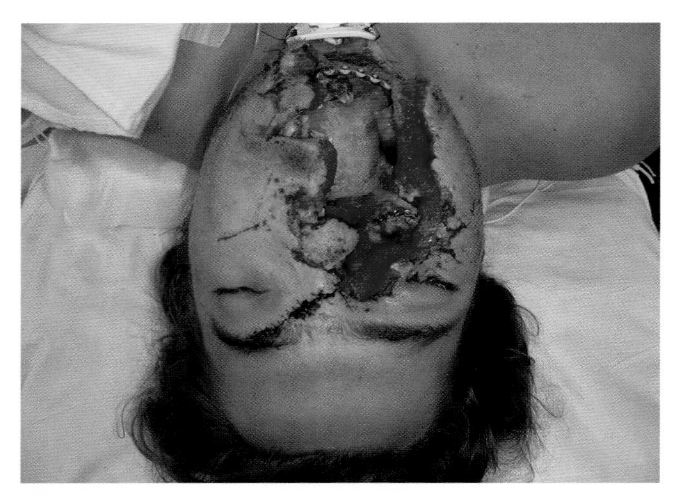

• **Fig. 10.53** Another intraoperative view showing the extent of soft tissue defects and facial fractures and bony gaps after initial wound debridement and bony fixations with miniplates and reconstruction plates.

several years for a suboptimal result. Preparation of the patient with extremely complex facial trauma for future face transplant can be considered when the extent of the injury is beyond conventional reconstructive limits. For this case, the option of a future face transplant was considered and offered to the patient at the beginning of his reconstructive care after his psychological evaluation because of the extent of the ballistic injury. He was determined to be a competent patient who desired to look "normal" after reconstruction to his face. His psychiatric condition was under control with medications and we believed that he could be a reasonably good candidate for a future face transplant. In preparation for a future face transplantation, only skin flaps such as free ALT perforator flap or pedicled supraclavicular artery flap would be selected for soft tissue coverage once "definitive" bony reconstructions are completed with only titanium plates. The goal for his "definitive" bony reconstruction would be to restore this patient's nearly normal facial skeleton in terms of the height, width, and projection. Reliable soft tissue reconstruction was essential so that his facial soft tissue wounds could heal and he could be placed on the face transplant list after being discharged from hospital.

Operative Procedures

Under general anesthesia, the procedure started by debriding the entire middle and lower facial wounds, including some of the fragments of the bone and colonized soft tissue wounds. Pulsavac irrigation was also performed.

The first step of "definitive reconstruction" involved plating the entire panfacial fractures. Both significant displaced fractures of the frontozygomatic suture were explored with the lateral brow incision, manually reduced, and fixed with 1.0-mm miniplates. Both zygomatic fractures were explored, previously placed miniplates were removed, and fractures were manually reduced to maintain his facial width. All these fractures were fixed again with new 1.0-mm miniplates. For the left orbital floor, the medial orbital wall and the left orbital rim were plated with a 1.0-mm miniplate. The right orbital rim was completely destroyed. A 1.0-mm curved miniplate was used to reconstruct the right orbital rim from the lateral orbital rim to extend to the medial portion of the left side of the nasal bone. In this way, both sides of the orbital rim were reconstructed.

The additional midface fracture reduction was performed. The fracture of the maxilla, which had an approximately 7-cm bony gap, was reduced and a 2.0-mm plate was used to stabilize the zygomatic bony defect and to restore the projection. Both sides of the lateral buttress were reconstructed with 2.0-mm miniplates.

The previous mandibular plate was removed. Based on a 3-D dental model, the new reconstruction plate was placed to bridge both sides of the residual mandibles and to restore the reasonably good lower face width. This was performed with a 3.0-mm reconstruction plate. A 2 × 3 cm fragment of the mandible was also placed as a bone graft, secured with a 1.0-mm box miniplate. All facial fractures were reduced, fixed with multiple miniplates, and bridged with stronger reconstruction plates. The patient's original facial height, width, and projection were restored as closely as possible (Fig. 10.55).

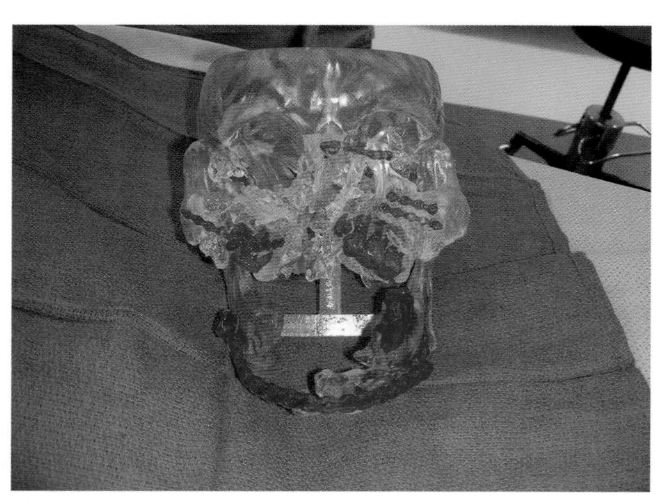

• **Fig. 10.54** A facial 3-D model showing the extensive facial fractures and placed multiple miniplates and a reconstruction plate after initial wound debridement and bony fixations.

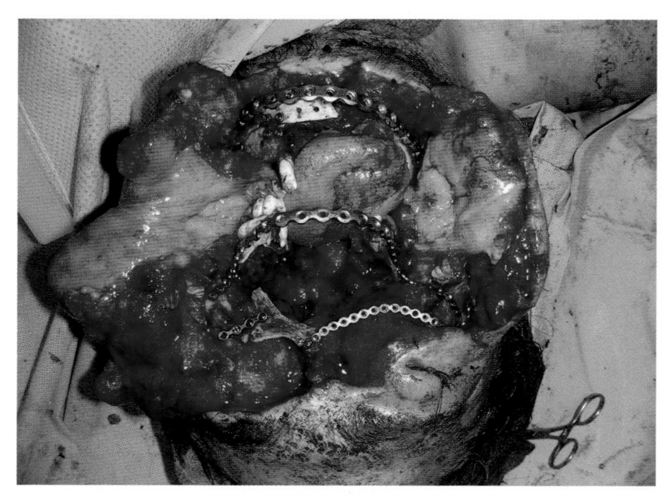

• **Fig. 10.55** Intraoperative view showing completion of redone multiple facial fracture fixations. The infraorbital rims, maxilla, and mandible were restored with miniplates and reconstruction plates.

The second step of "definitive reconstruction" was soft tissue coverage for all open areas and exposed plates or miniplates of the face after facial skeletal reconstructions. A 20 × 8 cm ALT perforator flap was marked on the right thigh, based on duplex scan findings, where there was a better and dominant perforator in the right thigh. The skin paddle was elevated and the fascia was included with the flap.

A perforator dissection was performed. After a brief intramuscular dissection, the perforator dissection was completed. By further dissection following the perforator, the descending branch of the circumflex femoral vessels was exposed. After the distal end was divided, the flap's pedicle dissection was performed following the descending branch of the circumflex femoral vessels retrogradely to reach the profunda vessels. When the pedicle length and the diameter of the pedicle were considered to be satisfactory, the artery and vein were divided with hemoclips (Fig. 10.56).

Under loupe magnification, the artery and vein were prepared with microsurgical instruments. The flap was temporarily inserted into the midface. The proximal portion of the palate wound was closed with the proximal portion of the ALT free flap with interrupted 2-0 Vicryl sutures and the rest of the flap was wrapped around the maxillary plate to keep in the midface so that the dead space could be obliterated. A portion of the flap was de-epithelialized for better approximation with the adjacent tissues. The flap's pedicle was then placed close to the left fascial artery and vein.

The left facial artery and vein were explored and dissected free through a separate incision. They were also prepared under loupe magnification. The microvascular anastomosis was performed under microscope after further preparation of those vessels. For the arterial microvascular anastomosis, an end-to-end anastomosis was performed with 8-0 nylon sutures, in an interrupted fashion. For the venous microvascular anastomosis, a 3.0 coupler device was also used in an end-to-end fashion. The flap appeared to be well perfused with a good Doppler signal within the flap after the release of the clamps (Fig. 10.57).

The design of the left supraclavicular artery flap was marked on the patient's left shoulder. The pedicle was identified with Doppler. The widest portion was 7 cm and the pedicle portion was relatively narrow, about 4 cm. The flap was extended to the proximal one-third of the deltoid region and elevated subfascially

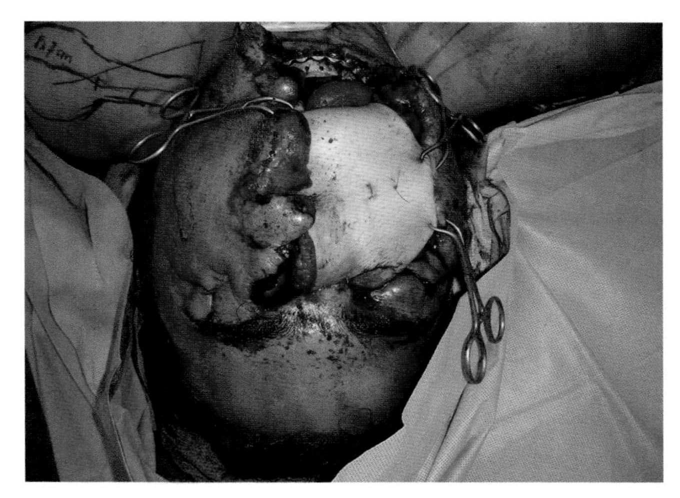

• **Fig. 10.57** Intraoperative views showing completion of preliminary free ALT flap inset to the middle face after microvascular anastomoses.

under direct vision toward the pedicle. A tunnel of the left neck was created under the neck skin. The tunneled portion of the flap was de-epithelialized. The final inset of the flap was performed. The flap was wrapped around the entire exposed mandible and the reconstructed plate. The flap was somewhat short on the right side and a 10 × 6 cm right neck skin flap, including platysma, was therefore elevated and approximated to the distal portion of the supraclavicular flap in two layers (Fig. 10.58).

The final inset of the right free ALT perforator flap was performed. Several areas of the flap were de-epithelialized, and tissue closure was approximated in two layers, where possible. The deep tissue layer was approximated with several interrupted 3-0 Vicryl sutures and the skin was then closed with either 3-0 Monocryl or 4-0 chromic sutures. The remnants of the left nasal skin, left upper lip, and left lower lip were sutured to the ALT flap. Two Penrose drains were inserted, one in the midface and one in the lower face under the mandible (Figs. 10.59 and 10.60).

The left supraclavicular island flap donor site was closed in two layers after significant undermining. For the most part, it was approximated with 3-0 Monocryl suture in simple interrupted

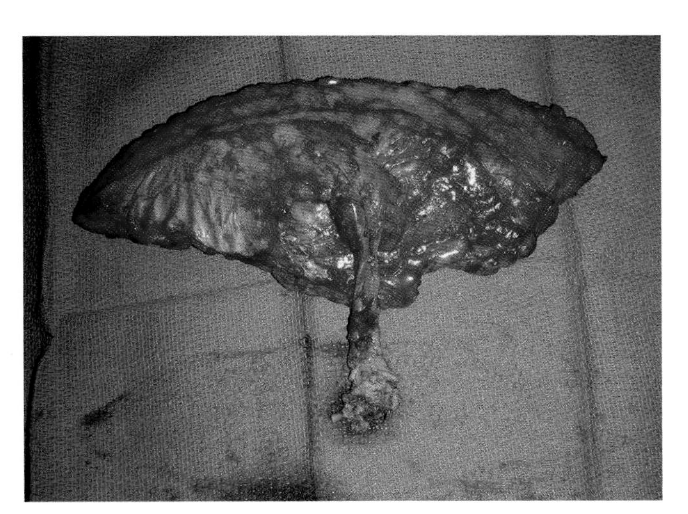

• **Fig. 10.56** Intraoperative view showing completion of the right free ALT perforator flap dissection.

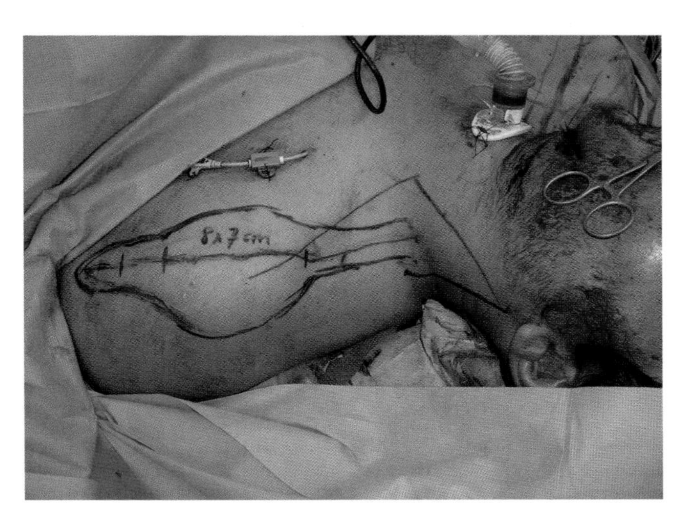

• **Fig. 10.58** Intraoperative view showing the design of the left supraclavicular artery flap.

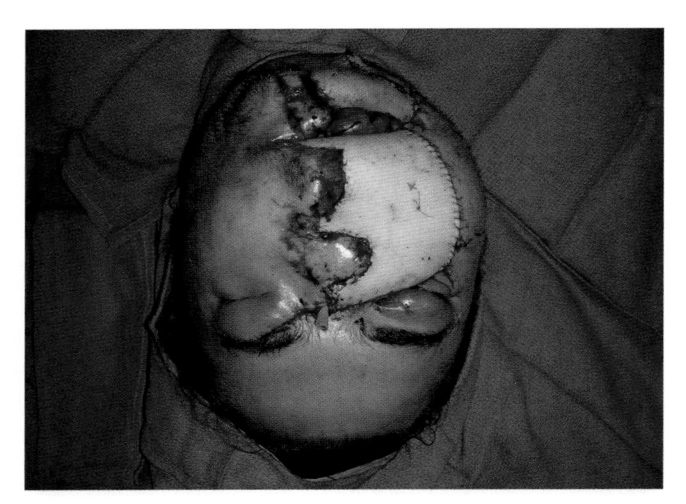

• **Fig. 10.59** Intraoperative view showing completion of both free ALT flap and left supraclavicular artery flap inset. All facial fracture wounds and miniplates or reconstruction plates were covered with these flaps.

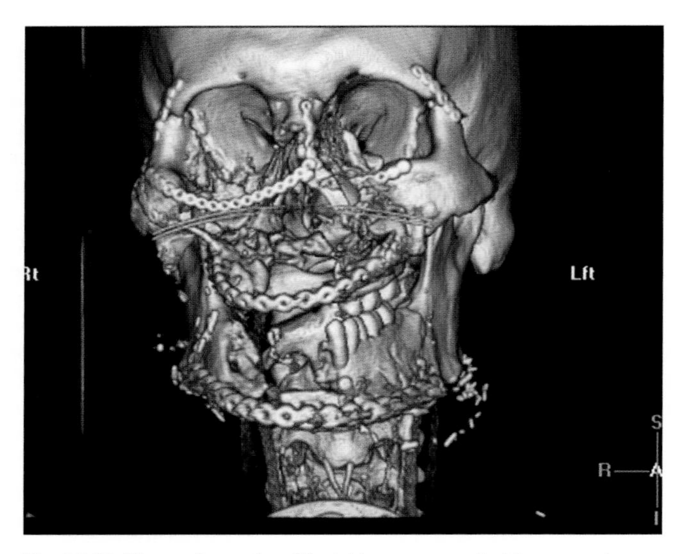

• **Fig. 10.60** Three-dimensional facial bone computed tomography scan image showing open reduction and internal fixation of multiple comminuted facial fractures after "definitive" restoration of the facial skeletal structures.

fashion, followed by 4- 0 Monocryl suture in a running subcuticular fashion. An 8 × 12 cm area was covered with a sheet split-thickness skin graft harvested from the right thigh. The right thigh ALT flap donor site was closed in three layers. The fascial layer closure was approximated with several interrupted 2-0 PDS sutures in simple interrupted fashion. The deep dermal closure was performed with several interrupted 3-0 Monocryl sutures in interrupted fashion. The skin was closed with 3-0 V-Loc suture in a running subcuticular fashion.

Management of Complications

The patient did well postoperatively without general complications related to the airway, pulmonary system, and infections. He had adequate supportive care from our surgical critical care service.

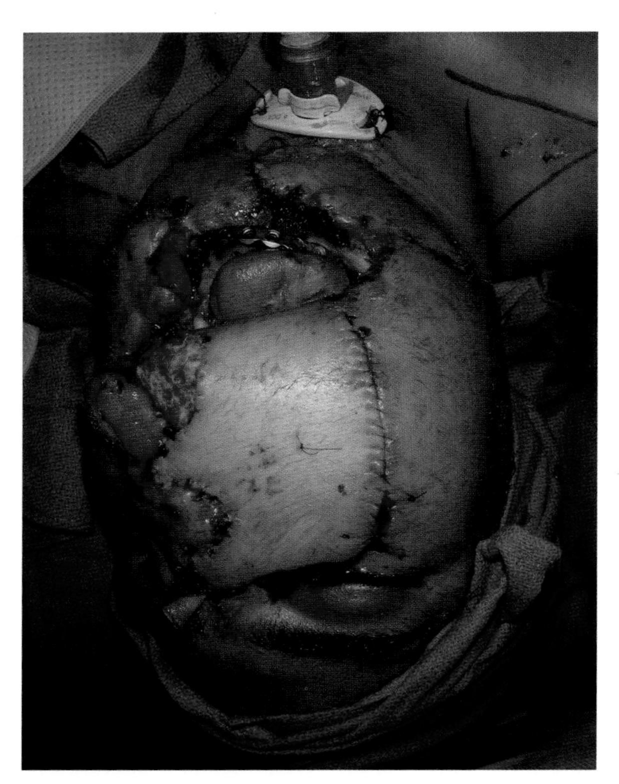

• **Fig. 10.61** Intraoperative view showing the lower face soft tissue defect with the exposed mandibular reconstruction plate after debridement of necrotic left supraclavicular artery flap.

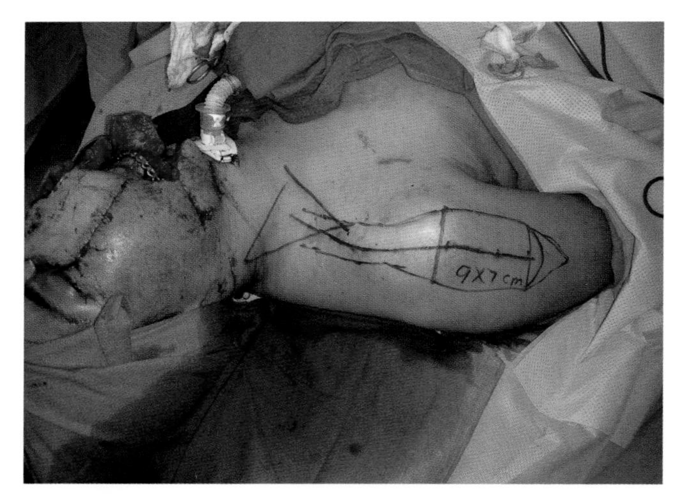

• **Fig. 10.62** Intraoperative view showing the design of the right supraclavicular artery flap.

Unfortunately, he developed a flap dehiscence of the supraclavicular artery flap as a result of distal flap necrosis and there was exposure of the mandibular reconstructive plate (Fig. 10.61). He was taken back to the operating room 8 days later for wound debridement and additional flap reconstruction. During this time, a second supraclavicular artery flap from his right shoulder was harvested and transferred to cover the exposed mandibular reconstruction plate (Fig. 10.62). The flap was directly placed and not tunneled this time to avoid any possible direct compression to the flap (Fig. 10.63).

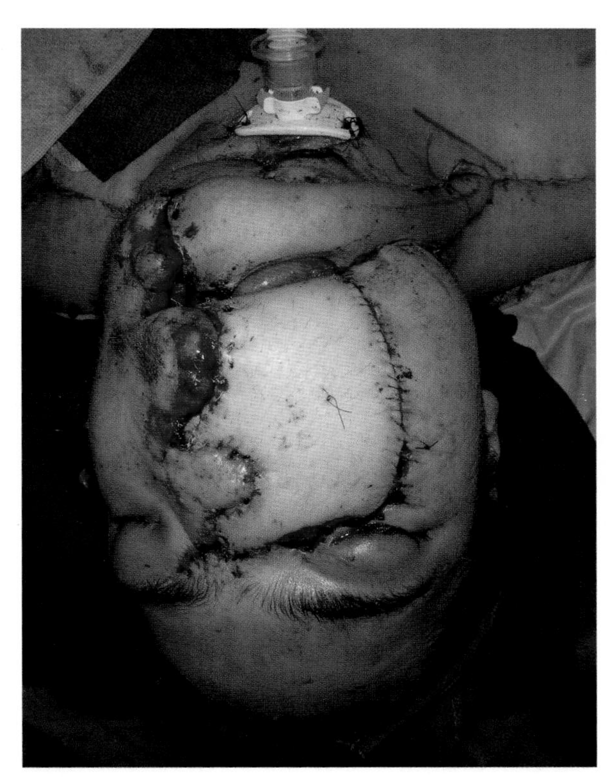

• **Fig. 10.63** Intraoperative view showing completion of the right supraclavicular artery flap direct inset.

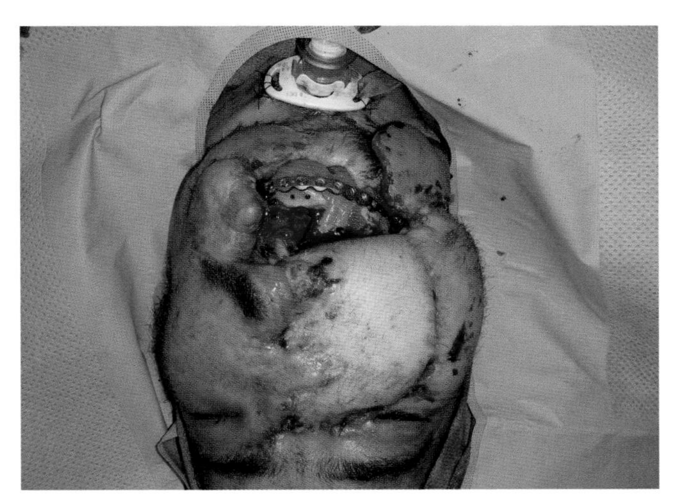

• **Fig. 10.64** Intraoperative view again showing the lower face soft tissue defect with the exposed mandibular reconstruction plate after debridement of necrotic right supraclavicular artery flap.

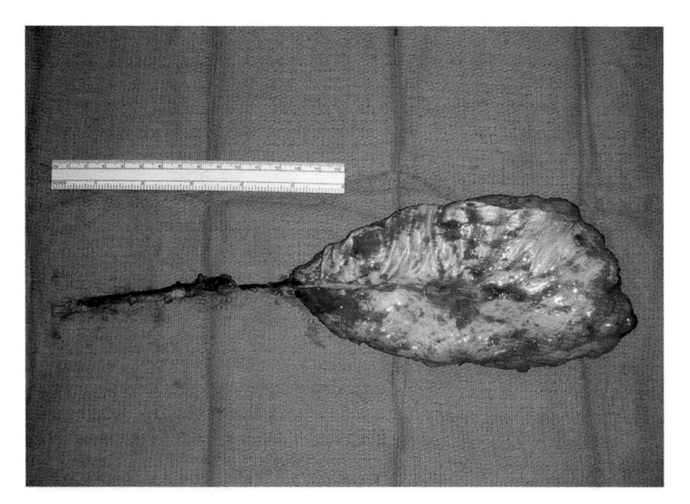

• **Fig. 10.65** Intraoperative view showing completion of the left free anterolateral thigh perforator flap dissection.

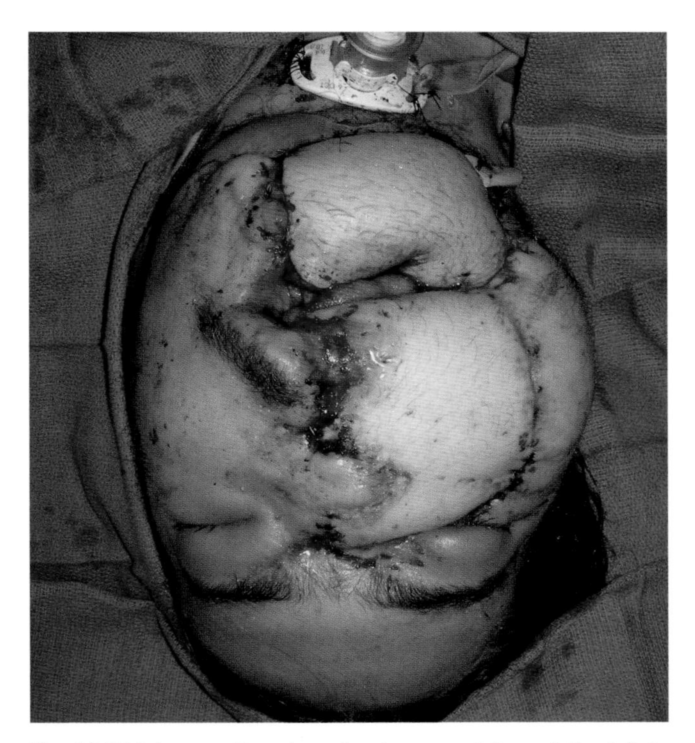

• **Fig. 10.66** Intraoperative view showing completion of the left free anterolateral thigh flap inset. The lower face soft tissue defect with the exposed mandibular reconstruction plate was covered with the flap.

The patient unfortunately developed a distal flap necrosis and again had an exposed mandibular reconstructed plate for an unknown reason (Fig. 10.64). He was taken back to the operating room 2 weeks later and this time, a second free ALT flap from his left thigh was harvested and transferred successfully to cover the exposed mandibular reconstruction plate after microvascular anastomoses to the right facial artery and vein (Figs. 10.65 and 10.66). The flap survived well and all his facial "definitive" reconstruction sites healed well except a small wound dehiscence between the upper ALT flap and native midfacial skin and between the lower ALT flap and native mandibular skin (Fig. 10.67). This was thought to be caused by saliva leakage from his oral cavity. He was placed on a medication to limit his saliva production and a repair was attempted in the operating room (Fig. 10.68). The dehiscence sites finally healed and the patient was discharged from the hospital after nearly 5 months (Fig. 10.69).

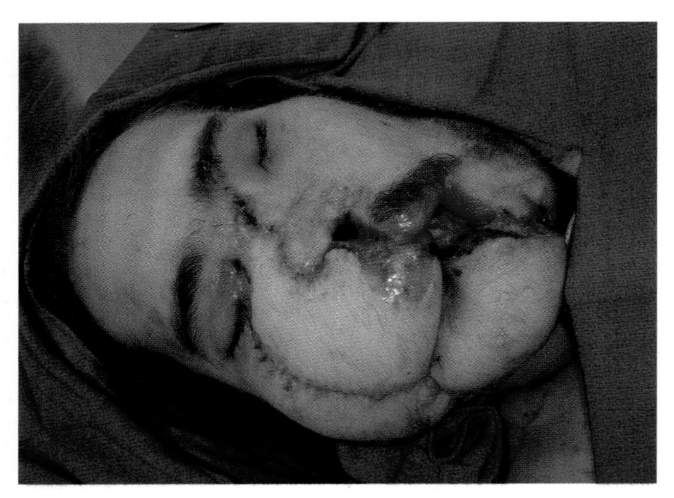

• **Fig. 10.67** Intraoperative view showing wound dehiscence of both free anterolateral thigh flap closure sites on the left.

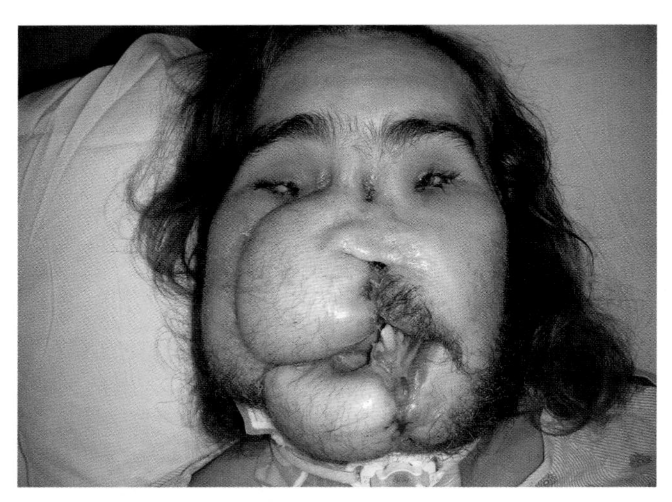

• **Fig. 10.69** The result 3 months after "definitive" reconstruction while the patient was still in the hospital.

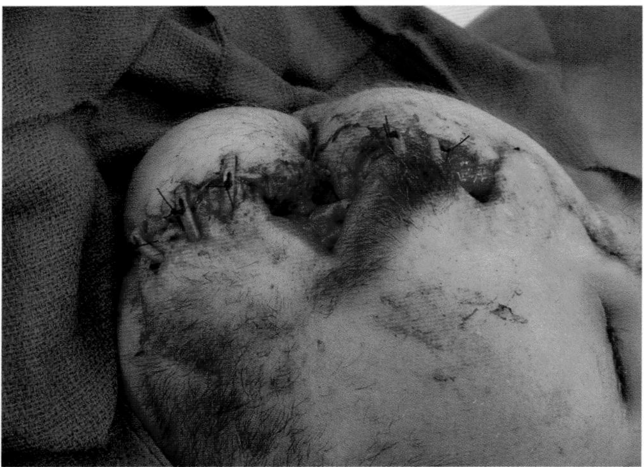

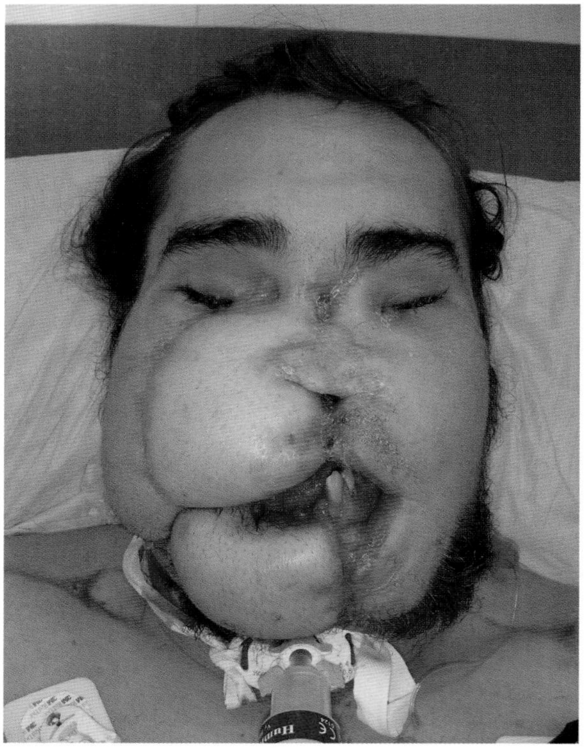

• **Fig. 10.68** Intraoperative view showing completion of wound closure on both free anterolateral thigh flap closure sites on the left.

Follow-Up Results

The patient was followed as an outpatient. He had an additional outpatient procedure for his right orbital floor repair with a Medpor implant (Figs. 10.70 and 10.71). He did well after this procedure but unfortunately developed recurrent wound dehiscence between the upper ALT flap and his native midfacial skin (Fig. 10.72). This was repaired again in the operating room as an outpatient procedure and all the facial reconstruction sites have remained intact since then (Fig. 10.73).

Final Outcome

After a hospital stay of almost 5 months and seven operations under the author's care, the patient was able to resume some of his normal life as a young adult in his hometown (Fig. 10.74). He was able to travel to New York City and was evaluated by the world-renowned face transplant team at New York University under the leadership of Dr. Eduardo D. Rodriguez. He was placed on the transplant's waiting list and underwent vigorous pre-face transplant assessments and preparations. On January 5, 2018, he underwent a very successful face transplant surgery led by Dr. Rodriguez's team. The operation took nearly 25 hours and the surgery has been an amazing success. Now the patient lives a normal life in his hometown and has been regularly followed by the transplant team at New York University. A special ABC 20/20 program was broadcast about him, "Brave New Face," on November 16, 2018.

• **Fig. 10.70** Preoperative view 4 months after "definitive" reconstruction before his right orbital floor reconstruction.

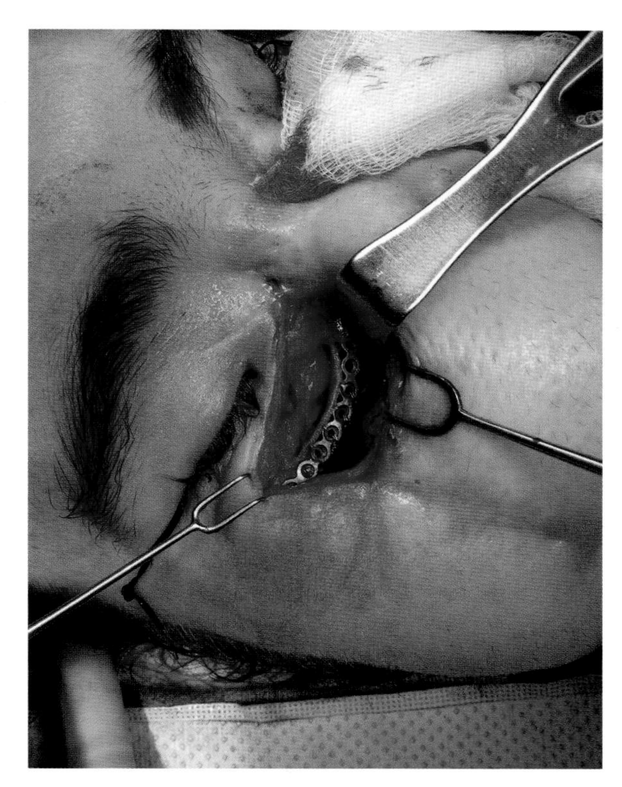

• **Fig. 10.71** Intraoperative view showing completion of his right orbital floor reconstruction with a Medpor implant.

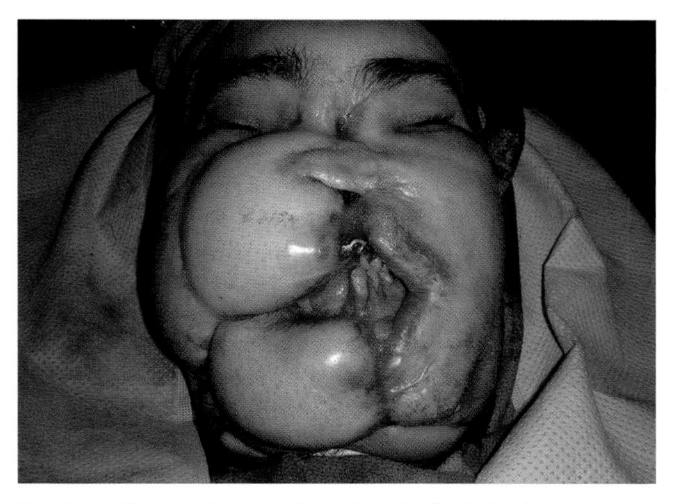

• **Fig. 10.72** Preoperative view 5 months after "definitive" reconstruction showing wound dehiscence between the upper anterolateral thigh flap and the native middle face skin with the exposed reconstruction plate.

Pearls for Success

Preparation of the patient with extremely complex facial trauma for a future face transplant can be considered when the extent of the injury is beyond conventional reconstructive limits. This is particularly true when the central face has a significant ballistic injury, which is also associated with comminuted fractures of the nasal and palatal bones and ethmoid. Therefore, face transplantation is indicated for this patient because of his "irreparable

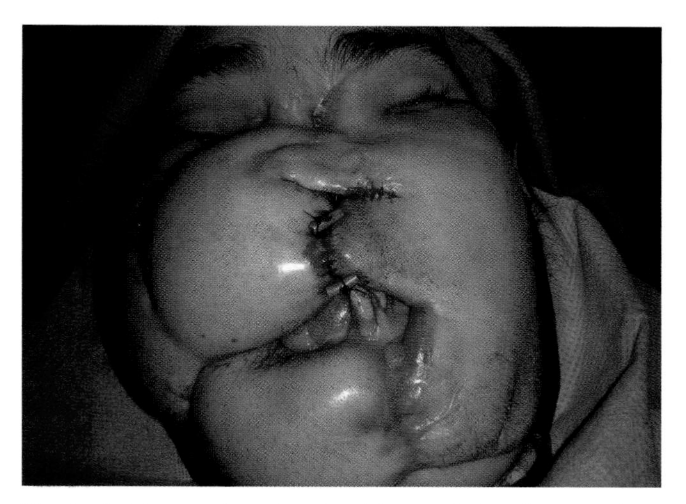

• **Fig. 10.73** Intraoperative view showing completion of wound closure between the upper anterolateral thigh flap and the native middle face skin.

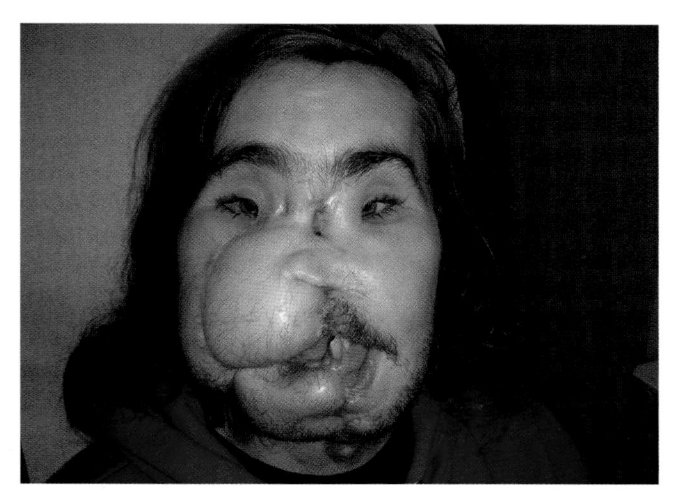

• **Fig. 10.74** The result 6 months after definitive reconstruction and 1 month after the patient's final surgical procedure for closure of the wound dehiscence after he was discharged home. All procedures were performed to prepare this patient for a possible future face transplant.

facial injury" and because both anatomic structures and functional rehabilitations can be provided by the face transplant. In this case, the option of a future face transplant was considered and offered to the patient at the beginning of his surgical care. An intraoperative evaluation under general anesthesia is necessary to provide more accurate and detailed assessment of soft tissue and bony injuries and would allow the surgeon to make a more appropriate surgical plan for ultimate reconstruction. The "definitive" reconstruction for this patient would include restoring close to normal facial skeleton in 3-D dimension with miniplates to reduce and stabilize facial fractures and with a reconstruction plate to bridge large bony gaps. The selections for soft tissue reconstruction would include both free and adjacent pedicled skin flaps. These flaps all have minimal donor site morbidity or functional loss except a surgical scar. A free ALT flap can be an excellent choice for such a reconstruction. The flap itself can be used to wrap around the reconstruction plate and to provide a good intraoral coverage. Although a supraclavicular artery flap can be a good choice to provide adequate soft tissue coverage, the partial flap necrosis in this patient may be an issue for this particular patient because the distal portion of the flap below the shoulder may not be reliable. Flap dehiscence can be a real problem because the patient does not have a normal swallow function. Attempted wound closure should be performed once saliva production is under control by medication. Attempted closure can be challenging because of poor tissue condition and potential saliva soaking over the suture line. Nevertheless, when caring for the patient with extensive facial trauma, especially involving the central face, a face transplant can be offered to the patient and should be considered a long-term goal for the patient. Initial reconstruction should minimize donor site morbidity if a face transplant is a viable option for the patient and appropriate reconstructive procedures should be selected to achieve restoration of facial skeleton and healing of the soft tissue wound.

Recommended Readings

Ali RS, Bluebond-Langner R, Rodriguez ED, Cheng MH. The versatility of the anterolateral thigh flap. *Plast Reconstr Surg*. 2009;124:395e–407e.

Chiu ES, Liu PH, Friedlander PL. Supraclavicular artery island flap for head and neck oncologic reconstruction: indications, complications, and outcomes. *Plast Reconstr Surg*. 2009;124:115–123.

Guo L, Pribaz J. Clinical flap prefabrication. *Plast Reconstr Surg*. 2009;124:340e–350e.

Jaiswal R, Pu LLQ. Reconstruction after complex facial trauma achieving optimal outcome through multiple contemporary surgeries. *Ann Plast Surg*. 2013;70:406–409.

Kantar RS, Ceradini DJ, Gelb BE, et al. Facial transplantation for an irreparable central and lower face injury: a modernized approach to a classic challenge. *Plast Reconstr Surg*. 2019;144:264e–283e.

Pribaz JJ, Caterson EJ. Evolution and limitations of conventional autologous reconstruction of the head and neck. *J Craniofacial Surgery*. 2013;24:99–107.

Walton RL, Cohn AB, Beahm EK. Epidermal overgrafting improves coloration in remote flaps and grafts applied to the face for reconstruction. *Plast Reconstr Surg*. 2008;121:1606–1613.

Wei FC, Jain V, Celik N, Chen HC, Chuang DCC, Lin CH. Have we found an ideal soft-tissue flap? An experience with 672 anterolateral thigh flaps. *Plast Reconstr Surg*. 2002;109:2219–2226.

Zeiderman MR, Pu LLQ. Contemporary reconstruction after complex facial trauma. *Burns and Trauma*. 2020;8:1–10.

Zeiderman MR, Firriolo JM, Dave DR, Pu LLQ. Should we consider preparing patients for future face transplant when managing complex facial trauma? *Plast Reconstr Surg Global Open*. 2020;8:e2962.

12
Lateral Neck Reconstruction

Clinical Presentation

An 89-year-old White male developed a recurrent squamous cell cancer (SCC) over his right upper lateral neck with a large, ulcerated lesion. He had an SCC resection in the same area many years before. The patient was referred by the surgical oncology service for soft tissue reconstruction after a planned wide local excision of this recurrent SCC lesion. He also had a planned postoperative radiation after surgical resection (Fig. 12.1).

Operative Plan and Special Considerations

For an anticipated large soft tissue defect down to the underlying bone and future postoperative radiation, a reliable soft tissue reconstruction should be performed. Based on the anticipated location and size of the soft tissue defect, a distant flap with a relatively long pedicle should be selected. The pectoralis major myocutaneous flap is a reliable flap and can reach the level of the zygomatic arch. It would be an ideal distant flap to be selected for the reconstruction. The flap can be elevated with a skin paddle and tunneled through the neck to reach the soft tissue defect and provide a good soft tissue coverage following the wide local resection. Other options such as a supraclavicular artery island flap, trapezius myocutaneous flap, or submental island flap can also be considered. However, those flaps are less consistent and reliable than the pectoralis major myocutaneous flap for this type of reconstruction.

Operative Procedures

Under general anesthesia, a wide local resection of the recurrent SCC in the area was performed by the surgical oncology service without difficulty. There was an 8 × 5 cm soft tissue defect down to the underlying the mastoid and ear canal (Figs. 12.2 and 12.3). The results from an intraoperative frozen section showed all soft tissue margins to be negative.

The design of the right pectoralis major myocutaneous flap was marked and its pedicle, the thoracoacromial artery, was also marked with the skin paddle (Fig. 12.4). The flap was designed to ensure it could reach the soft tissue defect. After an oblique skin incision had been made, the dissection of the pectoral fascia was performed. The suprafascial dissection was performed both medially and laterally until the entire outline of the muscle could be visualized. The muscle attachment was divided from laterally to inferiorly and then medially. The area inferior to the muscle, the pectoral fascia, was elevated in continuity with the muscle. Once the pedicle was visualized under the muscle, the flap was elevated from the chest wall and the dissection was continued to release a major portion of the muscle attachment to the clavicle both medial and lateral to the flap's pedicle. In this way, the flap could be mobilized freely with only minimal muscle attachment to prevent kicking of the pedicle. The neck subcutaneous tunnel was made and care was taken to ensure the tunnel was wide enough to let the muscle pass through easily. The flap was tunneled through subcutaneously and inserted into the defect without any tension.

The flap was inserted into the defect and sutured in two layers after a JP drain had been inserted under the flap. The flap donor site was also closed in two layers. One JP drain was placed under the skin in the donor site (Fig. 12.5).

Follow-Up Results

The patient did well postoperatively without any complications related to the pectoralis major myocutaneous flap reconstruction to the upper lateral neck wound. He was discharged from the

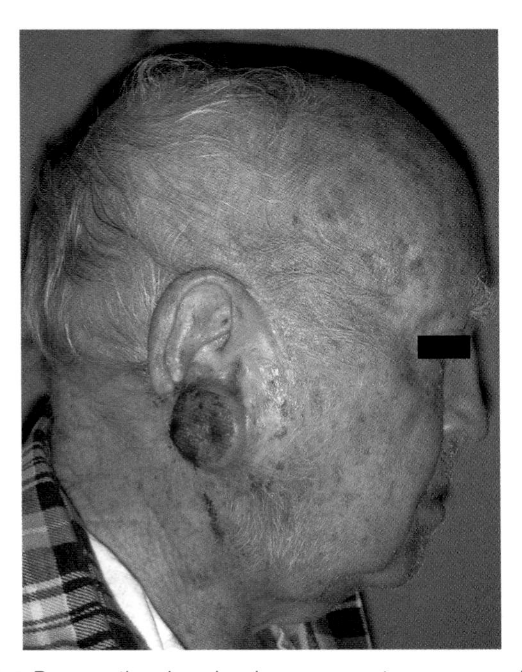

• **Fig. 12.1** Preoperative view showing a recurrent squamous cell cancer in the right upper lateral neck involving a portion of the ear.

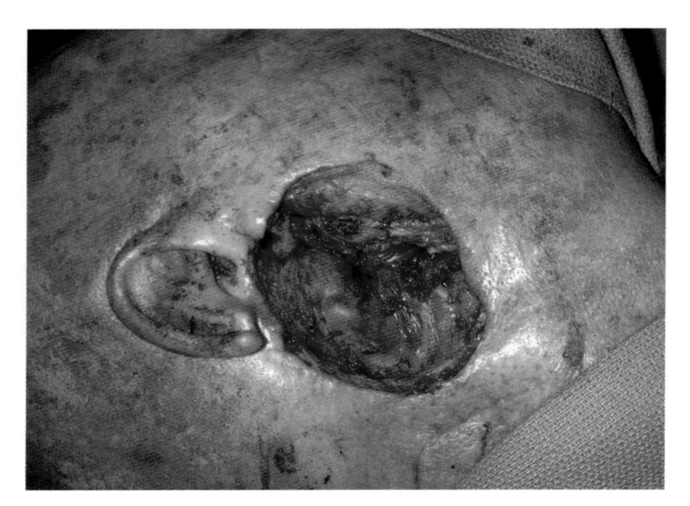

• **Fig. 12.2** Preoperative view showing a large soft tissue defect with the exposed mastoid and ear canal after wide local resection of the recurrent squamous cell cancer.

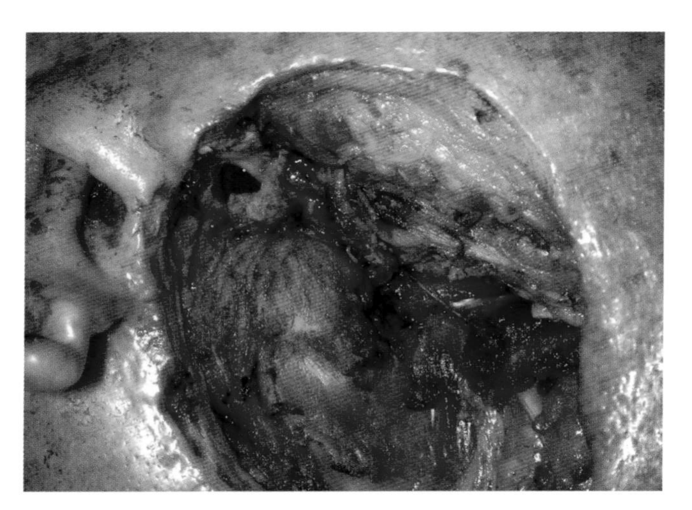

• **Fig. 12.3** Preoperative close-up view showing the soft tissue defect.

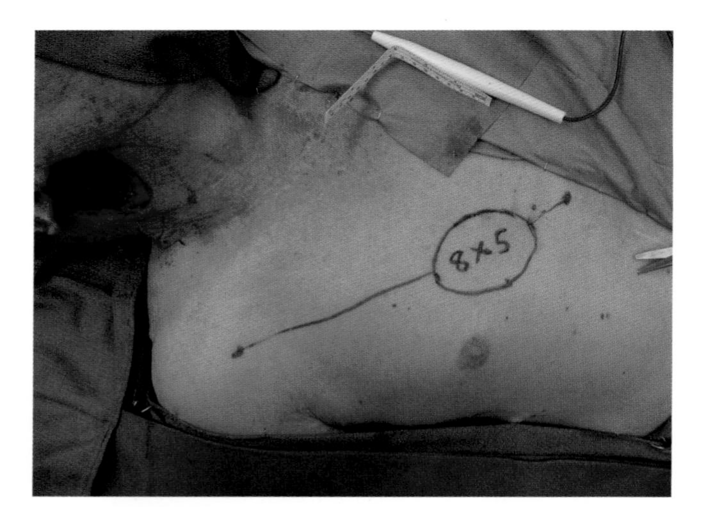

• **Fig. 12.4** Intraoperative view showing the design of a right pectoralis major myocutaneous flap. The design of the skin paddle was also clearly marked.

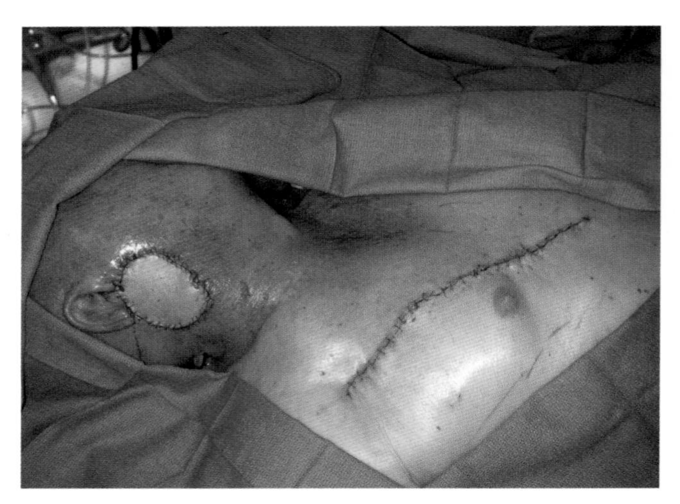

• **Figs. 12.5** Intraoperative view showing completion of the flap inset and closure as well as the donor site closure.

hospital on postoperative day 7. The drain was removed before discharge. During immediate follow-ups, the skin paddle of the flap healed well. The patient then underwent the planned postoperative radiation to the operative field (Fig. 12.6).

Final Outcome

The patient underwent postoperative radiation treatment to the resection area. The flap remained well-healed and tolerated the radiation well (Fig. 12.7). He has had no issues of recurrent SCC and has resumed his normal life. He has been followed by the surgical oncology service primarily for the cancer follow-up.

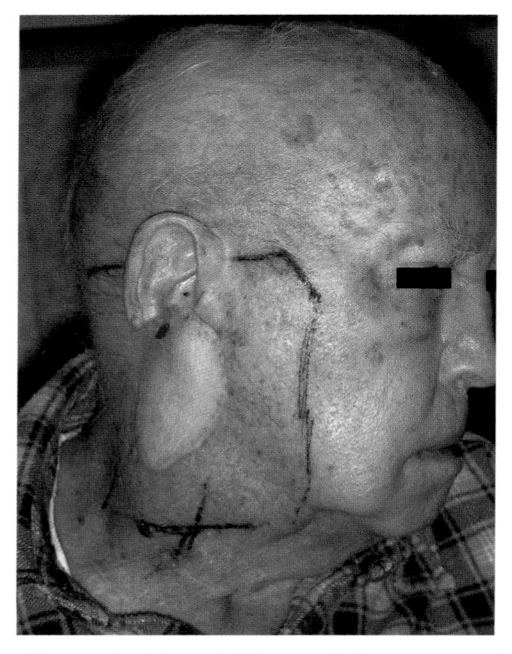

• **Fig. 12.6** The result at 6-week follow-up before postoperative radiation. The flap site healed nicely.

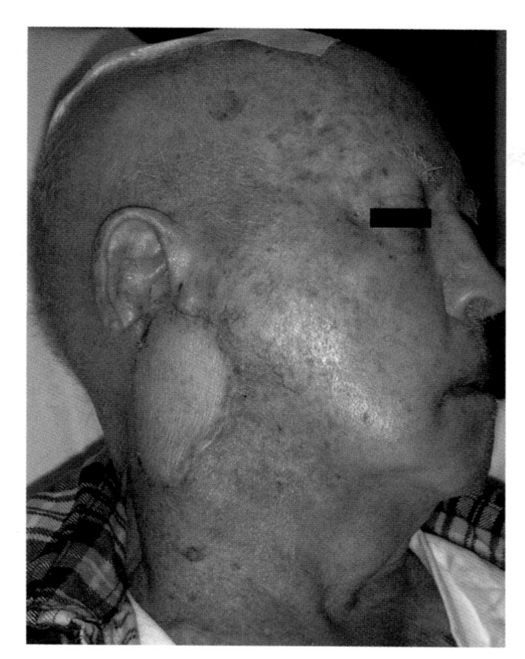

• **Fig. 12.7** The result at 3-month follow-up after postoperative radiation. Again, the flap site remained well-healed.

Pearls for Success

A pectoralis major myocutaneous flap can be a good option to provide relabel soft tissue coverage for an upper lateral neck soft tissue defect. The design of the skin paddle is based on the size and location of the soft tissue defect in the area. If the skin paddle has to be designed below the level of the inferior insertion of the muscle, a portion of the pectoral fascia should be incorporated into the flap. The dissection around the pedicle vessels should be performed relatively aggressively to free most of the muscle attachment to the clavicle so that the flap can be easily rotated superiorly. However, a small portion of the muscle attachment to the clavicle should be kept so that kicking of the pedicle can be prevented. The neck subcutaneous tunnel should be made large enough so that the muscle and/or the pedicle are not compressed by any adjacent tissues. In addition, incorporating a skin paddle to the flap would definitely be better than a skin-grafted muscle flap with anticipation of future postoperative radiation.

Recommended Readings

Koh KS, Eom JS, Kirk I, Kim SY, Nam S. Pectoralis major musculocutaneous flap in oropharyngeal reconstruction: revisited. *Plast Reconstr Surg*. 2006;118:1145–1149.

Ramirez CA, Fernandes RP. The supraclavicular artery island and trapezius myocutaneous flaps in head and neck reconstruction. *Oral Maxillofac Surg Clin*. 2014;26:411–420.

Rikimaru H, Kiyokawa K, Watanabe K, Koga N, Nishi Y, Sakamoto A. New method of preparing a pectoralis major myocutaneous flap with a skin paddle that includes the third intercostal perforating branch of the internal thoracic artery. *Plastic Reconstr Surg*. 2009;123:1220–1228.

Zenga J, Emerick KS, Deschler DG. Submental island flap: a technical update. *Ann Otol Rhinol Laryngol*. 2019;128:1177–1181.

13

Posterior Neck Reconstruction

Clinical Presentation

A 52-year-old White male underwent C4–C7 posterior cervical fusion 4 months previously. He was discharged home and subsequently had wound dehiscence and drainage from his neck wound. He was seen in outpatients by the orthopedic spine service and was admitted to the hospital directly for debridement, intravenous antibiotic treatment, and definitive wound closure. The plastic surgery service was consulted for this complex wound closure and after evaluating the wound, bilateral adjacent flaps for wound closure were planned (Fig. 13.1).

Operative Plan and Special Considerations

Before the definitive wound closure, the patent was brought to the operating room by the plastic surgery service for more definitive wound debridement and preparation of the wound bed for flap reconstruction. A vacuum-assisted closure was placed after the definitive wound debridement and an operative plan was made during this procedure. Based on the size and location of the skin defect in the area, bilateral trapezius myocutaneous advancement flaps could be an excellent option for soft tissue coverage. The cervical portion of the muscle flap can be raised as a myocutaneous flap from each side and approximated in the midline of the posterior neck. Bilateral trapezius myocutaneous flaps can provide a three-layer closure including the muscle, subcutaneous layer, and skin and can be an excellent option for a complex midline posterior neck wound reconstruction.

Operative Procedures

Under general anesthesia, the patient was placed in the prone position. The posterior neck wound was 4 cm in diameter (Fig. 13.2). The wound edges were sharply debrided to remove unhealthy-looking skin and subcutaneous tissue. The underlying exposed bone was also debrided along with surrounding nonviable tissue, with curette for the bone and electrocautery for the subcutaneous tissue and muscle.

The cervical portion of the trapezius muscle on each side was identified. Each side of the trapezius myocutaneous flap was

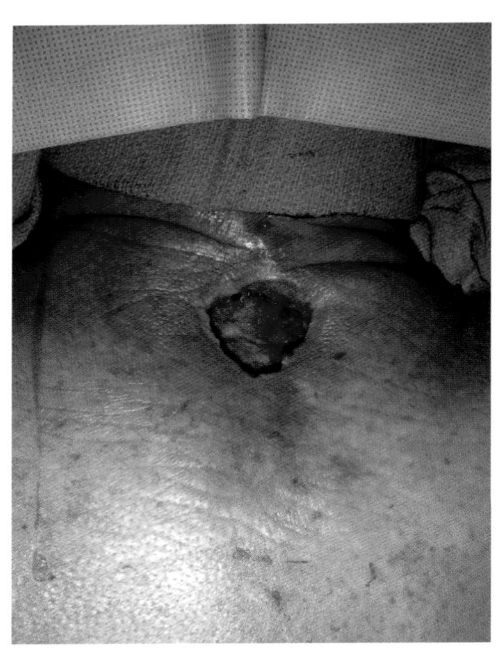

• **Fig. 13.1** A preoperative view showing a 4 × 4 cm open wound in the posterior neck with exposed cervical spinal processes.

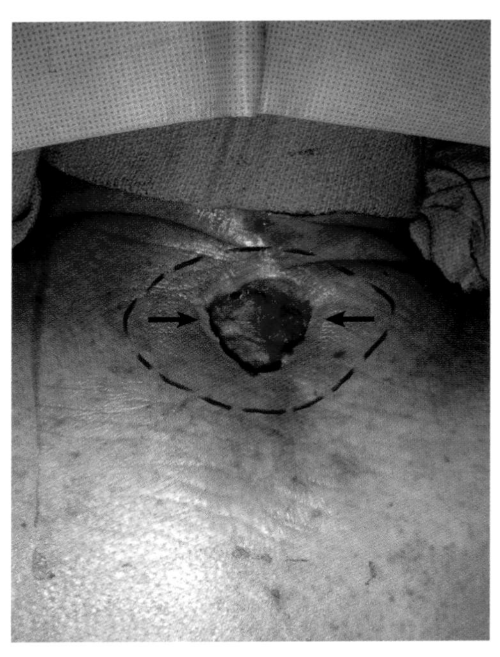

• **Fig. 13.2** An intraoperative view showing an outline of the flap dissection on each side and the direction of the flap advancement.

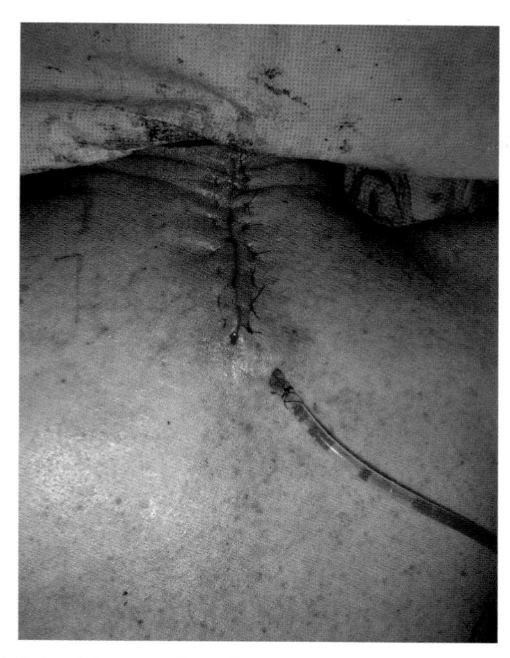

• **Fig. 13.3** An intraoperative view showing completion of bilateral trapezius myocutaneous advancement flaps for closure of the posterior neck wound.

elevated following the submuscular tissue plane and both flaps could easily be brought to the midline without tension once adequate flap dissection was completed. A 7-mm flat JP was placed under each side of the myocutaneous flap. The wound closure was accomplished in three layers, with 2-0 PDS

suture in an interrupted fashion for the trapezius muscle closure, 3-0 Monocryl in an interrupted fashion for the dermal layer, and a 3-0 nylon in an interrupted horizontal mattress fashion for the skin closure (Fig. 13.3). A sterile dressing was applied to the wound closure site.

Follow-Up Results

The patient did well postoperatively without any complications related to the bilateral trapezius myocutaneous advancement flap reconstruction. He was kept in hospital for 2 days and discharged home on postoperative day 3. The drain was removed during the 2-week follow-up visit. His posterior neck wound healed well after the flap closure (Fig. 13.4).

Final Outcome

His complex posterior neck wound healed well without any issues. He has a stable wound coverage over his posterior neck with a nicely faded scar. He has returned to his normal life and has been followed by the plastic surgery service as needed.

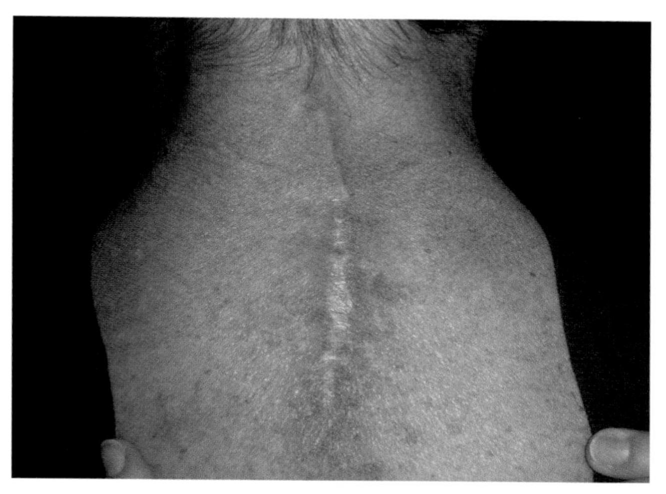

• **Fig. 13.4** Result at a 6-week follow-up showing well-healed midline posterior neck wound after bilateral trapezius myocutaneous flap advancement flaps for wound closure.

Pearls for Success

A midline posterior neck wound can be closed with bilateral adjacent tissue advancements. The cervical portion of the trapezius muscle can be used and elevated as a myocutaneous flap. Such bilateral advancement flaps can be approximated in the midline for a durable wound coverage after adequate flap dissection. Because the pedicle, the transverse cervical artery, is far from the flap dissection field, the trapezius myocutaneous flap elevation can be quickly and safely performed once the advancement of one side flap is beyond the midline. A three-layer closure with muscle, subcutaneous tissue, and skin can provide durable wound approximation and optimal healing.

Recommended Readings

Cohen LE, Fullerton N, Mundy LR, et al. Optimizing successful outcomes in complex spine reconstruction using local muscle flaps. *Plast Reconstr Surg.* 2016;137:295–301.

Lynch JR, Hansen JE, Chaffoo R, Seyfer AE. The lower trapezius musculocutaneous flap revisited: versatile coverage for complicated wounds to the posterior cervical and occipital regions based on the deep branch of the transverse cervical artery. *Plast Reconstr Surg.* 2002;109:444–450.

Mathes DW, Thornton JF, Rohrich RJ. Management of posterior trunk defects. *Plast Reconstr Surg.* 2006;118:73e–83e.

Mericli AF, Mirzabeigi MN, Moore Jr JH, Fox JW, Copit SE, Tuma GA. Reconstruction of complex posterior cervical spine wounds using the paraspinous muscle flap. *Plast Reconstr Surg.* 2011;128:148–153.

Wright MA, Weinstein AL, Bernstein JL, et al. Muscle flap closure following complex spine surgery: a decade of experience. *Plast Reconstr Surg.* 2020;146:642e–650e.

SECTION 2

Shoulder and Upper Extremity

14 Shoulder Reconstruction

Clinical Presentation

A 48-year-old White male with a large soft tissue mass over his right shoulder and upper chest had a wide local excision of dermatofibrosarcoma (Fig. 14.1). After the initial resection, he had a 20 × 18 cm soft tissue defect down to the clavicle and ribs as well as the adjacent deltoid and pectoralis major muscles (Fig. 14.2). Portions of those two muscles were also resected (Fig. 14.3). Alloskin grafts were used for temporarily wound closure. Six days later, the final pathology report conformed negative peripheral and deep margins of the sarcoma.

Operative Plan and Special Considerations

Because of the size and location of the soft tissue defect after wide local excision for the soft tissue sarcoma, a pedicle latissimus dorsi muscle flap from the same side can be selected for soft tissue coverage of this large shoulder and upper chest wound. The latissimus flap has a long pedicle and is reliable and large enough to cover a large defect in the shoulder and upper chest. It is a logical and distant flap to choose for soft tissue coverage in this case. The split-thickness skin graft can be added for the wound closure and better contour. The pectoralis major muscle cannot be selected because its pedicle was ligated during the tumor resection.

Operative Procedures

Under general anesthesia with the patient in the left lateral decubitus position, the right latissimus dorsi muscle was marked. With an oblique incision, the latissimus dorsi muscle was first exposed. Once the medial and lateral borders of the muscle had been identified, the dissection was performed to elevate the muscle from the chest wall. The muscle's attachment to the anterior chest wall, midline back, and posterior iliac crest were divided under direct vision. Once the pedicle vessels had been identified and marked, the muscle flap was dissected free toward the axilla. The muscle attachment to the humerus was divided. With proper traction and protection, the pedicle dissection was extended to the axilla. The surgical dissection of a pedicled latissimus dorsi flap was completed. The flap was then tunneled subcutaneously to the shoulder and upper chest under direct vision. The right back of the latissimus dorsi muscle flap donor site was closed in two layers after placement of 2 flat JP drains.

The patient was then turned to the supine position. The final inset of the latissimus dorsi muscle flap was performed after excess tissue of the flap had been excised. The flap was inserted into the shoulder and upper chest defect with 3-0 Vicryl sutures in a half-buried horizontal mattress fashion. A JP drain was placed under the flap (Fig. 14.4). A meshed split-thickness skin graft, harvested from the right lateral thigh with a dermatome,

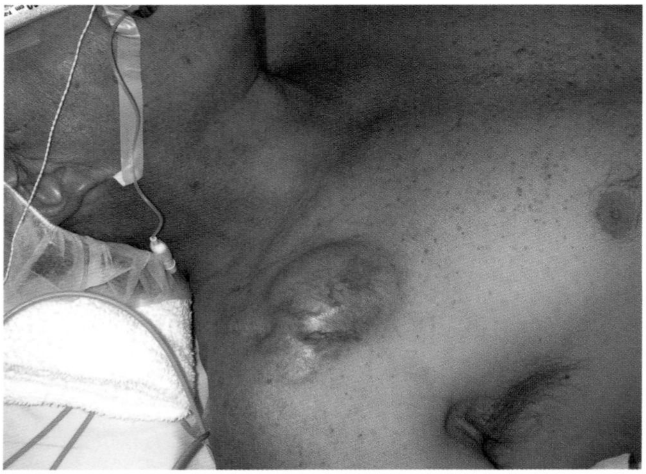

• **Fig. 14.1** Preoperative view showing a large dermatofibrosarcoma with its indurated area.

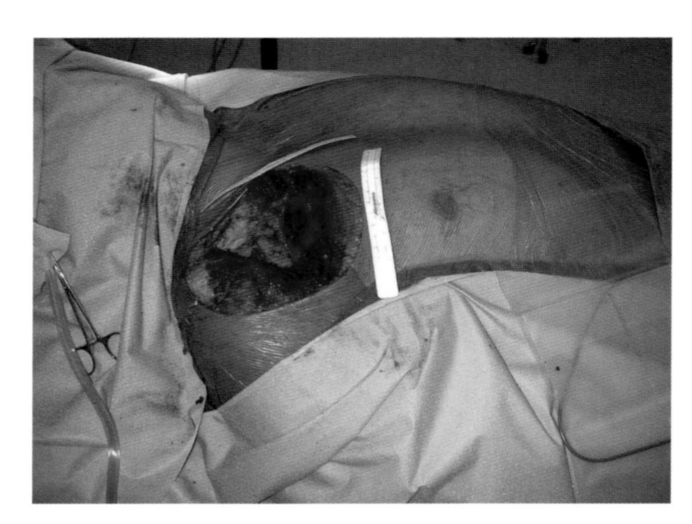

• **Fig. 14.2** Intraoperative view showing a large shoulder and upper chest soft tissue defect down to the clavicle and ribs. Portions of the deltoid and pectoralis major muscles were also transected.

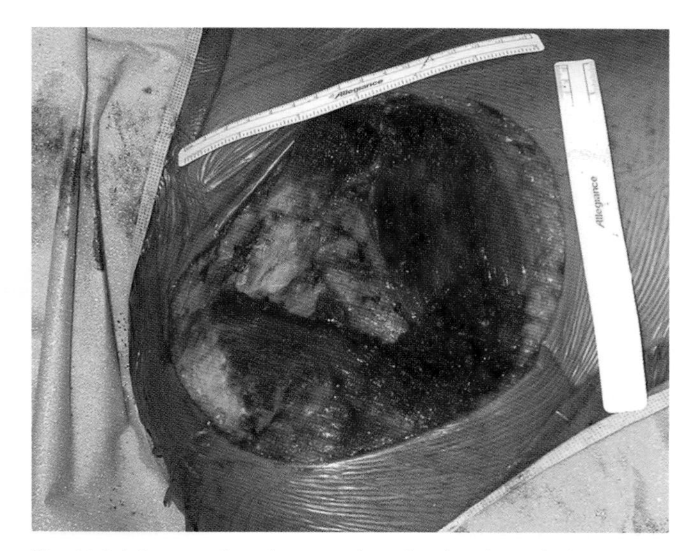
• **Fig. 14.3** Intraoperative close-up view showing the soft tissue defect.

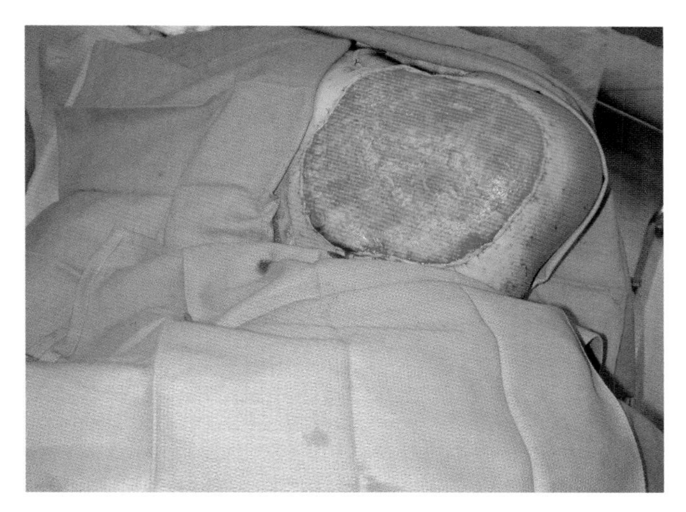
• **Fig. 14.4** Intraoperative view showing completion of the right pedicled latissimus dorsi muscle flap inset to the right shoulder and upper chest defect before placement of a skin graft.

was placed over the muscle flap and secured with skin staples to the adject healthy edge.

Follow-Up Results

The patient did well postoperatively without any complications related to the pedicled latissimus dorsi muscle flap reconstruction. He was discharged from the hospital on postoperative day 5. The drain was removed during the 2-week follow-up visit. His shoulder and upper chest reconstruction site healed well (Fig. 14.5).

Final Outcome

His shoulder and upper chest latissimus dorsi muscle flap reconstruction site healed well. He resumed his normal activities and

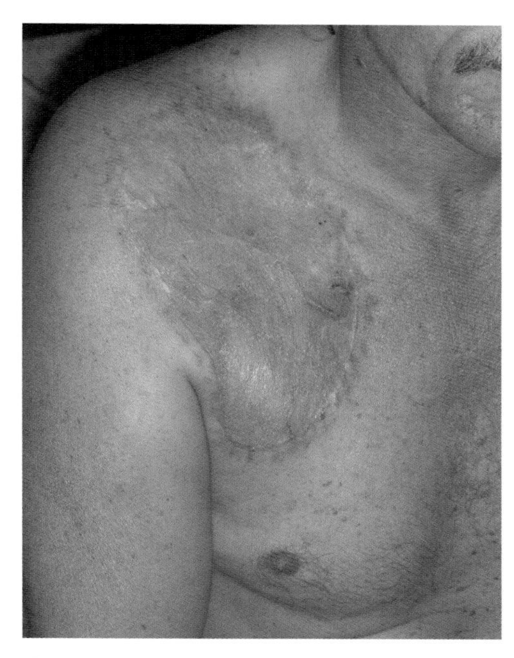
• **Fig. 14.5** The result at 2 months postoperative follow-up showing well-healed skin-grafted latissimus dorsi muscle flap site with an excellent contour.

remains tumor free. He has been followed by the surgical oncology service for routine follow-up.

Pearls for Success

A pedicled latissimus dorsi muscle is the distant flap of choice for the reconstruction of a large shoulder and upper chest wall defect. It is a large muscle flap with a long pedicle and reliable blood supply. It can be harvested relatively quickly and tunneled easily to the shoulder or upper chest location. Division of the muscle insertion to the humerus can increase the length of the flap advancement and allow more freedom for the flap inset. Selection of a split-thickness skin graft can improve the contour in the reconstruction site because a myocutaneous flap can be bulky and a skin graft to the back flap donor site for donor site closure can be avoided.

Recommended Readings

De La Torre JI, Griffin DW, Vasconez LO. Harvesting the latissimus dorsi muscle for cardiomyoplasty. *Plast Reconstr Surg*. 2000;105: 83–88.

Durkin AJ, Pierpont YN, Patel S, et al. An algorithmic approach to breast reconstruction using latissimus dorsi myocutaneous flaps. *Plast Reconstr Surg*. 2010;125:1318–1327.

Hammond DC. Latissimus dorsi flap breast reconstruction. *Plast Reconstr Surg*. 2009;124:1055–1063.

Spear SL, Hess CL. A review of the biomechanical and functional changes in the shoulder following transfer of the latissimus dorsi muscles. *Plast Reconstr Surg*. 2005;115:2070–2073.

15 Axillary Reconstruction

Clinical Presentation

A 67-year-old White male had a chronic wound in the right axilla secondary to previous radiation for treatment of his advanced metastatic lung cancer. He had responded incredibly well to chemotherapy for his lung cancer and had been cancer-free since the completion of the last chemotherapy. The patient was referred by his medical oncologist for possible closure of this longstanding wound in his right axilla. On initial examination, he had a 2 × 2 cm deep open wound with significant indurated and fibrotic surrounding tissues from his previous radiation (Figs. 15.1 and 15.2).

Operative Plan and Special Considerations

Adequate debridement was planned to excise all fibrotic tissues around and deep to the open wound. Such a debridement should be done to healthy and normal-looking tissue either around or at the base of the wound. Care should be taken to avoid injuries to neurovascular structures in the axilla while removing all deep fibrotic tissues. Because of the location of potential soft tissue defect after the debridement, a pedicled parascapular flap could be a good option for reconstruction of the axillary wound. The flap can be elevated and tunneled to the defect without any tension. In addition, the flap donor site can be closed primarily without any problems.

Operative Procedures

Under general anesthesia with the patient in the left lateral decubitus position, his right axillar wound was debrided and the wound excision was carefully done, under direct vision, to the healthy-looking tissue free of fibrosis. After debridement, the new wound measured 8 × 5 cm (Fig. 15.3). The wound was irrigated with Pulsavac.

The pedicled parascapular fasciocutaneous flap was designed over the right back (Fig. 15.4). A handheld Doppler was used to map the descending branch of the circumflex scapular vessel. An 8 × 5 cm skin paddle was marked on the back because it could easily reach to the right axilla without any tension. The proposed skin incision was infiltrated with 1% lidocaine with 1:100,000 epinephrine.

The skin paddle was elevated in the subfascial plane. During the dissection, the pedicle of the flap was identified by a handheld Doppler and marked with a marker pen. The skin paddle dissection was quickly performed down to the proximal flap near the main pedicle. Although the pedicle was not visualized during the procedure, the arterial signal of the circumflex scapular artery was confirmed by Doppler throughout. The pedicle dissection was then completed within the triangular space. The tunnel was made between the right axillary wound and the right back donor site. The flap was tunneled subcutaneously and temporarily placed over the right axilla wound. The hidden area of the flap was deepithelialized with a knife and the extra distal portion of the flap was excised.

The skin paddle of the flap appeared to be well-perfused. The 7-mm flat JP was inserted under the right axillary wound and the 10-mm flat JP was placed in the flap donor site. The flap was inset into the axillary defect and closed in two layers. The subcutaneous tissue layer was approximated with interrupted 3-0 Monocryl sutures. The skin was closed with a 3-0 Monocryl suture in a half-buried interrupted horizontal mattress fashion (Fig. 15.5).

The back donor site was closed without very much tension. The deep layer tissue was approximated with several interrupted 2-0 PDS sutures. The deep dermal closure was approximated with several interrupted 3-0 Monocryl sutures. The skin was closed with a 3-0 V-Loc suture in a running subcuticular fashion. A pressure dressing was applied to the right back donor site.

Follow-Up Results

The patient did well postoperatively without any complications related to his parascapular flap reconstruction. He was discharged from the hospital on postoperative day 3. The drain was removed during subsequent follow-up visits. His axillary wound after the flap reconstruction healed well (Figs. 15.6 and 15.7).

Final Outcome

His axillary wound after the parascapular flap reconstruction healed well (Figs. 15.8 and 15.9). He has no recurrent open wound in the area, has resumed his normal activities, and is followed by the medical oncology service for his lung cancer.

Pearls for Success

A pedicled parascapular fasciocutaneous flap can be a good choice for axial soft tissue reconstruction if only skin coverage is needed such as in this case. The key for successful dissection of the flap is to identify the descending branch of the circumflex scapular vessel, the pedicle of the flap. The flap

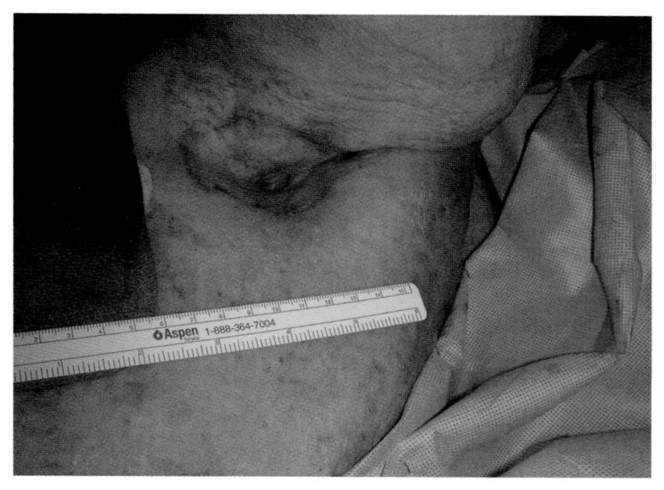

• **Fig. 15.1** Preoperative view showing a chronic and radiated deep axillary wound with surrounding fibrotic and scarred tissues.

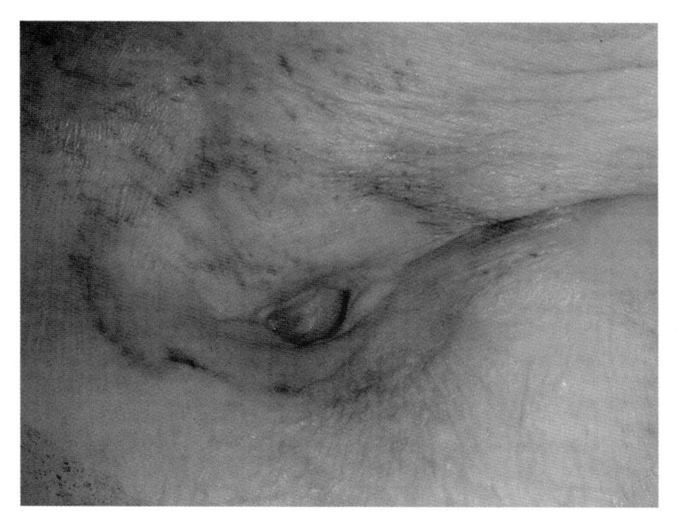

• **Fig. 15.2** Preoperative close-up view showing this deep axillary wound with surrounding fibrotic and scarred tissues.

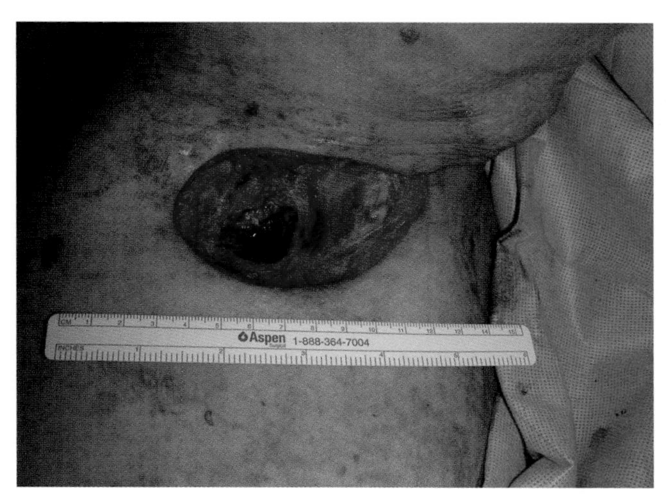

• **Fig. 15.3** Intraoperative view showing the extent of the debridement for this deep axillary wound.

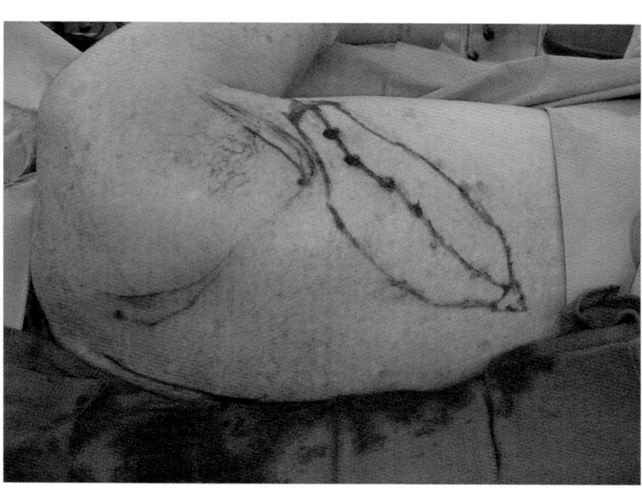

• **Fig. 15.4** Intraoperative view showing the design of the parascapular fasciocutaneous flap. The pedicle, the descending branch of the circumflex subscapular artery, was mapped for this flap.

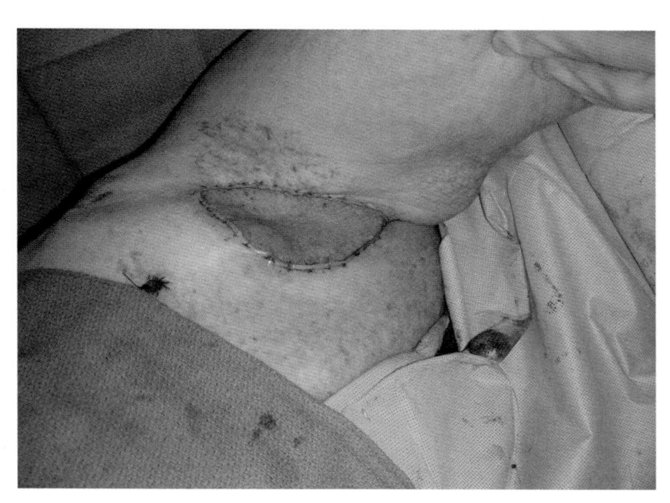

• **Fig. 15.5** Intraoperative view showing completion of the parascapular flap inset in the axilla.

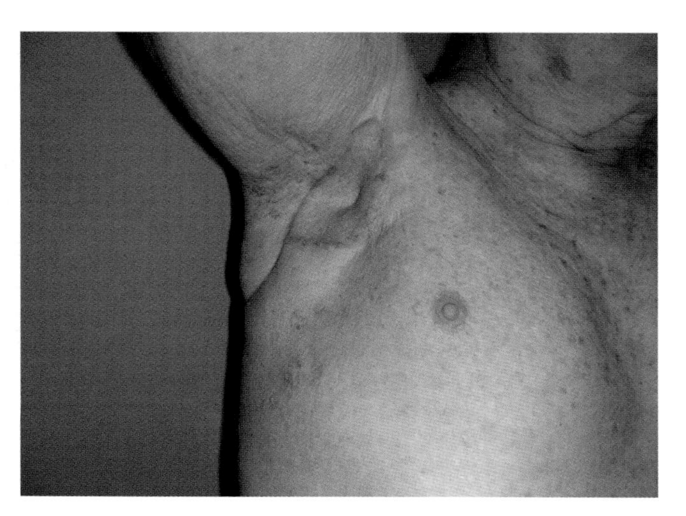

• **Fig. 15.6** The result at 6-week follow-up showing well healed right axillary wound.

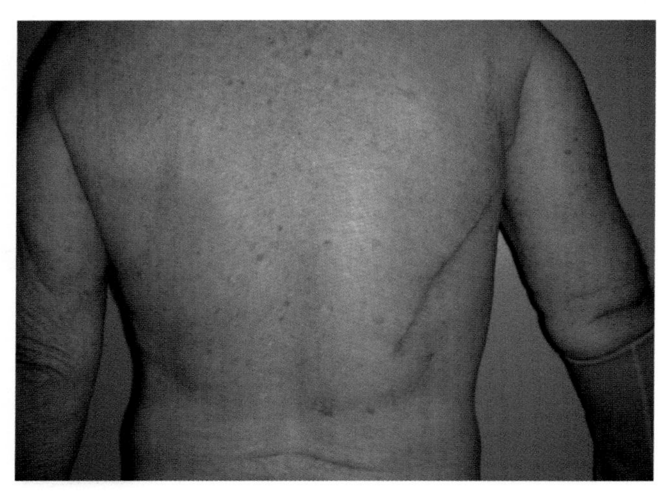

• **Fig. 15.7** The result at 6-week follow-up showing the flap's donor site after primary closue.

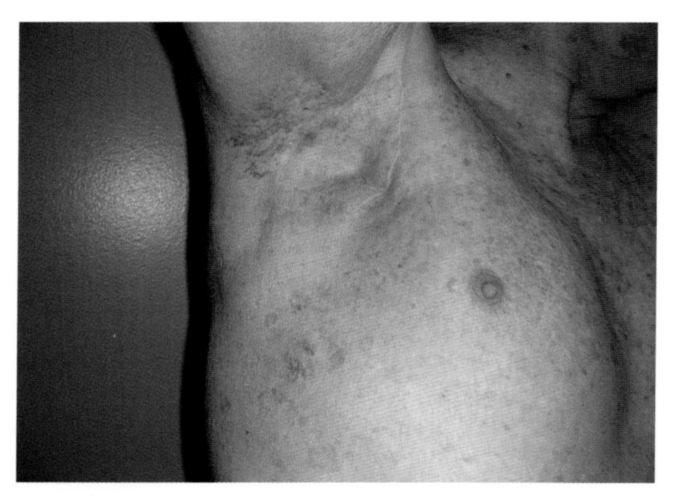

• **Fig. 15.8** The result at 9-month follow-up showing stable and well-healed right axillary wound.

dissection should be in the subfascial plane because the pedicle vessels are located within the subcutaneous tissue layer. The pedicle can usually be visualized through the fascia. Additional

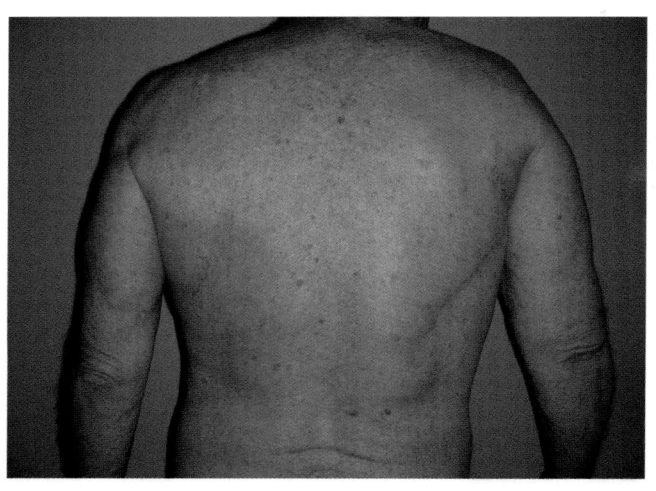

• **Fig. 15.9** The result at 9-month follow-up showing the flap's donor site after primary closure.

dissection around the pedicle within the triangular space can add more freedom to the flap's arc of rotation. An island flap can be made, which can facilitate the flap inset. Postoperatively, the upper arm should be placed abductively to avoid direct compression to the flap.

Recommended Readings

Chen JT, Schmid DB, Israel JS, Siebert JW. A 26-year experience with microsurgical reconstruction of hemifacial atrophy and linear scleroderma. *Plast Reconstr Surg*. 2018;142:1275–1283.

Klinkenberg M, Fischer S, Kremer T, Hernekamp F, Lehnhardt M, Daigeler A. Comparison of anterolateral thigh, lateral arm, and parascapular free flaps with regard to donor-site morbidity and aesthetic and functional outcomes. *Plast Reconstr Surg*. 2013;131:293–302.

Nisanci M, Altiparmak M, Sahin I, Kasap S. A wise surgical approach for reconstruction of postburn axillary contractures and versatility of perforator flaps. *J Burn Care Res*. 2018;39:332–338.

Nisanci M, Isik EES, Sengezer M. Treatment modalities for post-burn axillary contractures and the versatility of the scapular flap. *Burns*. 2002;28:177–180.

16 Upper Arm Reconstruction

Clinical Presentation

A 55-year-old White female had residual sarcoma over her left upper arm after previous resection. She underwent a wide local excision of the sarcoma by the surgical oncology service. The plastic surgery service was asked to perform a soft tissue reconstruction after additional resection of residual sarcome. After the wide local excision, there was an 11 × 8 cm full-thickness skin and subcutaneous tissue defect down to the underlying muscles (Fig. 16.1).

Operative Plan and Special Considerations

Based on the size and location of the skin defect over the lateral upper arm, a large adjacent skin rotational flap could be planned. The portion of the soft tissue defect could be closed directly after significant undermining and the rest of the defect would be reconstructed by the skin rotational flap. In this way, the most critical part of the wound could be covered by the more reliable tissue and the patient would have better overall reconstructive outcome. Although a skin graft-only procedure can be selected to close this defect, the resulting contour of the reconstruction would probably not be optimal. In addition, a direct skin graft to the underlying muscles may result in tethering, which would compromise the function of those muscles.

Operative Procedures

Under general anesthesia with the patient in a supine position, the soft tissue defect was assessed and the intraoperative decision was made to perform a large adjacent skin rotational flap to cover the defect and a skin graft to close the flap donor site. After significant undermining, the lateral soft tissue defect was closed. A large adjacent skin rotational flap was designed (Fig. 16.2). The proposed skin incision was then infiltrated with 1% lidocaine with 1:100,000 epinephrine. Once the skin incision had been made, the flap was elevated in the suprafascial plane. The flap was rotated and advanced into the defect without very much tension. The temporary inset of the flap was performed with towel clips and skin staples. This left an 8 × 5 cm skin defect over the flap donor site. The donor site defect was closed with a split-thickness skin graft harvested from the left lateral thigh. This was a sheet graft, which was placed on the flap donor site and secured with skin staples. The skin graft site was covered with Xeroform and VAC dressing. There was a small portion of dog ear along the inferolateral aspect of the closure that was corrected by a direct excision (Fig. 16.3).

A 10 flat JP was inserted under the flap. The flap was inserted and closed in two layers. The deep dermal layer was approximated with several interrupted 3-0 PDS sutures. The skin was closed

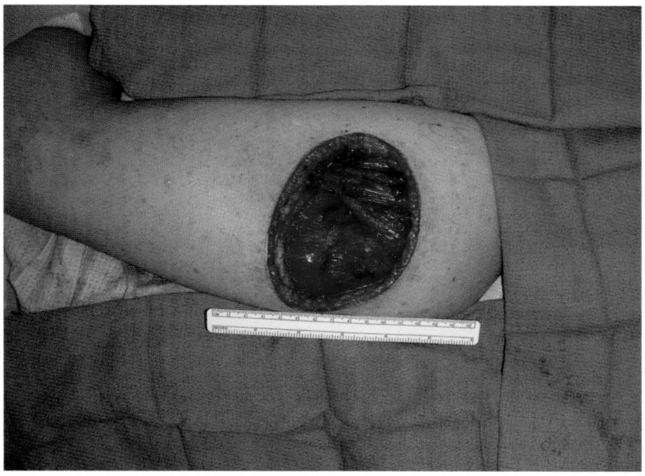

• **Fig. 16.1** An intraoperative view showing a large skin defect over the patient's left upper arm after a wide local excision of residual sarcoma. The underlying muscles were visible.

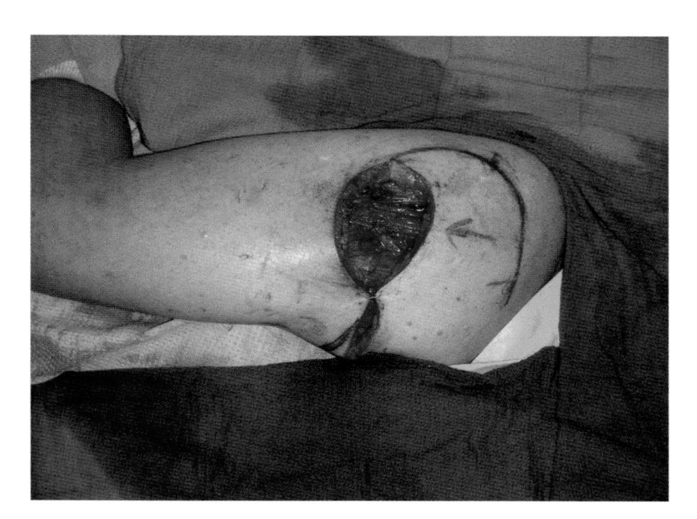

• **Fig. 16.2** An intraoperative view showing design of the large adjacent skin rotational flap and a temporary closure of the portion of the skin defect.

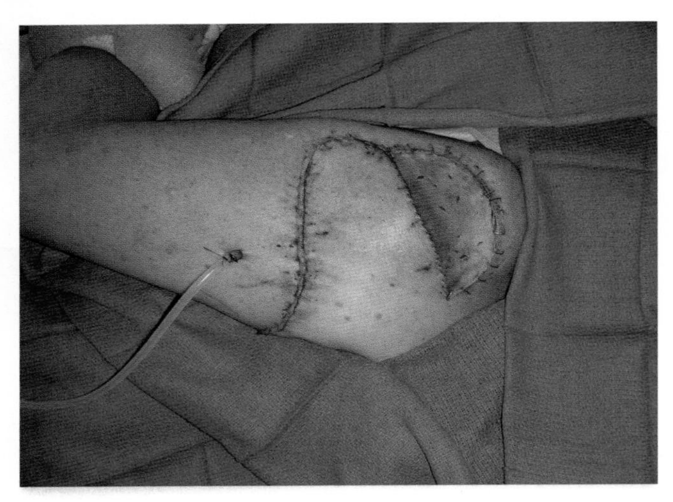

• **Fig. 16.3** An intraoperative view showing immediate result of the adjacent skin rotational flap inset and a split-thickness skin graft for the flap donor site's closure.

with several interrupted 3-0 Monocryl suture in half-buried mattress fashion.

Follow-Up Results

The patient did well postoperatively without any complications related to the skin rotational flap reconstruction. She was observed overnight in the hospital and discharged home next day. The drain was removed during the 1-week follow-up visit. The flap site and skin graft sites healed well.

Final Outcome

The adjacent skin rotational flap site well healed without any problems. (She returned to her normal life and was initially followed by our surgical oncology service for routine cancer follow-up. She then relocated to aother state.

Pearls for Success

A large skin defect of the lateral arm can be reconstructed with a large skin rotational flap from the adjacent area. The portion of such a defect can be closed primarily with significant undermining and the rest of the defect is closed with an adjacent skin rotational flap. Because it is a random flap, its base should be designed wide enough so that it is more reliable. If a robust perforator can be identified, the flap can be designed less wide and can even be elevated as an island flap. A split-thickness skin graft is selected for closure of the flap's donor site. A sheet skin graft may provide a better cosmetic outcome once it heals.

Recommended Readings

Cayci C, Carlsen BT, Saint-Cyr M. Optimizing functional and aesthetic outcomes of upper limb soft tissue reconstruction. *Hand Clinic*. 2014;30:225–238.

Jordan SW, Wayne JD, Dumanian GA. The pedicled lateral arm flap for oncologic reconstruction near the shoulder. *Ann Plast Surg*. 2015; 74:30–33.

Knaus WJ, Alluri R, Bakri K, Iorio ML. Oncologic reconstruction of the hand and upper extremity: maximizing functional outcomes. *J Surg Onco*. 2016;113:946–954.

Sabapathy SR, Bajantri B. Indications, selection, and use of distant pedicled flap for upper limb reconstruction. *Hand Clinic*. 2014;30:185–199.

17 Elbow Reconstruction

Clinical Presentation

An 18-year-old White male had multiple subcutaneous rheumatoid nodules over his left elbow. He complained about pain and discomfort in the area and agreed to surgical resection to remove the subcutaneous lesions. Because of the large area affected, a large soft tissue defect was anticipated after surgical resection for these lesions (Fig. 17.1).

Operative Plan and Special Considerations

Based on the size and location of the skin defect in the lateral elbow over the weight-bearing area, a more durable soft tissue reconstruction should be performed. The size of the soft tissue defect is too large for a lateral arm skin rotational flap. A pedicled radial forearm fasciocutaneous flap would be a good option for such a reconstruction. The flap is reliable and has a long pedicle for easy flap inset. It can provide durable soft tissue coverage to this weight-bearing area of the elbow. The Allen test should be done preoperatively to evaluate the patency and adequacy of the ulnar artery system when the radial artery is sacrificed during the flap elevation to ensure an adequate blood supply to the hand.

Operative Procedures

Under general anesthesia, the resection of rheumatoid nodules was done under a tourniquet control (Fig. 17.2). All lesions and the affected skins were excised, which resulted in a 10 × 6 cm skin defect (Fig. 17.3). A proximally based pedicled radial forearm flap was designed in the same forearm, oriented longitudinally, based on the distance from the defect to the distal tip of the flap (Fig. 17.4). The flap dissection was again under tourniquet control. Once the skin incision had been made through the fascia, subfascial dissection was performed to elevate the skin paddle including the pedicle vessels. Once the distal radial artery and its venae comitantes as well as the cephalic vein were divided with hemoclips, the skin paddle was elevated freely. With a zigzag incision proximally to the skin paddle, the dissection of the pedicle in the forearm was performed between the flexor carpi radialis and brachioradialis muscles to the antecubital fossa. The flap was tunneled, based on the radial vessels proximally, through a skin bridge between the forearm and the elbow defect and was easily inset into the elbow defect. The flap was approximated to the adjacent skin with interrupted 3-0 nylon in half-buried horizontal mattress fashion. A drain was placed under the flap before final closure (Fig. 17.5).

The forearm donor site skin incision was closed in two layers. An unmeshed split-thickness skin graft, harvested from the lateral thigh, was placed on the flap donor site, approximated to the adjacent skin with skin staples, and secured with a tie-over dressing.

Follow-Up Results

The patient did well postoperatively without any complications related to the pedicled radial forearm flap reconstruction to the

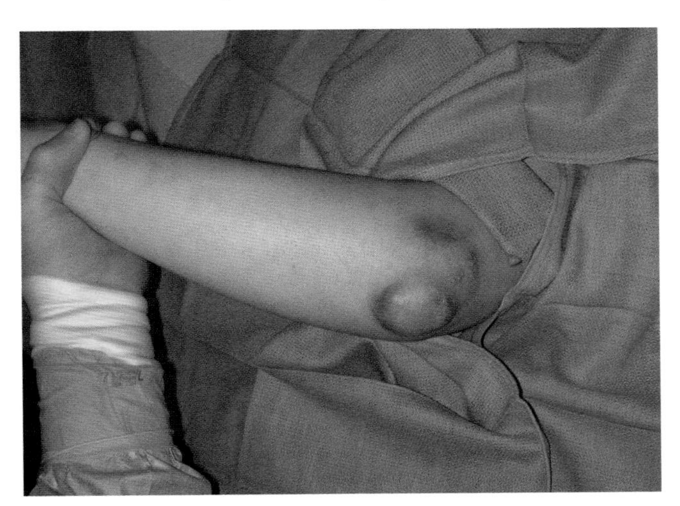

• **Fig. 17.1** A preoperative view showing multiple subcutaneous rheumatoid nodules in the left elbow.

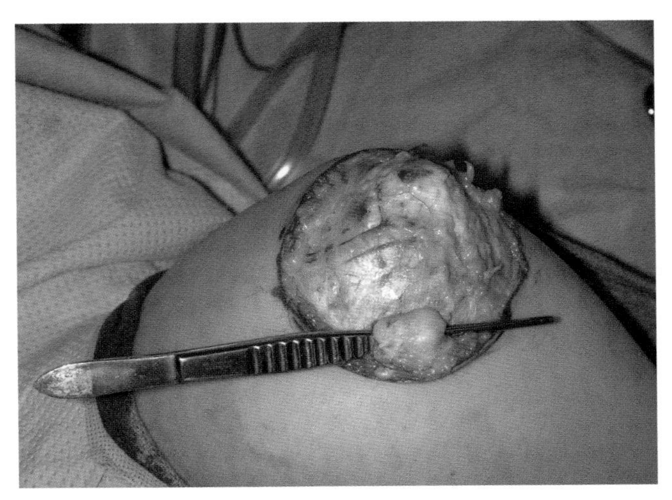

• **Fig. 17.2** An intraoperative view showing a rheumatoid nodule during the resection under tourniquet control.

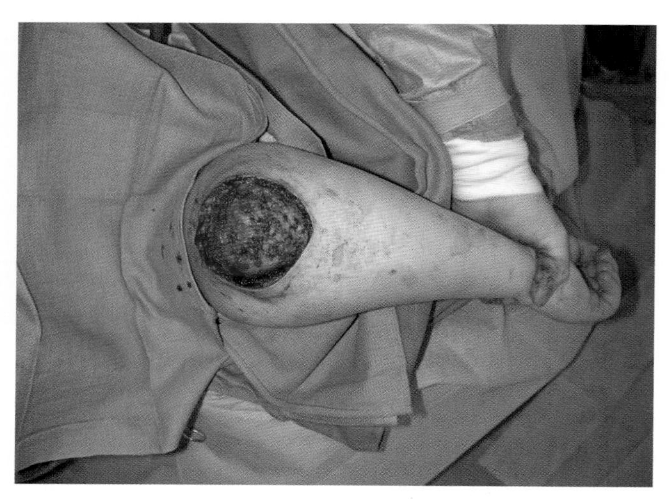

• **Fig. 17.3** An intraoperative view showing a 10 × 6 cm soft tissue defect after excision of multiple rheumatoid nodules.

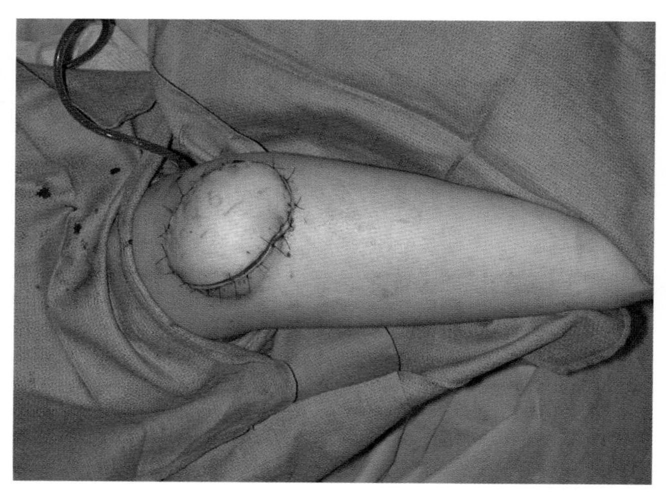

• **Fig. 17.5** An intraoperative view showing immediate result after placement of the pedicled radial forearm flap for closure of a large elbow soft tissue wound.

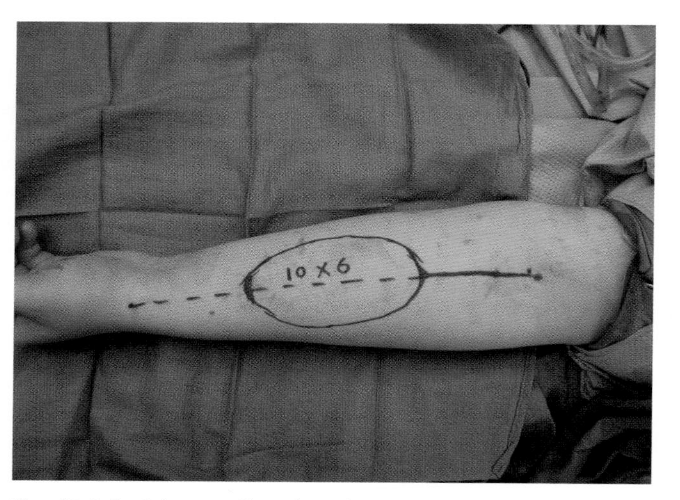

• **Fig. 17.4** An intraoperative view showing design of the proximally based pedicled radial forearm flap.

elbow. He was observed overnight in the hospital and discharged home next day. The drain was removed during the 1-week follow-up visit. His elbow flap site and the flap donor site wound healed well.

Final Outcome

The left elbow flap reconstruction site healed well without any problems. He has had durable soft tissue coverage over his elbow after excision of multiple rheumatoid nodules. He resumed his normal activities and has been followed by the plastic surgery service as needed.

Pearls for Success

A proximally based pedicle radial forearm flap can be used to cover a sizable elbow wound. The flap's dissection is relatively fast and the flap's inset is also relatively easy following a standard arc of the rotation to the elbow. Because the flap has two venous drainage systems, venous congestion may occur if the cephalic vein is not included in the flap. An intraoperative decision is needed to decide whether the cephalic vein should be included in the flap. A bloodless flap dissection can be performed under tourniquet control. The flap donor site is usually closed with an unmeshed skin graft.

Recommended Readings

Choudry UH, Moran SL, Li S, Khan S. Soft-tissue coverage of the elbow: an outcome analysis and reconstructive algorithm. *Plast Reconstr Surg.* 2007;119:1852–1857.

Giovanni di Summa P, Sapino G, Guillier D, Dash J, Hart A, Raffoul W. Reverse-flow versus perforator propeller lateral arm flap for elbow reconstruction. *Ann Plast Surg.* 2020;84:535–554.

Jones NF, Jarrahy R, Kaufman MR. Pedicled and free radial forearm flaps for reconstruction of the elbow, wrist, and hand. *Plast Reconstr Surg.* 2008;121:887–898.

Megarle K, Sauerbier M, German G. The evolution of the pedicled radial forearm flap. *Hand.* 2010;5:7–42.

Murakami M, Ono S, Ishii N, Hyakusoku H. Reconstruction of elbow region defects using radial collateral artery perforator (RCAP)-based propeller flaps. *J Plast Reconstr Aesthetic Surg.* 2012;65:1418–1421.

Stevanovic M, Sharpe F. Soft-tissue coverage of the elbow. *Plast Reconstr Surg.* 2013;132:387e–402e.

18

Forearm Reconstruction

Clinical Presentation

A 24-year-old Black American female sustained an avulsion injury to her left forearm wound secondary to a motor vehicle accident. She sustained a large complex soft tissue wound, measuring 18 × 8 cm, in the left volar forearm with multiple flexor digitorum superficialis muscle injuries and a transection of the median nerve with a 5-cm gap. The radial artery and its accompanied veins within the wound were also transected (Figs. 18.1 and 18.2). The plastic surgery service was consulted to provide a soft tissue reconstruction for her forearm as well as the medial nerve reconstruction once she was cleared by the trauma service.

Operative Plan and Special Considerations

Based on the location and size of the soft tissue defect in the forearm as well as the nature of the reconstruction to provide a good skin coverage to the forearm, a free anterolateral thigh (ALT) perforator flap was offered to this patient for the reconstruction of such a large forearm wound. The ulnar artery system was also evaluated for its patency and adequacy to ensure an adequate blood supply to the hand. In addition, perforators in each thigh's potential donor site were mapped by duplex scan so that a preferred site for free ALT perforator flap harvest could be chosen. The sural nerve from the left leg was prepared as a nerve graft donor site for the cable nerve grafting of the medial nerve gap.

Operative Procedures

Under general anesthesia, the procedure started by debriding the left forearm wound followed by Pulsavac irrigation. After debridement, all flexor digitorum superficialis muscles were repaired accordingly with 3-0 vicryl suture and both proximal and distal ends of the median nerve in the forearm were identified after further dissection. Both nerve ends were tagged with a 4-0 Prolene suture. The zigzag incisions were made proximally toward the antecubital fossa. The stump of the radial artery was identified and dissected further proximally toward the bifurcation of the radial artery and the ulnar artery in order to make sure the artery microvascular anastomosis would be outside the zone of injury. The vena comitans and the radial artery appeared to be very small. However, the superficial medial antecubital vein appeared to be a good size and could be used as a recipient vein for venous microvascular anastomosis.

An 18 × 8 cm skin paddle was marked within the left ALT territory. Three perforators were identified by preoperative duplex scan (Fig. 18.3). With suprafascial dissection, two perforators were identified but only one appeared to be large with a strong arterial signal. Therefore, the flap could be based on this larger perforator. The fascia was incised around the perforator. After a course of septocutaneous dissection, the descending branch of the lateral circumplex femoral vessel was identified. The end of the descending branch distal to the junction of the perforator was divided and two visible motor nerves were preserved. The pedicle dissection was performed between the vastus lateralis and rectus femoris muscles toward the profunda vessels. The pedicle vessels were individually separated and divided with hemoclips and the flap dissection was completed (Fig. 18.4).

The pedicle was prepared under loop magnification. One artery and two veins were identified. The artery was flushed with heparinized saline solution. One good vein was selected for microvascular anastomosis. Both microvascular anastomoses were performed under a microscope. The arterial microanastomosis to the radial artery stump was performed in an end-to-end fashion with interrupted 8-0 nylon sutures (Fig. 18.5). The venous microanastomosis to the superficial antecubital vein was also performed in an end-to-end fashion with a 2-mm coupler (Fig. 18.6). Once all the clamps had been released, the flap appeared to be well perfused. The flap was temporarily inset into the forearm wound.

A skin incision was made on the left lateral foot from the level of the lateral malleolus to the middle leg. The sural nerve was identified. Two 7-cm nerve grafts were taken and used as cable grafts. Each proximal end of the sural nerve was buried into the adjacent muscle and secured with a purse string suture to prevent neuroma formation. Each distal end was secured with hemoclips. The sural nerve donor site was closed in two layers.

The cable nerve grafting was performed under a microscope. An 11 blade was used for wound-freshening of the median nerve stump and each cable nerve graft was prepared under a microscope (Fig. 18.7). Each nerve graft was sutured to the median nerve stump with six or seven interrupted 8-0 nylon epineural repairs for each end. A total of two cable grafts were used to reconstruct the nerve gap (Fig. 18.8).

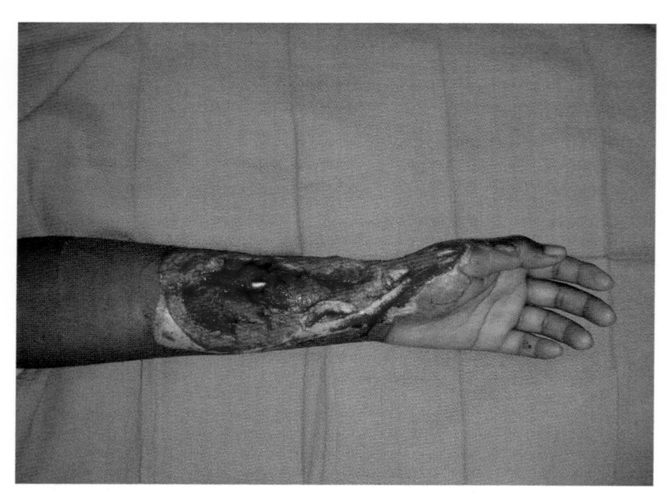

• **Fig. 18.1** Intraoperative view showing a large left forearm wound with the exposed forearm muscles, bone, and medial nerve.

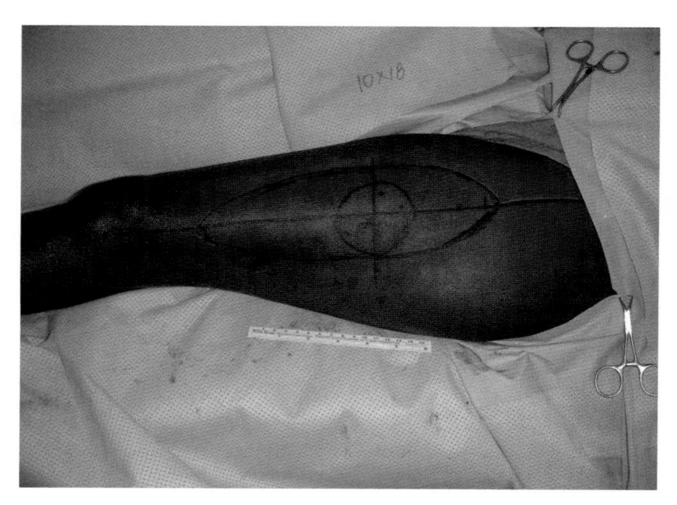

• **Fig. 18.3** Intraoperative view showing the design of a left anterolateral thigh perforator flap. Three perforators were identified during preoperative duplex scanning.

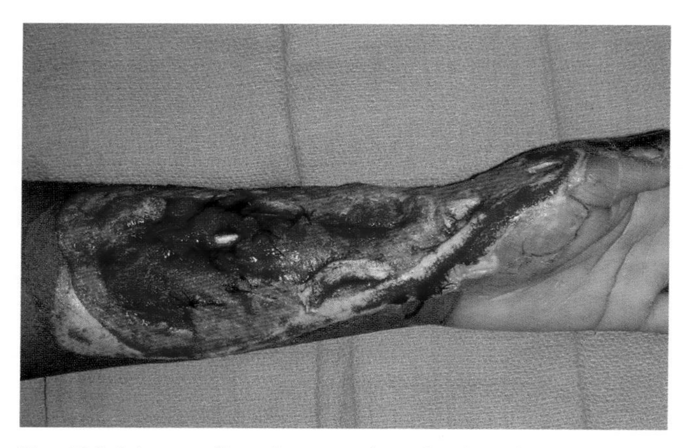

• **Fig. 18.2** Intraoperative close-up view showing the large forearm wound.

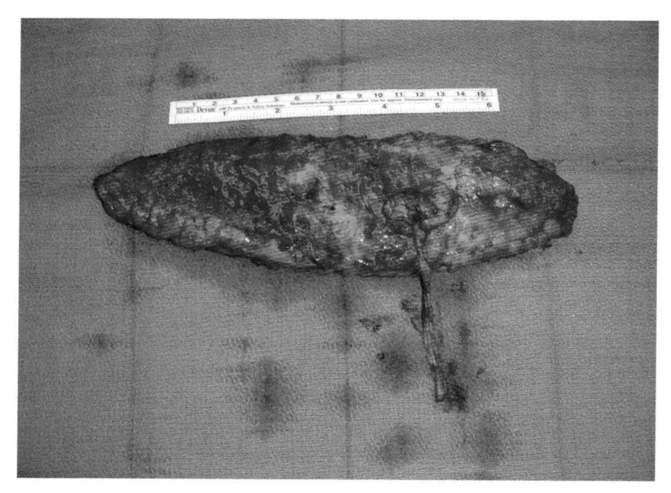

• **Fig. 18.4** Intraoperative view showing completion of a free anterolateral thigh perforator flap dissection.

The two Penrose drains were inserted under each side of the flap and the entire flap was inset into the forearm wound with several interrupted 3-0 Monocryl sutures in a half-buried horizontal mattress fashion (Fig. 18.9).

The left ALT flap donor site was approximated in three layers. The fascial repair was approximated with several interrupted 2-0 PDS sutures. The deep dermal layer repair was approximated with several interrupted 3-0 Monocryl sutures. The skin closure was reinforced with Dermabond.

Management of Complications

Although the ALT flap appeared to be viable for the first few weeks postoperatively, the patient unfortunately developed distal flap necrosis, possibly because of the direct pressure from the splint used postoperatively to immobilize her forearm (Fig. 18.10). She was taken back to the operating room about 2 months later for debridement of necrotic tissue and additional skin grafting for the wound closure. The full-thickness skin graft was harvested from the extension of the left thigh incision for the previous ALT flap harvest. The harvested skin graft was defatted and several small stab wounds were made with a 15 blade. The skin graft was placed on the left forearm wound and secured with 5-0 chromic sutures (Fig. 18.11).

Follow-Up Results

The patient did well postoperatively after the second operation. Both the ALT flap and full-thickness skin graft sites healed well without additional complications (Fig. 18.12). She underwent extensive physical therapy for her left forearm and hand.

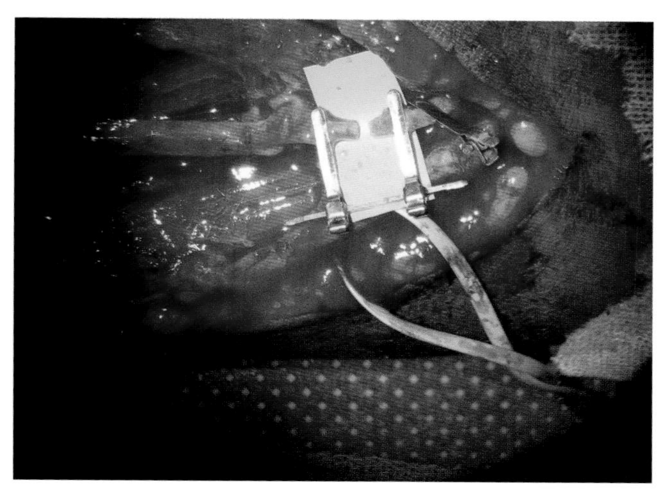

• **Fig. 18.5** Intraoperative view showing the preparation and readiness of an end-to-end arterial microvascular anastomosis under a microscope.

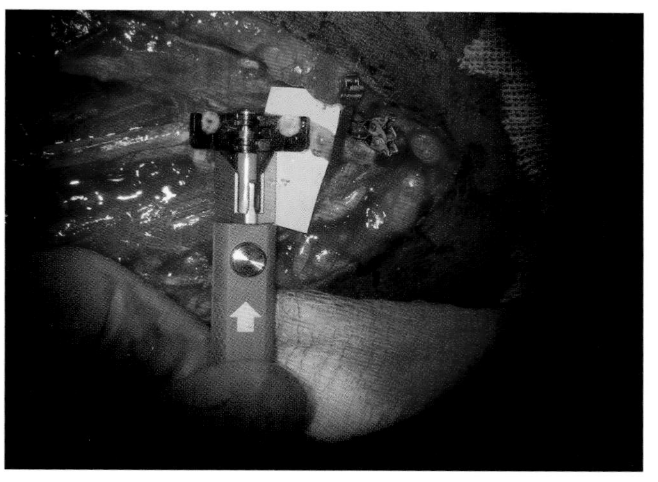

• **Fig. 18.6** Intraoperative view showing the preparation and readiness of an end-to-end venous microvascular anastomosis with a coupling device under a microscope.

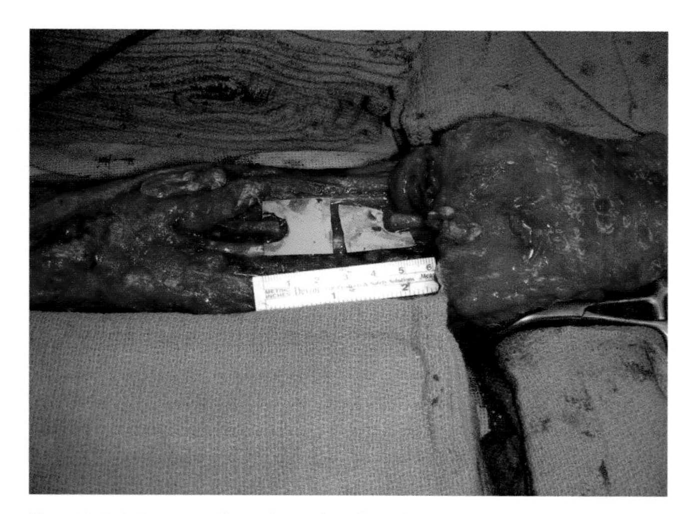

• **Fig. 18.7** Intraoperative view showing the preparation of the median nerve reconstruction under a microscope.

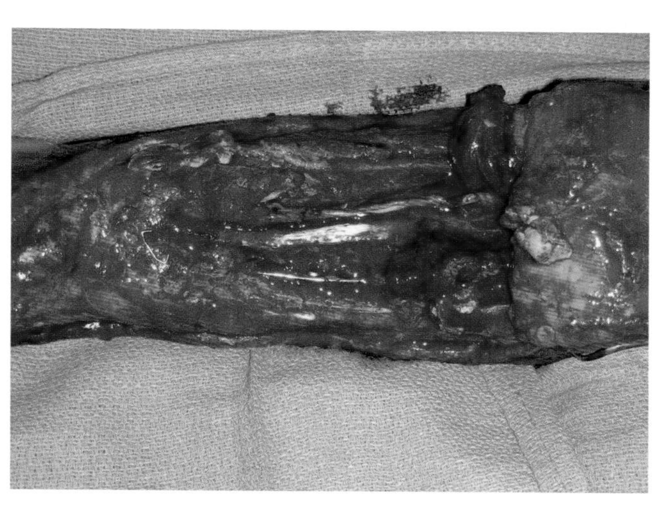

• **Fig. 18.8** Intraoperative view showing the completion of the median nerve reconstruction with capable nerve grafts under a microscope.

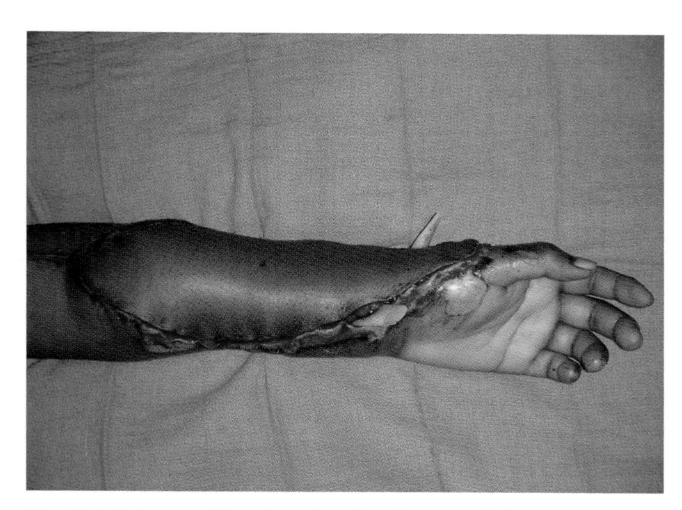

• **Fig. 18.9** Intraoperative view showing the completion of a free anterolateral thigh flap reconstruction for the forearm wound coverage.

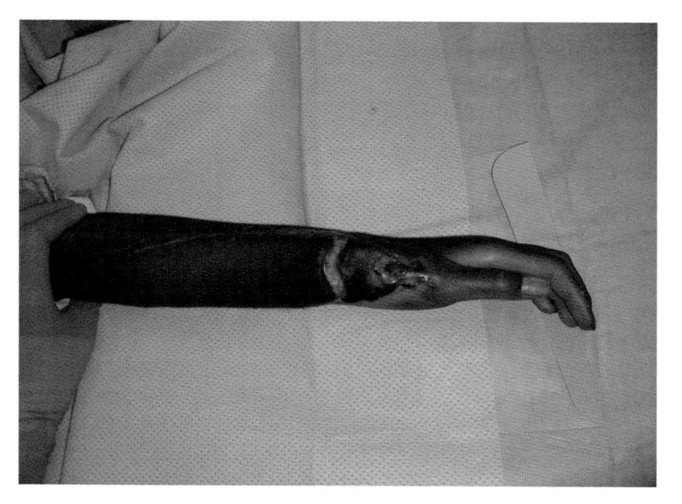

• **Fig. 18.10** The result at 2-month follow-up showing distal flap necrosis of the anterolateral thigh flap.

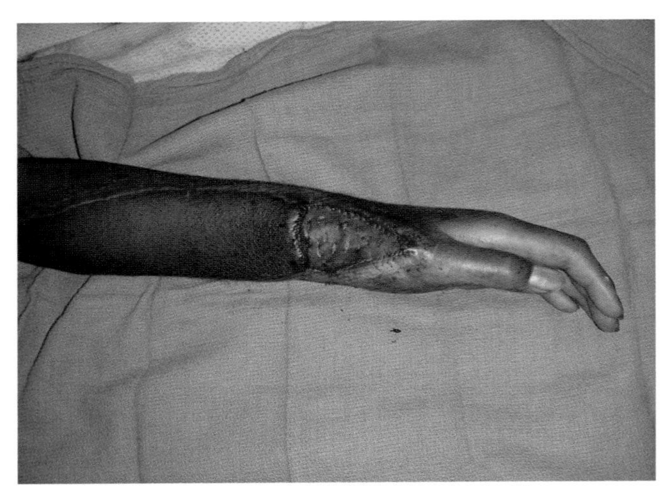

• **Fig. 18.11** Intraoperative views showing the placement of a full-thickness skin graft to the distal forearm wound after debridement.

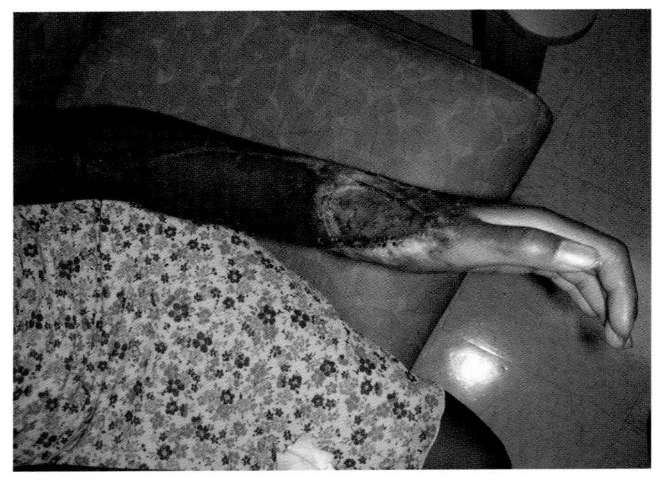

• **Fig. 18.12** The result at 2-week follow-up after reoperation showing well-healed skin graft site in the distal forearm.

Final Outcome

Her forearm reconstruction site healed well and the final contour of her left forearm appeared to be quite good (Figs. 18.13 and 18.14). The ALT flap donor site also had minimal scarring (Fig. 18.15). She has resumed her normal activities and there are signs of medial nerve regeneration. She has been followed by the plastic surgery service as needed.

Pearls for Success

A free ALT perforator flap can be a good option for reconstruction of a large forearm wound. In this case, an 18 × 8 cm soft tissue wound in the forearm can be reconstructed based on a single perforator. The ALT flap donor site can often be closed primarily without a skin graft. However, its flap dissection does have a learning curve and can be time-consuming. Perforator mapping with duplex scan can be helpful in selecting an easy side for perforator flap dissection. Either the radial artery or the ulnar artery stump can be used as a recipient artery, but careful intraoperative assessment should be made to ensure the recipient artery

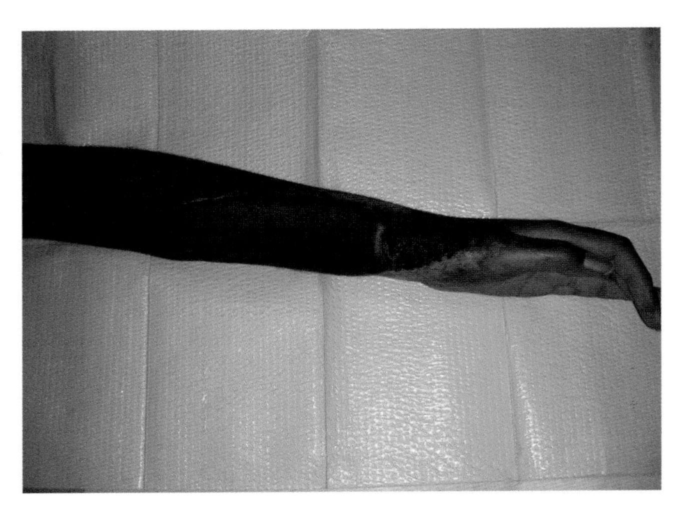

• **Fig. 18.13** The result at 4-week follow-up after reoperation showing well-healed flap and skin graft sites.

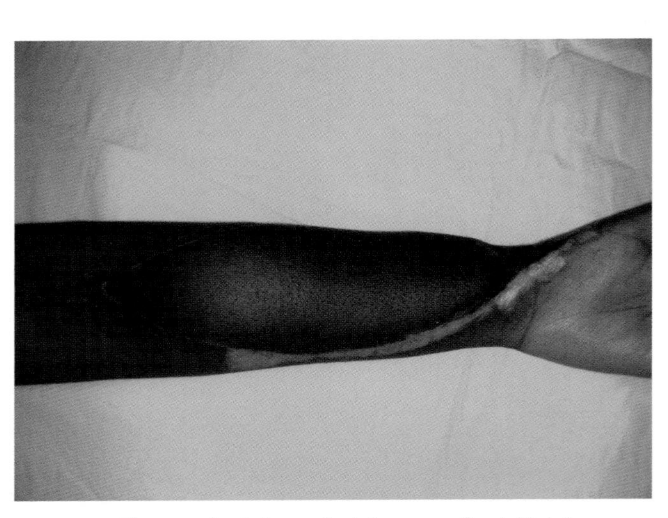

• **Fig. 18.14** The result at 6-month follow-up after initial flap reconstruction showing well-healed flap and skin graft sites.

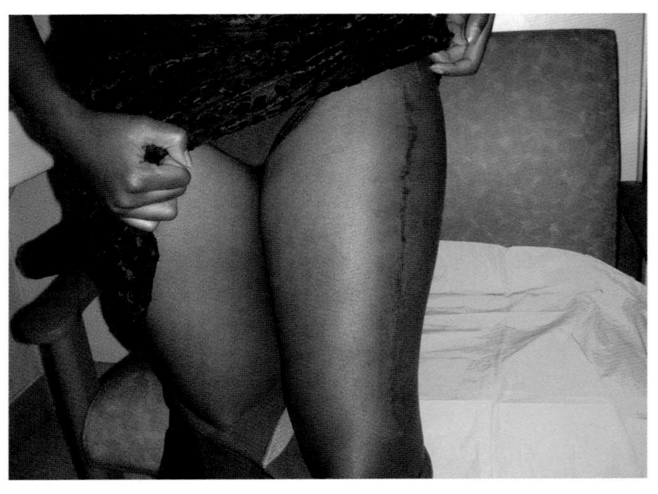

• **Fig. 18.15** The result at 6-month follow-up after initial flap reconstruction showing minimal scarring from the anterolateral thigh flap donor site.

is not within the zone of the injury. A splint, used to immobilize the forearm and hand postoperatively, should be placed carefully and care should be taken not to compress any part of the flap.

Recommended Readings

Engel H, Gazyakan E, Cheng MH, Piel D, German G, Giessler G. Customized reconstruction with the free anterolateral thigh perforator flap. *Microsurgery*. 2008;28:489–494.

Sabapathy SR, Bajantri B. Indications, selection, and use of distant pedicled flap for upper limb reconstruction. *Hand Clin*. 2014;30: 185–199.

Spindler N, Al-Benna S, Ring A, et al. *GMS Interdisciplinary Plast Recon Surg*. 2015;4:1–8.

Wei FC, Jain W, Celik N, Chen HC, Chuang DCC, Lin CH. Have we found an ideal soft- tissue flap? An experience with 672 anterolateral thigh flaps. *Plast Recon Surg*. 2002;109:2219–2226.

19 Dorsal Hand Reconstruction

Clinical Presentation

A 41-year-old White male had a degloving injury of his right hand as a result of a motor vehicle accident. He sustained a large soft tissue open wound, measuring 9 × 8 cm, over his dorsal hand with the underlying bones and extensor tendons exposed. He was managed initially by the trauma service and the plastic surgery service was consulted for soft tissue reconstruction of the dorsal hand wound (Fig. 19.1). Preoperative evaluation using the Allen test confirmed an adequate blood supply to the right hand.

Operative Plan and Special Considerations

Based on the size and location of the soft tissue defect over the dorsal hand, a reversed radial forearm fasciocutaneous flap can be a good option. The flap is reliable and has a long pedicle for easy flap inset. It can provide durable soft tissue coverage to a dorsal hand wound. The Allen test should be performed preoperatively to evaluate the ulnar artery system to ensure there is an adequate blood supply to the hand when the radial artery is sacrificed after the flap elevation. A suprafascial flap dissection can be performed to improve donor site cosmesis after a skin graft procedure for the donor site closure.

Operative Procedures

Under general anesthesia, the dorsal hand wound was debrided (Fig. 19.2). A reversed radial forearm flap was designed and oriented longitudinally and a 10 × 9 cm skin paddle was marked. The proximal incision was determined based on the flap's arc of turnover to cover the dorsal hand wound (Fig. 19.3). The flap dissection was performed under a tourniquet control.

Once the skin incision had been made to the fascia, suprafascial dissection was performed for elevation of the skin paddle. When the dissection was about 1 cm from the pedicle vessels in both medial and lateral directions, subfascial dissection was performed to free the pedicle vessels. Once the proximal radial artery and its venae comitantes and the cephalic vein had been divided with hemoclips, the skin paddle was elevated freely. With a zigzag incision distal to the skin paddle, the dissection of the pedicle in the distal forearm was made between the flexor carpi radialis and brachioradialis to the wrist line. The flap was turned over, based on the radial vessels but in a reverse fashion, through a skin tunnel between the dorsal hand defect and the distal forearm. It was easily inserted into the dorsal hand wound in a reverse fashion without any tension. The flap was approximated to the adjacent skin with interrupted 3-0 Monocryl in half-buried horizontal mattress fashion. A drain was placed under the flap before the final closure (Fig. 19.4).

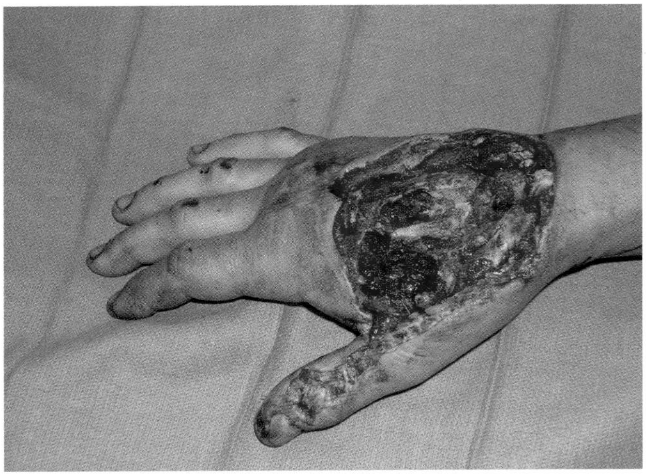

• **Fig. 19.1** A preoperative view showing a large dorsal hand wound after degloving injury.

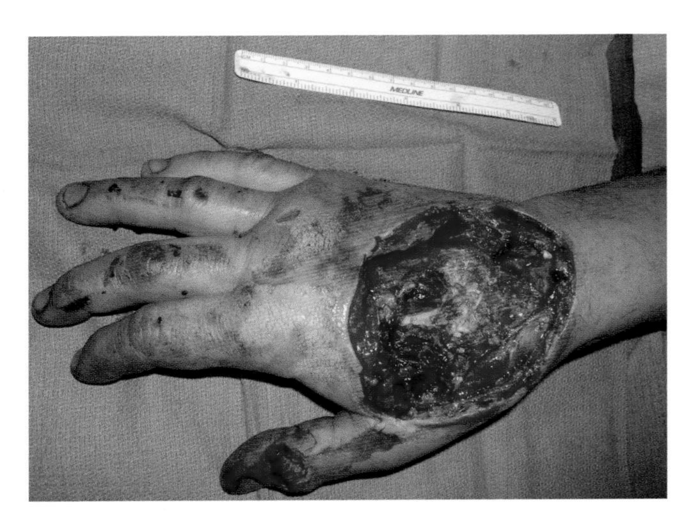

• **Fig. 19.2** An intraoperative view showing a 9 × 8 cm dorsal hand wound after debridement in the operating room.

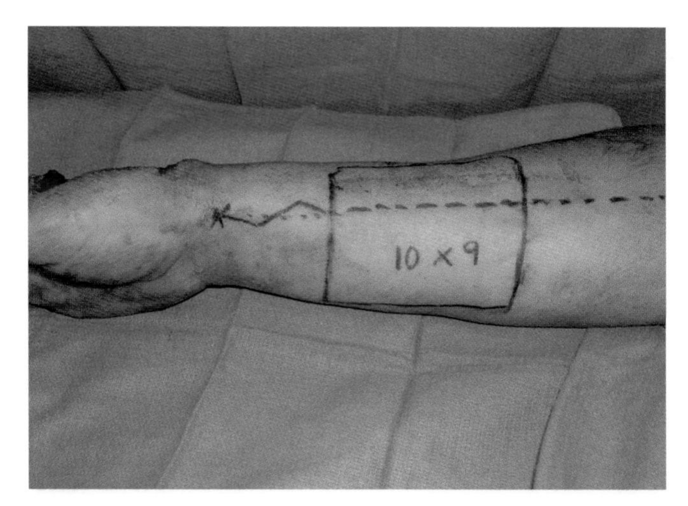

• **Fig. 19.3** An intraoperative view showing design of the reversed radial forearm flap.

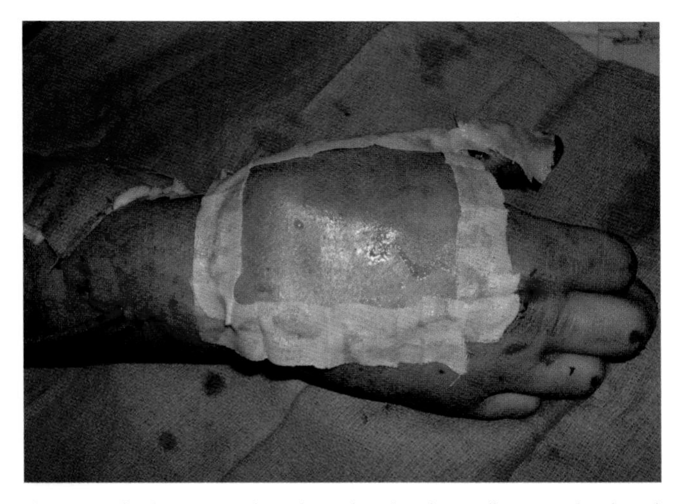

• **Fig. 19.4** An intraoperative view showing immediate result after the reversed radial forearm flap for coverage of a large dorsal hand soft tissue wound. In this case, mild venous congestion of the flap was noticed initially.

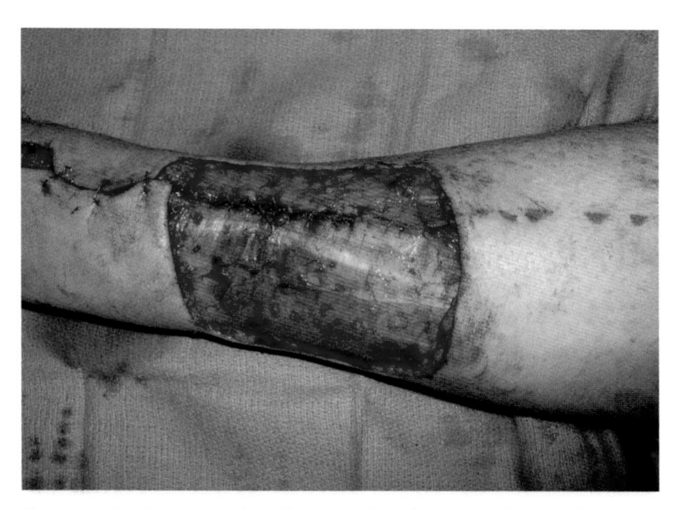

• **Fig. 19.5** An intraoperative view showing the approximated fascia after suprafascial dissection of the reversed radial forearm flap for coverage of a large dorsal hand soft tissue wound.

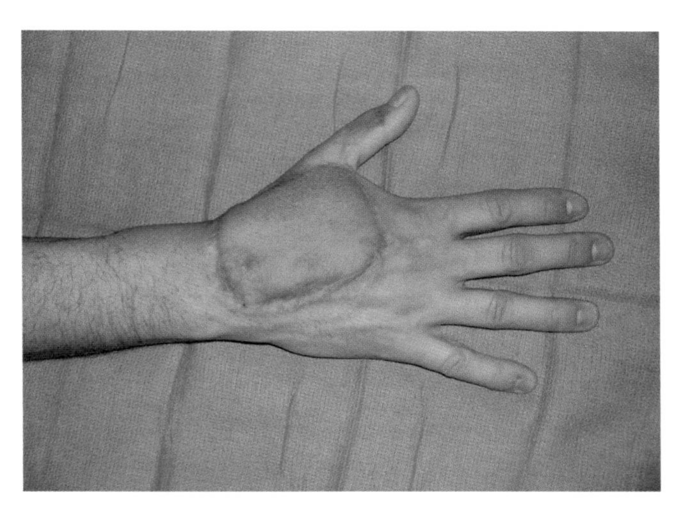

• **Fig. 19.6** The results at 1-year follow-up showing a well-healed durable soft tissue reconstruction for the dorsal hand wound.

The distal forearm donor site skin incision was closed in two layers. The fascial defect in the mid-forearm was approximated with a 3-0 Vicryl suture (Fig. 19.5). An unmeshed split-thickness skin graft, harvested from the lateral thigh, was placed on the flap donor site, approximated to the adjacent normal skin with skin staples, and secured with a tie-over dressing.

Follow-Up Results

The patient did well postoperatively. However, the flap appeared to be congested after the completion of the flap inset but no direct compression or kicking of the pedicle was found. Fortunately, venous congestion was resolved with hand elevation and time. The patient was observed in the hospital for 3 days and discharged home on postoperative day 4. The drain was removed during the 2-week follow-up visit. The dorsal hand flap site and the flap donor site skin graft both healed well.

Final Outcome

The dorsal hand flap reconstruction site healed well without any issues (Fig. 19.6). The patient had durable soft tissue coverage over his dorsal hand. His radial forearm donor site also healed well with minimal scarring (Fig. 19.7). His hand function has almost returned to normal (Fig. 19.8). He resumed his normal activities and has been followed by the plastic surgery service as needed.

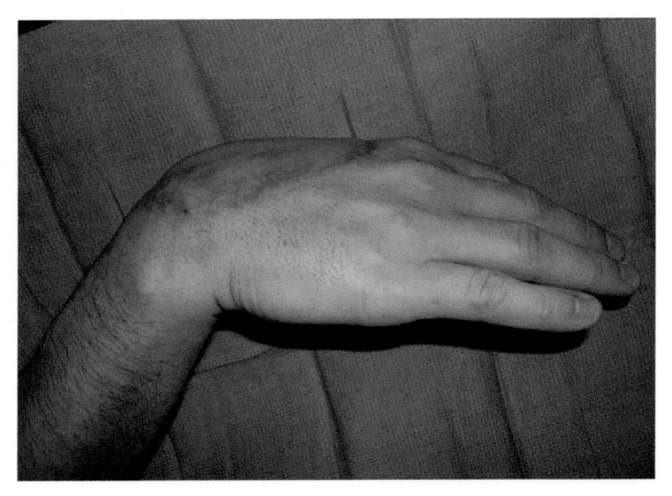

• **Fig. 19.7** The results at 1-year follow-up showing a good range of motion for the patient's right hand after a reversed radial forearm reconstruction for the dorsal hand wound.

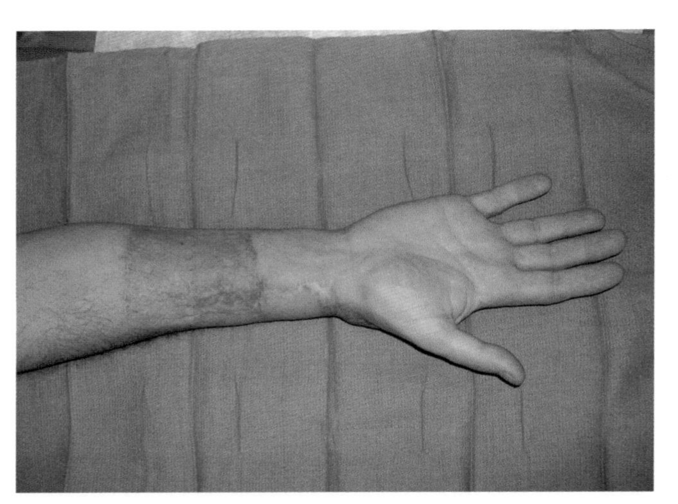

• **Fig. 19.8** The results at 1-year follow-up showing a well-healed flap donor site with minimal scarring and good cosmesis.

Pearls for Success

A reverse radial forearm flap can be a good option for soft tissue coverage of a dorsal hand wound. The flap's dissection is relatively fast and the flap's inset is also relatively easy following a standard arc of the turnover to the dorsal hand. Because the flap is reversed, venous congestion may occur even if the cephalic vein is included within the flap. However, such venous congestion is usually temporary and can be resolved with effective hand elevation postoperatively. Nitropaste or Leech therapy can be added to speed up the resolution of venous congestion. If venous congestion becomes persistent, a supercharge procedure can be added from the cephalic vein within the distal flap to an adjacent vein in the dorsal hand. A bloodless flap dissection can be performed under a tourniquet control. Because suprafascial dissection of the flap is performed, the flap donor site is closed with an unmeshed split-thickness skin graft over the fascia and its cosmetic outcome can be improved.

Recommended Readings

Jones NF, Jarrahy R, Kaufman MR. Pedicled and free radial forearm flaps for reconstruction of the elbow, wrist, and hand. *Plast Reconstr Surg.* 2008;121:887–898.

Lutz BS, Wei FC, Chang SCN, Yang KH, Chen IH. Donor site morbidity after suprafascial elevation of the radial forearm flap: a prospective study in 95 consecutive cases. *Plast Reconstr Surg.* 1999;103:132–137.

Megerle K, Sauerbier M, Germann G. The evolution of the pedicled radial forearm flap. *Hand.* 2010;5:37–42.

Page R, Chang J. Reconstruction of hand soft-tissue defects: alternatives to the radial forearm fasciocutaneous flap. *J Hand Surg.* 2006;31A: 847–856.

Saint-Cyr M, Mujadzic M, Wong C, Hatef D, Lajoie AS, Rohrich RJ. The radial artery pedicle perforator flap: vascular analysis and clinical implications. *Plast Reconstr Surg.* 2010;125:1469–1478.

White CP, Steve Jr AK, Buchel EW, Hayakawa TE, Morris SF. Reverse radial artery flap perforator anatomy and clinical applications. *Ann Plast Surg.* 2016;77:345–349.

20 Palmar Hand Reconstruction

Clinical Presentation

A 29-year-old White female had a thermal burn injury to her right hand. She sustained a large soft tissue open wound, measuring 9 × 6 cm, over her palmar hand with the underlying bones and flexor tendons exposed. The palmar wound also extended to the volar thumb. She was managed initially by the burn service and the plastic surgery service was consulted for soft tissue reconstruction (Fig. 20.1). A preoperative Allen test confirmed an adequate blood supply to the right hand via the ulnar artery system.

Operative Plan and Special Considerations

Based on the location and size of the soft tissue defect over the palmar hand, a reverse radial forearm fasciocutaneous flap could also be a good option. The flap is reliable and has a long pedicle for an easy flap inset. It can provide durable soft tissue coverage to a palmar hand wound. The Allen test should be performed preoperatively to evaluate the ulnar artery system to ensure there is an adequate blood supply to the hand when the radial artery is sacrificed after the flap elevation. A suprafascial rather than subfascial flap dissection can be performed to improve donor site cosmesis after a skin graft procedure for the donor site closure.

Operative Procedures

Under general anesthesia, the entire palmar hand wound was debrided. A reverse radial forearm flap was designed and oriented horizontally. A large skin paddle, measuring 6 × 9 cm, was marked. The proximal incision was determined based on the flap's arc of turnover to cover the entire palmar hand wound including the thumb (Fig. 20.2). The flap dissection was performed under a tourniquet control.

Once the skin incision had been made to the fascia, suprafascial dissection was performed for elevation of the skin paddle. When the dissection was about 1 cm from the pedicle vessels in both medial and lateral directions, subfascial dissection was performed to free the pedicle vessels. The proximal radial artery and its venae comitantes and the cephalic vein were divided with hemoclips and the skin paddle was elevated freely. With a zigzag incision distal to the skin paddle, the dissection of the pedicle in the distal forearm was performed between the flexor carpi radialis and brachioradialis as far as to the wrist line. The flap was turned over, based on the radial vessels in a reverse fashion, through the skin bridge between the palmar hand defect and the distal forearm. The flap was easily inset into the palmar hand wound in a reverse fashion without any tension. The flap was approximated to the adjacent skin with interrupted 3-0 Monocryl sutures in half-buried horizontal

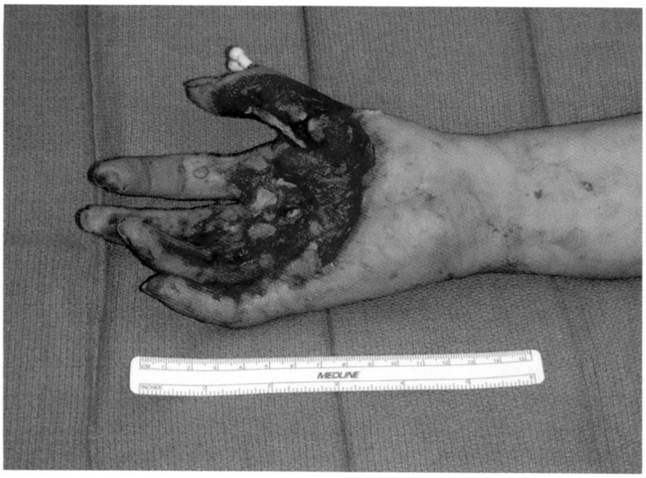

• **Fig. 20.1** A preoperative view showing a large palmar hand wound including volar aspect of the thumb.

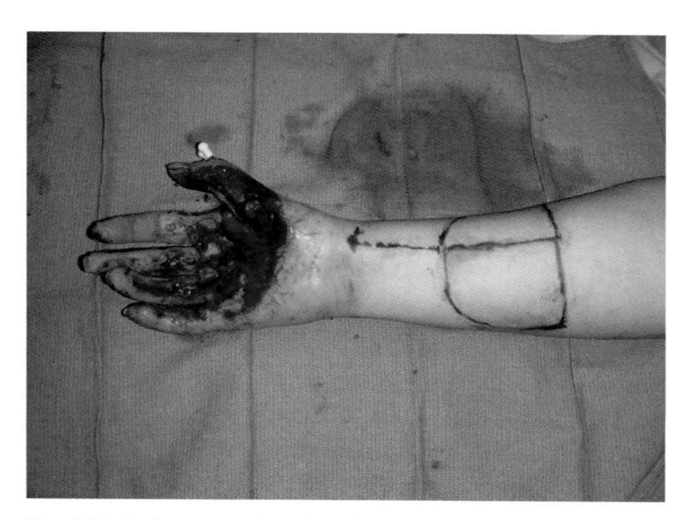

• **Fig. 20.2** An intraoperative view showing a 9 × 6 cm palmar hand wound after debridement in the operating room and design of the reverse radial forearm flap.

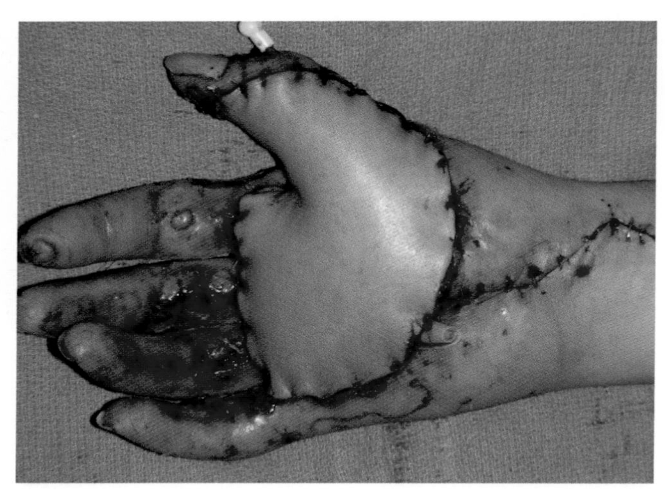

• **Fig. 20.3** An intraoperative view showing immediate result after the reverse radial forearm flap for closure of a large palmar hand soft tissue wound involving the thumb.

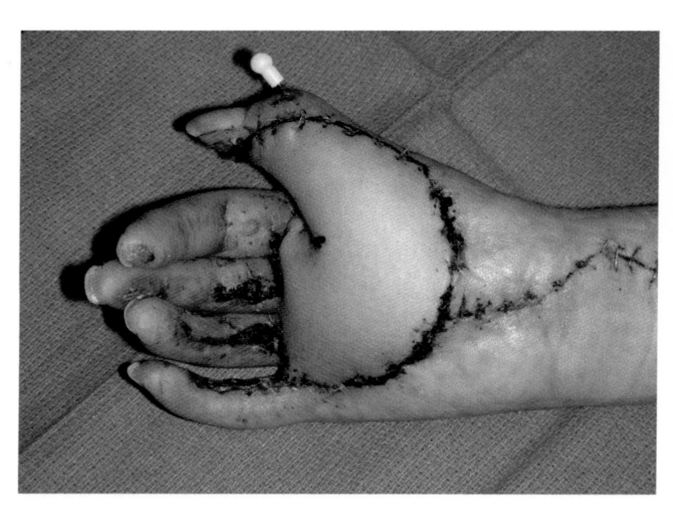

• **Fig. 20.5** The results at 10-day follow-up showing good healing of the durable soft tissue coverage for the palmar hand wound.

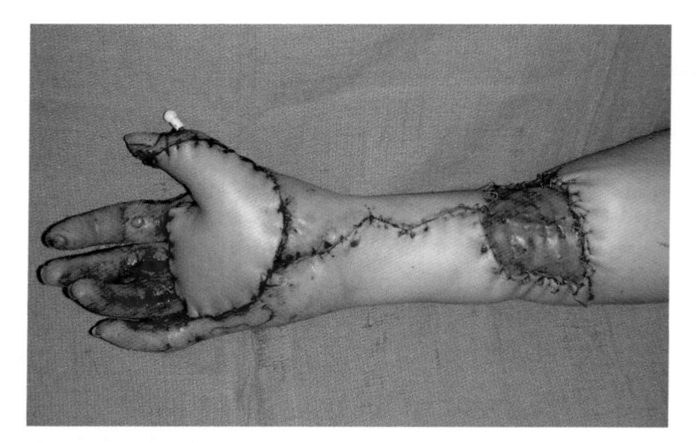

• **Fig. 20.4** An intraoperative view showing the placement of a sheet split-thickness skin graft to the approximated fascia for closure of the flap donor site skin defect.

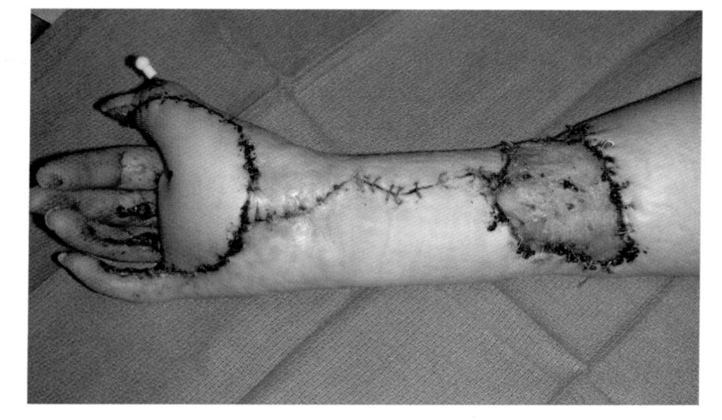

• **Fig. 20.6** The results at 10-day follow-up showing good healing of the flap donor site after split-thickness skin graft.

mattress fashion. A Penrose drain was placed under the flap before the final closure (Fig. 20.3).

The distal forearm donor site skin incision was closed in one layer either with skin staples or 3-0 Monocryl sutures. The fascial defect in the mid-forearm was approximated with a running 3-0 Vicryl suture. An unmeshed split-thickness skin graft, harvested from the lateral thigh, was placed on the flap donor site, approximated to the adjacent normal skin with skin staples, and secured with a tie-over dressing (Fig. 20.4).

Follow-Up Results

The patient did well postoperatively without any complications related to the reverse radial forearm flap reconstruction for the palmar hand wound. She was observed in hospital for 3 days and discharged home on postoperative day 4. The Penrose drain was removed during the first week follow-up visit. The palmar hand flap site and the flap donor site skin graft healed well (Figs. 20.5 and 20.6).

Final Outcome

The palmar hand flap reconstruction site healed well without any complications. The patient has durable soft tissue coverage over her palmar hand including the thumb. Her radial forearm donor site has also healed well with minimal scarring. She underwent vigorous hand therapy and has been followed by the plastic surgery service as needed.

Pearls for Success

A reverse radial forearm flap can also be a good option for soft tissue coverage of a palmar hand wound. The flap's dissection is relatively fast and the flap's inset is also relatively easy following a standard arc of the turnover to the palmar hand. Some degree of venous congestion may occur in the beginning but it can be resolved with effective hand elevation. However, Nitropaste or leech therapy can be added to speed up the resolution of venous congestion. If venous congestion becomes persistent, a supercharge procedure can be applied. A bloodless flap dissection can be performed under a tourniquet control. Because suprafascial dissection of the flap is performed, the flap donor site can be closed with a sheet split-thickness skin graft over the fascia with good long-term cosmetic outcome.

Recommended Readings

Chang SM, Hou CL, Zhang F, Lineaweaver WC, Chen ZW, Gu YD. Distally based radial forearm flap with preservation of the radial artery: anatomic, experimental, and clinical studies. *Microsurgery*. 2003;23:328–337.

Jones NF, Jarrahy R, Kaufman MR. Pedicled and free radial forearm flaps for reconstruction of the elbow, wrist, and hand. *Plast Reconstr Surg*. 2008;121:887–898.

Lo S, Sebastin S, Tsai L, Pin PY. Reverse radial forearm flap perforator used in digital revascularization. *Hand*. 2007;2:155–158.

Saint-Cyr M, Mujadzic M, Wong C, Hatef D, Lajoie AS, Rohrich RJ. The radial artery pedicle perforator flap: vascular analysis and clinical implications. *Plast Reconstr Surg*. 2010;125:1469–1478.

SECTION 3

Chest, Abdomen, and Back

21 Sternal Reconstruction

CASE 1

Clinical Presentation

A 72-year-old Iranian male with multiple medical problems, including coronary artery disease, severe aortic valve stenosis, chronic occlusive pulmonary disease, and congestive heart failure, underwent coronary artery bypass grafting and aortic valve replacement as part of the preparation for a total gastrectomy because of a newly diagnosed large gastric carcinoma. He had a complicated postoperative course with prolonged treatment in the intensive care unit. He developed a dehiscence of the lower sternal wound and was urgently taken to the operating room by the cardiothoracic service for sternal wound debridement (Fig. 21.1). All wires were removed during the initial debridement. The plastic surgery service was asked to provide soft tissue coverage to his sternal wound.

Operative Plan and Special Considerations

Additional more aggressive debridement should be performed first to control local infection and good sternal soft tissue condition. The goal of reconstruction would include obliteration of the sternal dead space with a well-vascularized tissue and the sternal wound closure. Bilateral pectoral major myocutaneous advancement flaps are a good option for this kind of sternal reconstruction. Each side of the pectoral major myocutaneous flap can be elevated individually and advanced toward the midline of the sternal wound so that the sternal soft tissue wound can be approximated without tension. The anterior rectus sheath can also be elevated with each side of the pectoral major muscle to provide additional tissue coverage for better lower sternal wound closure. Such combined bilateral flap reconstructions provide a durable soft tissue reconstruction for the sternal region with maximal obliteration of the underlying sternal dead space.

Operative Procedures

Under general anesthesia with the patient in a supine position, additional aggressive bony and soft tissue debridement was performed by both the cardiothoracic surgery service and the plastic surgery service. The wound was irrigated with warm antibiotic solution. At completion of the additional wound debridement, all wound edges appeared to be fresh and healthy (Fig. 21.2).

The left pectoral major myocutaneous flap was elevated first. Under direct vision, the flap was elevated from the chest wall as a single unit. The submuscular space was entered and dissection was carried out in this tissue plane with the aid of a mammary light retractor. The flap dissection was performed toward the anterior axillary line and the lateral board of the muscle was released. Inferiorly, the muscle was elevated in conjunction with the anterior rectus sheath. The entire flap could easily be advanced across the midline of the sternal wound and the flap dissection was completed (Fig. 21.3A). The right pectoral major myocutaneous flap was dissected in the same way (Fig. 21.3B).

Both flaps were advanced and approximated in the midline of the sternal wound and final closure was performed in three layers after hemostasis and placement of a drain under each muscle flap. The muscle layer was approximated with interrupted 2-0 PDS sutures. The deep dermal layer was approximated with interrupted 3-0 Monocryl sutures. The skin closure was performed with skin staples (Fig. 21.4).

Follow-Up Results

The patient had a slow recovery with a complicated postoperative course. His sternal wound eventually healed well without any major issues related to the sternal wound reconstruction. He was discharged from the hospital 49 days after the open-heart surgery and 26 days after the sternal flap reconstruction. The drain was removed about 3 weeks after the sternal wound closure (Fig. 21.5).

The patient was readmitted to the hospital 1 month later and a total gastrectomy with a Roux-en-Y esophageal jejunostomy and feeding jejunostomy was performed by the surgical oncology service. His postoperative course was complicated by prosthetic valve bacterial endocarditis, sepsis, and multisystem organ failure. He was also found to have a seroma under the intact closure of the upper sternal flap reconstruction (Fig. 21.6). The sternal flap site was stable and there was no cellulitis. The etiology of this fluid collection was thought to be an infiltration after a central line placement. Approximately 100 cc of cloudy fluid was aspirated and a pressure dressing was applied to the sternal area. The final culture showed *Candida albicans*. Follow-up chest CT scans showed a healed sternal soft tissue closure with no substernal fluid collection (Figs. 21.7 and 21.8).

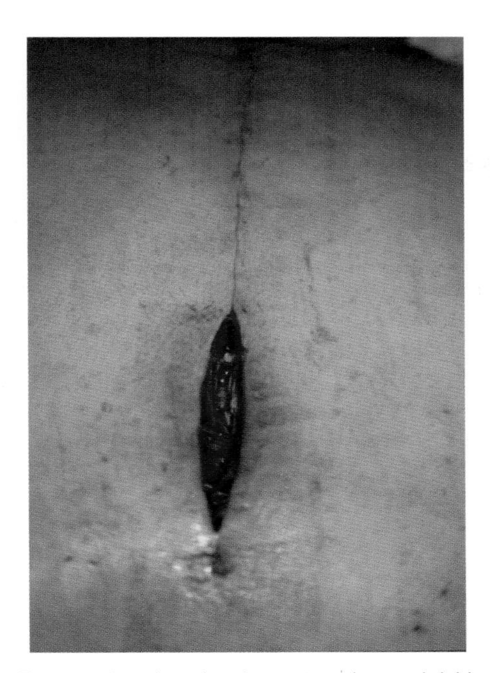

• **Fig. 21.1** Preoperative view showing a sternal wound dehiscence with exposed wires.

• **Fig. 21.2** Intraoperative view showing the appearance of the sternal wound after additional aggressive debridement of infected bone and soft tissue.

Final Outcome

The patient had a well-healed sternal wound after bilateral pectoral major myocutaneous advancement flap reconstructions for sternal wound dehiscence (Fig. 21.9). His postoperative course after total gastrectomy was complicated by prosthetic valve endocarditis, sepsis, and multisystem organ failure. He eventually died 2 months after the total gastrectomy.

Pearls for Success

Bilateral pectoral major myocutaneous advancement flaps are a good option for closure of a sternal wound. In general, the amount of the sternal bony defect after debridement does not warrant a rigid reconstruction and the potential dead space would need attention for soft tissue filling in addition to a reliable soft tissue wound closure. The pectoral major myocutaneous flap can be elevated as a single unit and both flaps can be approximated in the midline of the anterior chest in three layers, including the pectoral major muscle from each side. This option can be an excellent choice to fill the defect and obliterate the dead space and can provide a durable soft tissue reconstruction. Each flap can be elevated through the existing sternal wound. Once the lateral and inferior attachments of the pectoral major muscle are released, each flap can be advanced to the midline of the anterior chest without difficulty. If needed, the anterior rectus fascia can be incorporated with the inferior portion of the pectoral major muscle. During the

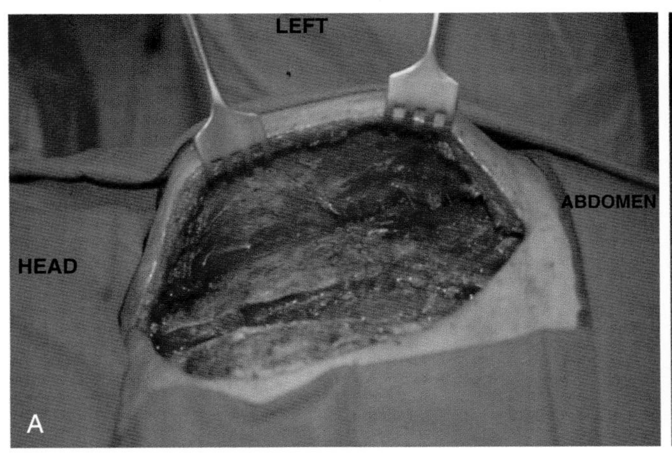

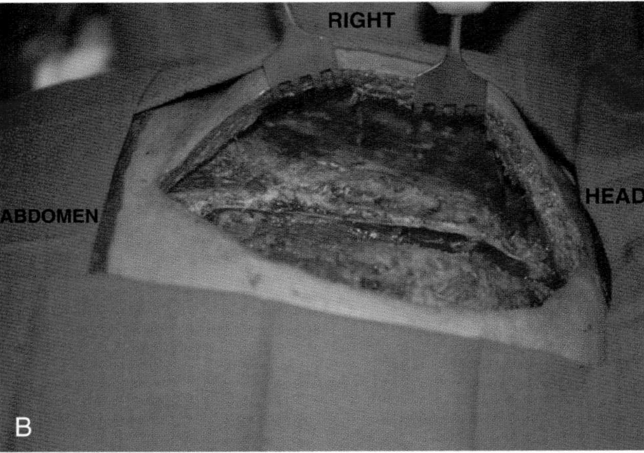

• **Fig. 21.3** (A) Intraoperative view showing completed elevation of the left pectoral major myocutaneous flap. (B) Intraoperative view showing completed elevation of the right pectoral major myocutaneous flap.

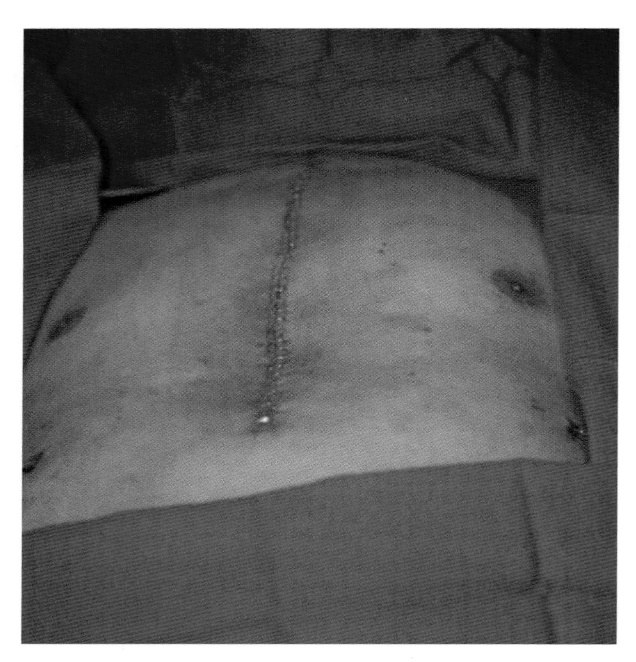

• **Fig. 21.4** Intraoperative view showing the final appearance after bilateral pectoral major myocutaneous advancement flap for this sternal wound closure.

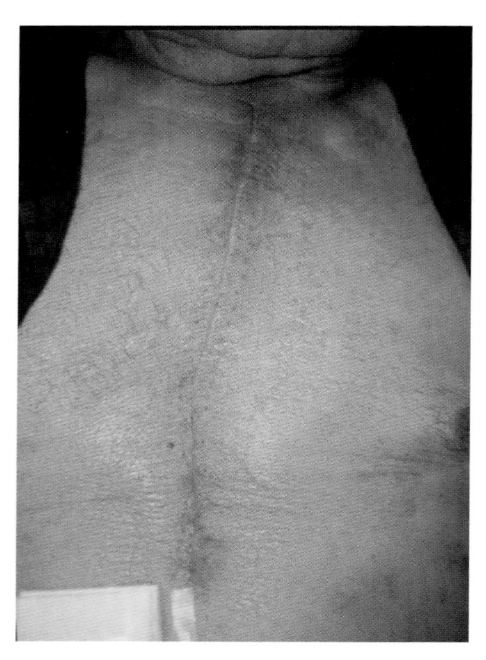

• **Fig. 21.5** The result at 5-week follow-up showing stable and well-healed sternal wound.

flap dissection, the thoracoacromial vessels should be visualized and protected. Seroma under the lower third of the flap closure can occur and can be managed with needle aspiration. If more bony debridement in the lower sternum is anticipated, the right rectus abdominis muscle turnover flap may be added to provide better obliteration of the dead space in the area because the internal mammary vessels are usually intact on that side.

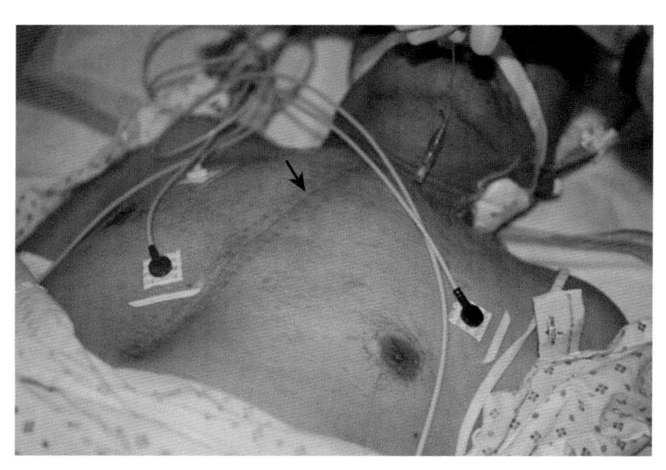

• **Fig. 21.6** The result at 8-week follow-up showing a seroma *(arrow)* under the upper intact sternal wound closure.

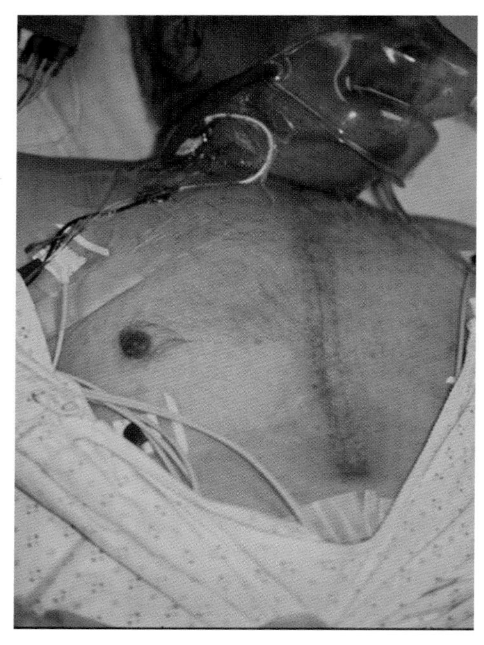

• **Fig. 21.7** The result 1 week after needle aspiration for seroma under the upper third of the sternal wound closure.

CASE 2

Clinical Presentation

A 43-year-old incarcerated male developed an infection of his sternum caused by coccidioidomycosis. This was widely debrided by the cardiothoracic service to remove all infected tissues. He was left with a large sternal defect, measuring 20 × 12 cm, with exposed right lung and mediastinal structures (Figs. 21.10 and 21.11). The patient remained hemodynamically stable once his systemic infection was under control. The plastic surgery service was asked to close the defect in conjunction with further surgical debridement by the primary service.

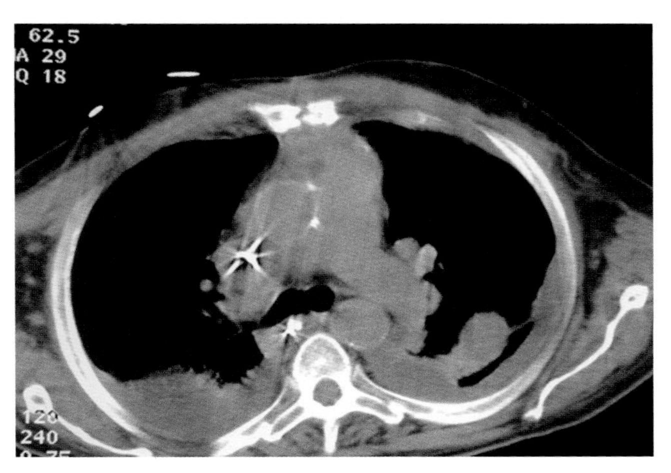

• **Fig. 21.8** Chest CT scan after 2 months showing well-healed and stable sternal wound closure in the mid sternum.

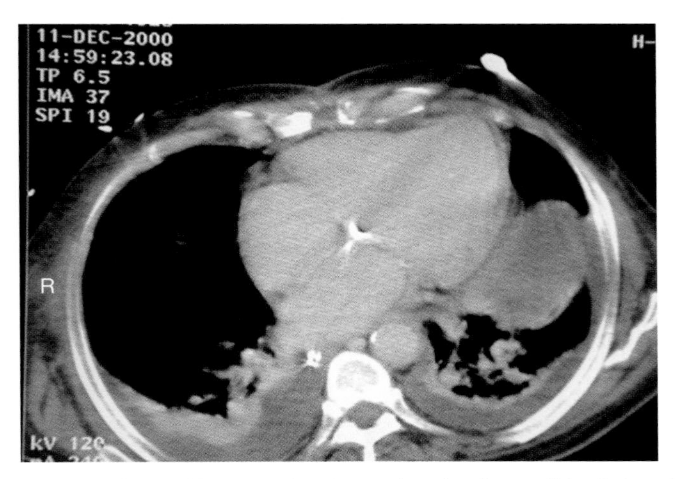

• **Fig. 21.9** Chest CT scan after 2 months showing well-healed and stable sternal wound closure in the lower sternum.

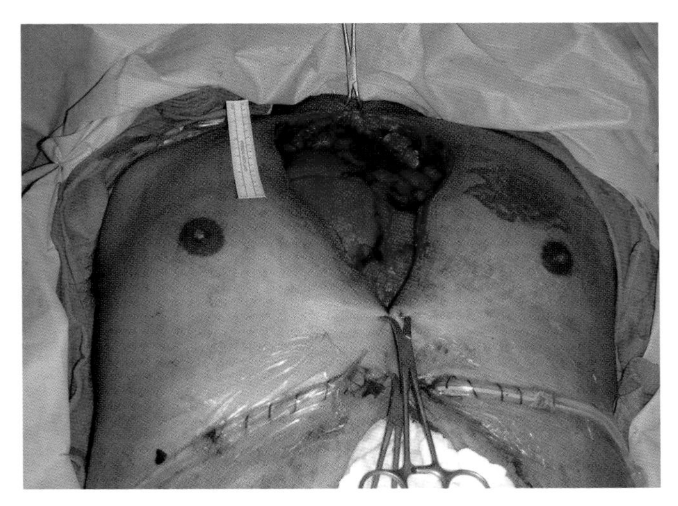

• **Fig. 21.10** Preoperative view showing a large sternal wound after extensive composite surgical debridement of the infected sternum and its surrounding tissues by the primary service.

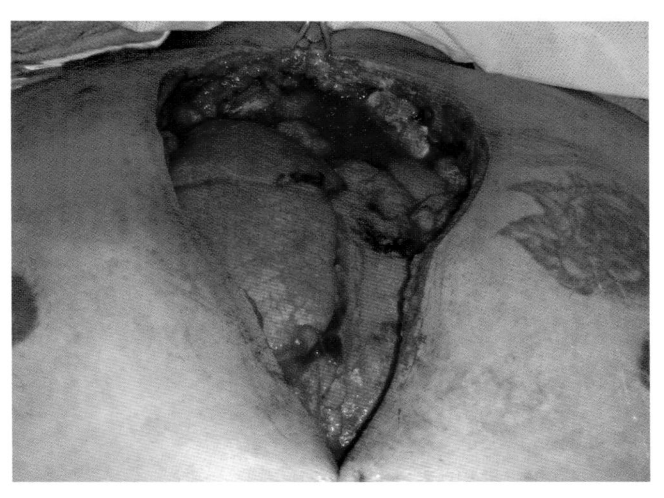

• **Fig. 21.11** Preoperative close-up view showing the exposed underlying lung and mediastinal structures after additional surgical debridement.

Operative Plan and Special Considerations

Once adequate debridement had been accomplished, a reconstructive plan was made to close this large sternal wound with a pedicled omental flap in addition to bilateral pectoral major myocutaneous advancement flaps. An omental flap can provide a large amount of vascularized tissue to obliterate a dead space and to cover most of the sternal defect. The omental flap will be covered with a skin graft. Bilateral pectoral major advancement flaps can also cover a portion of the sternal defect through a flap advancement from each side toward the midline sternum. Such a combination of multiple flap reconstructions could provide a stable soft tissue reconstruction of the sternal region without need for rigid support.

Operative Procedures

Under general anesthesia with the patient in the supine position, the sternal wound was debrided by the cardiothoracic surgery service to the healthy-looking tissue free of infection. Additional debridement was performed by the plastic surgery service and the wound was irrigated with Pulsavac.

The omental flap was dissected out via a midline laparotomy. The flap was designed based on the left gastroepiploic vessels. Once the omentum had been identified, its anterior attachment to the stomach was divided followed by the division of its posterior attachment to the colon. For this case, a large amount of flap tissue was placed over the sternal area for further flap inset (Fig. 21.12). The abdominal incision was closed in two layers.

Bilateral pectoralis major myocutaneous advancement flaps were then elevated. Each side of the pectoralis major myocutaneous flap was dissected from the chest wall leaving the pectoralis minor intact. Its inferior insertion was elevated along with the anterior rectus sheath. Dissection was carried out laterally to free the lateral border of the pectoralis major muscle (Fig. 21.13). The thoracoacromial pedicle was noted to be intact on each side during the flap dissection. Both flaps were advanced toward the midline, which markedly decreased the size of the defect from 22 × 12 cm to 12 × 7 cm. Two 10-mm flat drains were placed under each

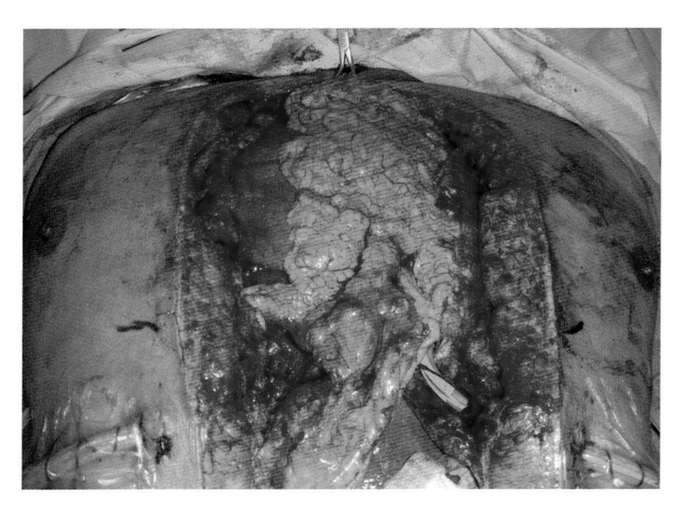

• **Fig. 21.12** Intraoperative view showing the omental flap that was brought out and placed in the sternal wound before the final closure.

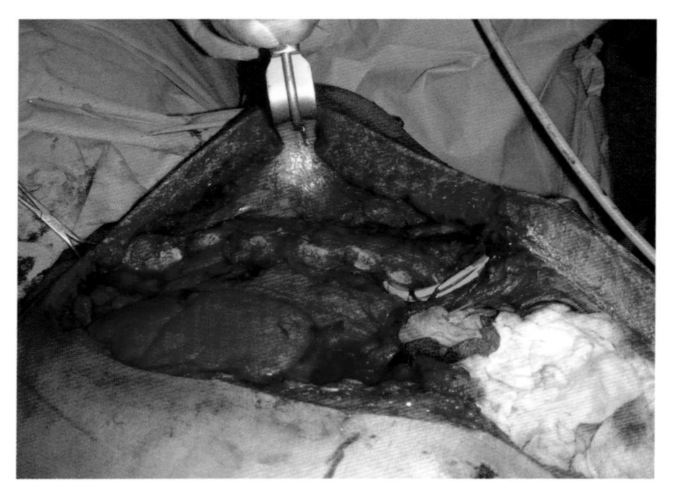

• **Fig. 21.13** Intraoperative view showing completion of the left pectoral major myocutaneous flap elevation. The flap was elevated as a single unit and advanced toward the midline anterior chest.

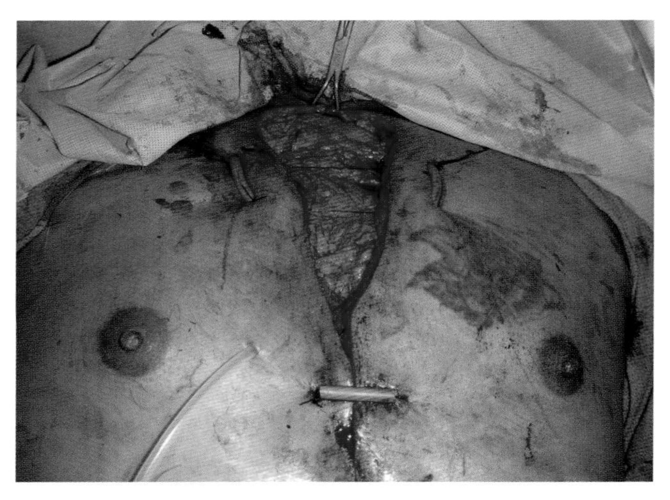

• **Fig. 21.14** Intraoperative view showing completion of the omental flap inset after approximation of bilateral pectoral major myocutaneous advancement flaps toward the midline of the anterior chest.

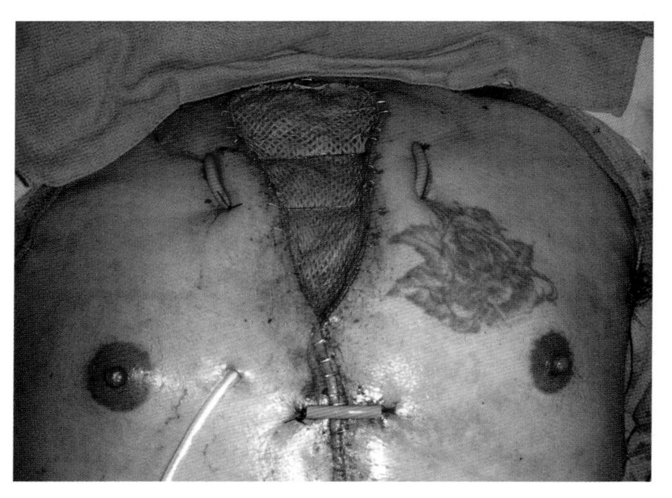

• **Fig. 21.15** Intraoperative view showing completion of the skin graft placement to the omental flap after approximation of bilateral pectoral major myocutaneous advancement flaps toward the midline of the anterior chest.

side of the pectoral major myocutaneous flap through separate stab incisions.

The inferior aspect of the chest wound was reapproximated primarily using 2-0 PDS sutures for the deep tissue closure. The skin was ultimately closed using skin staples. Several retention sutures were used. A horizontal mattress bolster was placed through the midportion of the wound to bring both pectoral major flaps into position. The omental flap was inset into the chest defect, filling the defect almost entirely (Fig. 21.14). The Doppler signals within the flap were good after the closure of the inferior portion of the chest as well as the abdomen. One additional drain was placed under the omental flap. Two anterior chest tubes were placed by the cardiothoracic surgery service. A split-thickness skin graft was harvested from the left anterior thigh. The skin graft was meshed and placed over the omentum within the sternal defect with skin staples (Fig. 21.15) and secured with a bolster dressing. The remainder of the skin incisions were closed using skin staples (Fig. 21.16).

Follow-Up Results

The patient did well postoperatively without any complications related to the omental flap or bilateral pectoral major myocutaneous advancement flap reconstructions. He was discharged from the hospital on postoperative day 10. The drain was removed during the subsequent follow-up visit. The sternal wound after above flap reconstructions healed well and appeared to be stable (Fig. 21.17).

Final Outcome

This large sternal wound healed well after successful combined reconstruction with a pedicled omental flap and bilateral pectoral major myocutaneous advancement flaps (Fig. 21.18). The patient has no recurrent infection or open wound in the area and his sternal reconstruction site reamains stable. He has resumed his

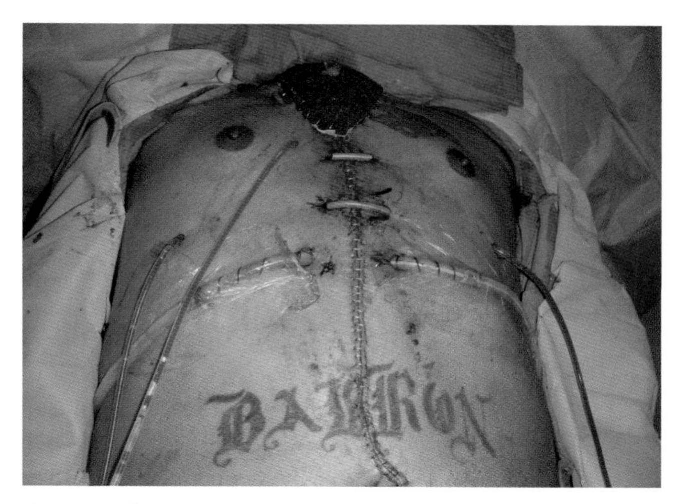

• **Fig. 21.16** Intraoperative view showing the final appearance after completion of the omental flap and bilateral pectoral major myocutaneous advancement flaps reconstruction for this large sternal wound.

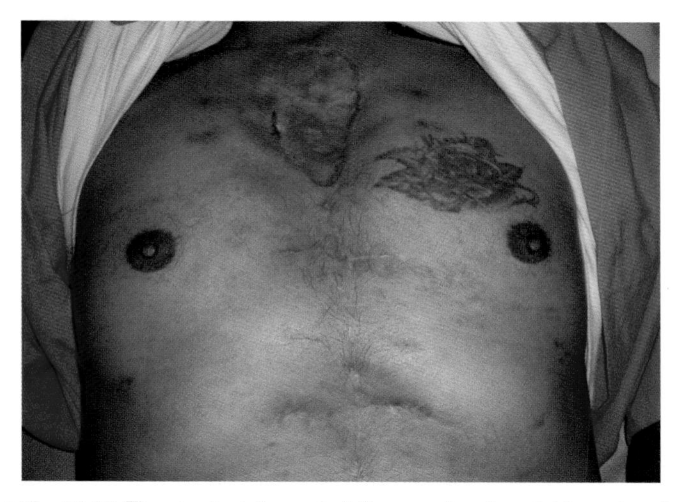

• **Fig. 21.17** The result at 3-month follow-up showing stable and well-healed sternal wound.

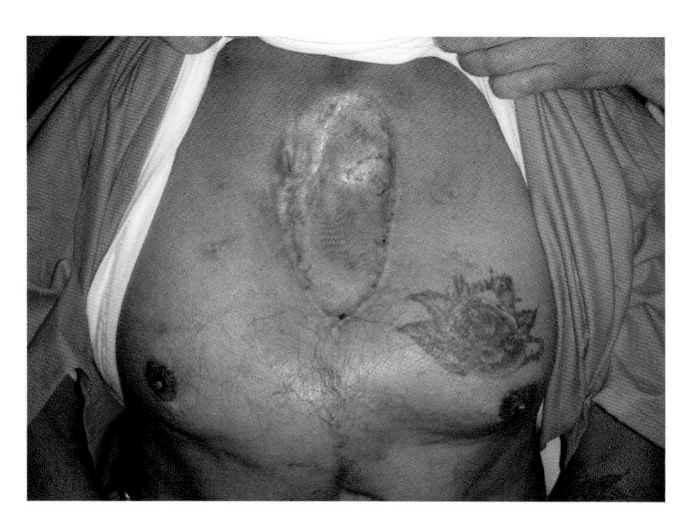

• **Fig. 21.18** The result at 8-month follow-up showing stable and well-healed sternal wound.

normal activities and is followed by the cardiothoracic surgery service for routine follow-up.

Pearls for Success

Bilateral pectoral major myocutaneous advancement flaps are the flaps of choice for closure of a sternal wound that typically follows sternal wound debridement after open-heart surgery. However, if a medial portion of the flap has been debrided significantly such as in this case, the two advancement flaps would not be able to approximate in the midline of the anterior chest. Therefore, a pedicled omental flap can be selected to provide the rest of soft tissue coverage in the midline of the sternal area. Care should be taken to decrease the risk of contamination from the sternal wound to the abdominal cavity. Each pectoral major myocutaneous flap should be elevated as a single unit and the lateral and inferior attachments of the pectoral major muscle should be released. If needed, the anterior rectus fascia can be incorporated with the inferior portion of the pectoral major muscle. One or more retention sutures can be placed to provide more stable approximation to the midline of the anterior chest. Attention should be made to identify the thoracoacromial vessels during the pectoral major myocutaneous flap elevation or the gastroepiploic vessels during the omental flap dissection.

CASE 3

Clinical Presentation

A 54-year-old White male had suffered a gunshot wound to his right upper chest several years previously. He subsequently developed a chronic infection of the upper sternum that required a radical debridement including resection of the upper portion of the sternum by the thoracic surgery service. This left a large sternal defect in the upper sternum, measuring 15 × 15 cm. The extensive sternal soft tissue wound measured 24 × 10 cm. The plastic surgery service was asked to provide the sternal wound coverage in the area for a composite sternal defect (Figs. 21.19 and 21.20).

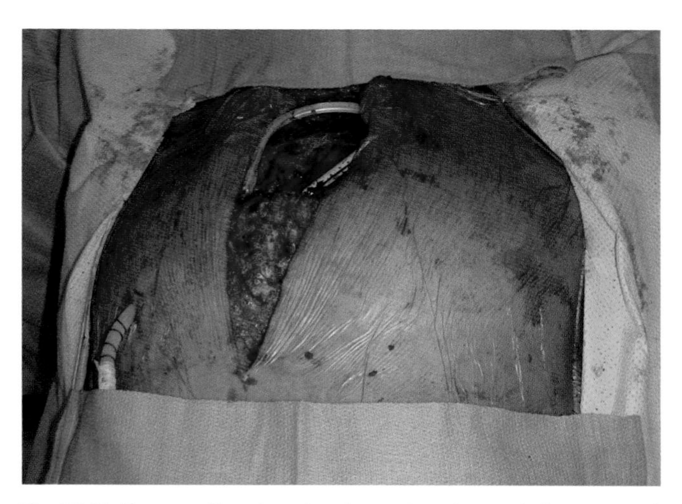

• **Fig. 21.19** Preoperative view showing a sternal wound after composite surgical debridement of the infected upper sternum and its surrounding soft tissues by the primary service.

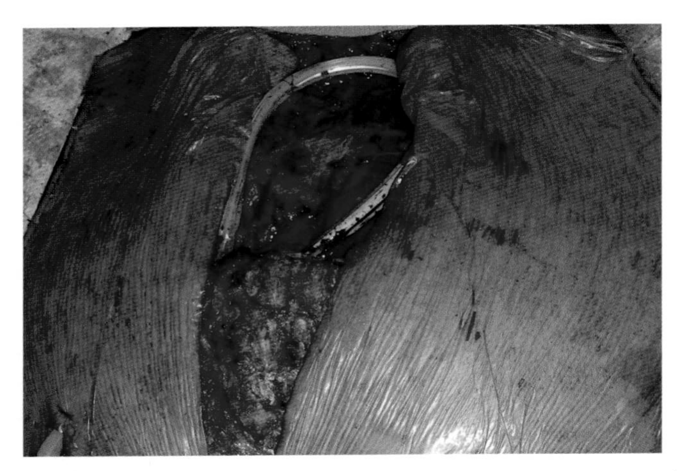

• **Fig. 21.20** Preoperative close-up view showing the upper sternal defect and open sternal wound.

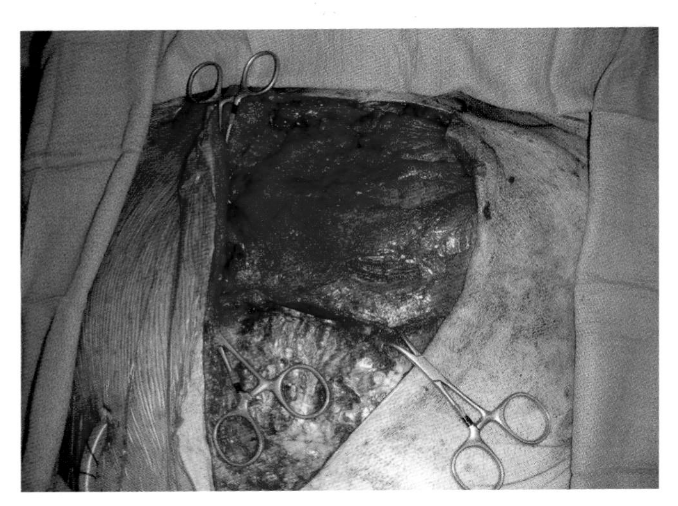

• **Fig. 21.21** Intraoperative view showing the left pectoral major muscle flap that was brought out and placed to cover the upper sternal defect.

Operative Plan and Special Considerations

The reconstruction plan should include obliteration of the sternal dead space with well-vascularized tissue and sternal wound closure with the right pectoral major myocutaneous advancement flap. In this case, additional left pectoral major muscle flap would be needed and can be harvested through the existing sternal wound. The muscle flap can be used to fill the sternal dead space. Once the muscle is mobilized, the left chest skin can be automatically advanced to the midline of the sternal wound. The right pectoral major myocutaneous flap can be elevated and advanced as a single unit to achieve the sternal soft tissue wound closure. Such combined flap reconstructions provide a durable soft tissue reconstruction of the sternal region with obliteration of the underlying sternal dead space.

Operative Procedures

Under general anesthesia with the patient in a supine position, radical bony and soft tissue debridement were completed by the thoracic surgery service. Additional soft tissue debridement was performed by the plastic surgery service and all wound edges appeared to be healthy. The left pectoral major muscle was identified first. Biplane dissections were performed above and below the muscle. The dissection was first done above the muscle and the skin over the muscle was elevated. The anterior muscle was dissected completely free. The submuscular dissection was then performed until the lateral boarder of the muscle was released. The inferior insertion of the pectoral major muscle was divided and the medial superior aspect attachment of the muscle to the clavicle was divided. The major portion of the pectoral major muscle attachment to the humerus was also divided. During the flap dissection, the pedicle vessels were visualized and protected. The left pectoral major muscle was dissected free and rotated into the sternal bony defect, filling well without tension (Fig. 21.21).

The right pectoral major myocutaneous flap was elevated as a single unit along the submuscular space under direct vision. The flap dissection was done toward the anterior axillary line and the lateral board of the muscle was released. The flap could easily be advanced across the midline of the sternal wound and approximated with the left chest skin flap for definitive wound closure (Fig. 21.22).

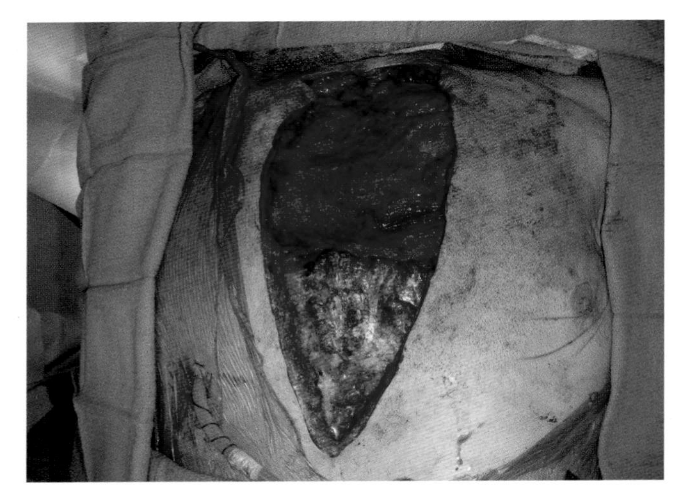

• **Fig. 21.22** Intraoperative view showing completion of the left pectoral major muscle flap inset and complete elevation of the right pectoral major myocutaneous flap.

The left pectoral major muscle flap was inset into the sternal bony defect and secured to its adjacent soft tissue with multiple 2-0 PDS sutures in a figure-of-eight fashion. A Blake drain was placed under the muscle flap. Several air leak sites were repaired by the thoracic surgery service. Two JP drains were inserted, one under the left chest skin flap and the other under the right pectoral major myocutaneous flap.

The final skin closure was performed in three layers. The deep tissue was approximated with several interrupted 2-0 PDS sutures and the deep dermal closure was approximated with interrupted 3-0 Monocryl sutures. The final skin closure was performed with skin staples (Fig. 21.23).

Follow-Up Results

The patient did well postoperatively without any complications related to the sternal wound reconstruction. He was discharged from hospital on postoperative day 3. The drain was removed

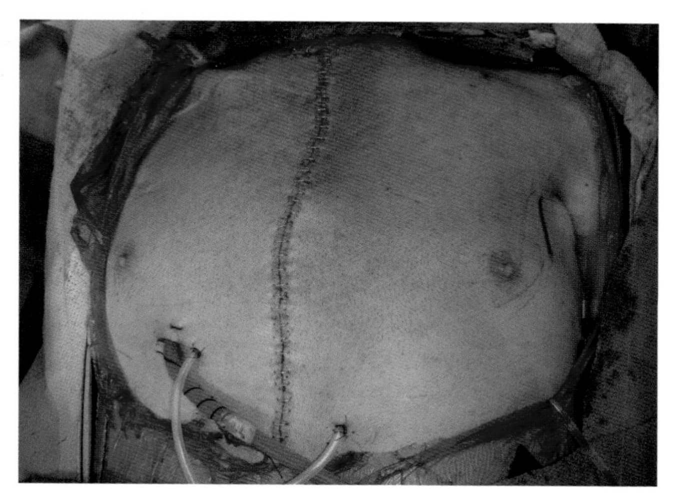

• **Fig. 21.23** Intraoperative view showing the final appearance after completion of the left pectoral major muscle flap and right pectoral major myocutaneous advancement flap reconstructions for this sternal wound closure.

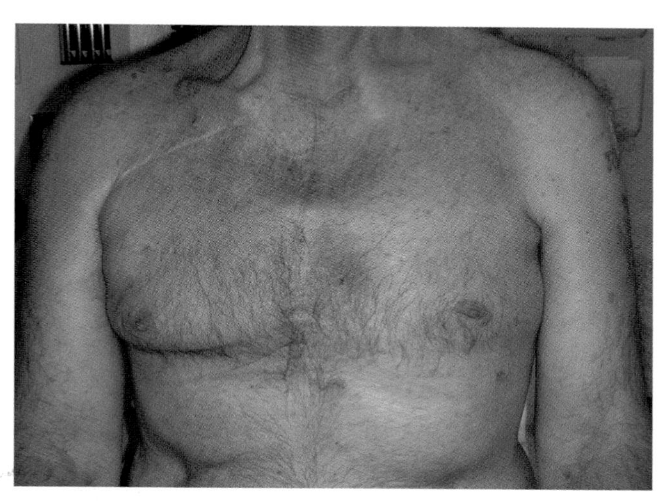

• **Fig. 21.24** The result at 3-month follow-up showing stable and well-healed sternal wound.

during subsequent follow-up visits. The sternal wound healed well after the flap reconstructions.

Final Outcome

The combined reconstructions with a left pectoral major muscle rotation flap and right pectoral major myocutaneous advancement flap were successful and the sternal wound healed well (Figs. 21.24). The patient has no recurrent infection or wound breakdown in the area, has resumed his normal activities, and is followed by the thoracic surgery service for routine follow-up.

Pearls for Success

The pectoral major myocutaneous advancement flap, even unilateral, is a reliable procedure for closure of a sternal wound. Although the amount of the sternal bony defect after debridement does not warrant a rigid reconstruction in this case, the potential dead space would need attention for soft tissue reconstruction. The pectoral major muscle flap can be an excellent choice to fill the defect and obliterate the dead space after the flap inset. The flap can be dissected through the existing sternal wound and can be elevated with minimal muscle attachment to the clavicle. During the flap dissection, the thoracoacromial vessels should be visualized and traction injury to the flap's pedicle should be avoided during the flap inset. Once again, the pectoral major myocutaneous flap should be elevated as a single unit and the lateral and inferior attachments of the pectoral major muscle should be released. If needed, the anterior rectus fascia can be incorporated with the inferior portion of the pectoral major muscle. Such combined flap reconstructions could provide durable soft tissue coverage in the area.

Recommended Readings

Ascherman JA, Patel SM, Malhotra SM, Smith CR. Management of sternal wounds with bilateral pectoralis major myocutaneous advancement flaps in 114 consecutively treated patients: refinements in technique and outcomes analysis. *Plast Reconstr Surg*. 2004;114:676–683.

Davison SP, Clemens MW, Armstrong D, Newton ED, Swartz W. Sternotomy wounds: rectus flap versus modified pectoral reconstruction. *Plast Reconstr Surg*. 2007;120:929–934.

Izaddoost S, Withers EH. Sternal reconstruction with omental and pectoralis flaps: a review of 415 consecutive cases. *Ann Plast Surg*. 2012;69:296–300.

Preminger BA, Yaghoobzadeh Y, Ascherman JA. Management of sternal wounds by limited debridement and partial bilateral pectoralis major myocutaneous advancement flaps in 25 patients. *Ann Plast Surg*. 2014;72:446–450.

Pu LLQ, O'Connell JB, Takei T, Restifo RJ, Newton CG, Sandberg GR. Closure of infected sternal wounds with a unilateral rectus abdominis muscle flap in addition to bilateral pectoralis major myocutaneous advancement flaps. *Eur J Plast Surg*. 1999;22:313–317.

Vyas RM, Prsic A, Orgill DP. Transdiaphragmatic omental harvest: a simple, efficient method for sternal wound coverage. *Plast Reconstr Surg*. 2013;131:544–552.

Yasuura K, Okamoto H, Morita S, et al. Results of omental flap transposition for deep sternal wound infection after cardiovascular surgery. *Ann Plast Surg*. 1998;227:455–459.

22 Lateral Chest Reconstruction

Clinical Presentation

A 74-year-old White female suffered a lateral chest wound and had a partial breast defect secondary to wound debridement, complicated by the previous minimally invasive right lobectomy. Apparently, she had a seroma formation in the area, which had been managed by the thoracic surgery service. The plastic surgery service was asked to provide soft tissue coverage for the wound and to facilitate healing of the complicated wound. The lateral chest wound also involved part of the axilla and the superior lateral quadrant of the breast (Fig. 22.1). Prior to the procedure the wound had been treated with local wound care.

Operative Plan and Special Considerations

Additional debridement was planned to excise all fibrotic tissues around and deep to the open wound. Such debridement should be done to healthy and normal-looking tissue either around or at the base of the wound. Attention should be paid to avoid injuries to neurovascular structures in the axilla. Because of the location and size of the soft tissue defect after debridement, a pedicled latissimus dorsi myocutaneous flap can be selected to cover this wound in one stage. The flap can be elevated from the patient's right back and tunneled to the defect without any difficulty. In addition, a portion of the breast defect can be reconstructed at the same time. If the skin paddle of the flap is not too wide, the flap donor site can also be closed primarily.

Operative Procedures

Under general anesthesia with patient initially in the supine position, the procedure started by removing all the colonized and necrotic tissues within the right axilla and chest wound. After debridement, the wound showed exposed ribs. The wound, measuring 9 × 6 cm, was irrigated thoroughly with Pulse-Vac (Fig. 22.2).

The patient was then placed in the left lateral decubitus position. The right latissimus dorsi myocutaneous flap with a 9 × 6 cm skin paddle was designed and marked. (Fig. 22.3). About 10 cc of 1% lidocaine with 1:100,000 epinepherin was administered to the proposed skin incision. After the incision had been made around the skin paddle, the dissection was performed around the skin paddle down to the latissimus dorsi muscle. Once the muscle had been identified, the muscle flap was dissected more superiorly to identify the superior border of the latissimus dorsi muscle. Once the superior border had been identified, the muscle was dissected free from the chest wall superiorly, then medially, then inferiorly, and then laterally. In this way the muscle flap with its skin paddle was elevated from the chest wall. The thoracodorsal vessels were identified with a handheld Doppler. A further dissection was done around the pedicle toward the muscle's insertion. The flap was tunneled through the lateral chest subcutaneous tissue and then placed inside the right chest wound.

Additional release of the scar around the wound was performed under direct vision. The skin paddle of the latissimus dorsi flap was oriented and easily inset into the defect without tension. One drain was placed under the flap and the muscle was approximated to the lateral part of the breast tissue with several interrupted 3-0 PDS sutures. The rest of the skin paddle inset was performed with 3-0 Monocryl sutures to the adjacent skin edge. The skin paddle was also inserted into the right breast wound filling the superolateral aspect of the breast defect. Skin closure was performed with several interrupted 3-0 Monocryl sutures in half-buried horizontal mattress fashion (Fig. 22.4).

The right back flap donor site was closed in two layers after placing two drains. The deep tissue layer was approximated with several interrupted 2-0 PDS sutures. The skin closure was performed with 3-0 Monocryl sutures in simple running fashion.

Follow-Up Results

The patient did well postoperatively without any complications related to the latissimus dorsi myocutaneous flap reconstruction. She was discharged from hospital on postoperative day 3. All drains were removed during subsequent follow-up visits. The lateral chest wound healed well after the flap reconstruction (Fig. 22.5). In addition, her breast symmetry appeared to be satisfactory (Fig. 22.6).

Final Outcome

The lateral chest wound healed well after the latissimus dorsi flap reconstruction. The patient has no recurrent open wound in the area, has resumed her normal activities, and is followed by the thoracic surgery service for additional follow-up.

Pearls for Success

A pedicled latissimus dorsi myocutaneous flap can be an excellent choice for lateral chest soft tissue reconstruction. It may also improve breast symmetry in a female patient. The flap dissection

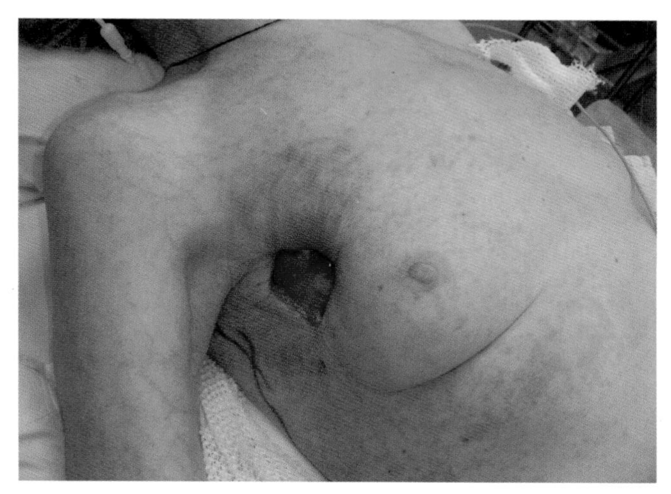

• **Fig. 22.1** Preoperative view showing a right chronic lateral chest wound involving a portion of the breast and surrounded by fibrotic and scarred tissues.

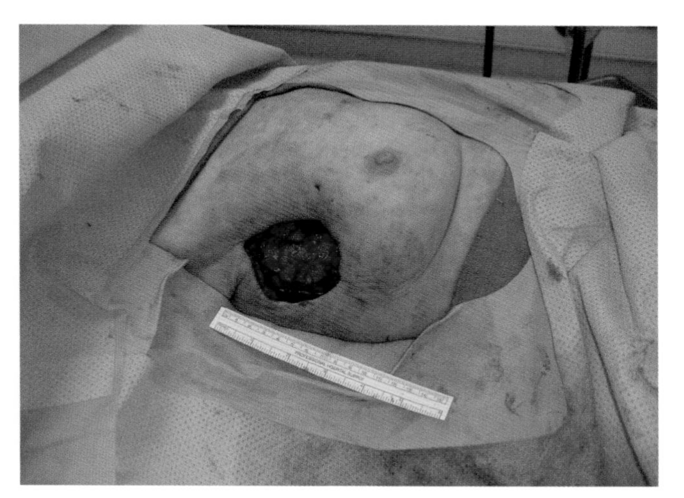

• **Fig. 22.2** Intraoperative view showing a large lateral chest wound with fresh- and healthy-looking tissue after additional debridement.

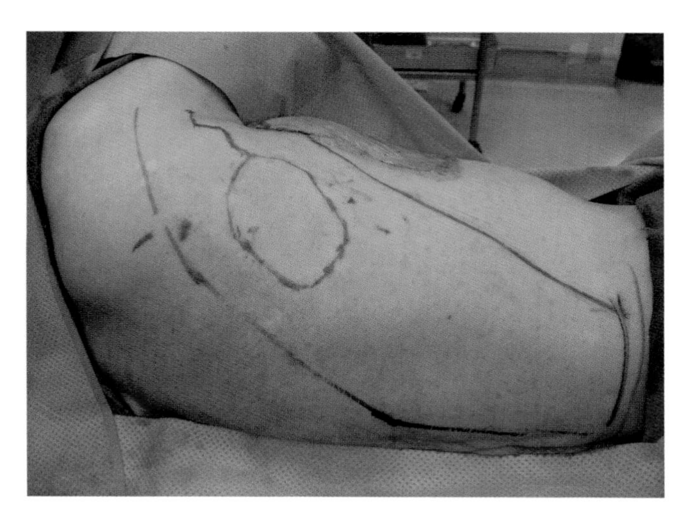

• **Fig. 22.3** Intraoperative view showing the design of the right latissimus dorsi myocutaneous flap with a skin paddle.

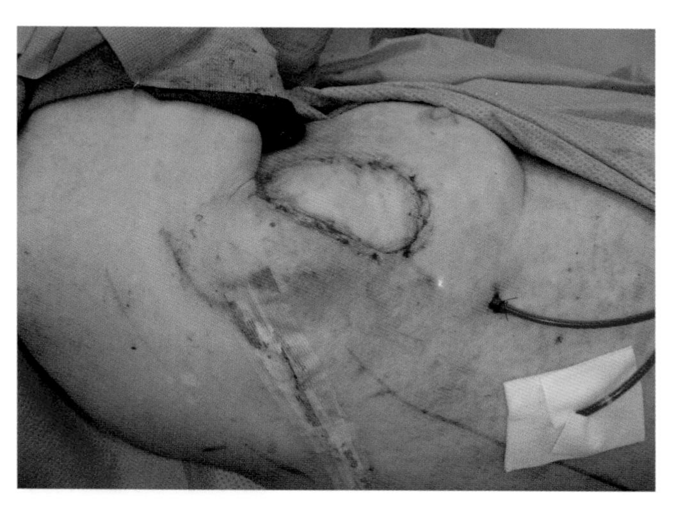

• **Fig. 22.4** Intraoperative view showing completion of the right latissimus dorsi myocutaneous flap inset over the lateral chest wound and the right breast.

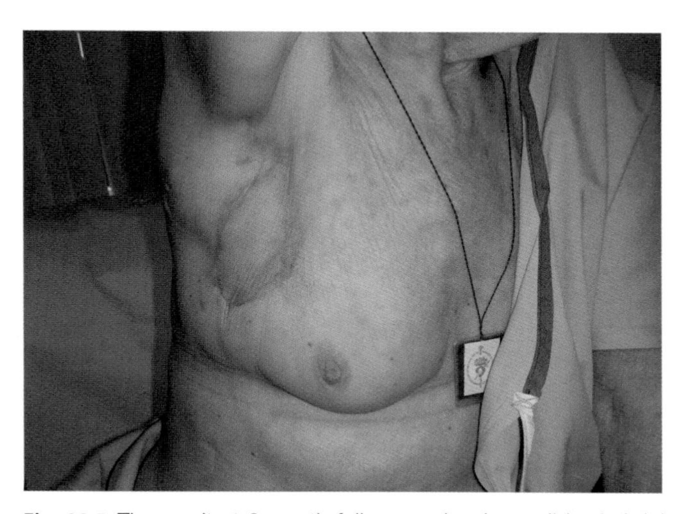

• **Fig. 22.5** The result at 2-month follow-up showing well healed right lateral chest wound.

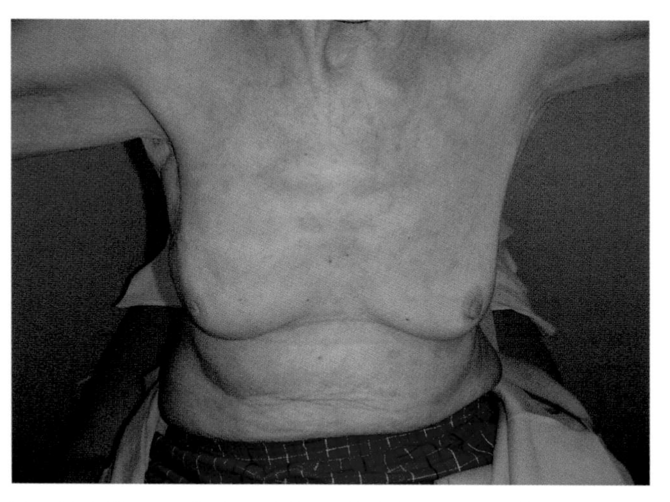

• **Fig. 22.6** The result also at 2-month follow-up showing good symmetry between breasts.

is relatively straightforward and the flap donor site can be closed primarily in most cases. The division of the muscle insertion to the humerus is usually not necessary but can be done if more arc of the flap rotation is needed. Postoperatively, the upper arm should be placed abductively to avoid a direct compression to the pedicle vessels of the flap.

Recommended Readings

Basta MN, Fischer JP, Lotano VE, Kovach SJ. The thoracoplastic approach to chest wall reconstruction: preliminary results of a multidisciplinary approach to minimize morbidity. *Plast Reconstr Surg.* 2014;134:959e–967e.

Corkum JP, Garvey PB, Baumann DP, et al. Reconstruction of massive chest wall defects: a 20-year experience. *J Plast Reconstr Aesthet Surg.* 2020;73:1091–1098.

Growth AK, Pazio ALB, Kusano LDC, et al. Thoracic wall reconstruction surgical planning in extended malignant resections. *Ann Plast Surg.* 2020;85:531–538.

Munhoz AM, Montag E, Arruda E, et al. Immediate locally advanced breast cancer and chest wall reconstruction: surgical planning and reconstruction strategies with extended V-Y latissimus dorsi myocutaneous flap. *Plast Reconstr Surg.* 2011;127:2186–2197.

Netscher DT, Baumholz MA. Chest reconstruction: I. anterior and anterolateral chest wall and wounds affecting respiratory function. *Plast Reconstr Surg.* 2009;124:240e–252e.

23 Lower Chest Reconstruction

Clinical Presentation

A 19-year-old White female had a large soft tissue mass in her lower chest and sternal area. Preoperative biopsy showed desmoid type of fibromatosis. She underwent resection of this soft tissue mass by the pediatric cardiothoracic surgery service and the plastic surgery service was asked to provide lower chest wall reconstruction after the tumor resection. After resection, the entire skin defect of the lower sternal and upper abdominal areas measured 18 × 14 cm to the rectus abdominis muscles on both sides. Both sides of the anterior rectus sheath were also resected (Fig. 23.1). The lower sternal bony defect measured 13 × 6 cm (Fig. 23.2). Two chest tubes were placed by the primary service. The left superior epigastric vessels were apparently transected during the resection. However, the right superior epigastric vessels remained intact.

Operative Plan and Special Considerations

This was a large composite defect of the lower chest and upper abdomen with a sizable sternal bony defect. Only a small portion of the skin defect could be closed primarily after undermining. The sternal bony defect should be reconstructed with at least semirigid material. In this case, Strattice, a relatively rigid biological mesh was selected for the sternal bony reconstruction. A right rectus abdominis muscle could be used as a turnover flap to provide reliable soft tissue coverage to the Strattice. The muscle flap, based on the right superior epigastric vessels, could be elevated from the abdominal wall on the right side. It reached to at least midsternal level and was covered with a split-thickness skin graft for definitive wound closure. This composite defect could be reconstructed with a semirigid biological mesh and a well-vascularized skin grafted muscle flap with almost no donor site morbidities because the rectus abdominis muscle flap donor site could be closed primarily.

Operative Procedures

Under general anesthesia with the patient in the supine position, the reconstructive procedure started after an adequate tumor resection. A 5-cm posterior rectus sheath defect over the upper abdomen was repaired with 2-0 PDS sutures in a figure-of-eight. The lower sternal bony defect, measuring 13 × 6 cm, was reconstructed with Strattice. The selected Strattice had several perforated holes. Scissors were used to prepare a 13 × 6 cm Strattice, which was placed onto the lower sternal bony defect while the dermal side was facing up, approximated with several interrupted 2-0 PDS sutures followed by 2-0 PDS sutures in simple running fashion (Fig. 23.3).

A right paramedian skin incision was designed in the right abdomen (Fig. 23.4). The proposed incision was infiltrated with 1% lidocaine with 1:100,000 epinephrine. The procedure was started by making a paramedian incision to the anterior rectus sheath. Once the anterior rectus sheath was opened, the dissection was performed around the rectus abdominis muscle. During dissection, several tendious intersections were dissected free. The rectus abdominis muscle was identified and after further dissection around the muscle, its entire length was dissected free. The right inferior epigastric vessels were identified and divided with hemoclips near the muscle's origin. The muscle was then divided with electrocautery very close to the suprapubic symphysis area and the muscle flap was completely dissected free from the posterior rectus sheath. Before further dissection of the muscle, the superior epigastric vessels were identified. The flap was then turned over to cover the soft tissue defect in the lower sternal area (Fig. 23.5). The muscle flap was completely inset into the defect to cover the entire exposed Strattice and was approximated to the adjacent tissue with several interrupted 3-0 Vicryl sutures (Fig. 23.6).

The entire lower sternal and upper abdominal skin wound, measuring 25 cm in length, was approximated superiorly and inferiorly after simple suprafascial undermining for skin closure (Fig. 23.7). The skin edge of the rest of the wound was tacked to the deep muscle with 3-0 Monocryl sutures. The rest of the open wound with a good muscle coverage measured 14 × 9 cm. The skin graft was harvested from the patient's left lateral thigh. The skin graft was meshed to 1 to 1.5 ratio and sutured to the wound edge with 5-0 chromic sutures in simple running fashion (Fig. 23.8). A vacuum-assisted closure (VAC) dressing was applied over the skin graft site and connected to the VAC machine.

The abdominal incision was then closed. The anterior rectus sheath was approximated with several interrupted 3-0 Monocryl sutures. The deep dermal was approximated with several interrupted 4-0 Monocryl sutures. The skin was closed with a running subcuticular 4-0 Monocryl suture (Fig. 23.9).

Follow-Up Results

The patient did well postoperatively without any complications related to the lower chest and sternal reconstruction with Strattice

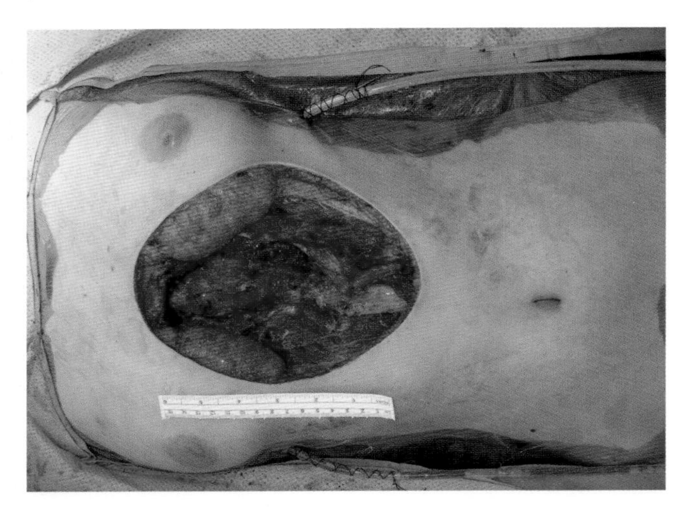

• **Fig. 23.1** Preoperative view showing a large soft tissue defect after the tumor resection involving the lower chest and sternal area and upper abdomen associated with a lower sternal bony defect.

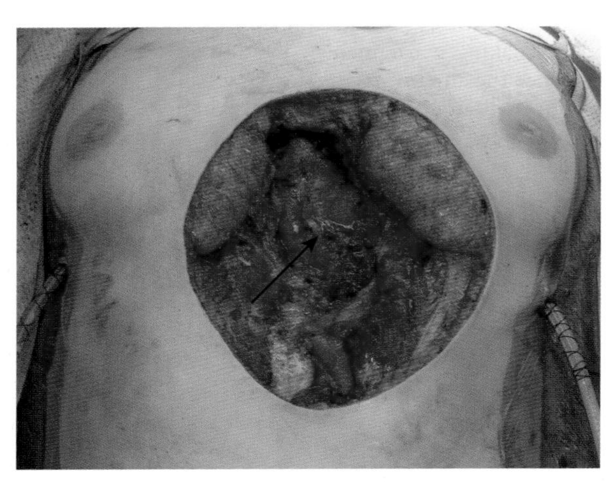

• **Fig. 23.2** Intraoperative close-up view showing a large composite tissue defect involving the central lower chest and upper abdomen.

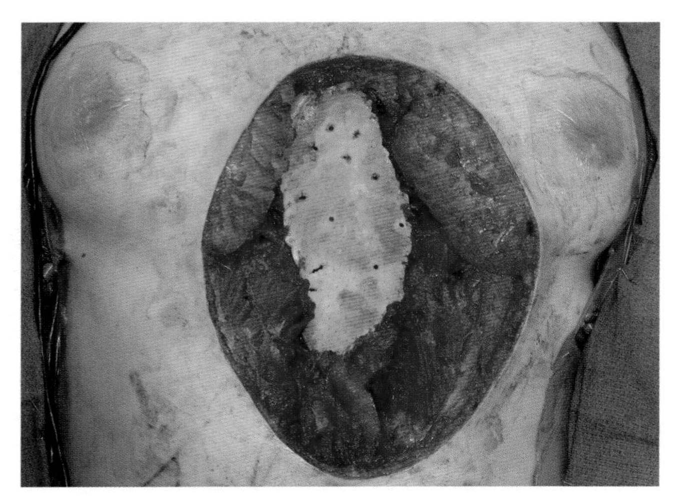

• **Fig. 23.3** Intraoperative view showing completion of Strattice placement for reconstruction of the lower sternal bony defect.

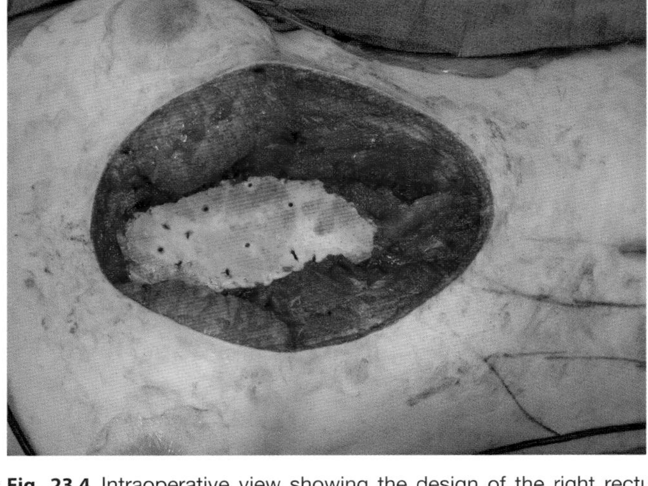

• **Fig. 23.4** Intraoperative view showing the design of the right rectus abdominis muscle turnover flap.

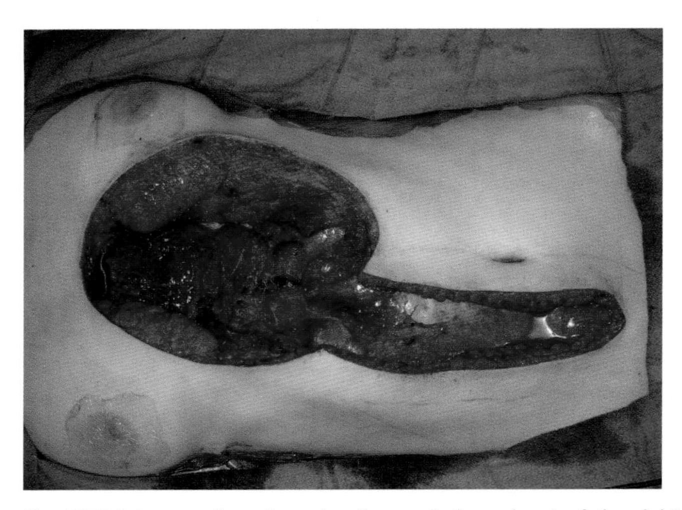

• **Fig. 23.5** Intraoperative view showing preliminary inset of the right rectus abdominis muscle turnover flap for soft tissue coverage over the Strattice and lower sternal wound.

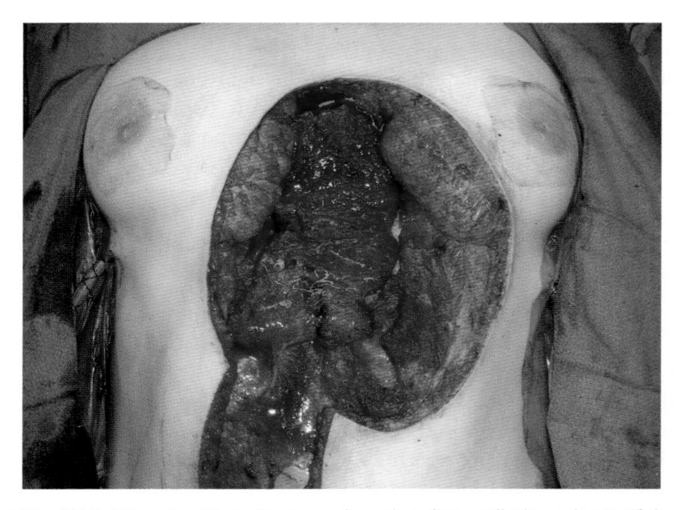

• **Fig. 23.6** Intraoperative close-up view showing preliminary inset of the right rectus abdominis muscle turnover flap for the soft tissue coverage over the deep lower sternal wound.

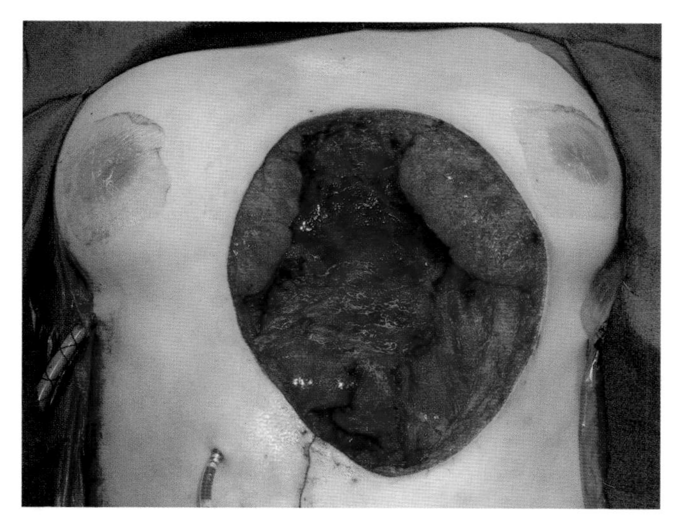

• **Fig. 23.7** Intraoperative close-up view showing completion of the right rectus abdominis muscle turnover flap inset for soft tissue coverage over the lower sternal wound.

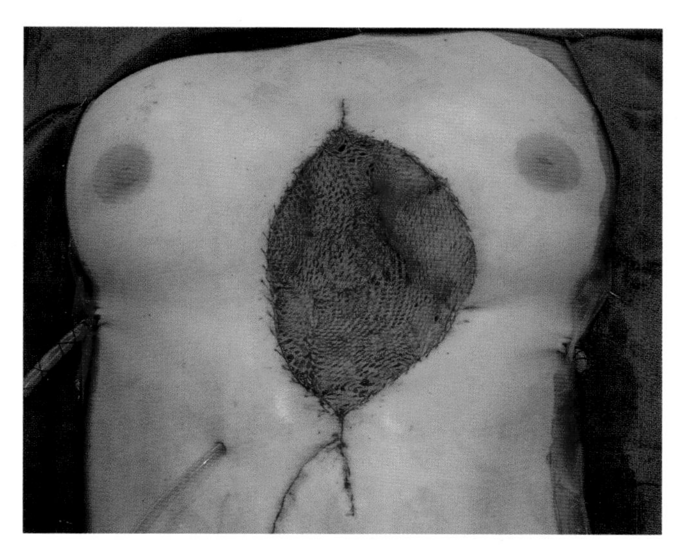

• **Fig. 23.8** Intraoperative close-up view showing completion of a skin graft placement over the right rectus abdominis muscle turnover flap for soft tissue coverage over the lower sternal wound.

and the rectus abdominis muscle flap. She was discharged from hospital on postoperative day 5. The chest tubes and drains were removed during subsequent follow-up visits. The lower chest wound healed well after the composite reconstruction (Fig. 23.10). The patient's breast symmetry also appeared to be satisfactory (Fig. 23.11).

Final Outcome

The lower chest wound after Strattice placement for the sternal reconstruction and the rectus abdominis muscle turnover flap reconstruction healed well. The patient has had a stable reconstruction without recurrent open wound or infection in the area. She has resumed her normal activities and is

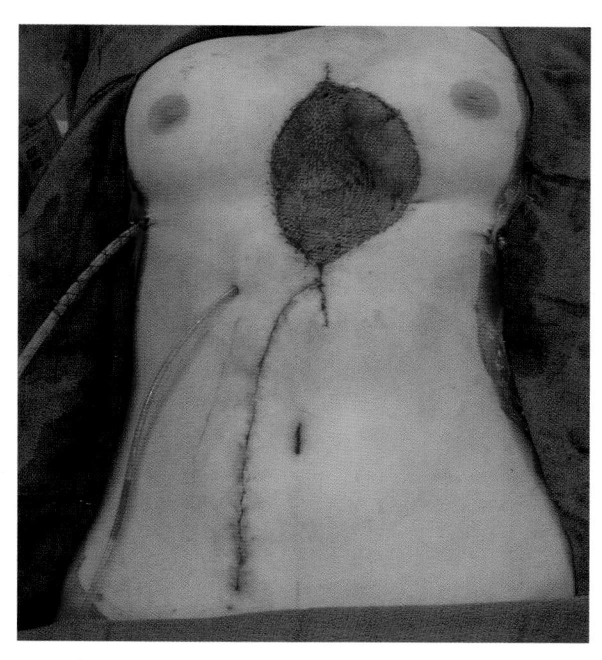

• **Fig. 23.9** Intraoperative view showing completion of the right rectus abdominis muscle turnover flap reconstruction and closure of its donor site.

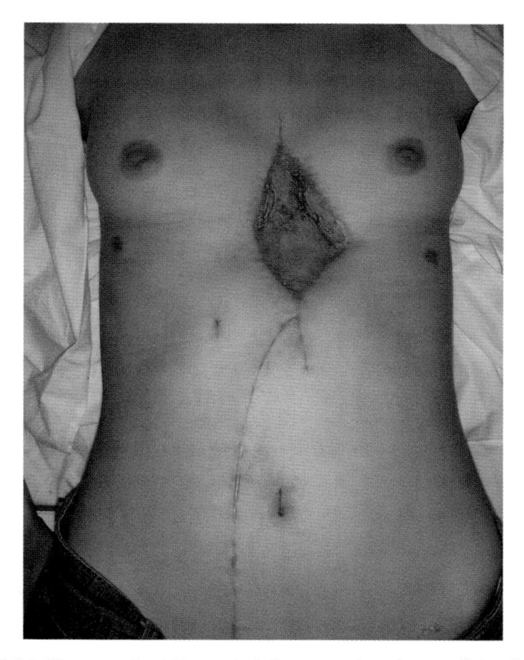

• **Fig. 23.10** The result at 7-week follow-up showing well-healed lower chest sternal wound and right abdominal flap donor site.

followed by the pediatric cardiothoracic surgery service for routine follow-up.

Pearls for Success

A rectus abdominis muscle turnover flap, based on the superior epigastric vessels, can be an excellent choice for lower chest soft tissue reconstruction associated with a sternal bony defect.

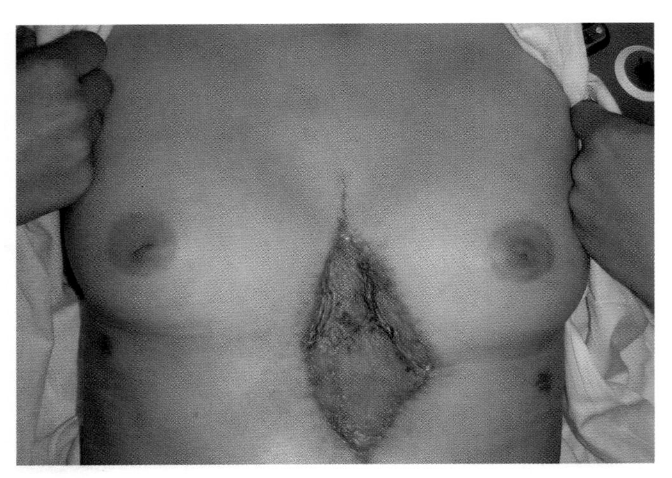

• **Fig. 23.11** A close-up view of the result at 7-week follow-up showing stable wound healing after composite reconstructions and good symmetry between breasts.

Strattice, a semirigid biological mesh, can be used to reconstruct such a bony defect. The surgical dissection of a rectus abdominis muscle flap is relatively straightforward as long as the superior epigastric vessels remain patent after the tumor resection. During the muscle flap disssection, the anterior rectus sheath can be preserved completely so that the flap donor site can be closed with a relatively intact anterior abdominal wall structure. Such a composite reconstruction of the lower chest appears to be strong enough and adequate for stabilization of the lower sternal area.

Recommended Readings

Althubaiti G, Butler CE. Abdominal wall and chest wall reconstruction. *Plast Reconstr Surg*. 2014;133:688e−701e.

Growth AK, Pazio ALB, Kusano LDC, et al. Thoracic wall reconstruction surgical planning in extended malignant resections. *Ann Plast Surg*. 2020;85:531−538.

Momeni A, Kovach SJ. Important considerations in chest wall reconstruction. *J Surg Oncol*. 2016;113:913−922.

Netscher DT, Baumholz MA. Chest reconstruction: I. anterior and anterolateral chest wall and wounds affecting respiratory function. *Plast Reconstr Surg*. 2009;124:240e−252e.

Seder CW, Rocco G. Chest wall reconstruction after extended resection. *J Thoracic Disease*. 2016;8:S863−S871.

Villa MT, Chang DW. Muscle and omental flaps for chest wall reconstruction. *Thorac Surg Clin*. 2010;20:543−550.

24

Intrathoracic Reconstruction

CASE 1

Clinical Presentation

A 49-year-old White female underwent right total pneumonectomy for stage IIIA nonsmall cell lung cancer. She had preoperative radiation and chemotherapy for treatment of her advanced cancer. About 2 weeks postoperatively, she was found to have right bronchopleural fistula with air leak and vancomycin-resistant enterococcus infection as well as methicillin-resistant *Staphylococcus aureus* infection. A right thoracoplasty was performed initially by the thoracic surgeon to control the bronchopleural fistula. She had a very complicated hospital course including emergent cardiopulmonary bypass to control the bleeding from the right pulmonary artery stump. The plastic surgery service was asked by the thoracic surgery service to help the chest wound closure after repair of the bronchopleural fistula site (Fig. 24.1). The primary service determined that the patient was stable enough to proceed to a more definitive operation to control the bronchopleural fistula and to close the right chest wound.

Operative Plan and Special Considerations

After examining the open wound over the right lateral chest, it appeared that the most part of the open chest cavity was located in the lower chest and the actual fistula site was in the middle chest. A midabdominal transverse rectus abdominis musculocutaneous (TRAM) flap could be selected based on the right superior epigastric vessels. The reason for selecting a midabdominal TRAM flap was because of her previous lower abdominal midline scar and to ensure the near-total survival of the midabdominal TRAM flap based on its large periumbilical perforators. This myocutaneous flap, after de-epithelization of it skin paddle, might provide a large amount of vascularized tissue to seal the bronchopleural fistula site and to obliterate a large part of the pleural cavity. The midabdominal TRAM flap may be more reliable than a standard lower abdominal TRAM flap. It might be possible that all four zones of flap tissue could survive and the flap could be tunneled and placed entirely into the chest.

Operative Procedures

The patient was brought to the operating room by the plastic surgery service about 5 weeks after the right total pneumonectomy. Under general anesthesia with the patient in the left lateral decubitus position, careful debridement was performed to remove all necrotic, infected, or colonized tissues within the right chest. The patient was then placed in the supine position and a midabdominal TRAM flap was designed based on the right superior epigastric vessels (Fig. 24.2). The skin paddle (30 × 12 cm) was elevated first. Once the incisions had been made through the anterior rectus sheath over the muscle, it was dissected free and its inferior insertion was divided. The entire flap was elevated, tunneled through the right subcostal area (Fig. 24.3) and placed inside the right chest without tension after the skin paddle of the flap was de-epithelized. The flap donor site was closed in a standard fashion over two drains.

The patient was then placed in the left lateral decubitus position again. For an intrathoracic placement of the entire de-epithelized right midabdominal TRAM flap, zones 1 and 2 of the flap faced the site of the bronchopleural fistula and the stump of the pulmonary vessels and zones 3 and 4 faced outward. A chest tube was placed inside the chest. The muscle portion of the flap was wrapped around the repaired bronchopleural fistula site and sutured and the rest of the flap was then placed inside the chest with interrupted sutures (Fig. 24.4). After some skin undermining and local tissue rearrangement, the right chest open wound was closed in two layers after intrathoracic placement of the midabdominal TRAM flap (Fig. 24.5).

Follow-Up Results

Postoperatively the patient did well except she developed a deep venous thrombosis of the right upper extremity, which was treated accordingly. The air leak and infection appeared to be resolved. Repeated chest CT scans showed a good filling of vascularized soft tissue to the right middle and lower chest (Fig. 24.6). The right chest wound repair site remained closed. She was discharged from the hospital 2 months later.

Management of Complications

She unfortunately developed recurrent bronchopleural fistula about 4 months after the first flap surgery, with a small open wound on her right chest and a persistent air leak. She was otherwise doing well with no evidence of infection (Fig. 24.7). Repeated chest CT scans showed a less optimal filling of the pleural cavity (Fig. 24.8). At this point, it became clear that additional well-vascularized tissue would be required not only to seal the recurrent bronchopleural fistula but also to obliterate the remaining dead space within the thoracic cavity. She was brought to the operating room for the second intrathoracic flap

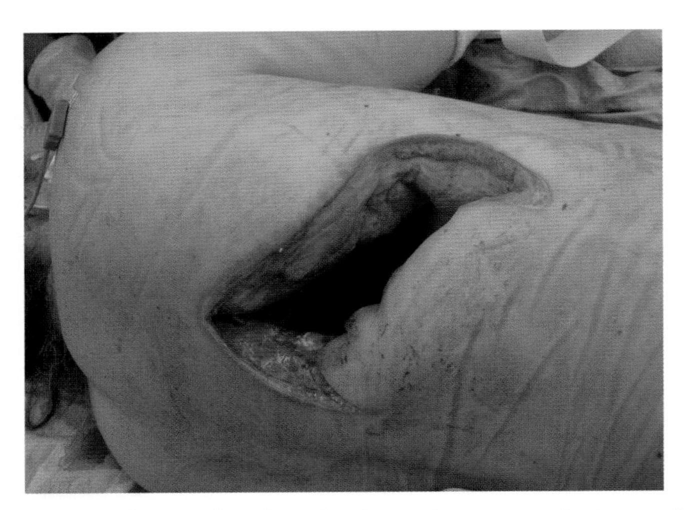

• **Fig. 24.1** Preoperative view showing a large open chest wound associated with right bronchopleural fistula.

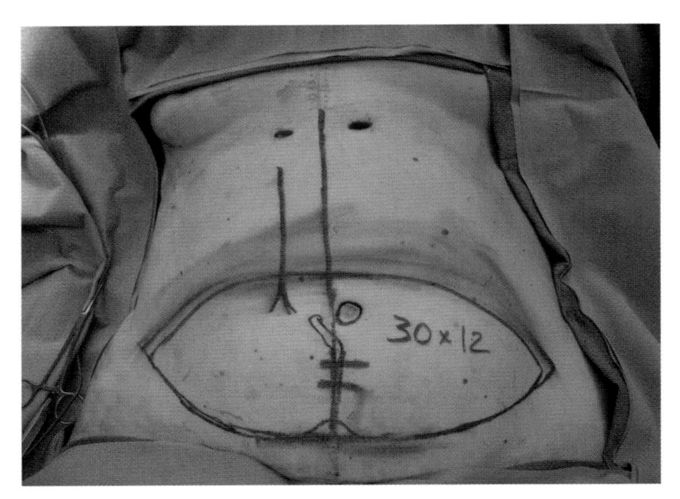

• **Fig. 24.2** Intraoperative view showing the design of a midabdominal transverse rectus abdominis musculocutaneous flap based on the right superior epigastric vessels.

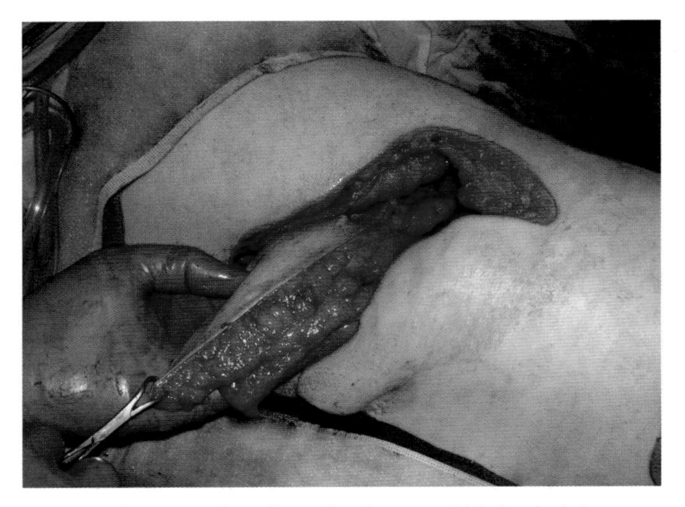

• **Fig. 24.3** Intraoperative view showing a midabdominal transverse rectus abdominis musculocutaneous flap that was elevated and tunneled through the right subcostal area.

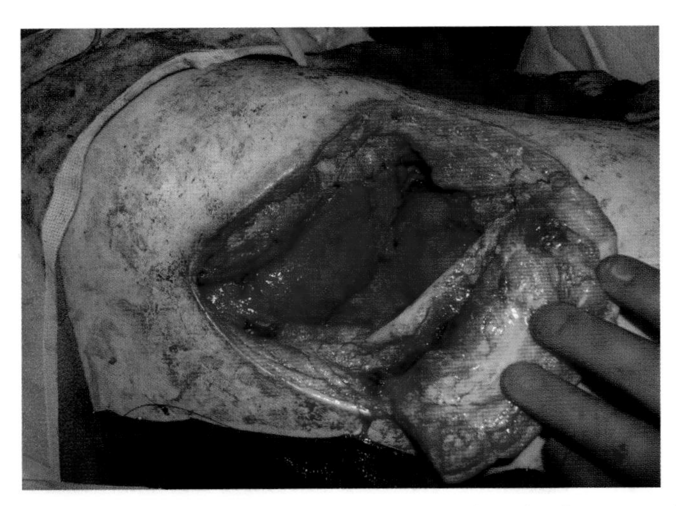

• **Fig. 24.4** Intraoperative view showing an intrathoracic placement of the entire de-epithelialized right midabdominal transverse rectus abdominis musculocutaneous flap. The muscle portion of the flap was sutured to wrap around the repaired bronchopleural fistula site and the rest of the flap was then placed inside the chest with interrupted sutures.

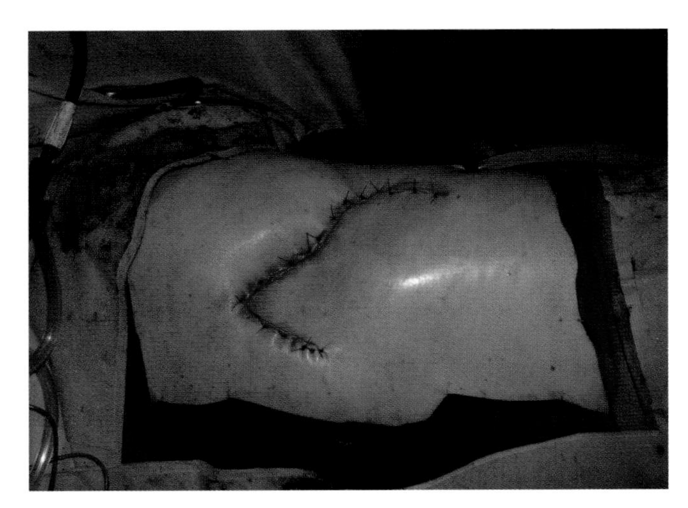

• **Fig. 24.5** Intraoperative view showing closure of the entire chest wound after intrathoracic placement of the midabdominal transverse rectus abdominis musculocutaneous flap.

transfer. During exploration, the recurrent bronchopleural fistula was identified (Figs. 24.9 and 24.10) and repaired again by the thoracic surgery service with additional suture and fascial patch graft (Fig. 24.11). Because of the previous right thoracotomy, the left latissimus dorsi myocutaneous flap was selected and elevated as a free flap (Fig. 24.12). The right thoracodorsal vessels were explored for the recipient vessels. After successful end-to-end microvascular anastomoses for both artery and vein, the entire flap appeared to be well perfused (Fig. 24.13). The de-epithelialized flap could be placed freely anywhere inside the pleural cavity. The repair site of the recurrent fistula was covered with the muscular portion of the flap and the remaining dead space was completely obliterated by the flap with the de-epithelized portion facing out (Fig. 24.14). With concerns of the flap being buried inside the chest, it was observed for an hour in the operating room after

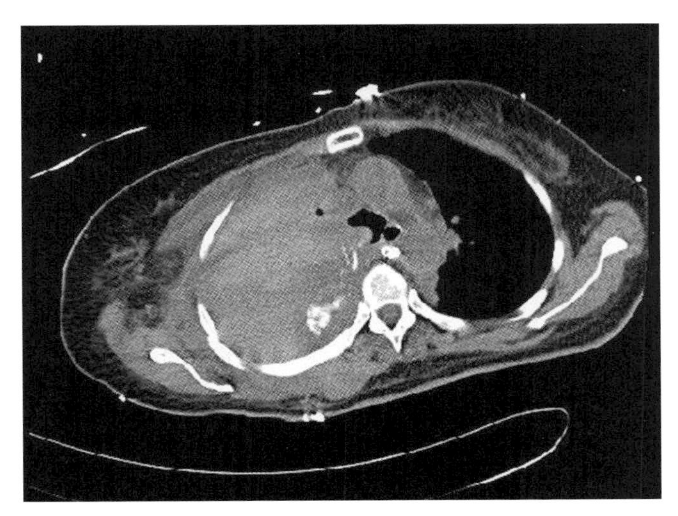

• **Fig. 24.6** Postoperative chest CT scan showing adequate filling of the vascularized soft tissue to the right middle and lower chest.

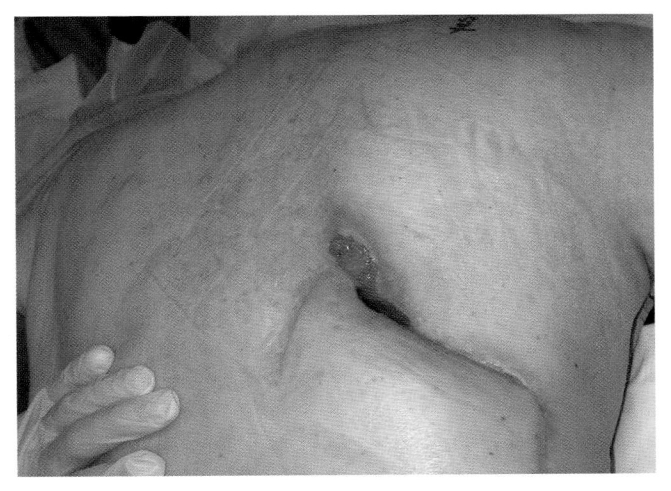

• **Fig. 24.7** Preoperative view showing recurrent bronchopleural fistula with small open chest wound 4 months after the initial flap surgery.

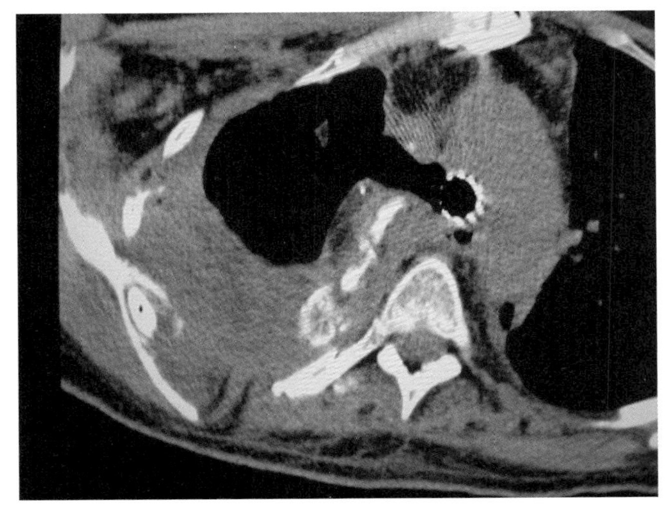

• **Fig. 24.8** Preoperative repeated chest CT scan showing a less complete obliteration of pleural cavity after the first flap surgery.

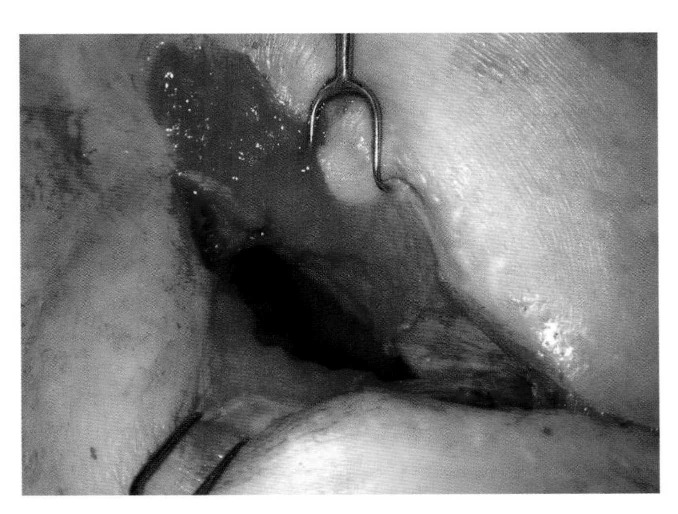

• **Fig. 24.9** Intraoperative view showing the recurrent bronchopleural fistula and open chest wound.

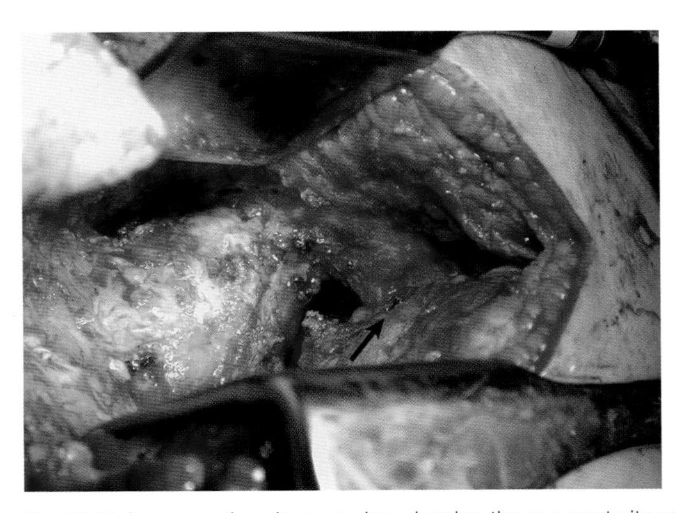

• **Fig. 24.10** Intraoperative close-up view showing the recurrent site of bronchopleural fistula.

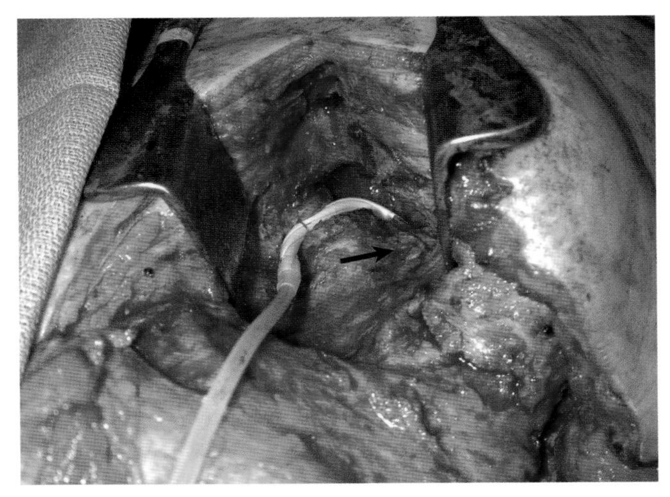

• **Fig. 24.11** Intraoperative view showing successful repair of the recurrent bronchopleural fistula and a drain placement near the repair site.

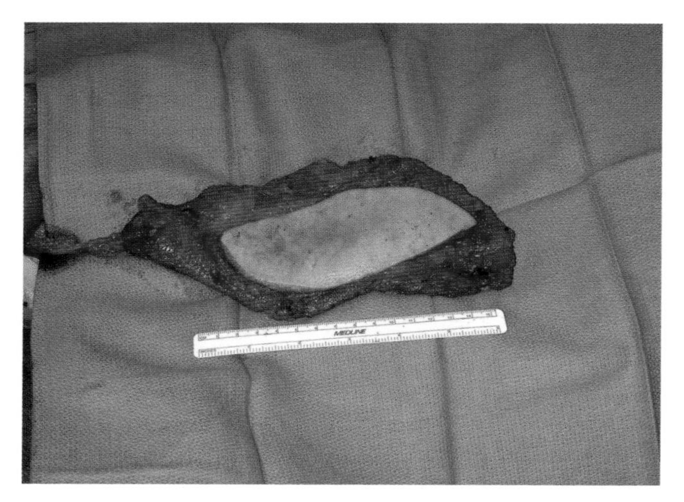

• **Fig. 24.12** Intraoperative view showing a successfully elevated contralateral latissimus dorsi myocutaneous flap before division of the pedicle vessels.

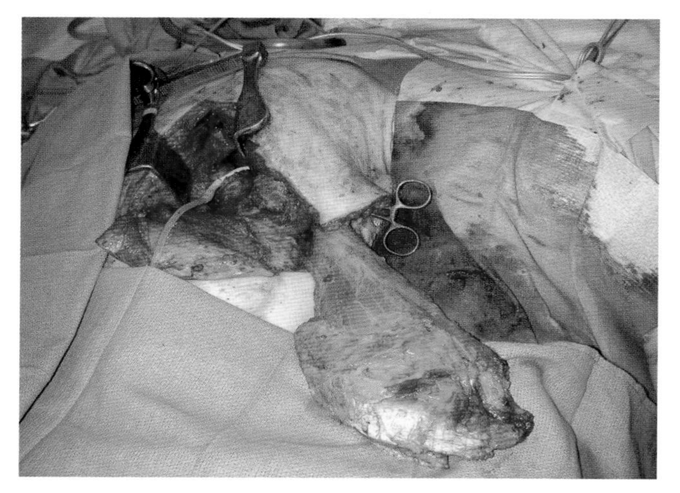

• **Fig. 24.13** Intraoperative view showing a successfully transferred free latissimus dorsi myocutaneous flap after microvascular anastomoses.

both microvascular anastomoses before the chest wound was closed. It reassured the surgeon that both microvascular anastomoses were patent and there were no technical errors in the free tissue transfer. The chest wound was closed again in two layers after local tissue rearrangement (Fig. 24.15). The patient tolerated the entire procedure well and was extubated the next day. She was found to have no further air leak after the second flap surgery and was discharged from the hospital 2 weeks postoperatively

Final Outcome

During subsequent follow-up visits, the patient had no recurrent bronchopleural fistula and the right chest wound healed well (Fig. 24.16). She has no recurrent bronchopleural fistula or open wound in the area, has resumed her normal activities, and is followed by the thoracic surgery service for routine follow-up.

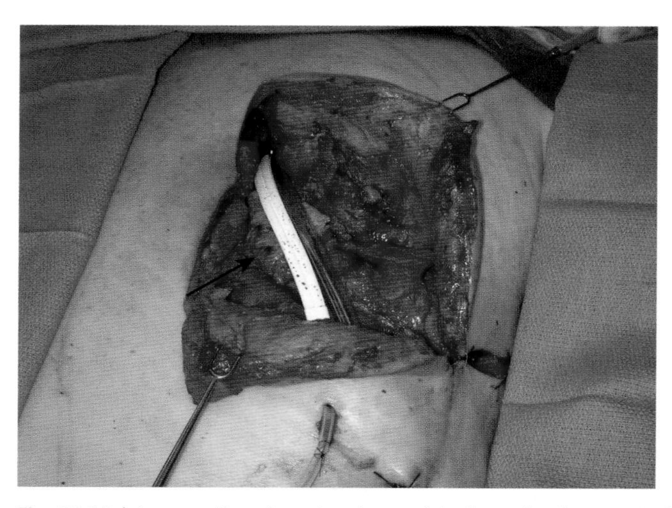

• **Fig. 24.14** Intraoperative view showing an intrathoracic placement of the de-epithelialized free flap *(arrow)*. The recurrent fistula repaired with additional suture and fascial patch graft were covered with the muscular portion of the flap and the remaining dead space was completely obliterated by the flap with the de-epithelialized portion facing outward.

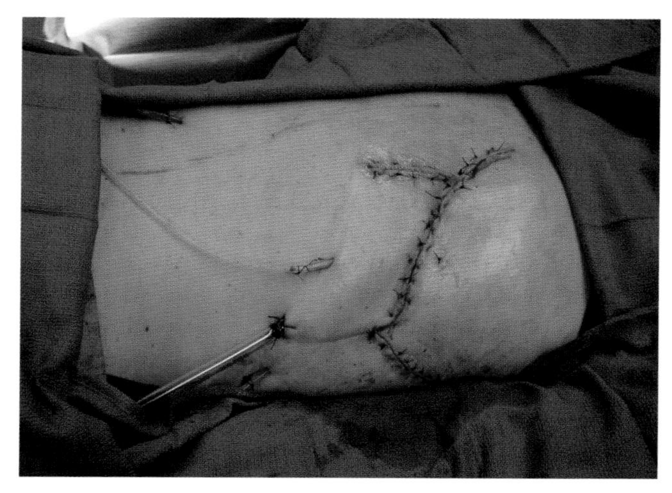

• **Fig. 24.15** Intraoperative view showing the closure of the entire chest wound after intrathoracic placement of a free latissimus dorsi myocutaneous flap.

Pearls for Success

Adequate debridement of infected or necrotic tissue in the thoracic cavity, closure of bronchopleural fistula, and minimization of the dead space with thoracoplasty and/or muscle flaps are the principles of the modern approach to bronchopleural fistula associated with infection after total pneumonectomy. However, management of a recalcitrant bronchopleural fistula associated with infection can be challenging and multiple flaps or procedures are often needed to close the air leak, to obliterate most of the dead space, and to eliminate the infection. Initial intrathoracic placement of a major large distant flap, such as a midabdominal TRAM flap, is often required to close the bronchopleural fistula and to obliterate a significant portion of the dead space within the chest. If such an effort fails, a major free tissue transfer, such as a contralateral latissimus dorsi myocutaneous, should be considered

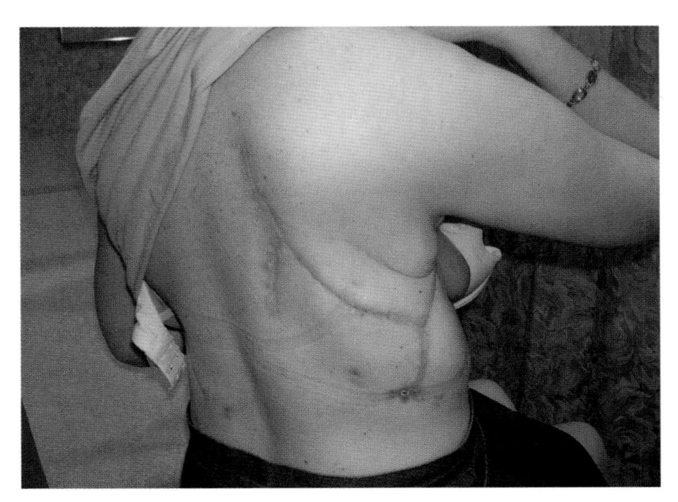

• **Fig. 24.16** The result at 3-month follow-up after the second intrathoracic flap placement showing well-healed right chest wound with no evidence of recurrent bronchopleural fistula.

as a second procedure. However, microvascular anastomoses can be difficult because the surgeon must perform the procedures within a deep hole of the axilla. This large free flap can provide additional well-vascularized tissue for a more sophisticated flap inset to close the fistula and to obliterate the dead space within the thoracic cavity. Such a combination may often be necessary and should be considered when managing this devastating postpneumonectomy complication.

CASE 2

Clinical Presentation

A 37-year-old White male with a history of left lobectomy and empyema subsequently developed a left bronchopleural fistula approximately 1 year ago. He had been treated with a chest tube drainage. He underwent a left thoracotomy 2 days earlier for exploration and drainage, at which time it was found he had an infection in the left chest. The infected pleural cavity was debrided by the thoracic surgery service. The plastic surgery service was asked to help the primary service to manage this complicated bronchopleural fistula. The definitive reconstruction of the bronchopleural fistula was planned 2 days later in conjunction with the primary service (Fig. 24.17).

Operative Plan and Special Considerations

Once accomplishing adequate debridement in the pleural cavity and attempting repair of the bronchopleural fistula site in the left chest, the planned reconstructive procedure would be to transfer well-vascularized flap tissue to the chest. Because a large amount of soft tissue would be needed to fill the large pleural cavity, a pedicled omental flap could provide large amount of well-vascularized tissue to the pleural cavity. Such a well-vascularized tissue could not only seal the bronchopleural fistula repair site but also obliterate any dead space in the remaining pleural cavity. The flap can be tunneled through the diaphragm and placed into the left pleural cavity without any problems.

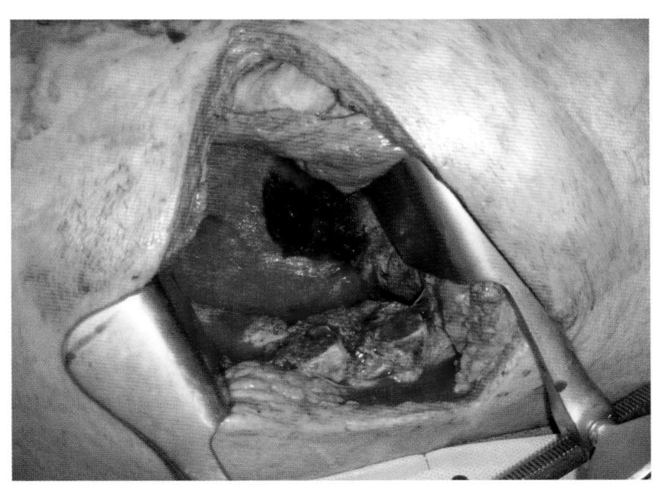

• **Fig. 24.17** Preoperative view showing a large left chest open wound associated with a bronchopleural fistula.

Operative Procedures

Under general anesthesia, the initial laparotomy and exposure of the omentum were performed by the general surgery service. The pedicled omental flap was dissected and elevated by the general surgery and plastic surgery services. The left and right gastroepiploic arteries were identified with a handheld Doppler and direct palpation. The left gastroepiploic vessels and vascular arcade attachments to the splenic artery were divided. The omentum was freed and had a considerable length at this point (Fig. 24.18). The upper surface of the right gastroepiploic vessels was marked to prevent the pedicle from getting twisted while tunneling through the diaphragm.

A partial resection of the left hemidiaphragm was performed by the thoracic surgery service to create a tunnel for the flap transfer from the abdomen to the chest (Fig. 24.19). Hemostasis was controlled adequately at conclusion of the flap harvest. The flap was passed gently through the left diaphragm. Care was taken to ensure that there was no twisting of the pedicle and the flap was

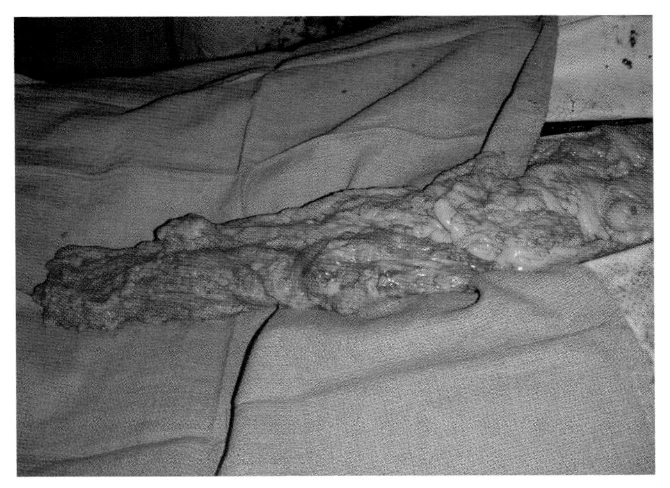

• **Fig. 24.18** Intraoperative view showing a pedicled omental flap that was harvested from the abdomen. The flap had a large amount of vascularized tissue.

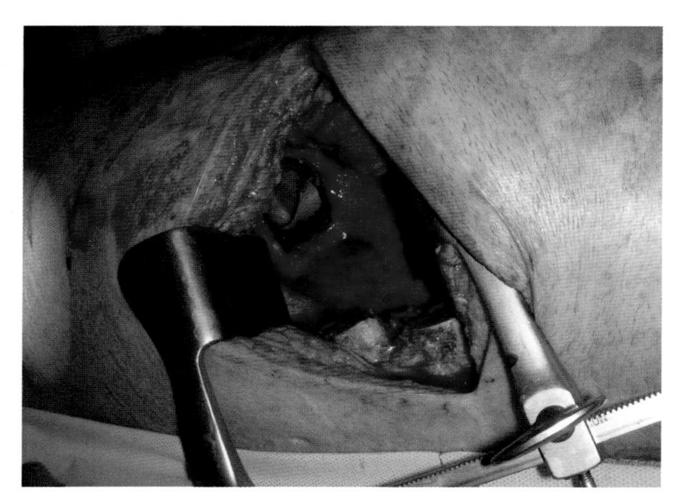

• **Fig. 24.19** Intraoperative view showing a tunnel that was made through the left diaphragm.

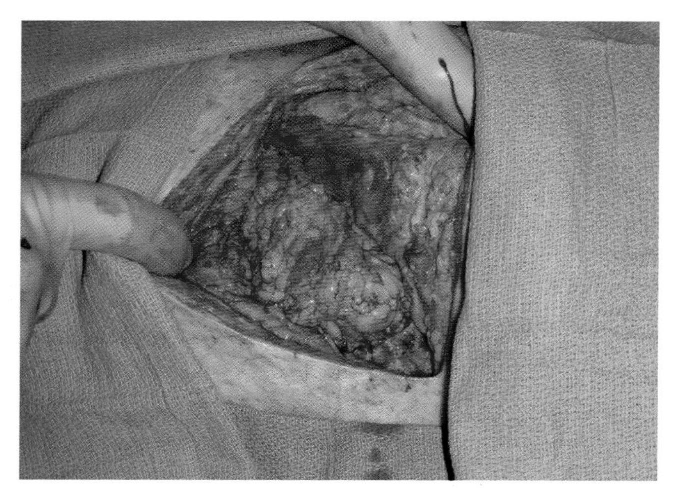

• **Fig. 24.20** Intraoperative view showing the well-vascularized omental tissue inside the left chest wound by the omental flap before the flap inset.

then inset into the left chest with interrupted 2-0 PDS sutures to the underlying surface of the serratus and latissimus (Fig. 24.20).

The flap appeared to be well perfused and there was a good Doppler signal at the distal portion of the flap. A 19-Fr round drain was placed just under the flap in the left chest and brought out through a stab incision. The flap filled the left lower chest completely. The flap was placed to cover the area where the left bronchopleural fistula repair was performed (Fig. 24.21). The chest and abdominal wounds were closed by the thoracic and general surgery services accordingly.

Follow-Up Results

The patient did well postoperatively without any complications related to the omental flap reconstruction. He was discharged from hospital on postoperative day 5. The drain was removed during subsequent follow-up visits. The chest wound and abdominal incision healed well and the bronchopleural fistula was under control (Fig. 24.22).

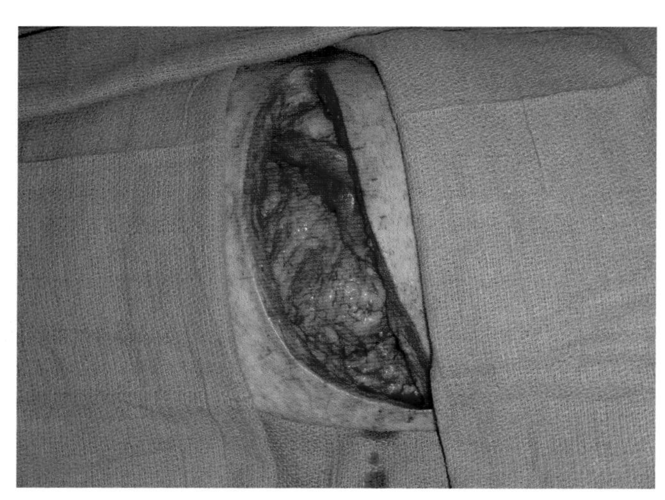

• **Fig. 24.21** Intraoperative view showing completely filled lower chest wound by the omental flap before the chest wound closure.

Final Outcome

The left chest wound after the omental flap reconstruction healed well. Most importantly, the patient has not had a recurrent bronchopleural fistula or any issues related to the left chest reconstruction. He has resumed his normal activities and is followed by the thoracic surgery service for routine follow-up.

Pearls for Success

A bronchopleural fistula is a challenging complication after lobectomy or pneumonectomy for any thoracic surgery service. After surgical repair of the fistula site, a large amount of well-vascularized tissue will be needed to seal it and to obliterate the dead space in the pleural cavity. A pedicled omental flap, based on either side of the gastroepiploic vessels, can be selected to provide soft tissue fill and coverage in the chest if there is enough omental tissue. Attention should be paid to decrease the risk of contamination from the chest wound to the abdominal cavity. Attention should also be paid to ensure that the pedicle vessels are not kinked or twisted during tunneling through a created diaphragm window. The amount of flap tissue is usually large enough to fill the lower chest cavity and the final chest wound closure can be accomplished after the flap has been completely buried inside the chest.

CASE 3

Clinical Presentation

A 73-year-old White male developed a complicated left bronchopleurocutaneous fistula secondary to chronic empyema. He had undergone a left upper lobectomy 3 years previously. He was managed by the thoracic surgery service for open chest debridement, which resulted in a left chest wound (Fig. 24.23). The vascular surgery service had also performed a ligation of the left

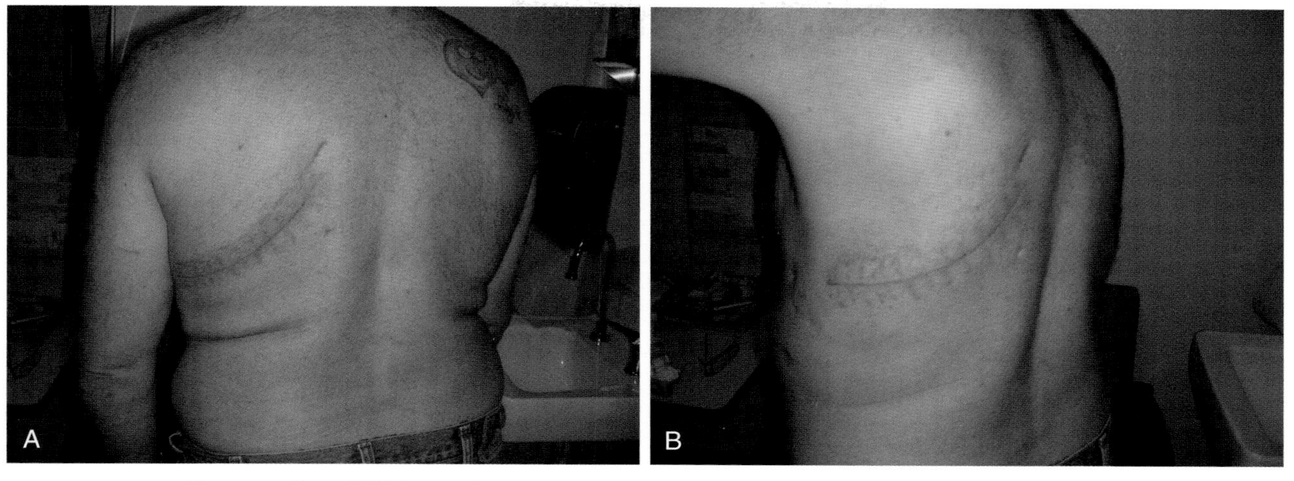

• **Fig. 24.22** (A and B) The result at 3-month follow-up showing stable and well-healed lower chest wound.

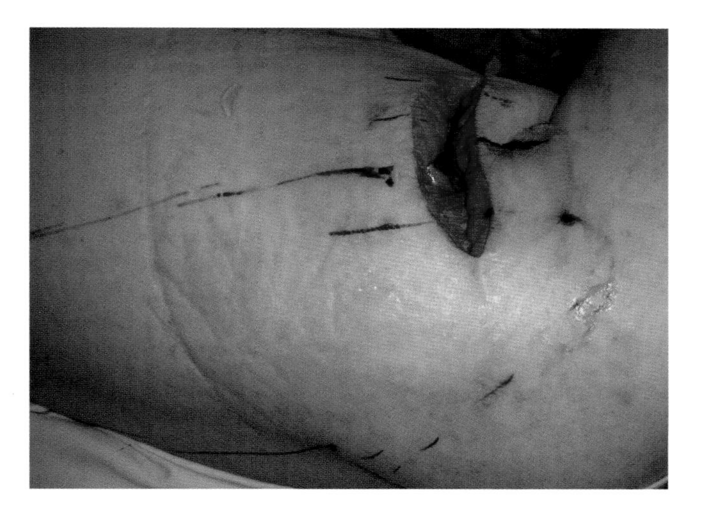

• **Fig. 24.23** Preoperative view showing a left upper chest open wound following initial debridement by the primary service.

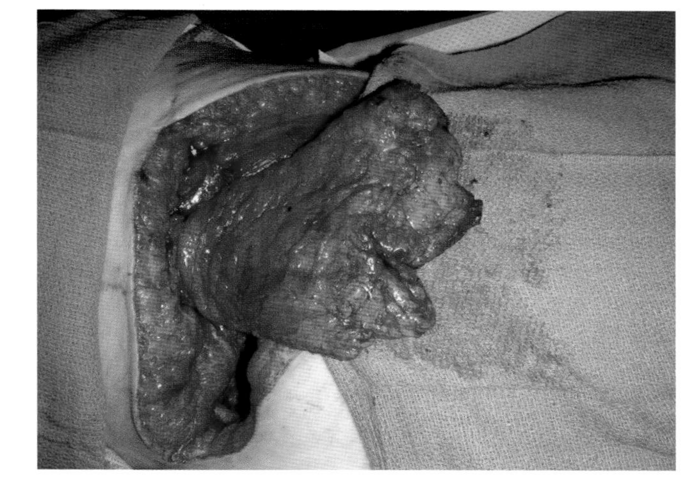

• **Fig. 24.24** Intraoperative view showing the amount of the latissimus dorsi muscle flap tissue that could be used to provide adequate soft tissue filling and sealing of a bronchopleural fistula wound.

distal subclavian artery and a carotid to axillary artery extra-anatomical bypass 2 days earlier. The plastic surgery service was asked to help the chest wound closure after repair of the bronchopleural fistula site. It was determined by the primary service that the patient was stable enough to proceed to another operation to close the bronchopleural fistula and the chest wound.

Operative Plan and Special Considerations

After examining the open wound over the left upper lateral chest for this patient, the latissimus dorsi muscle on this side is still largely intact and the muscle has only been transected at the level of the previous thoracotomy scar. Therefore, the pedicled latissimus dorsi muscle flap can still be used to fill the left chest cavity and to seal the bronchopleural fistula repair site by providing well-vascularized tissue. The flap can be elevated through an additional oblique incision and transposed into the chest wound. Prior to the procedure, the thoracodorsal vessels should be evaluated to make sure that they are still patent as the pedicel of the flap.

Operative Procedures

Under general anesthesia with the patient in right lateral decubitus position, an oblique incision was made over the left upper back between his chest wound and the previous thoracotomy incision. The skin and subcutaneous tissue were incised to the latissimus dorsi muscle.

Once the latissimus dorsi muscle had been elevated both anteriorly and posteriorly, most of the muscle could be seen. The anterior border of the muscle was released, followed by the release of the posterior boarder. Elevation of the muscle from the chest wall was then performed under direct vision. The muscle was found to be divided at the previous thoracotomy level. The latissimus muscle was then elevated after additional dissection both anteriorly and posteriorly. The flap was dissected from the serratus muscle and the teres major muscle toward the pedicle (Fig. 24.24). Dissection around the pedicle was carefully done under direct vision. During the flap dissection, the thoracodorsal vessels were identified and confirmed with a handheld Doppler.

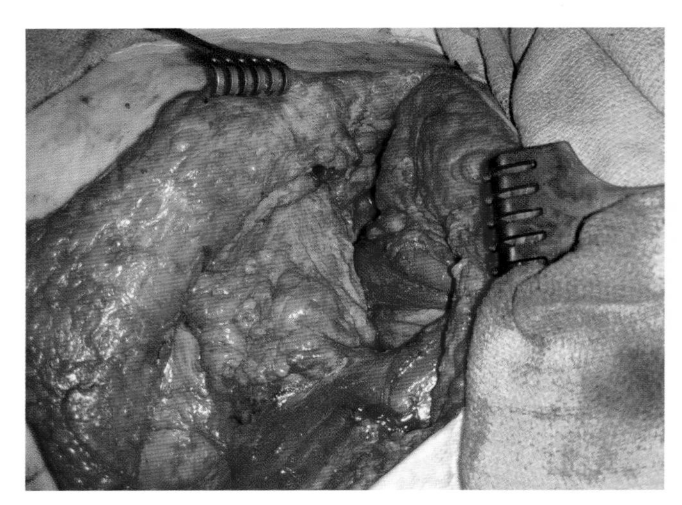

• **Fig. 24.25** Intraoperative view showing the amount of the fasciocutaneous tissue from the inferior chest wall that could be used to provide additional soft tissue filling within the chest wound.

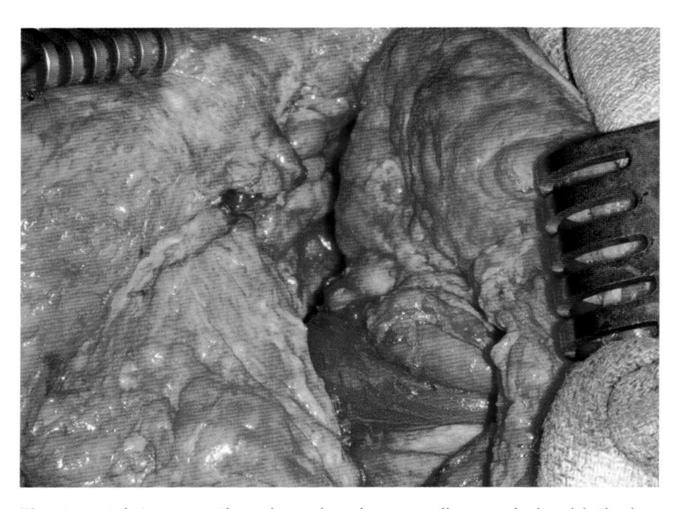

• **Fig. 24.26** Intraoperative view showing a well-vascularized latissimus dorsi muscle flap that was inset into the chest to fill and seal the bronchopleural fistula site.

Intraoperatively a well-perfused muscle flap was confirmed by intraoperative fluorescein test.

Intrathoracic flap inset was performed by the thoracic surgery service. The muscle flap was inset into the fistula site and filled the dead space of the chest. It was secured with interrupted 3-0 Vicryl sutures to maintain the proper position and placement of the flap.

The final chest wound closure, a 15 × 8 cm local fasciocutaneous flap, was elevated and mobilized off the skin from the inferior aspect of the chest wound. The flap was advanced to the wound (Fig. 24.25). The final chest wound was closed in three layers (Fig. 24.26). The deep tissue was approximated with several interrupted 2-0 PDS sutures. The deep dermal closure was performed with 3-0 Monocryl sutures in an interrupted fashion. The skin was then closed with skin staples. The latissimus dorsi muscle flap donor site was closed in three layers after placing two drains.

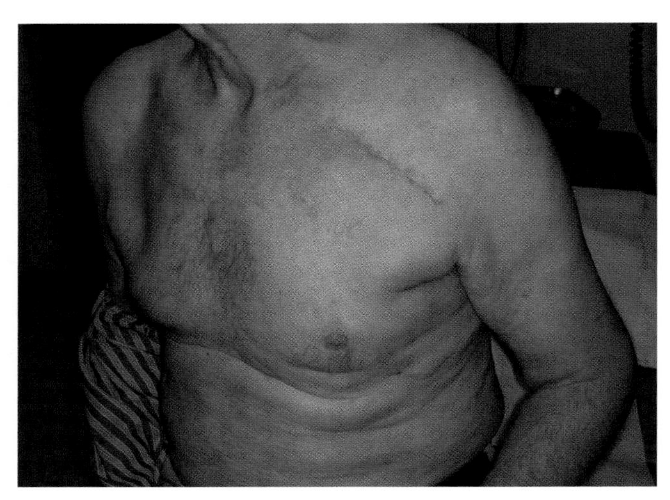

• **Fig. 24.27** The result at 4-month follow-up showing well-healed left chest wound.

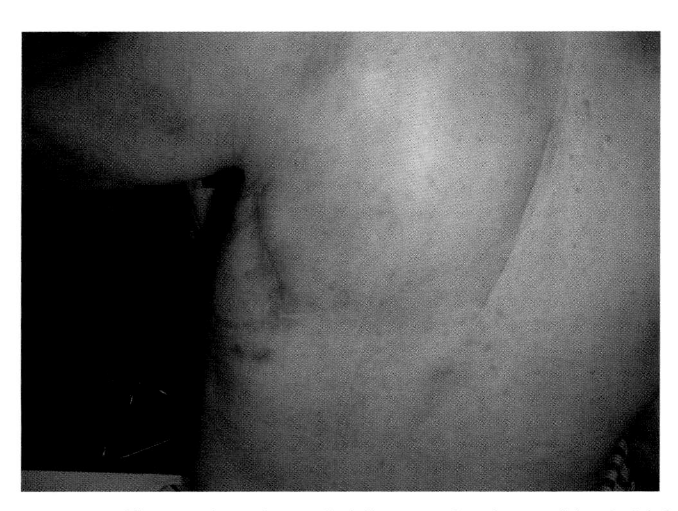

• **Fig. 24.28** The result at 4-month follow-up showing well-healed left chest wound with no evidence of recurrent bronchopleural fistula.

Follow-Up Results

The patient did well postoperatively without any complications related to the latissimus dorsi flap reconstruction. He was discharged from hospital on postoperative day 10. All drains were removed during subsequent follow-up visits. His left upper chest wound healed well after the flap reconstruction.

Final Outcome

The left chest bronchopleural fistula wound healed well after the latissimus dorsi flap reconstruction (Figs. 24.27 and 24.28). He has had no recurrent bronchopleural fistula or open wound in the area. He has resumed his normal activities and is followed by the thoracic surgery service for routine follow-up.

Pearls for Success

A pedicled latissimus dorsi muscle flap can be a good choice for intrathoracic placement when managing a relatively small bronchopleural fistula if a major portion of the flap still remains intact even after previous thoracotomy. The flap can be inset into the chest not only to seal the bronchopleural fistula repair site but also to fill the dead space within the pleural cavity. However, the surgeon should decide whether the amount of flap tissue is adequate to achieve both goals. With proper judgment, the flap can be selected for management of a less extensive bronchopleural fistula within a pleural space. Additional fasciocutaneous flap can also be mobilized to provide additional fill within the chest wound.

Recommended Readings

Asaad M, Van Handel A, Akhavan AA, et al. Muscle flap transposition for the management of intrathoracic fistulas. *Plast Reconstr Surg.* 2020;145:829e–838e.

Asaad M, Van Handel A, Akhavan AA, et al. Intrathoracic muscle flap transposition for the management of chronic pulmonary aspergillosis. *J Plast Reconstr Aesthet Surg.* 2020;73:1815–1824.

Botiau P. Current indications for the intrathoracic transposition of the omentum. *J Cardiothoracic Surg.* 2019;14:103.

Chen HC, Lo SJ, Kim JH. Management of intrathoracic defects. *Semin Plast Surg.* 2011;25:70–77.

Fricke A, Bannasch H, Klein HF, et al. Pedicled and free flaps for intrathoracic fistula management. *Euro J Cardiothoracic Surg.* 2017;52:1211–1217.

Gaucher S, Lococo F, Guinet C, et al. Indications and results of reconstructive techniques with flaps transposition in patients requiring complex thoracic surgery: a 12-year experience. *Lung.* 2016;194:855–863.

Mustala ST, Lempinen J, Saimanen E, Vilkko P. Efficacy of thoracic analgesia with or without intercostal nerve cryoanalgesia for post-thoracotomy pain. *Ann Thorac Surg.* 2011;91:869–873.

Pu LLQ. Successful management of a recalcitrant bronchopleural fistula associated with infection after total pneumonectomy. *J Plast Reconstr Aesthet Surg.* 2010;63:e180–e182.

25
Esophageal Reconstruction

CASE 1

Clinical Presentation

The plastic surgery service was asked by the surgical oncology service to evaluate a 53-year-old White male with esophageal discontinuity after esophagectomy for cancer and failure of two previous esophageal reconstructions. The patient's condition began 5 years ago when he was diagnosed with a thoracic esophageal cancer (stage III) during esophagogastroduodenoscopy (EGD). The EGD caused perforation of the cancer into the chest. He underwent an emergency thoracoabdominal esophagogastrectomy. The patient did reasonably well until he developed a gastric outlet obstruction and empyema 1 year later requiring further thoracic and abdominal surgery. Systemic chemotherapy and local radiation to his left neck completed the cancer treatment.

An anastomotic recurrence was revealed 2 years after his initial surgery. The patient underwent a thoracotomy with completion esophagectomy. Immediate gastrointestinal continuity was restored with a substernal colonic interposition utilizing the transverse colon and a portion of the descending colon supplied by the left colic artery. The distal half of the colon interposition was necrosed and was resected on postoperative day 1. A cervical tube esophagostomy was placed. The remaining colonic conduit was sutured to the anterior abdominal wall and a tube colostomy was created. The patient recovered over the next 2 years and remained cancer-free for at least 5 years after his initial esophagectomy. He strongly desired and sought a third attempt at esophageal reconstruction for restoration of gastrointestinal continuity in order to be able to eat and drink (Fig. 25.1). He was seen by many reconstructive surgeons in the region to find an option for the esophageal reconstruction.

Operative Plan and Special Considerations

During preoperative evaluation, the distance of discontinuity was estimated to span 22 cm prohibiting a safe, free jejunal transfer. Barium enema suggested the remaining ascending colon was also insufficient. In addition, the distance through a substernal tunnel between the cervical esophageal stump and the opening of the tube colostomy site within the remaining colonic conduit measured 15 cm. Because a preoperative noninvasive vascular study showed an adequate superficial palmar arch of the patient's right hand, a free right radial forearm flap could be selected and used to reconstruct a conduit and to bridge between the cervical esophageal stump and the opening of the tube colostomy site after a successful microvascular anastomosis of the flap to the neck recipient vessels. In addition, the left neck site would need additional soft tissue coverage because of previous radiation to the area. A right pedicled pectoral muscle flap could be used to provide adequate soft tissue coverage of the neck open area after surgical dissection of the neck recipient vessels and the esophageal reconstruction.

Operative Procedures

Under general anesthesia, abdominal exploration and dissection of the cervical esophagus were performed by the surgical oncology service to determine whether a retrosternal tunnel would even be feasible, given the patient's previous history of radiation, scarring, and operations. A retrosternal passage after careful dissection was obtained through neck and abdominal wounds.

The right radial forearm flap was harvested by the plastic surgery service. The flap was marked out on the volar surface of the forearm and measured 18 × 8.5 cm (Fig. 25.2). An intraoperative handheld Doppler was done to confirm pulses in the arch and the thumb with occlusion of the radial artery. The flap dissection was initially performed to the subcutaneous tissue. The suprafascial dissection was then performed and the cephalic vein, the radial artery, and its venae comitantes were identified and divided at the level of the wrist crease. The flap was raised from the ulnar to radial forearm and the septocutaneous perforators from the radial artery were preserved. This part of the flap dissection was performed under tourniquet control. The flap was raised from distal to proximal and the radial artery was dissected free to the level of the bifurcation of the brachial artery (Fig. 25.3). The flap was then tubularized over a Hegar dilator, putting the skin at the internal lining of the flap and constructing this with a running dermal 3-0 Vicryl suture for a watertight seal. The tube was approximately 3 cm in diameter and 18 cm long (Fig. 25.4).

Once the colon and cervical esophagus had been prepared by the surgical oncology service for an anastomosis, the pedicle vessels of the radial forearm flap were divided proximally as far as possible (Fig. 25.5). While waitfing for the flap inset and microvascular anastomoses, the fascial edges of the flexor carpi radialis and the brachial radialis were approximated with running 3-0 Vicryl suture and the loose skin around the periphery of the wound was fixed with 3-0 Vicryl suture, reducing the overall size of the wound to 17 × 7 cm for a skin graft placement (Fig. 25.6). A split-thickness skin graft at 0.015 thickness was harvested from the left thigh with a dermatome. It was placed on the forearm wound as a sheet graft and stapled to the periphery of the wound edge. A volar forearm splint was placed for immobilization.

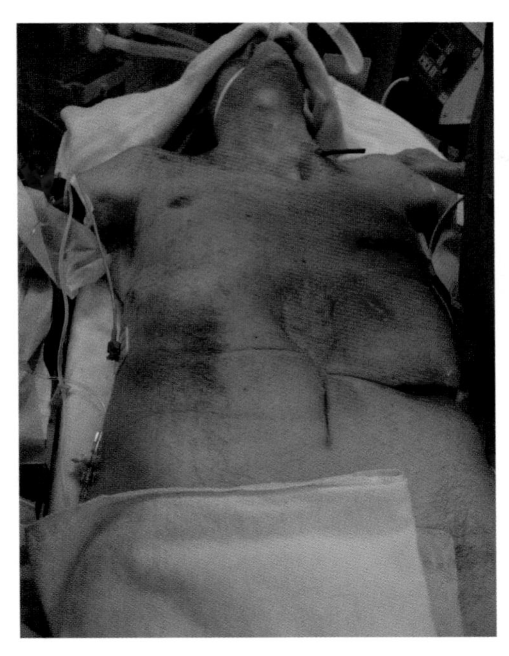

• **Fig. 25.1** A preoperative view showing the cervical esophageal fistula in the lower neck and multiple surgical scars in the abdomen.

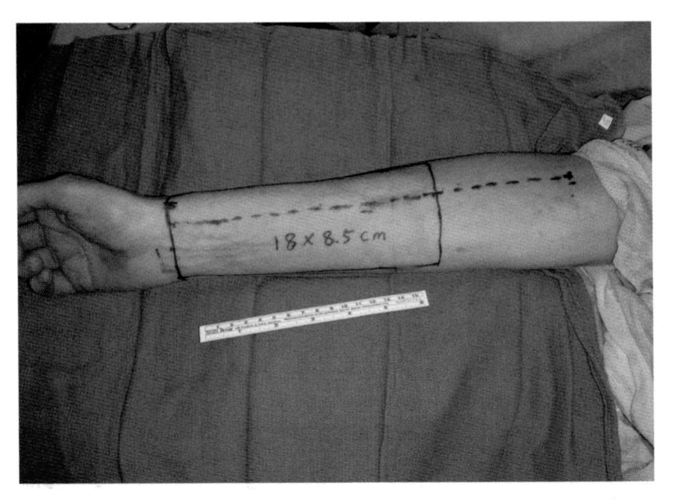

• **Fig. 25.2** Intraoperative view showing the design of the right free radial forearm flap. The size of the skin paddle was 18 × 8.5 cm.

The colonic stump to the flap was anastomosed by the surgical oncology service (Fig. 25.7). The flap was then tunneled under the sternum by the plastic surgery service and the flap to the cervical esophagus anastomosis was again performed by the surgical oncology service (Fig. 25.8). The right transverse cervical artery was dissected out. A branch of the right external jugular was also dissected out. Both vessels were prepared for microvascular anastomoses. However, the right transverse cervical artery was found to have poor blood flow and the right inferior thyroid artery was therefore selected instead and dissected out for microvascular anastomosis. The artery was also tunneled under the right external jugular vein. The arterial microanastomosis was performed with interrupted 8-0 nylons in an end-to-end fashion. The venous anastomosis was performed with a 3-mm coupler device in end-to-end fashion between the donor cephalic vein and a branch of the right external jugular vein (Fig. 25.9).

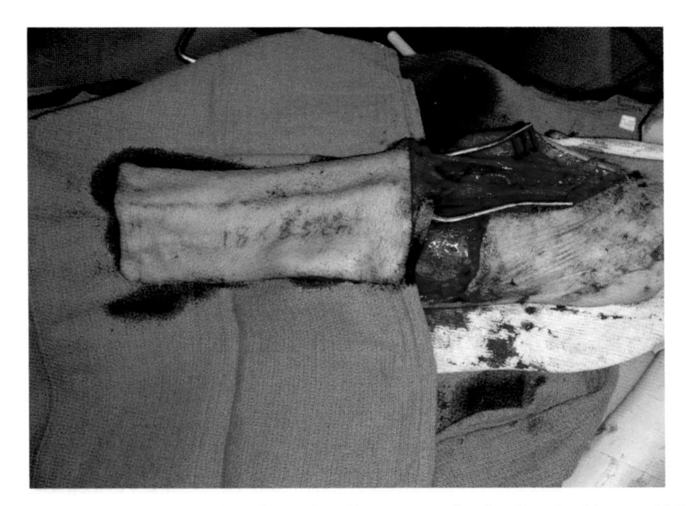

• **Fig. 25.3** Intraoperative view showing a completely elevated free radial forearm flap after release of the tourniquet.

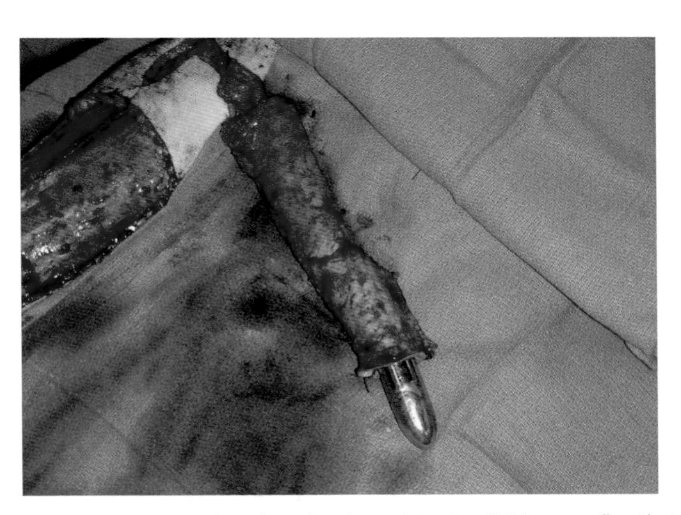

• **Fig. 25.4** Intraoperative view showing a tubed radial forearm flap that was made after two layers of water-tight closure longitudinally after release of the tourniquet.

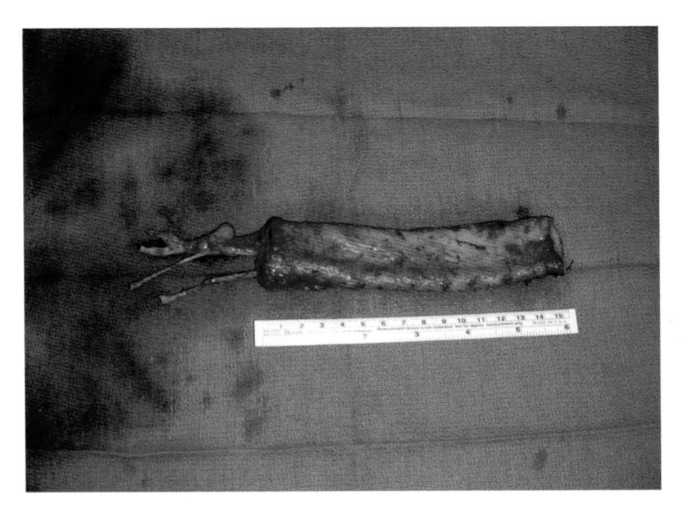

• **Fig. 25.5** Intraoperative view showing a tubed free right radial forearm flap that was ready for esophageal reconstruction. Only the cephalic vein was used for the venous microvascular anastomosis.

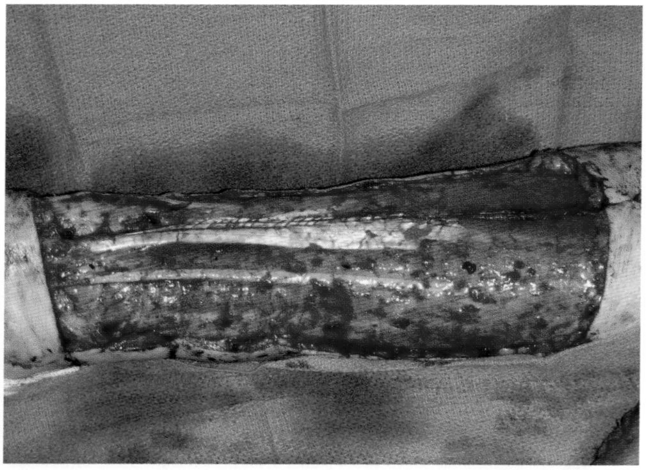

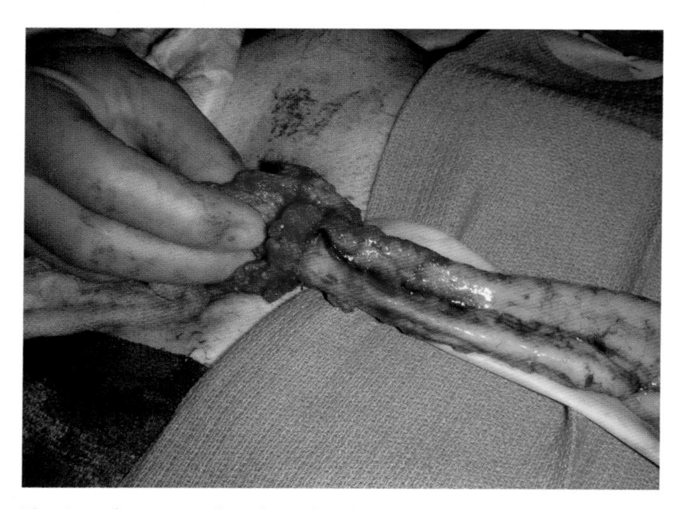

• **Fig. 25.6** Intraoperative view showing the surface area after the fascial approximation between the flexor carpi radialis and the brachial radialis. This might ensure a better cosmetic outcome in the radial forearm flap donor site.

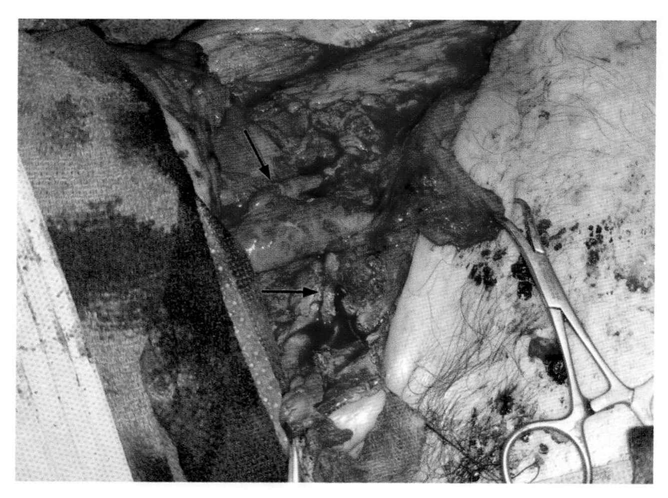

• **Fig. 25.9** Intraoperative view showing completion of microvascular anastomoses in the right neck. The arterial microvascular anastomosis was to the right inferior thyroid artery *(lower arrow)* and the venous microvascular anastomosis was to a branch of the right external jugular vein *(upper arrow)*.

The abdominal wound was closed and a feeding tube was inserted by the surgical oncology team. The right pectoral muscle flap was elevaeted to cover the exposed the radial forearm flap and the neck wound. An oblique incision was made in the right chest wall medial to the nipple extending from the level of the xiphoid to the level of the clavicle. The flap dissection was done in a suprafascial plane from medial to lateral. Once all of its attachments had been divided, the pedicle of the flap was confirmed by a handheld Doppler and marked (Fig. 25.10). The humeral attachment of the pectoralis major muscle was divided carefully. The flap was then completely mobilized on its pedicle and was advanced medially through a tunnel under the skin bridge to the neck wound. The flap was inset into the chest skin defect and approximated with interrupted 3-0 Vicryl sutures. A 15-Fr Blake drain was brought out through a stab incision in the right axilla. Additionally, a 10-Fr flat drain was placed between the muscle flap and the radial forearm flap in the neck wound. A 6 × 7 cm split-thickness skin graft, meshed 1 to 1.5 ratio at 0.015-inch thickness, was harvested from the left thigh with a dermatome and was placed over the muscle flap and secured with staples. The

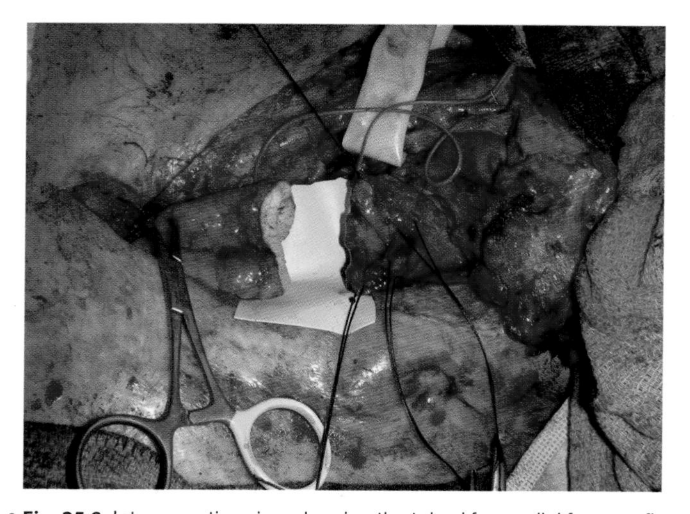

• **Fig. 25.7** Intraoperative view showing completion of the distal anastomosis between the colon and the tubed free radial forearm flap.

• **Fig. 25.8** Intraoperative view showing the tubed free radial forearm flap that was tunneled retrosternally and inserted within the created substernal space before the anastomosis to the cervical esophagus was performed by the surgical oncologist.

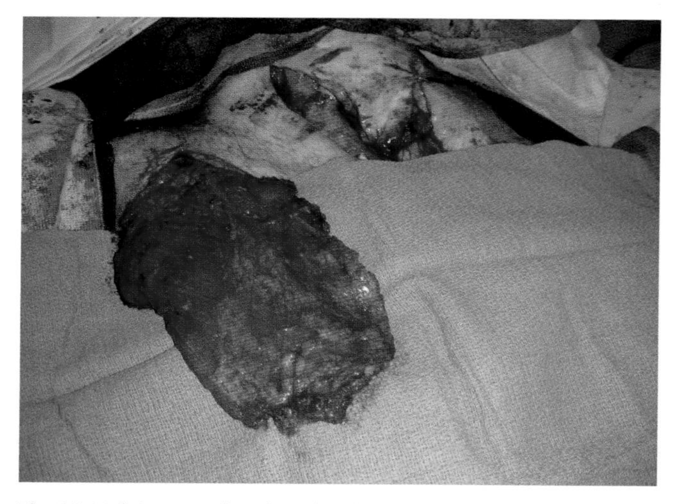

• **Fig. 25.10** Intraoperative view showing complete elevation of the right pectoral major muscle flap before inset.

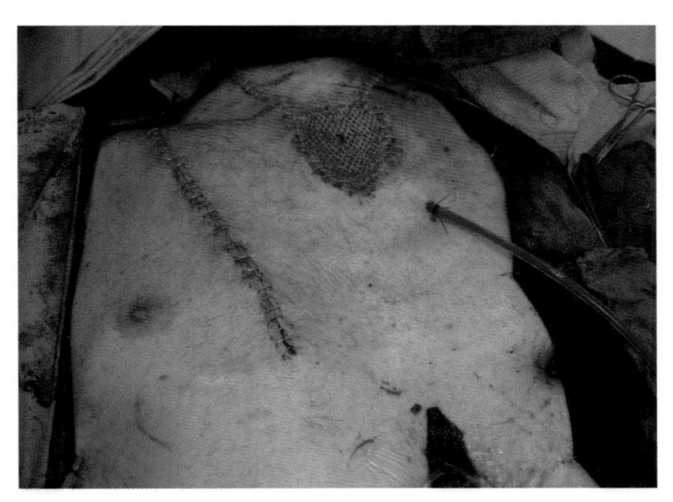

• **Fig. 25.11** Intraoperative view showing the skin-grafted right pectoralis major muscle flap used to cover an exposed portion of the free radial forearm flap and cervical esophagus at the end of the procedure. In this case, the tubed free radial forearm flap was buried completely.

pectoral muscle donor site was closed in layers with 3-0 Monocryl suture for the dermal closure and staples for the skin closure. The neck wounds were closed in a similar fashion (Fig. 25.11).

Management of Complications

The patient did well postoperatively and tolerated this long procedure well. While he was recovering on postoperative day 11, he developed excessive air from the drain and persistent cellulitis around the left side of his neck. Amylase from the drain fluid was approximately 12,000, which was consistent with a leak at the cervical anastomosis (Fig. 25.12). During reexploration in the operating room, a 1-cm anastomotic dehiscence with two 3-mm holes between the flap and the cervical esophageal stump were identified. The area had minimal local inflammation but a moderate degree of edema (Fig. 25.13). The distal edge of the radial forearm flap and remnant cervical esophagus were viable and did not require debridement. The buried radial forearm flap was completely viable and both arterial and venous microvascular anastomoses were patent.

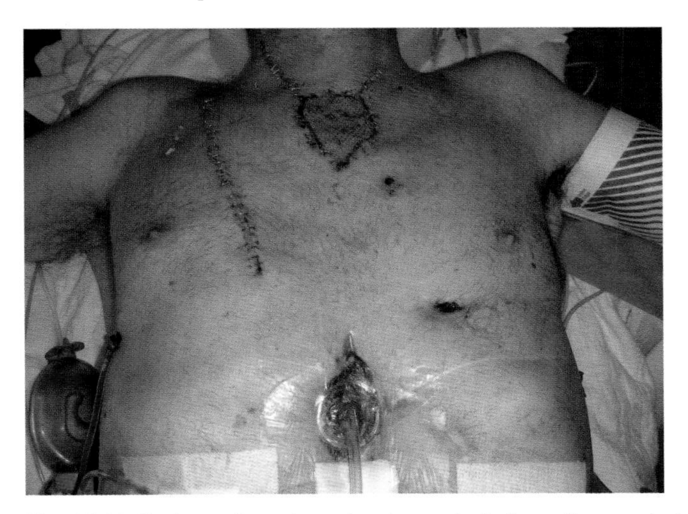

• **Fig. 25.12** Postoperative view showing a leak from the cervical anastomosis that was noted clinically on postoperative day 11.

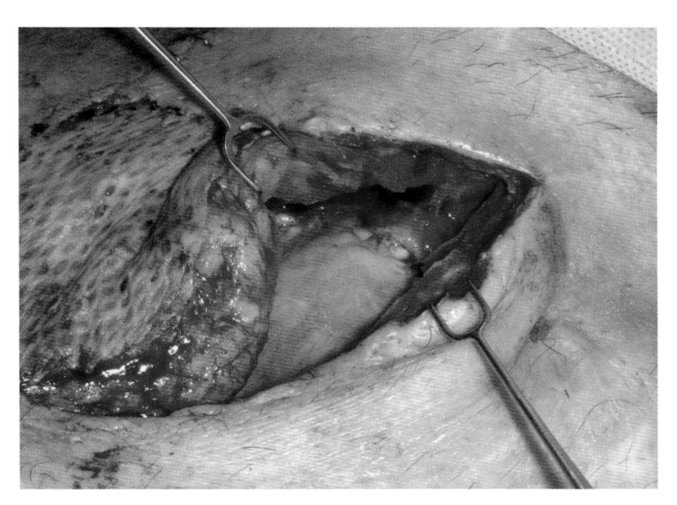

• **Fig. 25.13** Intraoperative view showing a 1-cm anastomotic dehiscence with two 3-mm holes of the proximal esophageal anastomosis. The leak site had minimal local inflammation but moderate degree of edema during reexploration. The distal edge of the radial forearm flap and remnant cervical esophagus were viable and did not require debridement.

Reanastomosis of the flap to the cervical esophageal stump was not performed because of the condition of the tissue near the anastomosis. It was strongly felt that any attempted reclosure of the anastomotic dehiscence would fail because of the poor condition of tissues at the cervical esophageal site. Instead, the adjacent lower sternocleidomastoid muscle was partially mobilized and sutured to the superior portion of the readvanced right pectoralis major muscle flap with interrupted 3-0 PDS sutures. Approximation of the adjacent muscles allowed complete coverage of the cervical anastomotic leak site with well-vascularized tissue. In addition, a 10-mm closed-suction drain was placed under the muscle flaps but away from the anastomotic leak site to provide adequate drainage (Fig. 25.14).

Follow-Up Results

The patient did well after reoperation without any complications related to the salvage procedure. He showed no signs of an anastomotic leak of the proximal anastomosis between the cervical esophageal stump and the radial forearm flap. He had a barium swallow test, which showed the patent anastomosis with no signs of a leak. He had no further issues related to his additional postoperative care. He underwent dilatation of his reconstructed esophagus and started to eat and drink 5 years after his esophagectomy for cancer. The neck and abdominal incisions healed well (Fig. 25.15), as did the right forearm flap donor site (Fig. 25.16).

Final Outcome

The patient underwent several dilatations of the reconstructed esophagus, especially the proximal anastomosis between the cervical esophageal stump and the radial forearm flap. He has maintained the ability to eat and drink freely. Most importantly, he has also remained cancer free. The neck and abdominal incisions healed well with minimal scarring (Fig. 25.17). The right forearm flap donor site also healed well with minimal scarring (Fig. 25.18). He has resumed his normal activities and has been followed by the surgical oncology service for routine follow-up.

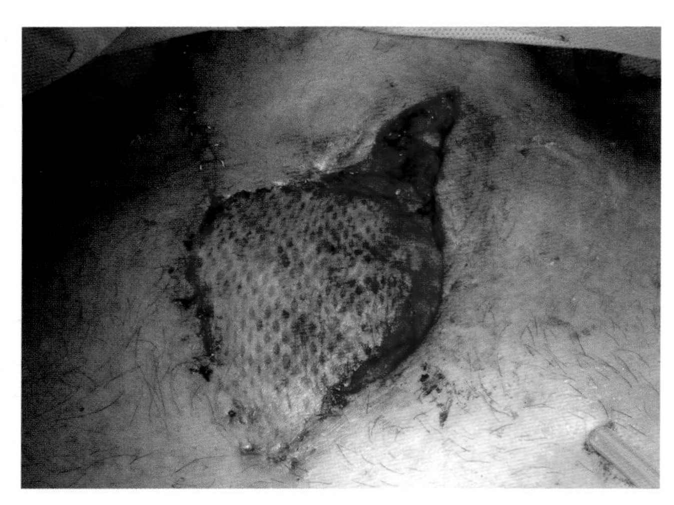

• **Fig. 25.14** Intraoperative view showing the adjacent sternocleidomastoid muscle was partially mobilized and sutured to the readvanced right pectoralis major muscle flap before the final skin closure. Approximation of the adjacent muscles allowed complete coverage of the cervical anastomotic leak site with well-vascularized tissue.

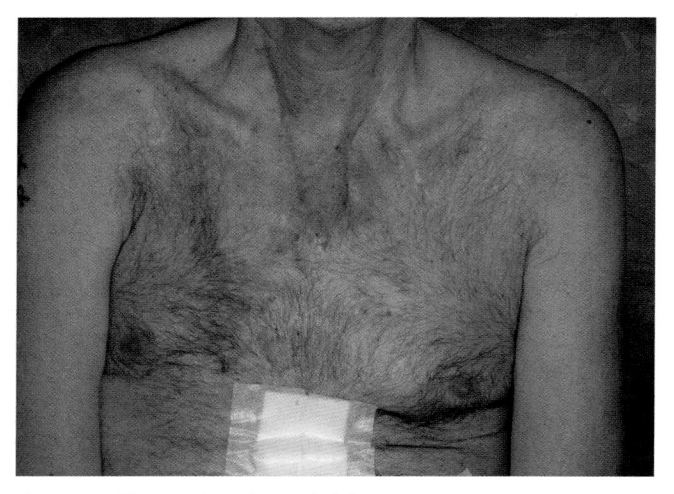

• **Fig. 25.15** The result at 1-month follow-up showing well-healed neck site and the right pectoral major muscle flap donor site.

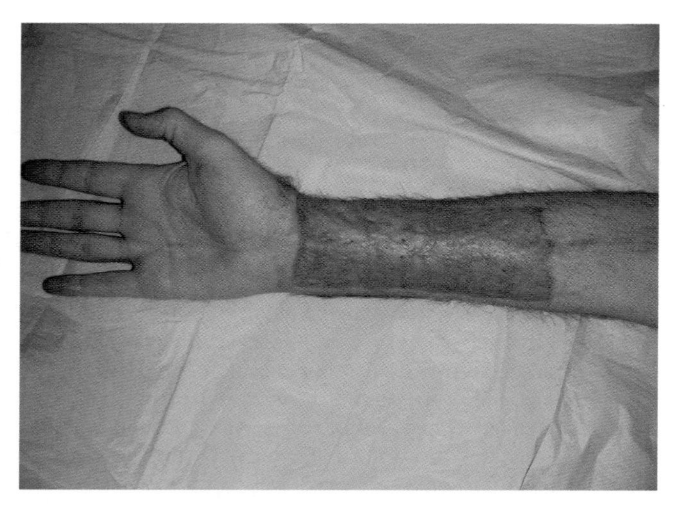

• **Fig. 25.16** The result at 1-month follow-up showing well-healed right radial forearm flap donor site.

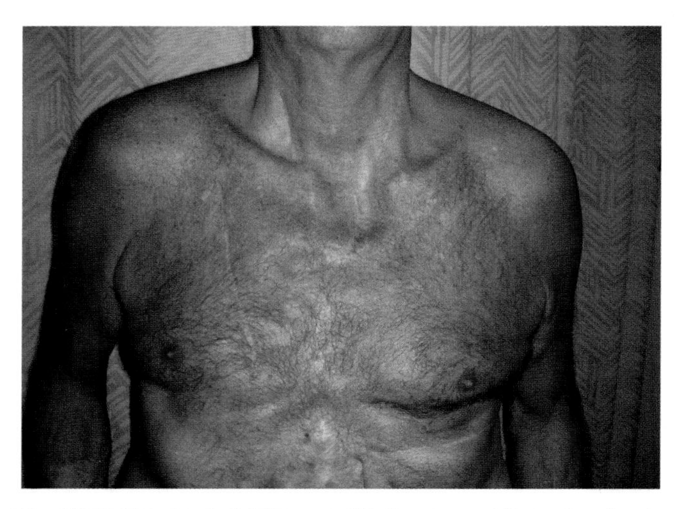

• **Fig. 25.17** The result at follow-up after 2 years and 8 months showing well-healed neck flap site and the right pectoral muscle flap donor site with good contour and minimal scarring.

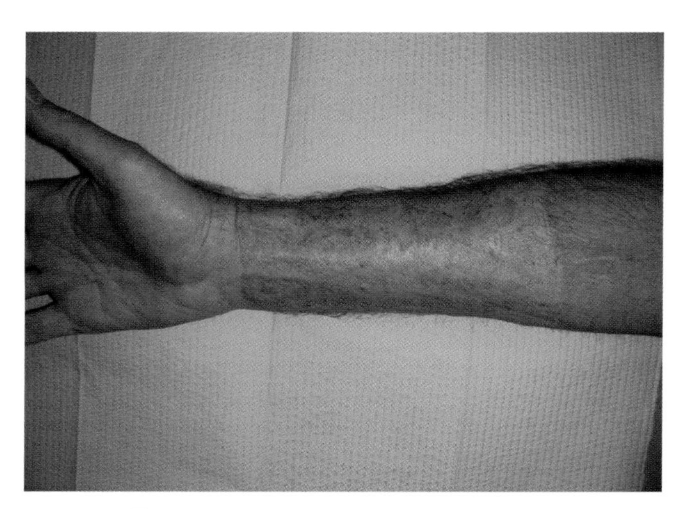

• **Fig. 25.18** The result at follow-up after 2 years and 8 months showing well-healed right radial forearm flap donor site with minimal scarring.

Pearls for Success

The free radial forearm flap has been used to reconstruct noncircumferential or short circumferential segments of the esophagus because it can provide a reliable well-vascularized conduit for esophageal reconstruction. As demonstrated in this case, an 18-cm long-tubed radial forearm flap can be used successfully to reconstruct a substernal esophagus. The flap can be harvested suprafascially for a better donor site closure after a skin graft and a long tube can be made while the flap is still connected with its pedicle after a two-layer, water-tight longitudinal closure. Microvascular anastomoses are usually not difficult to perform because of the flap's long pedicle and good caliber of the pedicle vessels. The cephalic vein should be selected as a primary pedicle vein.

The majority of cervical leaks after esophageal reconstruction result in local wounds with transient salivary fistula. However, the morbidity of cervical leaks should not be underestimated. Instead of causing more distal flap ischemia by attempting reanastomosis for the leak site, well-vascularized muscle flaps should be used to seal the leak and a closed suction drain should be placed to evacuate the contamination. The technique itself is relatively simple and reliable and works well in this clinical setting. This simple method potentially provides a quick solution for this complex clinical problem because of its sound reconstructive principle—the utilization of well-vascularized tissue to improve healing in a relatively ischemic environment. Simply covering a leak with vascularized tissue will avoid additional trauma and may result in fewer strictures because stricture formation is more likely from the greater tissue trauma during secondary revision and repair.

CASE 2

Clinical Presentation

A 68-year-old White male underwent total esophagectomy and end-esophagostomy (spit fistula) secondary to gangrenous para-esophageal hernia and strongly desired to have esophageal reconstruction to restore his esophageal continuity. The thoracic surgery service proposed a supercharged jejunal flap for total esophageal reconstruction. This procedure would need combined efforts from the thoracic surgery, general surgery, and plastic surgery services. The plastic surgery service was asked to perform microvascular anastomosis for a supercharged jejunal flap.

Operative Plan and Special Considerations

Pedicled jejunum has been used for esophageal reconstruction. However, it is generally unsuitable for reconstruction of the esophagus in the upper chest or neck because of the relatively short length of the mesentery and the lack of longitudinal vascular arcades. In addition, the curvature of the jejunum secondary to the fan-like foreshortening of its mesentery results in a sigmoidal conduit. Division of the mesentery to the mesenteric border of the jejunum allows the jejunum to unfurl, thus straightening the conduit and adding significant length, but this would create a devascularized segment of the jejunum proximally. However, the arterial and venous supply of this segment can be enhanced using microvascular techniques, anastomosing to vessels in the upper chest or neck. This results in a supercharged jejunal flap that can comfortably reach to the hypopharynx and more closely approximates the size of the native esophagus, retains peristalsis, and limits reflux (Fig. 25.19).

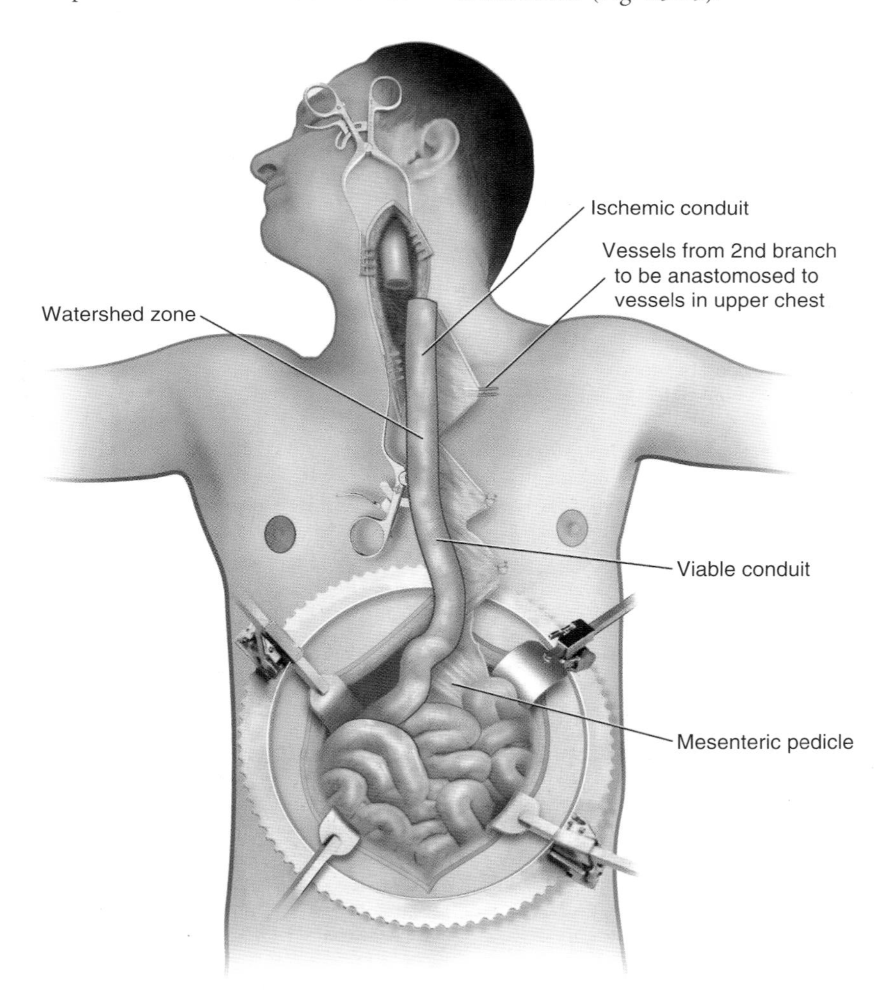

• **Fig. 25.19** A schematic diagram showing the design of a supercharged jejunal flap for total esophageal reconstruction. The lower portion of the jejunal flap receives blood supply from its mesenteric pedicle but the upper portion remains relatively ischemic and will receive additional blood supply through a supercharge by anastomosing the second branch to the proximal internal mammary vessel.

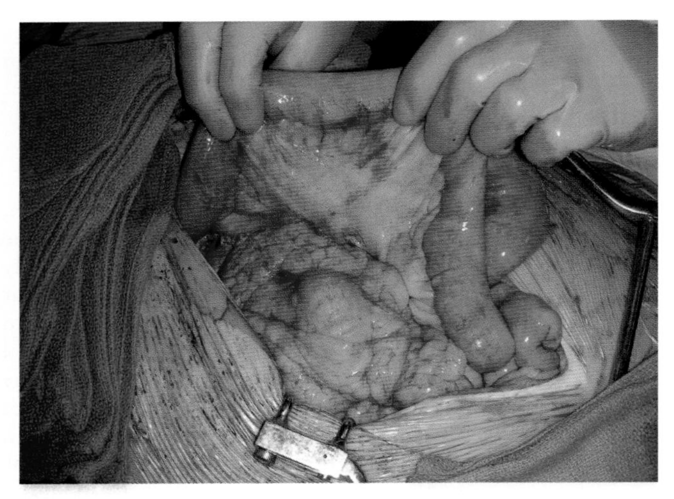

• **Fig. 25.20** Intraoperative view showing a suitable portion of the jejunum that could be used for total esophageal reconstruction.

Operative Procedures

Under general anesthesia with the patient in the supine position, the plastic surgery part of procedure started after the upper chest and abdominal incisions had been made and the exposure of the jejunum was performed by the thoracic and general surgery services. The suitable portion of the jejunum was identified (Fig. 25.20).

The second arcade of superior mesentery artery was identified. The jejunum was divided about 30 cm distal to the ligament of Treitz and a very long jejunal flap was developed after division of the proximal jejunum (Fig. 25.21). The second arcade vessel was preserved as the pedicle of the supercharged jejunum flap. The second and third arcades of the superior mesentery vessels were divided (Fig. 25.22).

The gastrojejunostomy was performed by the general surgery service. The proximal jejunum was tunneled under the sternum through this substernal space and placed on the neck area by the thoracic surgery service (Fig. 25.23). The left sternoclavicular joint and the head of the first rib were removed for better upper sternal exposure by the same service. Under direct vision, the proximal internal mammary artery and vein were dissected free and prepared for microvascular anastomoses under loupe magnification. Both artery and vein were divided distally and clamped with atraumatic microvascular clamps proximally.

Under microscope, both arterial and venous anastomoses were performed. The end-to-end arterial microanastomosis was performed between the second arcade artery and the internal mammary artery with interrupted 8-0 nylon sutures. The venous microanastomosis was performed also in an end-to-end fashion with a 3-mm coupler device (Fig. 25.24). Once all clamps had been removed, there was a good flow through both the arterial and the venous anastomosis and the supercharged jejunum flap

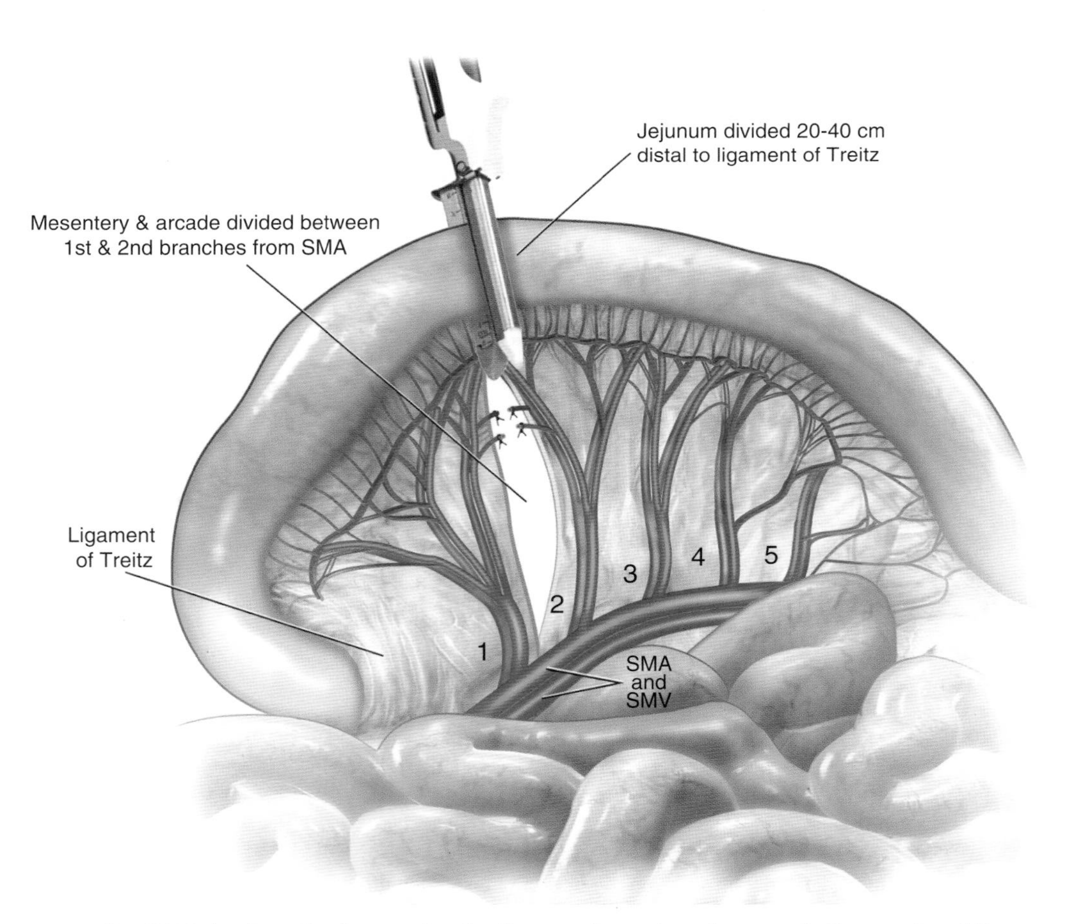

• **Fig. 25.21** A schematic diagram showing the vascular anatomy from one to five arcades of the superior mesentery vessels. The jejunum can be divided 30 cm distal to the ligament of Treitz.

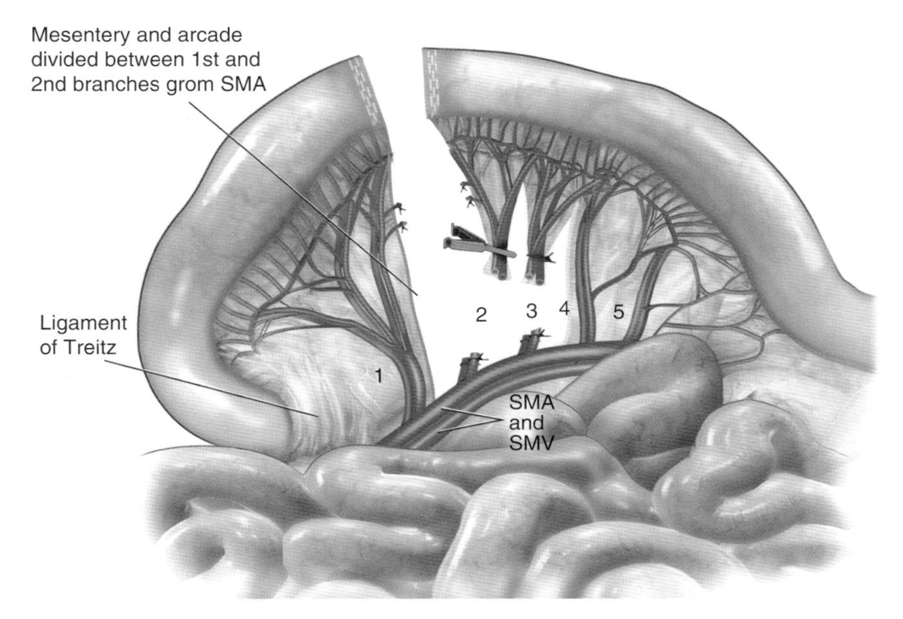

• **Fig. 25.22** A schematic diagram showing the division of the second and third branches from the superior mesentery vessels. If more length is needed, the fourth branch can also be divided. However, the fifth branch should be preserved to serve as a source for the pedicled jejunum flap.

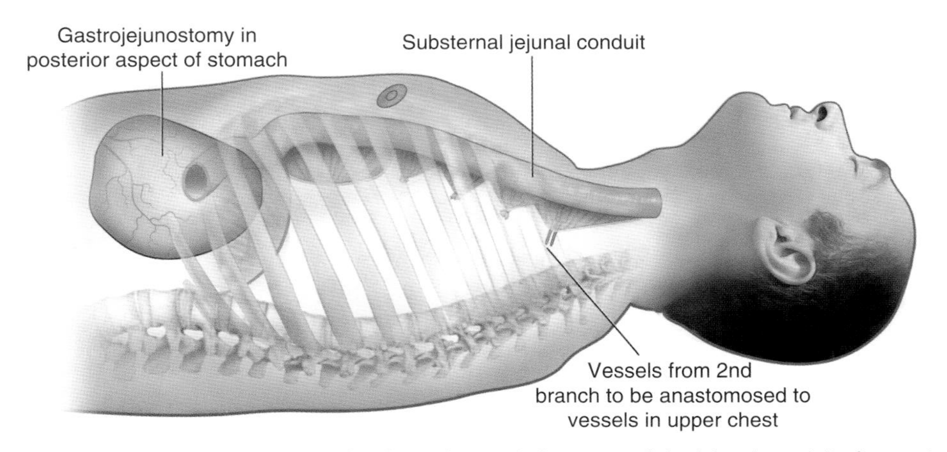

• **Fig. 25.23** A schematic diagram showing substernal placement of the jejunal conduit after gastrojejunostomy. The distal portion of the jejunal flap is placed on the lower neck and will be supercharged.

appeared to be well perfused (Fig. 25.25). A Cooke Doppler probe was wrapped around the distal arterial anastomosis for monitoring. The proximal anastomosis between the cervical esophageal stump and jejunum was then performed by the thoracic surgery service (Fig. 25.26). The distal end-to-end jejunojejunal anastomosis was performed by the general surgery service to restore small bowel continuity. The abdominal and upper chest and neck wounds were closed by thoracic surgery service and general surgery service separately.

Follow-Up Results

The patient did well postoperatively without any complications related to the supercharged jejunal flap for total esophageal reconstruction. The barium swallow test on postoperative day 7 showed a patent reconstructed esophagus with no evidence of anastomotic leak (Fig. 25.27). The patient resumed his oral intake and was discharged from hospital on postoperative day 10. His upper chest and neck as well as the abdominal incisions healed well.

Final Outcome

The left upper chest and neck wounds as well as the abdominal incision healed well with minimal scarring after supercharged jejunal flap for total esophageal reconstruction (Fig. 25.28). Most importantly, the patient has been able to eat freely. He has resumed his normal activities and is followed by the thoracic surgery service for routine follow-up.

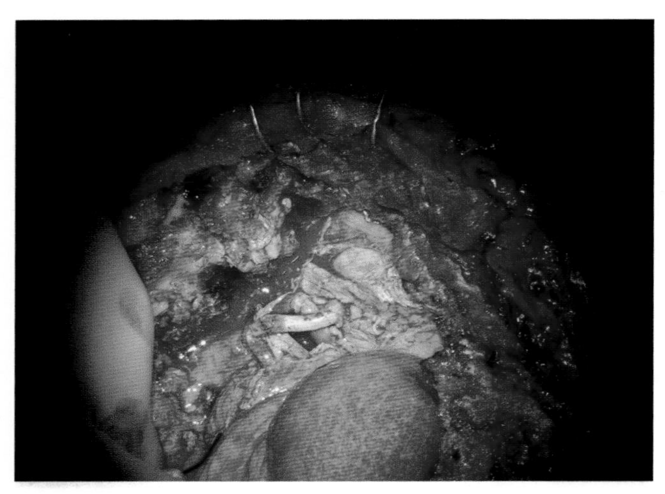

• **Fig. 25.24** Intraoperative view showing completion of arterial and venous microvascular anastomoses between the second branche and the proximal internal mammary vessel under microscope.

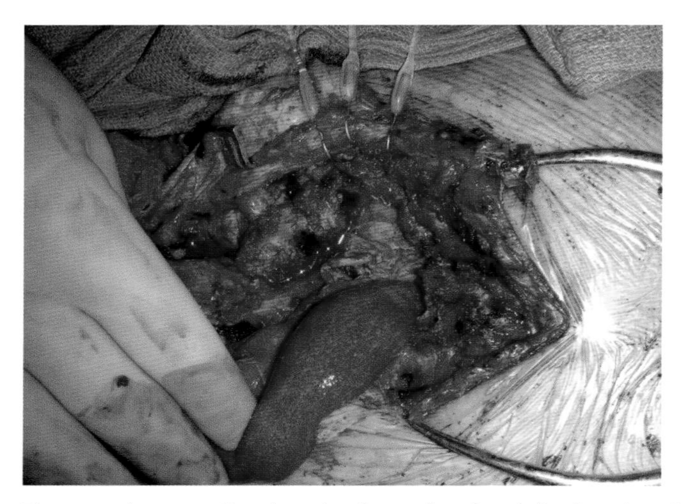

• **Fig. 25.25** Intraoperative view showing well-perfused distal portion of the jejunal flap after microvascular supercharge.

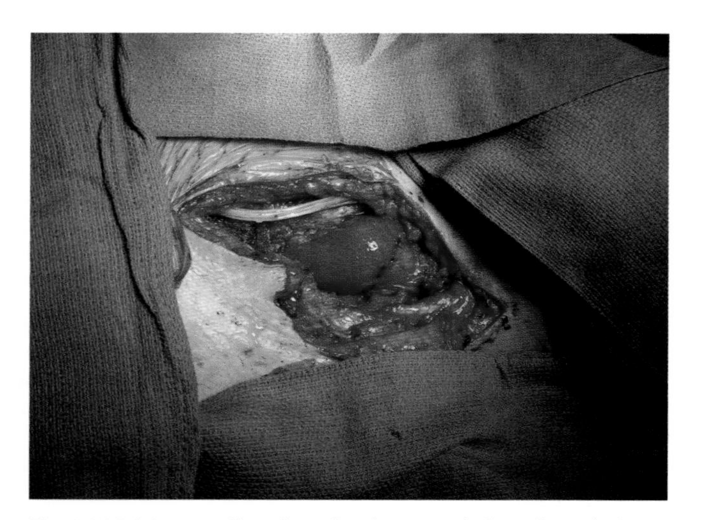

• **Fig. 25.26** Intraoperative view showing completion of cervical anastomosis between the cervical esophageal stump and the distal jejunal flap before the neck and upper chest incision closure.

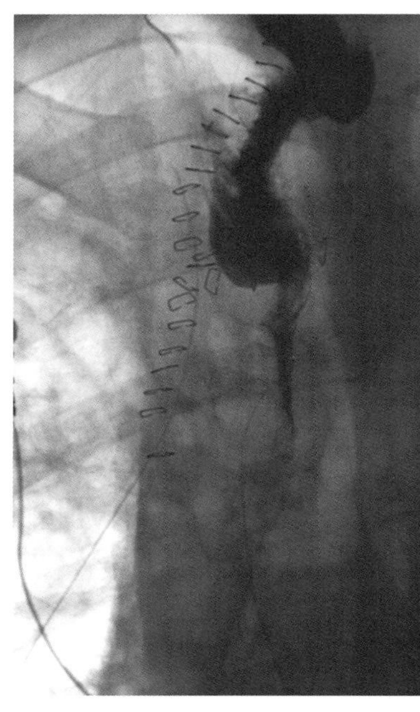

• **Fig. 25.27** Postoperative barium swallow test showing the patent esophageal reconstruction with no evidence of anastomotic leak.

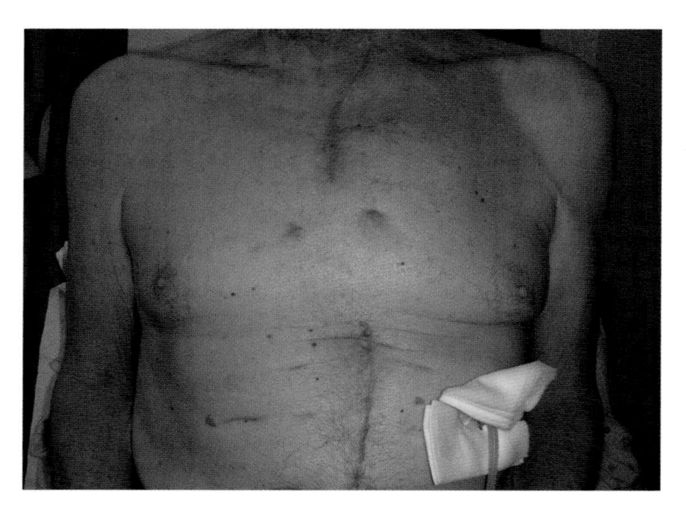

• **Fig. 25.28** The result at 10-week follow-up showing well-healed neck and chest incision as well as the abdominal incision.

Pearls for Success

Harvesting the jejunal segment is usually performed by the general surgery team and transillumination of the mesentery is critical for defining the vascular anatomy of mesentery arcade vessels. Great care should be taken when handling the pedicled section of the flap, particularly when delivering the conduit through the chest into the neck. Even slight excess tension may cause avulsion of the arcade vessels, causing devascularization of the midportion of the jejunal flap. Vessel mismatch can be a problem, especially for the second arcade vein from the superior mesentery vein because it can be much larger than the internal mammary vein. The surgeon should be well prepared to handle this problem. In addition, the surgeon should pay attention to the wound closure of the neck and upper chest incision because a tight closure might compress microvascular anastomoses and cause potential ischemia over the cervical anastomosis of the esophageal reconstruction.

CASE 3

Clinical Presentation

A 59-year-old Hispanic female had a very complicated history of esophageal injury. Gastroesophageal reconstruction had initially been performed by the thoracic surgery service but unfortunately, the anterior wall of the anastomosis was completely dehisced. She underwent several weeks of vacuum-assisted wound closure (VAC) dressing changes and subsequently had a pedicled vertical rectus abdominal myocutaneous flap for reconstruction of the anterior wall defect as a definitive cervical esophageal reconstruction. Unfortunately, the reconstruction failed because of partial flap necrosis and left an 8-cm circumferential cervical esophageal defect and an 11 × 8 cm complex neck wound (Fig. 25.29). The plastic surgery service was asked again by the primary service to provide a microvascular free flap reconstruction for cervical esophageal reconstruction (Fig. 25.30).

Operative Plan and Special Considerations

A microvascular free tissue transfer with a fasciocutaneous flap was considered and offered to this patient. Unfortunately, she had a previous A-line placement and both radial arteries were occluded. Therefore, a classic free radial forearm flap would not be an option for the esophageal reconstruction. However, a free anterolateral thigh (ALT) perforator flap could be an option for the cervical esophageal reconstruction as a one-stage reconstruction because she was relatively thin and the flap might not be bulky. The flap could be made as a tube for a lengthy circumferential esophageal reconstruction. With experience, a free ALT flap can be a reliable option in this setting. In addition, a skin-grafted pedicled pectoral muscle could be selected for the complex neck wound coverage including reconstructed cervical esophagus. A pectoral major muscle flap is reliable and can reach the neck area without difficulty.

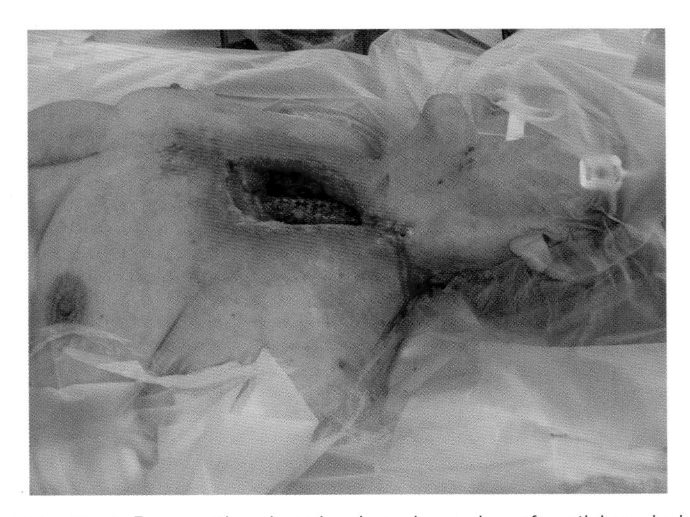

• **Fig. 25.29** Preoperative view showing a large circumferential cervical esophageal defect and large left neck open wound.

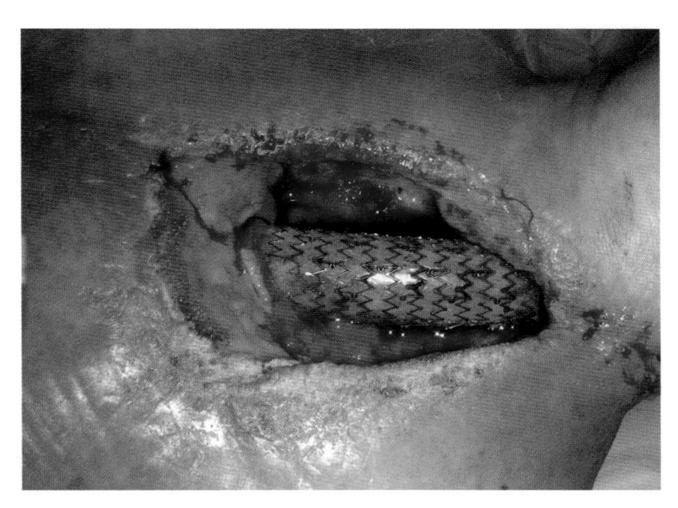

• **Fig. 25.30** Preoperative close-up view showing a large circumferential cervical esophageal defect and an exposed stent used to support cervical esophagus.

Operative Procedures

Under general anesthesia with the patient in supine position, the neck wound was debrided. All colonized tissues were removed and the skin edge of the wound was freshened with a blade. Based on the intraoperative duplex scan, the left ALT perforator flap was selected. A 11 × 9 cm skin paddle was marked and orientated based on those two perforators (Fig. 25.31). The flap was elevated using a subfascial dissection. During dissection, the superior perforator appeared to be more intramuscular and was divided during the flap dissection. Thus, the entire flap was based on the inferior perforator, which appeared to be quite good. After intramuscular dissection, the perforator was found to join the descending branch of the lateral circumflex femoral vessels. The distal end of the descending branch was divided and further pedicle dissection was done toward the profunda vessels. During dissection, the motor nerve branch to the vastus lateralis muscle was preserved. At this point, the flap pedicle dissection was completed and the entire flap appeared to be quite well perfused based on the single perforator (Fig. 25.32).

An 8 × 9 cm tube from an intact ALT flap was made using a 2.6 cm aortic dilator as a template. The tube flap was closed longitudinally with a two-layer watertight closure. Some defatting was performed on each edge of the flap in order to facilitate the contour of the reconstructed esophagus (Fig. 25.33). The pedicle of the flap was then divided (Fig. 25.34).

Both anastomoses of the cervical esophageal reconstruction were performed by the thoracic surgery service. Once the continuity of the cervical esophagus was established, the microvascular anastomosis of the flap was performed next. Both recipient artery and vein were explored by extending the neck incision prior to division of the flap's pedicle. The external jugular vein and the superior thyroid artery were identified and dissected free as the recipient vessels.

Once the pedicle vessels of the flap had been prepared under loupe magnification, the arterial microvascular anastomosis was performed with interrupted 8-0 nylon sutures in an end-to-end fashion. The venous microvascular anastomosis was performed with a 2.5-mm coupler device in an end-to-end fashion. Once all clamps had been removed, the flap appeared to have a good in or out flow. A Cook Doppler probe was wrapped around the arterial

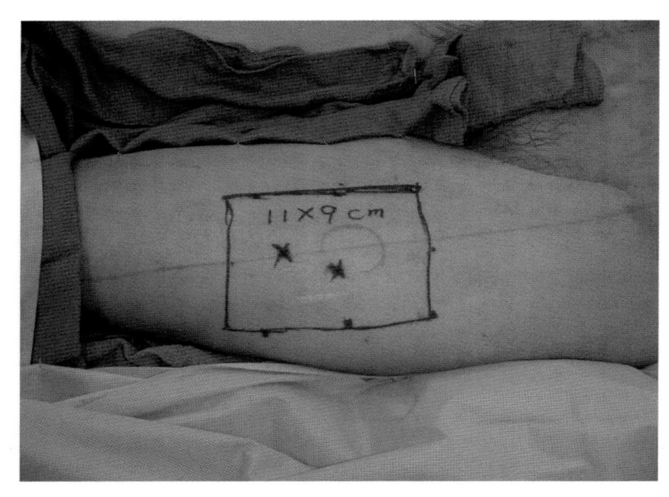

• **Fig. 25.31** Intraoperative view showing the design of the left anterolateral thigh flap. Two perforators, identified by preoperative Duplex scan, were clearly marked.

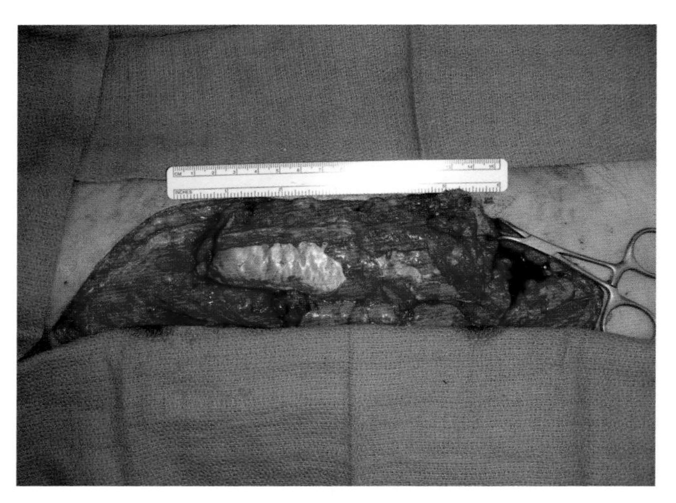

• **Fig. 25.33** Intraoperative view showing a tube that was made by the anterolateral thigh flap while the flap pedicle is still connected. An appropriate amount of the flap tissue was debulked to facilitate a tube formation for esophageal reconstruction.

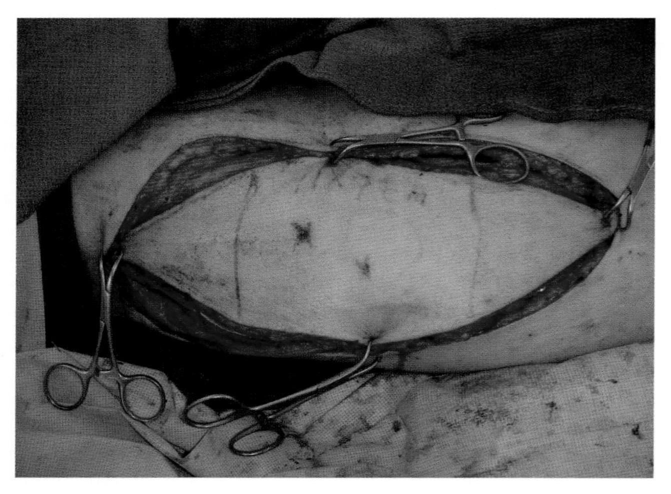

• **Fig. 25.32** Intraoperative view showing completion of the elevated left anterolateral thigh flap before division of the pedicle.

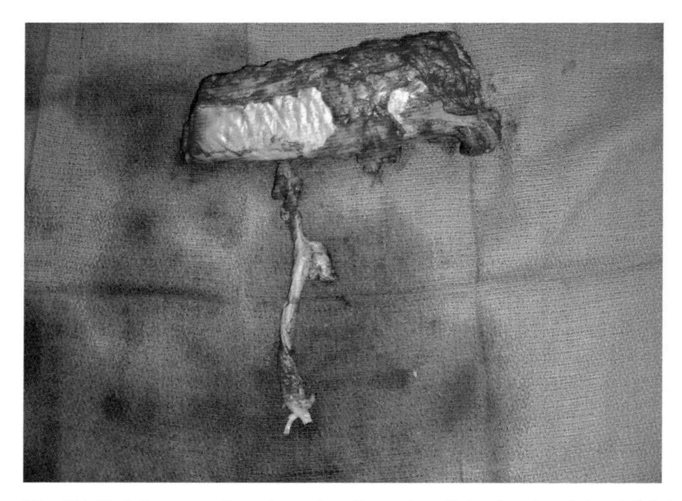

• **Fig. 25.34** Intraoperative view showing a free tubed anterolateral thigh flap that was ready for cervical esophageal reconstruction.

pedicle distal to the anastomosis for continue monitoring of the flap (Fig. 25.35).

The right pectoral major muscle flap was dissected through three incisions. One followed the inframammary fold, a second incision was over the superior lateral chest, and the third incision was just the extension of the left neck wound. The flap dissection was performed with the aid of a mammary light retractor. The subglandular dissection of the breast was done first, followed by a subpectoral dissection. Attachments of the pectoral muscle were released inferiorly, medially, laterally, and superiorly under direct vision. Some of the muscle attachment to the clavicle was preserved, leaving the pedicle with a cuff of muscle for protection. The muscle flap was rotated medially to cover the cervical esophageal reconstruction site and the left neck wound (Fig. 25.36).

The flap was inset into the neck wound with interrupted 3-0 Vicryl sutures in half-buried horizontal mattress fashion. A meshed split-thickness skin graft was harvested from the patient's right medial thigh with a dermatome and meshed to 1:1.5 ratio. The skin graft was placed over the muscle flap and secured with multiple skin staples (Fig. 25.37). A 7-mm JP was inserted around the medial aspect of the reconstructed esophagus. A Penrose drain was inserted over the lateral aspect of the reconstructed esophagus. Two JP drains were inserted into the right breast pocket. All chest incisions were closed in two layers.

The left thigh ALT flap donor site was closed in two layers after significant undermining. The deep dermal layer was closed with 2-0 PDS suture in an interrupted fashion. The skin was closed with 3-0 V-loc suture in running subcuticular fashion.

Follow-Up Results

The patient did well postoperatively without any complications related to the microsurgical esophageal reconstruction with a free ALT flap. The skin-grafted pectoral muscle flap also healed well. The barium swallow test on postoperative day 7 showed a patent reconstructed esophagus with no evidence of anastomotic leaks (Fig. 25.38). She was discharged from hospital on postoperative day 15. The neck and abdominal incisions also healed well

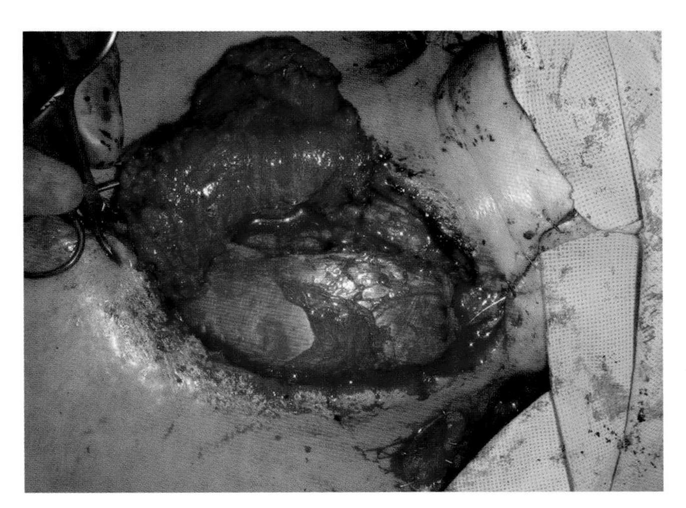

• **Fig. 25.35** Intraoperative view showing completion of cervical esophageal anastomoses and microvascular anastomoses of the flap before coverage with the pectoral major muscle flap.

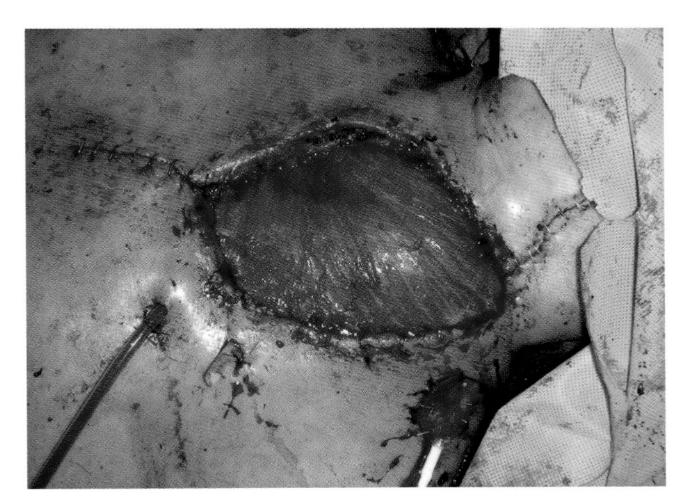

• **Fig. 25.36** Intraoperative view showing completion of coverage for the reconstructed esophagus and the rest of the neck wound with the right pectoral major muscle flap.

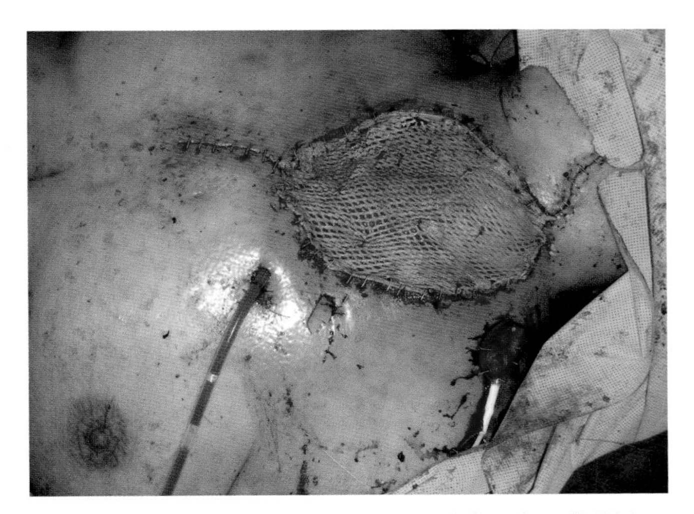

• **Fig. 25.37** Intraoperative view showing completion of a split-thickness skin graft placement over the right pectoral major muscle flap.

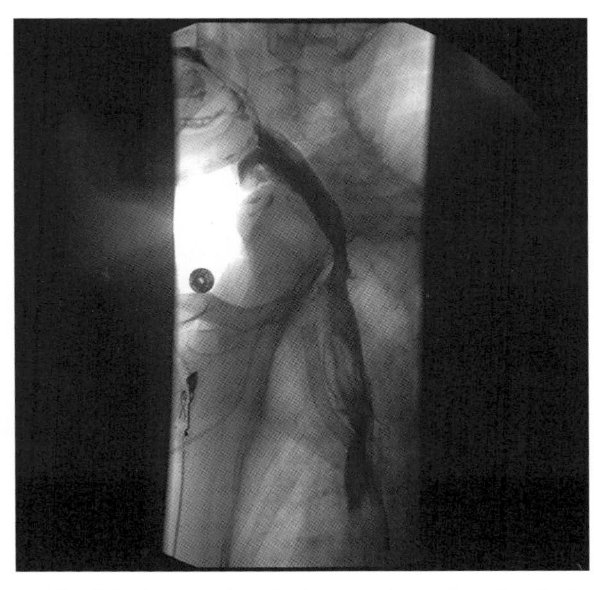

• **Fig. 25.38** A barium swallow test on postoperative day 7 showing patent reconstructed cervical esophagus with no evidence of the anastomotic leak.

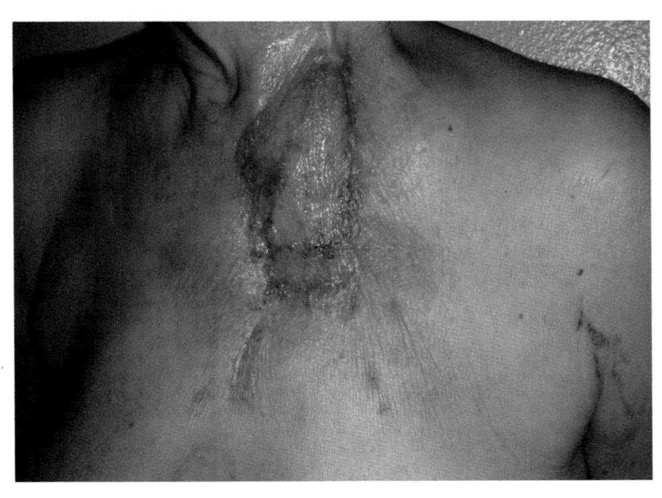

• **Fig. 25.39** The result at 7-week follow-up showing a completely healthy left neck wound after cervical esophageal reconstruction with a free anterolateral thigh flap and a right pectoral major muscle coverage to the left neck wound.

(Fig. 25.39). She started oral intake of clear liquid several weeks after the definitive esophageal reconstruction and tolerated it well.

Final Outcome

The left neck flap site and abdominal incision healed well after microsurgical free ALT flap for cervical esophageal reconstruction (Fig. 25.40). The patient has had dilation of her reconstructed cervical esophagus periodically and has been able to drink and eat freely. The ALT flap donor site also healed nicely (Fig. 25.41). She developed some degree of left neck scar contracture and underwent multiple Z-plasty procedures for scar release. She has slowly resumed her normal activities and has been followed by the thoracic surgery service for routine follow-up.

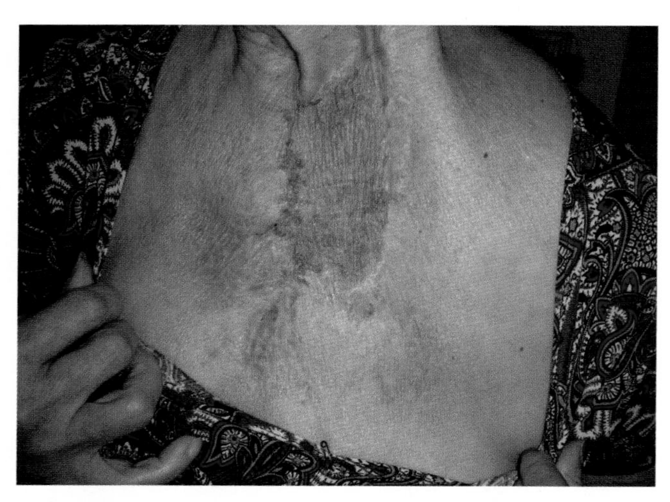

• **Fig. 25.40** The result at 5-month follow-up showing well-healed left neck wound after cervical esophageal reconstruction with a free anterolateral thigh flap and a right pectoral major muscle coverage to the left neck wound.

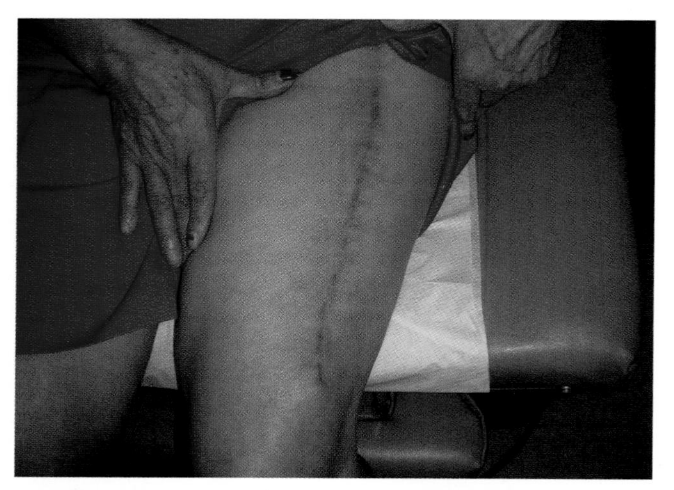

• **Fig. 25.41** The result at 5-month follow-up showing well-healed anterolateral thigh flap donor site in the left thigh with minimal scarring.

Pearls for Success

When a patient has a failed previous cervical esophageal reconstruction, it usually leaves a circumferential cervical esophageal defect and a large neck wound. An ALT flap can be used to reconstruct a circumferential defect of the cervical esophagus. In a relatively thin patient, the flap can be made as a tube after a watertight closure longitudinally. Proper amount of the flap thinning can be safely performed while the pedicle of the flap is still connected to facilitate tube formation. Because the ALT flap can tolerate a relatively long ischemic time (2–3 hours), esophageal anastomosis should be performed first before the flap's microvascular anastomoses. A contralateral pectoral major muscle flap can be selected to provide a reliable soft tissue coverage over the reconstructed esophagus and its microvascular anastomotic sites and the rest of the exposed neck wound. For a female patient, the pectoral muscle flap can be dissected via two separate and well-hidden incisions, an inframammary incision and upper lateral chest incision. An additional exposure for the flap dissection can be added by extending the neck open wound toward the flap's pedicle. A small cuff of the muscle attachment to the clavicle near the thoracoacromial pedicle should be preserved to prevent injury to the pedicle during the flap dissection and inset.

CASE 4

Clinic Presentation

A 46-year-old White female attempted to commit suicide by swallowing lye, which resulted in complete necrosis of the esophagus and stomach mucosa. She underwent a total gastrectomy, transhiatal esophagectomy and creation of an esophagocutaneous fistula. Three months later, a descending colon interpositional graft was placed in the substernal prepericardial orientation. The proximal anastomosis was a colojejunal anastomosis as part of a Roux-en-Y jejunal loop. Meanwhile, a prophylactic resection of the left sternal-clavicular joint was performed to widen the thoracic inlet. Unfortunately, she developed severe sepsis in the postoperative course and subsequent endoscopic findings confirmed that the proximal 5 cm of the colon conduit was necrotic. The necrotic tissue was resected. The colon was not removed entirely because it was viable. The most proximal colon was left as a mucous fistula. The open area between the esophageal spit fistula and the colonic mucous fistula was covered with a VAC dressing. Eventually, the wound bed became epithelialized after frequent VAC treatments. She had a 7 × 3 cm open wound over her left lower neck (Fig. 25.42). The plastic surgery service was asked by the thoracic surgery service to provide partial cervical esophageal reconstruction and closure of the neck wound.

Operative Plan and Special Considerations

Because this patient had only an anterior wall defect of the cervical esophagus and a neck wound, it would be ideal to design a single-stage reconstruction to reconstruct her partial esophageal defect and close the neck wound. The left pedicled pectoral major myocutaneous flap could potentially serve as a single-stage reconstruction. The skin paddle of the flap could be designed after its turnover to reconstruct the anterior cervical esophageal defect and to restore the continuity of the esophagus. The muscle portion of the flap was used to cover the neck wound after a skin graft and would possibly seal any potential wound seperation in the area. The flap has IV blood supply, is fairly reliable, and can be based on its main pedicle, the thoracoacromial vessels, as a turnover flap. It is located on the chest adjacent to the defect and its flap dissection is relatively standard with reduced operative time. Because the patient was a smoker and had poor nutritional status, a skin paddle designed above her breast would be more reliable. It is an innovative and effective local reconstruction option for such a complex reconstruction but without the need for free tissue transfer.

Operative Procedures

Under general anesthesia, the procedure was started by the thoracic surgery service to identify the proximal stump of the cervical esophagus and the distal stump of the pulled-up colon. An 8 × 5 cm skin paddle and the location and course of the

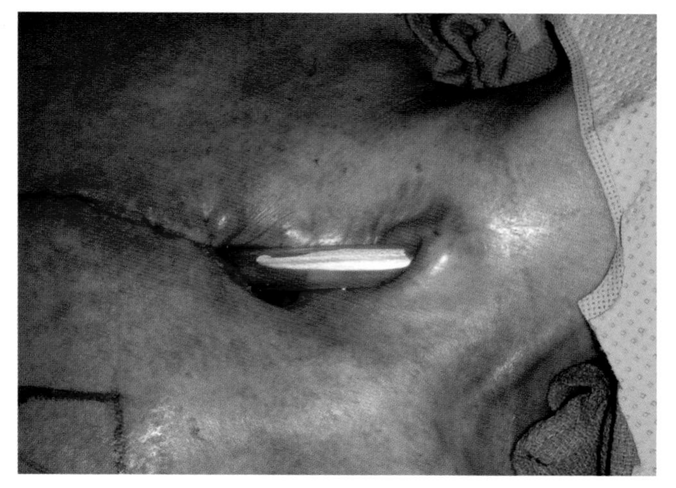

• **Fig. 25.42** Preoperative view showing an anterior wall discontinuity of the cervical esophagus due to the colon conduit necrosis.

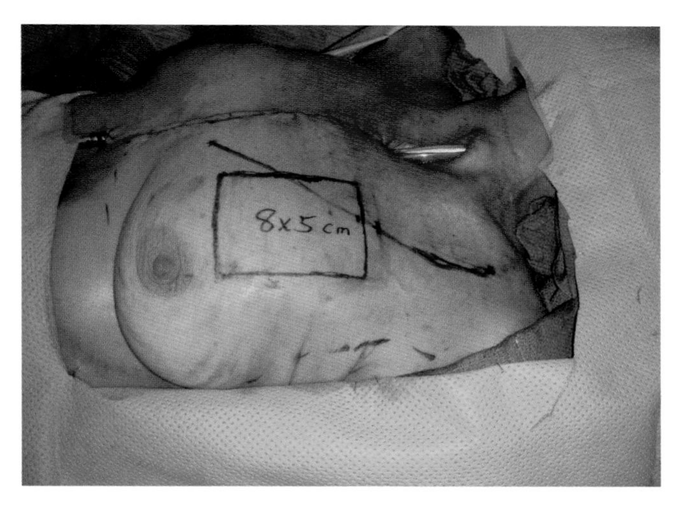

• **Fig. 25.43** Intraoperative view showing the design of an 8 × 5 cm skin paddle of the left pectoral major myocutaneous flap above the breast and the location of the thoracoacromial vessels.

thoracoacromial vessels were marked (Fig. 25.43). One perforator was identified within the skin paddle by a handheld Doppler. The skin and subcutaneous tissue of the flap was incised to the fascia of the pectoralis major muscle. The dissection was carried out to elevate the chest skin around the skin paddle of the flap and to identify the medial, inferior, and lateral borders of the pectoralis major muscle. The muscle was divided inferiorly, a submuscular dissection was performed to elevate the entire muscle. Once the muscle's medial and lateral borders had been divided, the flap could be elevated freely (Fig. 25.44). During the dissection, the thoracoacromial pedicles were identified and all efforts were made to avoid injury to the pedicles. The dissection was continued down toward the origin of the pedicle and a small cuff of the muscle around the pedicle was preserved. The skin paddle of the flap was easily aligned over the anterior portion of the cervical esophageal reconstruction and the muscle portion could be used to cover the anastomotic repair site (Fig. 25.45).

The repair of the anterior wall for cervical esophageal reconstruction was done by the thoracic surgery and plastic surgery services. The adequate de-epithelization was performed in the

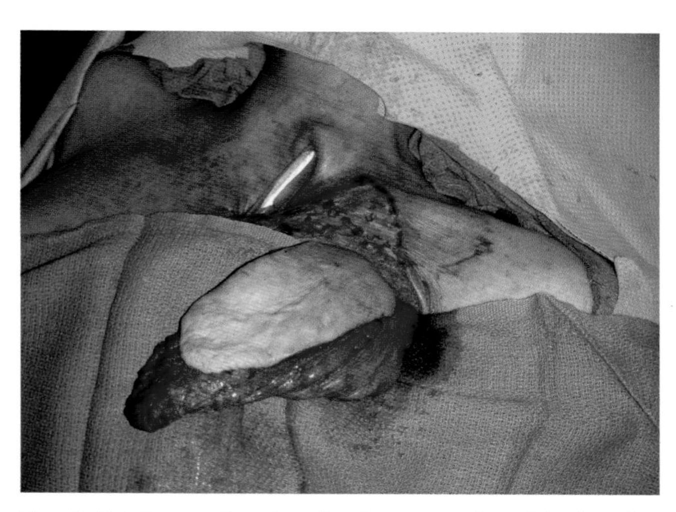

• **Fig. 25.44** Intraoperative view showing completion of the flap elevation off the chest wall.

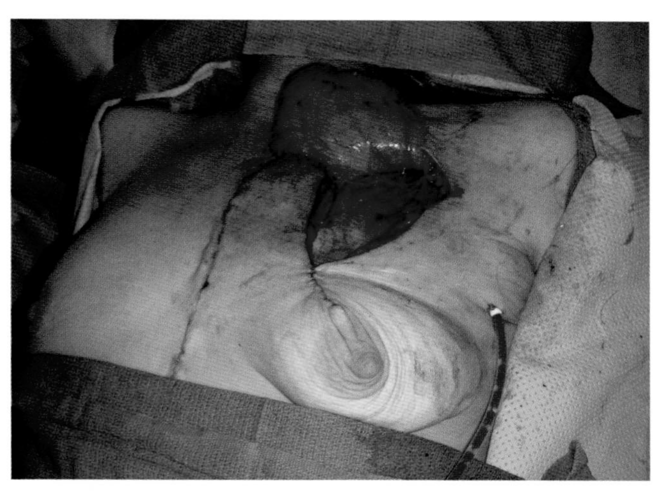

• **Fig. 25.45** Intraoperative view showing completion of the flap turnover to reconstruct the cervical esophagus and to close the neck wound before a skin graft placement.

adjacent areas of the posterior wall of the cervical esophagus in the neck. The flap was turned over to the posterior wall of the cervical esophagus and two longitudinal repairs were performed in two layers. Each skin edge of the flap was sutured to the full layer of the posterior wall of the remaining cervical esophagus with interrupted 3-0 Vicryl sutures. The muscle layer of the flap was sutured to the adjacent skin edge of the neck wound and a second layer closure was made with interrupted 3-0 Vicryl sutures. Both proximal and distal cervical esophageal anastomoses were then performed by the thoracic surgery service (Fig. 25.46). The excess tissue of the skin paddle was excised.

The rest of the breast wound was closed with local tissue arrangement. Both medial and lateral breast tissues were elevated and approximated in three layers to make sure there was no obvious deformity of the breast. The breast tissue and deep dermal layer were approximated with several interrupted 3-0 Vicryl sutures. The skin was then closed with 4-0 Monocryl in simple, running fashion.

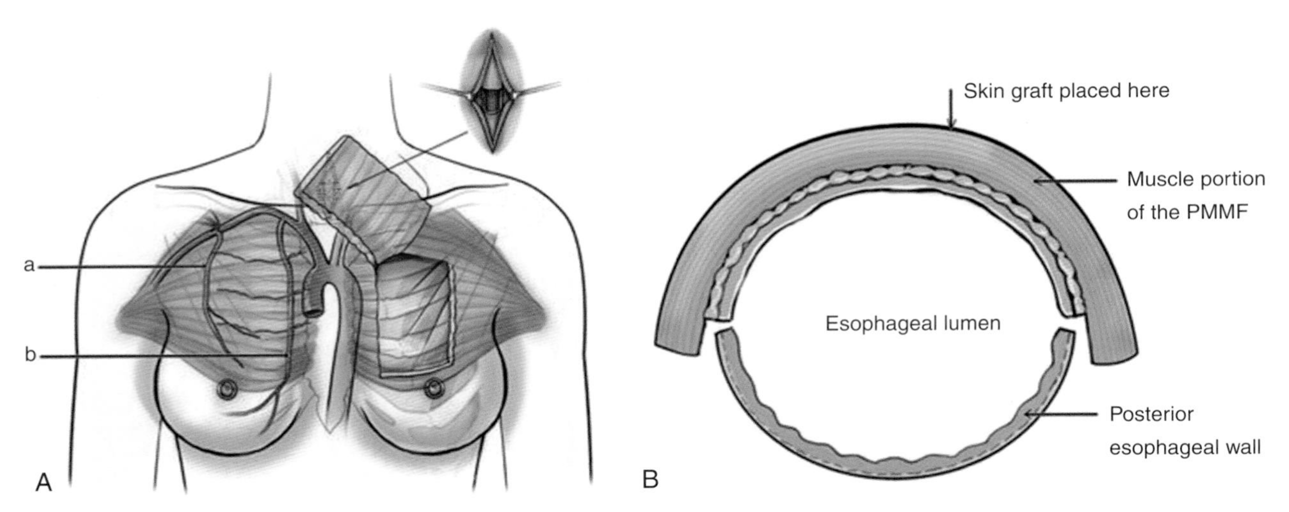

• **Fig. 25.46** Schematic diagrams showing (A) how the left pectoral major myocutaneous flap was turned over to reconstruct the cervical-esophageal defect; the major blood supply to the flap is shown on the opposite side and (B) the cross-sectional view of the reconstructed cervical esophagus and the neck wound closure. *PMMF*, Pectoral Major Myocutaneous Flap.

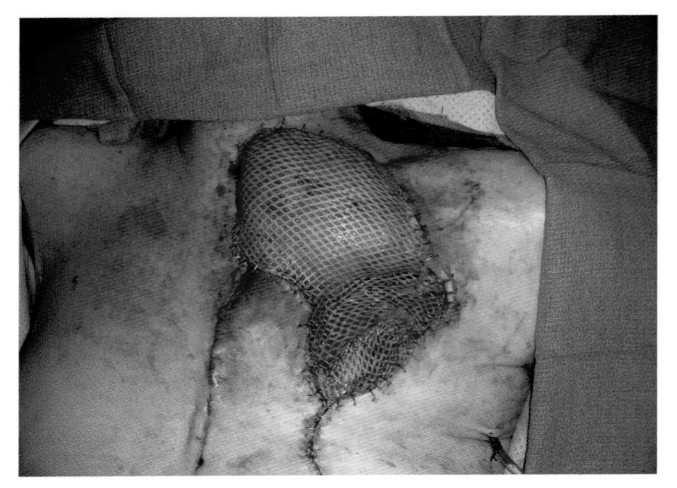

• **Fig. 25.47** Intraoperative view showing completion of the reconstruction for the cervical esophagus and neck wound with the left pectoral major myocutaneous flap as a one-stage procedure.

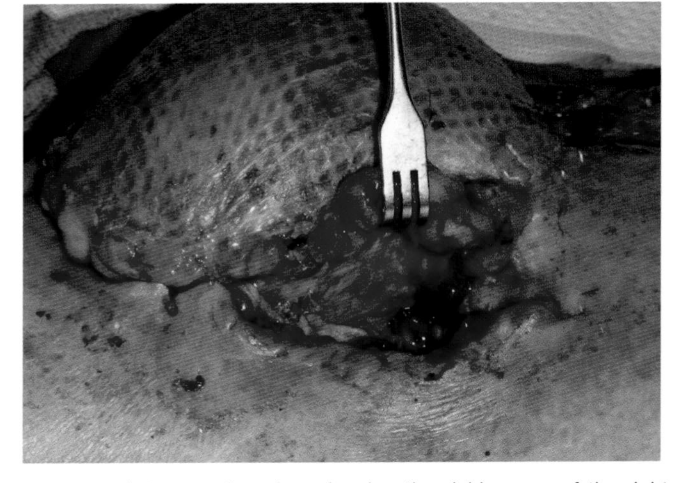

• **Fig. 25.48** Intraoperative view showing the dehiscence of the right-side repair for the cervical esophageal reconstruction.

A split-thickness skin graft was harvested from the left lateral thigh. The skin graft was harvested and meshed to 1:1.5 ratio. The skin graft was then placed on the entire muscle flap and on the chest wall donor site open area and secured with multiple skin staples. The pectoralis major muscle donor site was covered with a small VAC sponge and secured with multiple skin staples (Fig. 25.47).

Management of Complications

The patient was doing well initially after the reconstruction, the pectoral major myocutaneous flap survived completely, and the skin graft healed. Unfortunately, she developed a conduit leak on one side of the repair and distal anastomosis between the flap and the colon 10 days later (Fig. 25.48). She was brought to the operating room by the thoracic surgery service and the plastic surgery service was again asked to help the primary service to close the conduit leak.

During the intraoperative exploration, the leak appeared to be on the right side of the repair with a small leak between the flap and the colonic anastomosis. The skin paddle of the flap and the muscle portion of the flap appeared to be viable.

After irrigation, the unhealthy-looking skin edges of the flap were debrided. The edge of the pectoral major muscle was sutured to the edge of the neck and chest skins with interrupted 3-0 PDS sutures after the right chest skin was mobilized as an advancement flap (Fig. 25.49). The second layer repair between the flap and chest skin was performed with interrupted half-buried horizontal 3-0 PDS sutures. In addition, several retention sutures were placed to reinforce the skin closure. In this way, the right side of the leak was completely repaired. The distal anastomotic leak was repaired with several interrupted half-buried horizontal 3-0 PDS sutures (Fig. 25.50).

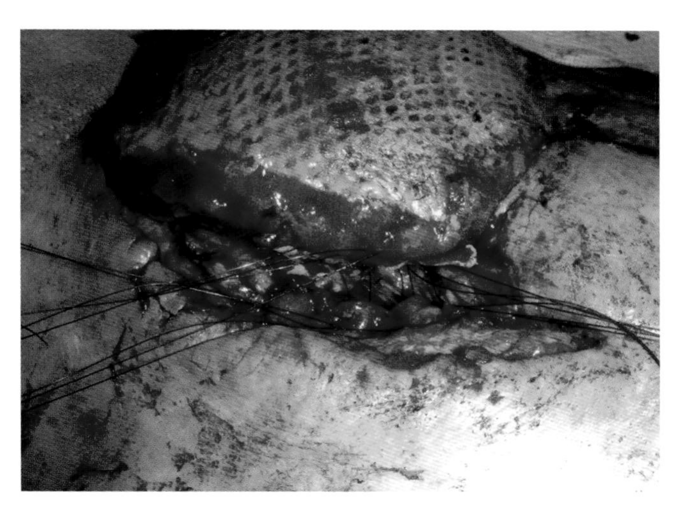

• **Fig. 25.49** Intraoperative view showing the first-layer repair between the muscle of the flap and the subcutaneous tissue of the neck and chest with interrupted PDS sutures.

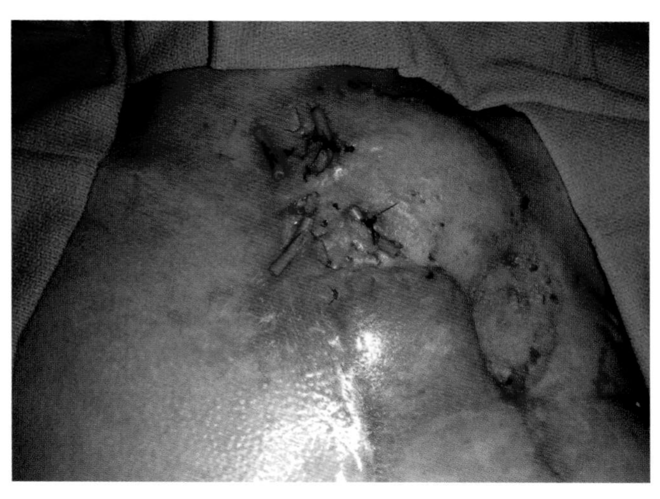

• **Fig. 25.51** The result at 3-week follow-up showing well-healed dehisced areas of the cervical esophageal reconstruction after repair.

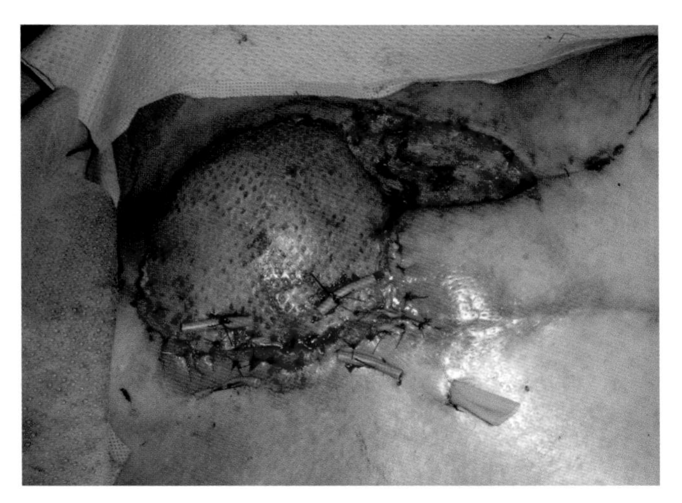

• **Fig. 25.50** Intraoperative view showing completion of two-layer repair for the dehisced areas of the cervical esophageal reconstruction and placement of retention sutures.

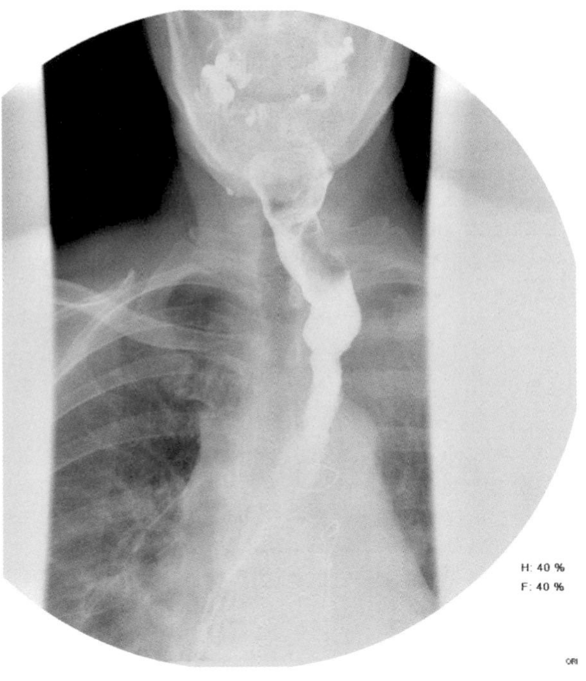

• **Fig. 25.52** Barium swallow test at 3 months showing wide patent reconstructed cervical esophagus with no evidence of leak.

Follow-Up Results

The patient did well postoperatively and there were no signs of leak from the repaired sites. She was discharged home uneventfully on postoperative day 22. The flap reconstruction site including the neck and chest wounds healed well (Fig. 25.51). During follow-up, the success of the cervical esophageal reconstruction was confirmed by a swallow test (Fig. 25.52).

Final Outcome

The patient was followed closely for at least 2 years after reconstruction. She was able to eat and drink and tolerated soft and solid foods. Her neck and chest flap sites healed well with minimal scarring (Fig. 25.53). The patient required episodic endoscopic dilatations for recurrent anastomotic stricture and some dysphagia. She was followed by the thoracic surgery service for routine follow-up.

Pearls for Success

Esophageal conduit necrosis after colonic reconstruction is a severe and emergent complication. As documented in this case, a pedicled pectoral major myocutaneous flap can be used not only to restore the cervical-esophageal colon conduit but also to reconstruct a neck wound in a single-stage operation. Compared with fasciocutaneous free flaps such as radial forearm and anterolateral thigh flaps, the pectoral major myocutaneous flap is an innovative and effective local reconstruction option without the need for free tissue transfer. In addition to its location on the chest being adjacent to the defect, a major advantage of the flap is its

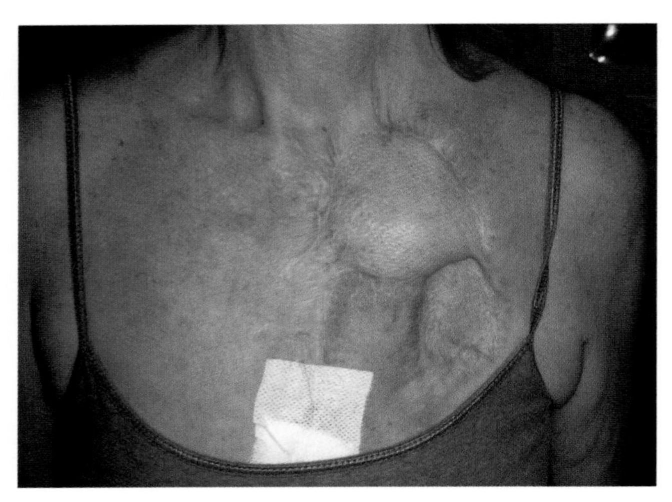

• **Fig. 25.53** The result at 7-month follow-up showing well-healed cervical esophageal reconstruction site and the rest of the chest wound with minimal scarring.

reliability and ease of harvesting, with reduced operative time. Therefore, no microsurgical flaps or specialized instruments are required. Two-layer closure can be performed for the anastomosis or repair and the muscle layer to the adjacent skin closure should be performed to reinforce the anastomosis or repair. In case of anastomotic or repair leak, the muscle layer can be readvanced to approximate the leak sites further. The main limitation of the flap is the bulkiness and rigidity of the entire flap including adipose layer and the skin. In this patient, the split-thickness skin graft that was placed over the muscle portion of the flap and the follow-up showed no sign of bulkiness or rigidity.

Recommended Readings

Archibald S, Young JEM, Thoma A. Pharyngo-cervical esophageal reconstruction. *Clin Plast Surg*. 2005;32:339–346.

Chang TY, Hsiao JR, Lee WT, et al. Esophageal reconstruction after oncological total laryngopharyngoesophagectomy: algorithmic approach. *Microsurgery*. 2019;39:6–13.

Dodd AR, Goodnight JE, Pu LLQ. Successful management of cervicoesophageal anastomosis leak after microsurgical esophageal reconstruction: a case report and review of the literature. *Ann Plast Surg*. 2010;65:110–114.

Komorowska-Timek E, Lee GK. Tube-in-a-tube anterolateral thigh flap for reconstruction of a complex esophageal and anterior neck defect. *Ann Plast Surg*. 2014;72:64–66.

LoGiudice JA, Wyler von Ballmoos MC, Gasparri MG, Lao WW. When the gastrointestinal conduit for total esophageal reconstruction is not an option review of the role of skin flaps and report of salvage with a single-stage tubed anterolateral thigh flap. *Ann Plast Surg*. 2016;76:463–467.

Rice DC, Yu P. Use of supercharged jejunal flap for esophageal reconstruction. *Oper Tech Thorac Cardiovasc Surg*. 2010;15:243–257.

Stile FL, Sud V, Zhang F, Angel MF, Anand V, Lineaweaver WC. Reconstruction of long cervical esophageal defects with the radial forearm flap. *J Craniofac Surg*. 2006;17:382–387.

Yin K, Xu H, Cooke DT, Pu LLQ. Successful management of oesophageal conduit necrosis by a single-stage reconstruction with the pedicled pectoralis major myocutaneous flap. *Interact Cardiovasc Thorac Surg*. 2015;21:124–126.

26 Upper Abdominal Wall Reconstruction

Clinical Presentation

A 36-year-old White male sustained extensive thermal burn and had excisions and skin graft procedures on his trunk, axilla, and upper extremity. He also developed compartment syndrome and subsequently underwent a decompression procedure for compartment syndrome release. He unfortunately developed a large ventral hernia and previous abdominal wall reconstructions by the general surgery service failed. The plastic surgery service was asked by the primary service to perform a soft tissue coverage to the potential upper abdominal defect with exposed mesh after abdominal wall reconstruction (Fig. 26.1). Because this patient had extensive burns over the trunk and had previously undergone a component separation procedure, there was no abdominal muscle or other flap that could safely be harvested to cover this potential soft tissue defect.

Operative Plan and Special Considerations

In this patient with a significantly large, healed skin graft over his trunk, a good soft tissue coverage to the upper abdomen after a mesh placement for abdominal wall ventral hernia repair was challenging because there was no local or distant flap that could be used for soft tissue reconstruction. A free latissimus dorsi myocutaneous flap could be selected to provide a good and reliable soft tissue coverage for potentially exposed mesh after abdominal wall reconstruction. The right internal mammary vessels at the third or fourth intercostal space could serve as recipient vessels for microvascular anastomoses. The right internal mammary vein is usually larger than the left, but a preoperative duplex scan could be performed to ensure good size and flow of those recipient vessels. The surgeons should anticipate some difficulties for the recipient vessel dissection.

Operative Procedures

Under general anesthesia with the patient in the supine position, the plastic surgery portion of the procedure started after the herniated bowels were taken back to the peritoneal cavity and the peritoneal closure was achieved with additional component separation technique and placement of Prolene mesh by the general surgery service. The upper abdominal soft tissue defect measured 15 × 7 cm with significant undermining and deep space (Fig. 26.2).

The right internal mammary vessels at the fourth intercostal space were explored first. After a skin incision and division of the medial portion of the pectoral major muscle, the fourth intercostal space was identified and a small portion of the rib connected to the sternum was resected. Both internal mammary artery and vein were identified and dissected out under loupe magnification.

The patient was then changed to the right lateral decubitus position. A 15 × 7 cm skin paddle was marked and an incision was made down to the latissimus dorsi muscle fascia. Once both medial and lateral borders of the latissimus muscle had been identified, the muscle was divided with electrocautery medially, inferiorly, and laterally. Under direct vision, the latissimus dorsi myocutaneous flap was elevated along with the skin paddle. It was elevated from the chest wall and the serratus muscle was preserved. Once the serratus branch of the artery had been divided, the muscle attachment to the humerus was also divided with electrocautery. The pedicle dissection was performed under direct vision with proper retraction. The thoracodorsal nerve was divided first and both thoracodorsal artery and vein were divided after further pedicle dissection (Fig. 26.3). The latissimus flap donor site was closed in three layers after placing two drains.

The patient was then returned to the supine position. The flap was prepared under loupe magnification. Both pedicle artery and vein were flushed with a heparinized saline solution. The additional preparation of both pedicle artery and vein was done under an operating microscope after the flap was temporarily inset into the upper abdomen. The arterial microvascular anastomosis was performed to the internal mammary artery with interrupted 8-0 nylon sutures in an end-to-end fashion. For the venous microvascular anastomosis, a 2.5-mm coupler device was selected in an end-to-end fashion. After all clamps were removed, the flap appeared to be well perfused (Fig. 26.4).

The flap was placed above the Prolene mesh. The muscle portion of the flap was tucked into the defect. The skin paddle of the flap was approximated to the adjacent abdominal skin with several interrupted 3-0 Monocryl sutures in half-buried horizontal mattress fashion. A small raw area over the tip of the flap was covered with a full-thickness skin graft harvested from the abdomen and secured with 5-0 chromic sutures. A Cook Doppler probe was wrapped in the distal part of the arterial anastomosis for

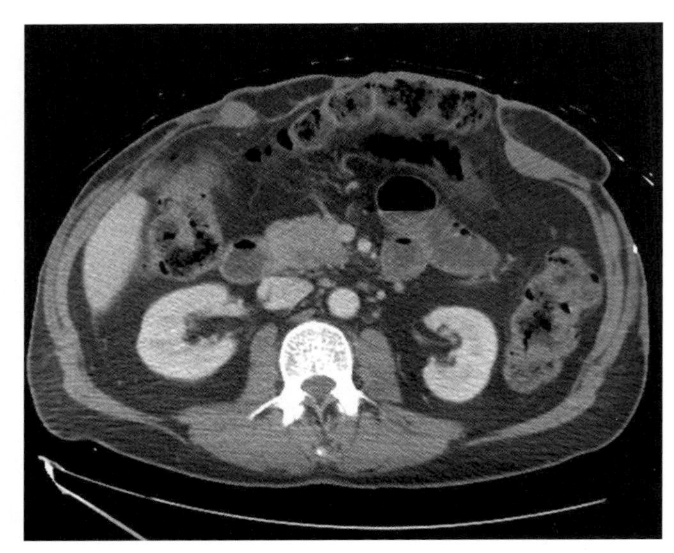

• **Fig. 26.1** Preoperative CT scan showing a large ventral hernia in the upper abdomen with significant separation of two rectus abdominis muscles.

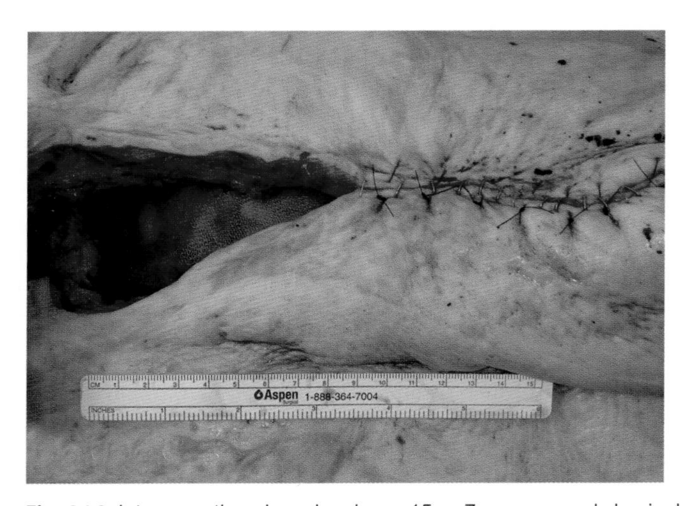

• **Fig. 26.2** Intraoperative view showing a 15 × 7 cm upper abdominal soft tissue wound after component separation and placement of Prolene mesh for ventral hernia repair.

continuous monitoring of the flap. The rest of the abdominal incision was closed by the general surgery service (Fig. 26.5).

Follow-Up Results

The patient did well postoperatively without any complications related to the free latissimus dorsi myocutaneous flap for the upper abdominal wall reconstruction. He was discharged from hospital on postoperative day 7. All drains were removed during subsequent follow-up visits. The upper abdominal flap reconstruction site healed well (Fig. 26.6).

Final Outcome

The upper abdominal free flap reconstruction site healed well with minimal scarring. There was no residual infection under the flap

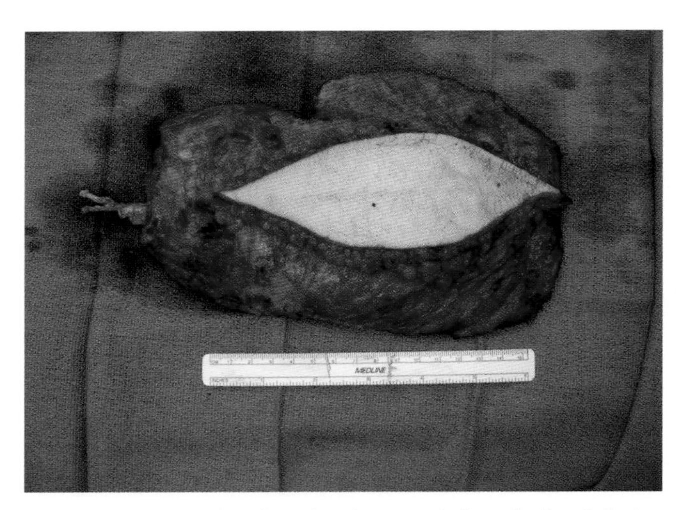

• **Fig. 26.3** Intraoperative view showing completion of a free latissimus dorsi myocutaneous flap dissection.

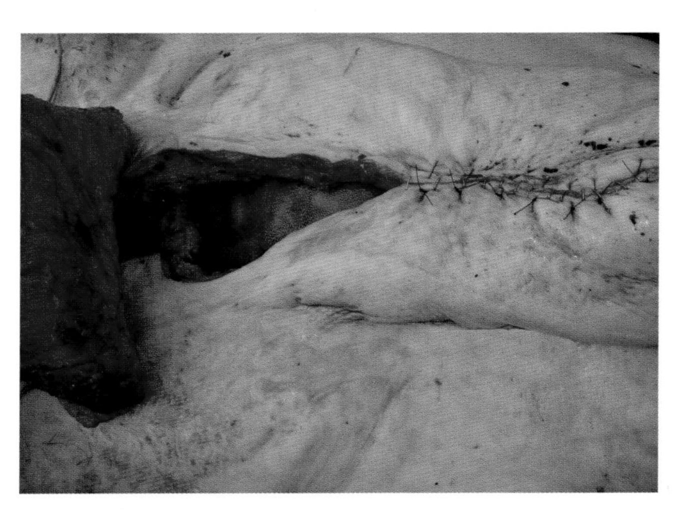

• **Fig. 26.4** Intraoperative view showing a well perfused free myocutaneous flap before it was inset into the upper abdominal wound.

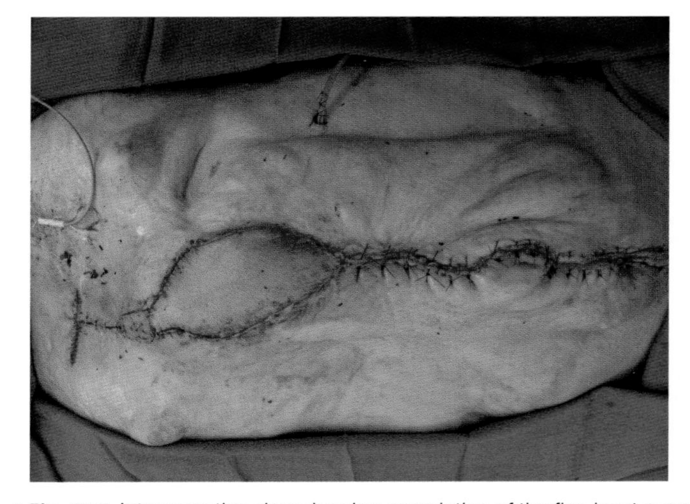

• **Fig. 26.5** Intraoperative view showing completion of the flap inset over the Prolene mesh.

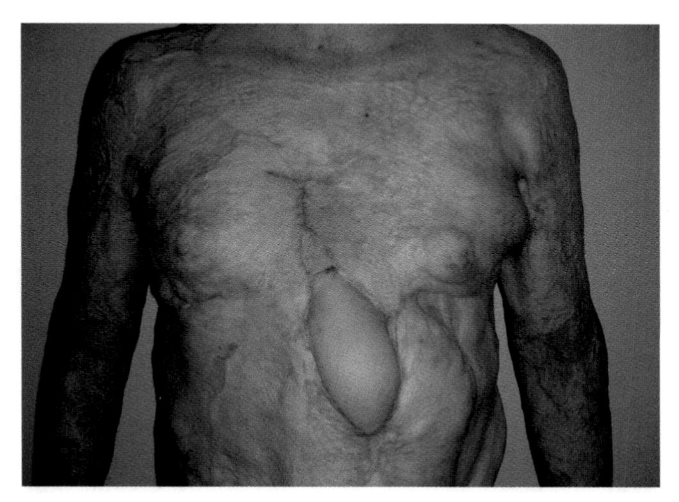

• **Fig. 26.6** The result at 7-week follow-up showing well-healed upper abdominal free flap site.

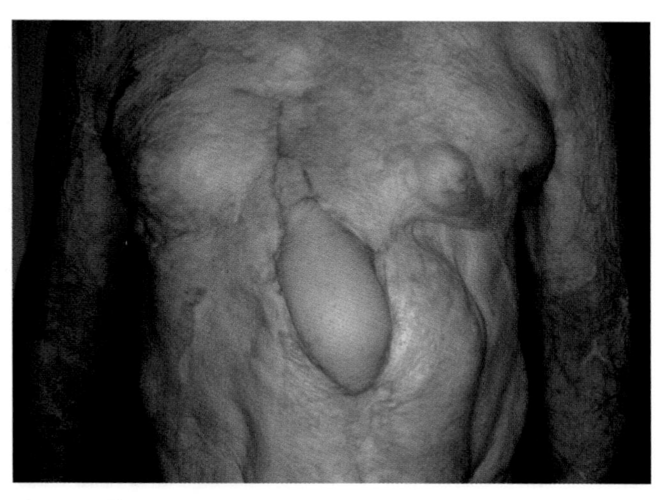

• **Fig. 26.7** The result at 4-month follow-up showing well-healed and stable upper abdominal free flap site with good contour and minimal scarring.

or recurrent ventral hernia (Fig. 26.7). The patient has resumed his normal activities and been followed by the general surgery service for routine follow-up.

Pearls for Success

For a large upper abdominal soft tissue wound with adjacent scar tissue, a free latissimus dorsi flap can be selected as a valid reconstructive option. The flap is large enough and can be harvested as a myocutaneous flap with a large skin paddle. It has a long pedicle and can reach the internal mammary vessels at the third or fourth intercostal space for easy end-to-end microvascular anastomoses. The muscle portion of the flap can be placed directly over the Prolene mesh and provide an excellent soft tissue coverage of the area. The combination of component separation, synthetic mesh placement, and free latissimus dorsi myocutaneous flap reconstruction provides the best possible chance for primary healing after ventral hernia repair in this patient.

Recommended Readings

Althubaiti G, Butler CE. Abdominal wall and chest wall reconstruction. *Plast Reconstr Surg*. 2014;133:688e–701e.

Bodin F, Dissaux C, Romain B, Rohr S, Brigand C, Bruant-Rodier C. Complex abdominal wall defect reconstruction using a latissimus dorsi free flap with mesh after malignant tumor resection. *Microsurgery*. 2017;37:38–43.

Mathes SJ, Steinwald PM, Foster RD, Hoffman WY, Anthony JP. Complex abdominal wall reconstruction: a comparison of flap and mesh closure. *Ann Surg*. 2000;232:586–596.

Roubaud MS, Baumann DP. Flap reconstruction of the abdominal wall. *Semin Plast Surg*. 2018;32:133–140.

Sinna R, Gianfermi M, Benhaim T, Qassemyar Q, Robbe M. Reconstruction of a full- thickness abdominal wall defect using an anterolateral thigh free flap. *J Visceral Surg*. 2010;147:e49–e53.

Tukiainen E, Leppaniemi A. Reconstruction of extensive abdominal wall defects with microvascular tensor fasciae latae flap. *Br J Surg*. 2011;98:880–884.

27
Lower Abdominal Wall Reconstruction

Clinical Presentation

A 66-year-old White male had a renal transplantation for end-stage renal disease secondary to polycystic kidney disease by the transplant surgery service. He also had 50 pack-year of smoking history. He had chronic hypoalbuminemia caused by peritoneal dialysis. Although he underwent successful deceased-donor transplantation, he required peritoneal dialysis because his early allograft function was delayed. One week after surgery, he was found to have an enlarging perigraft hematoma. He was taken to the operating room for hematoma evacuation. Over the following days, he continued to require dialysis and developed a superficial infection of lower abdominal incision, which was opened at the bedside and packed with gauze. He was discharged home with a vacuum-assisted closure dressing and continued ongoing peritoneal dialysis. One week later, it was noted that the superior pole of the transplanted kidney was extruding from the wound and the plastic surgery service was consulted for a soft tissue reconstruction of wound closure (Fig. 27.1).

Operative Plan and Special Considerations

After examining the open wound over the right lower quadrant of the abdomen, it appeared that the entire incision for the kidney transplant was dehisced. The surrounding wound edges were not healthy but the transplanted kidney, confirmed by biopsy, was still functioning (Fig. 27.2). A pedicled right rectus femoris muscle flap with a skin graft was selected for reconstruction of this right lower quadrant soft tissue wound. The flap has type II circulation pattern and receives blood supply dominantly from the descending branch of the lateral circumflex femoral artery and venae comitantes. It can be used as an alternative option for lower abdominal wall reconstruction. It is not an expandable muscle but approximation of the distal edges of the vastus medialis and lateralis muscles after the flap elevation may help to minimize impairment of full leg extension.

Operative Procedures

Under general anesthesia with the patient in the supine position, surgical debridement was performed to remove all necrotic, infected, or colonized tissues within the wound including the surface of the exposed transplanted kidney. The outline of the rectus femoris muscle flap and the planned incision for the flap elevation were marked in the right thigh (Fig. 27.3). The rectus femoris muscle was identified first after the skin incision had been made down to the fascia. The surgical dissection could be done quickly once the vastus lateralis and medialis muscles were dissected free from the rectus femoris muscle. The distal insertion of the muscle to the patella was divided and the muscle could be quickly elevated (Fig. 27.4). Once the pedicle had been identified, the proximal insertion was divided. The flap was now completely dissected free and tunneled to the right lower abdominal wound.

The flap was then placed onto the exposed kidney and approximated to the adjacent skin edges of the open wound with interrupted 3-0 Monocryl sutures in half-buried horizontal mattress fashion after drain placements (Fig. 27.5). A split-thickness skin graft was harvested from his right thigh and meshed to 1 to 1.5 ratio. It was placed over the muscle flap and secured with skin staples (Fig. 27.6). The donor site incision was closed in two layers over a drain (Fig. 27.7).

Follow-Up Results

Postoperatively the patient did well and the flap reconstruction site healed well. By coincidence, the renal allograft function afterward improved drastically, with serum creatinine levels reducing from 6–9 mg/dL previously to 1.2 mg/dL. The peritoneal dialysis catheter was removed by the transplant surgery service. The reconstructive procedure had reassuring good early results and the patient was discharged home 10 days postoperatively.

Management of Complications

One week later, the patient was seen at the transplant surgery clinic and readmitted to the hospital for the flap site dehiscence, with a small portion of the transplanted kidney that had become exposed (Fig. 27.8). The plastic surgery service was again asked for help in closing the wound. During exploration, the muscle flap had some superficial necrotic areas but was still essentially viable. There was a significant amount of ascites accumulated near the superior pole of the transplanted kidney (Fig. 27.9). It was believed that this was the reason the flap reconstruction was dehisced. Encouragingly, the renal allograft function was still good and the entire transplanted kidney remained viable based on the direct tissue biopsy. The dehisced portion of the wound edges was reapproximated after undermining the superior skin edge in the lower abdomen. Two new drains were also placed near the transplanted kidney (Fig. 27.10).

Unfortunately, reapproximation of the wound closure dehisced again after 6 days, which was thought to be caused by the tension on the closure (Fig. 27.11). Thus, a large V-to-Y cutaneous

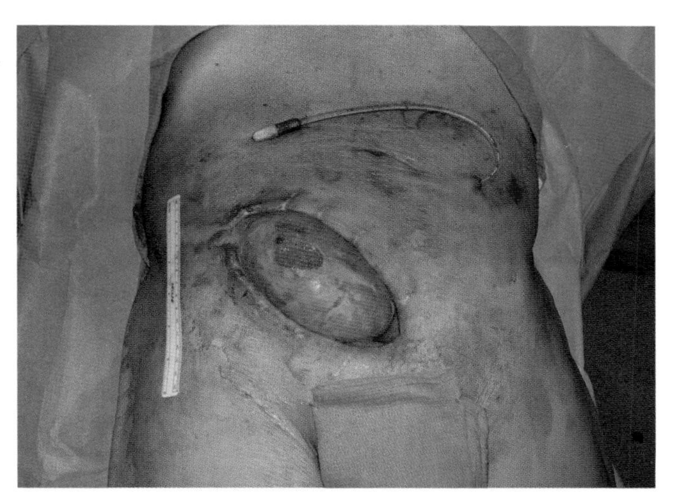

• **Fig. 27.1** Preoperative view showing the completely eviscerated renal allograft as a result of total wound dehiscence and fascial retraction.

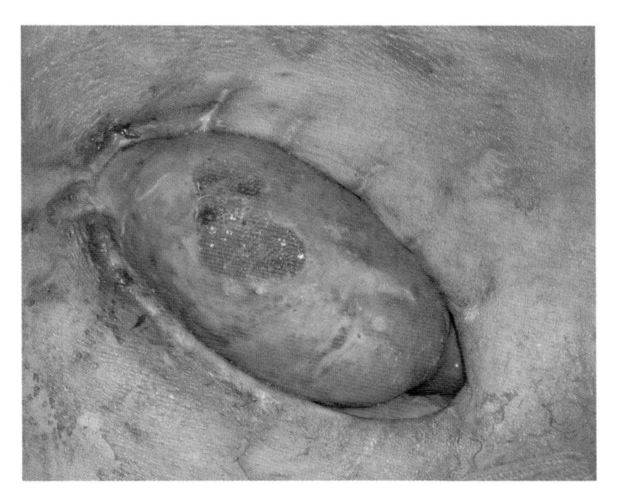

• **Fig. 27.2** Intraoperative close-up view showing the viable and functional transplanted kidney.

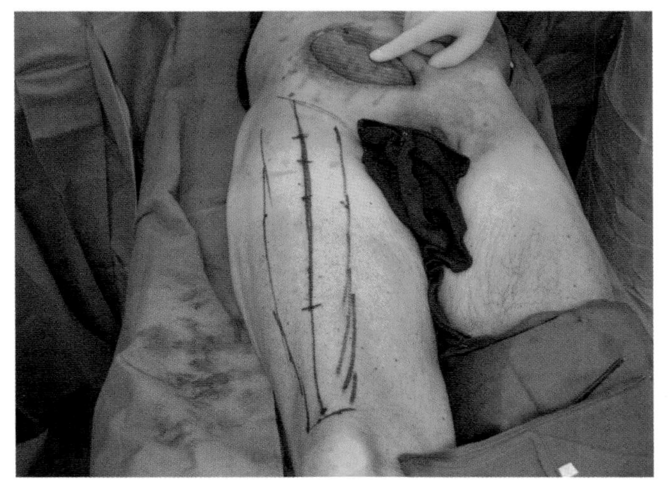

• **Fig. 27.3** Intraoperative view showing the design of the right rectus femoris muscle flap based on the descending branch of the lateral circumflex femoral vessels.

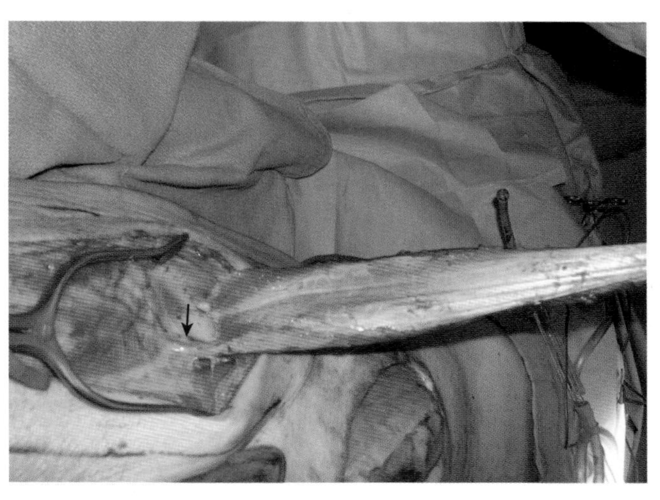

• **Fig. 27.4** Intraoperative view showing an elevated rectus femoris muscle flap. The pedicle of the flap is pointed by an *arrow*.

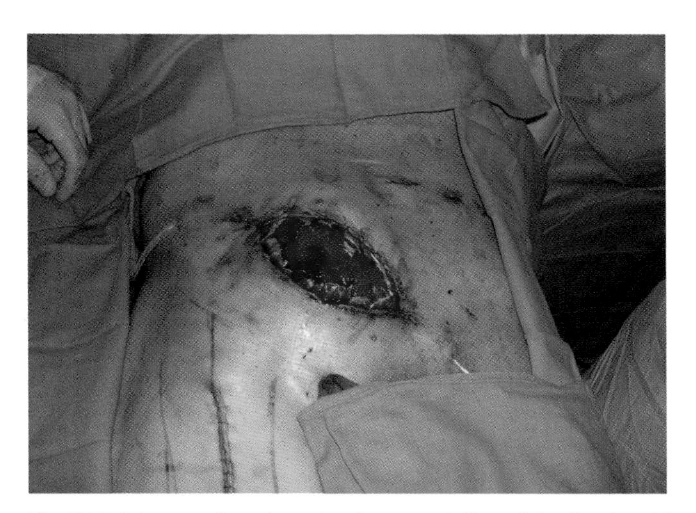

• **Fig. 27.5** Intraoperative view showing completion of the flap inset to cover an exposed transplanted kidney.

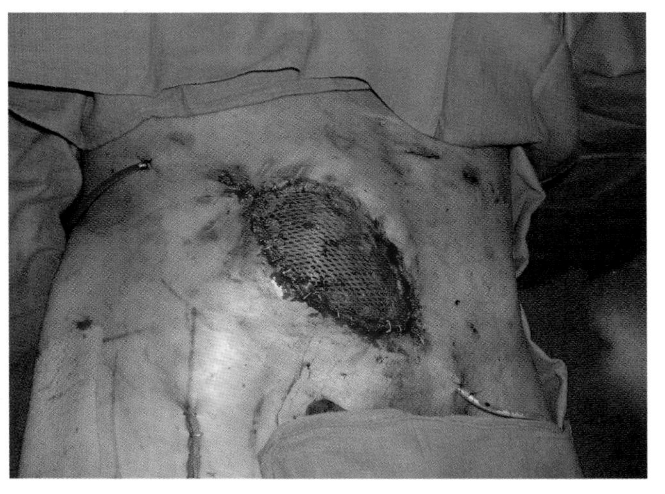

• **Fig. 27.6** Intraoperative view showing completion of a skin graft placement onto the muscle flap for coverage of an exposed transplanted kidney.

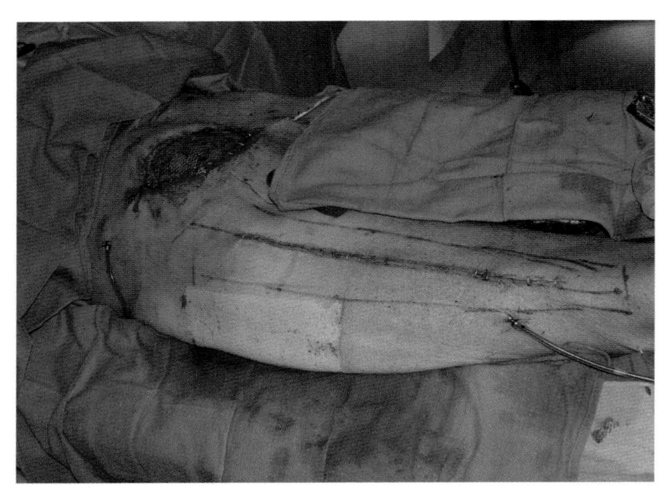

• **Fig. 27.7** Intraoperative view showing the closure of the rectus femoris muscle flap donor site in the thigh.

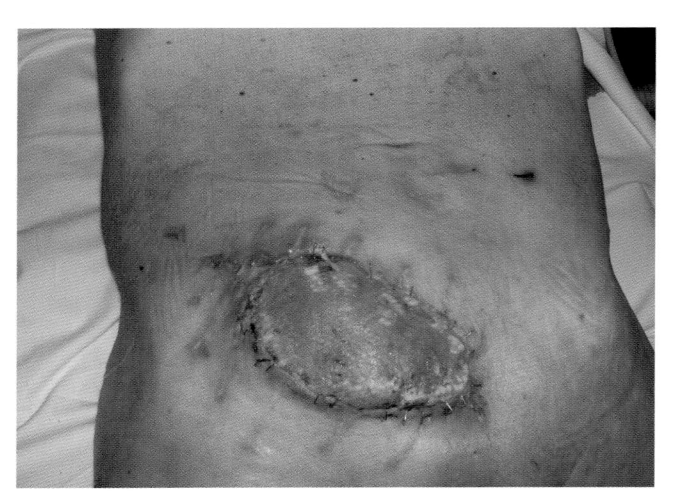

• **Fig. 27.8** Intraoperative view showing a superior wound dehiscence of the previous flap reconstruction site.

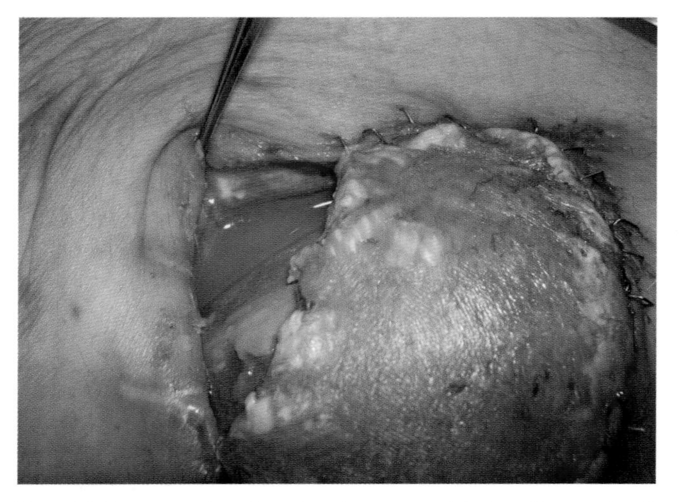

• **Fig. 27.9** Intraoperative view showing accumulated ascites next to the transplanted kidney.

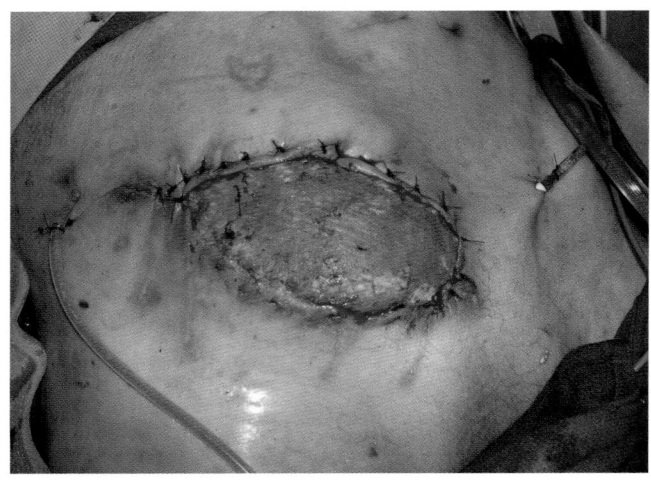

• **Fig. 27.10** Intraoperative view showing attempted primary closure after undermining of the superior skin edge in the lower abdomen.

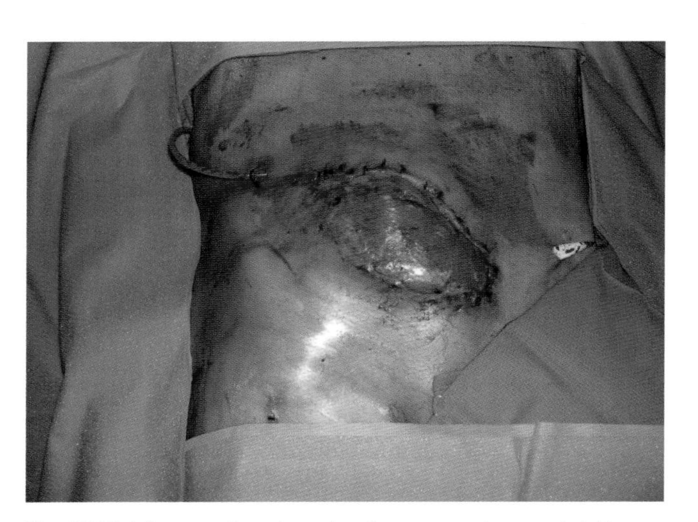

• **Fig. 27.11** Intraoperative view showing recurrent wound dehiscence after previous attempted wound closure.

periumbilical perforator-based advancement flap was designed after thorough debridement to remove the colonized tissue overlying the transplanted kidney. Several periumbilical perforators were identified and marked (Fig. 27.12). The flap was elevated with care being taken to preserve a few large perforators (Fig. 27.13). The flap was advanced easily to approximate the muscle flap for the wound closure without any tension (Fig. 27.14). A peritoneal dialysis catheter was also inserted by the transplant surgery service to prevent accumulation of ascites near the kidney. This V-to-Y cutaneous perforator-based advancement flap provided an effective and tension-free wound closure (Fig. 27.15). The remainder of the patient's hospitalization was unremarkable with serum creatinine levels between 1.3 and 1.6 mg/dL. He was discharged 5 days after the final operation and the flap reconstruction site healed completely (Fig. 27.16).

Final Outcome

During subsequent follow-up visits, the patient had no recurrent wound dehiscence. He had good and stable healing of the

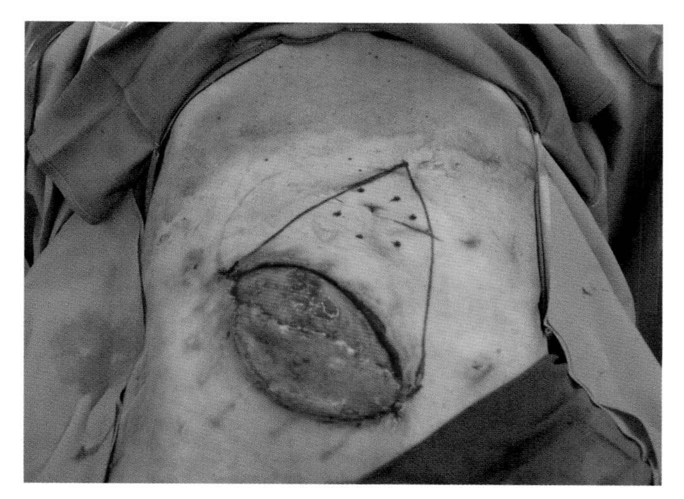

• **Fig. 27.12** Intraoperative view showing the design of a large V-to-Y periumbilical perforator-based cutaneous advancement flap.

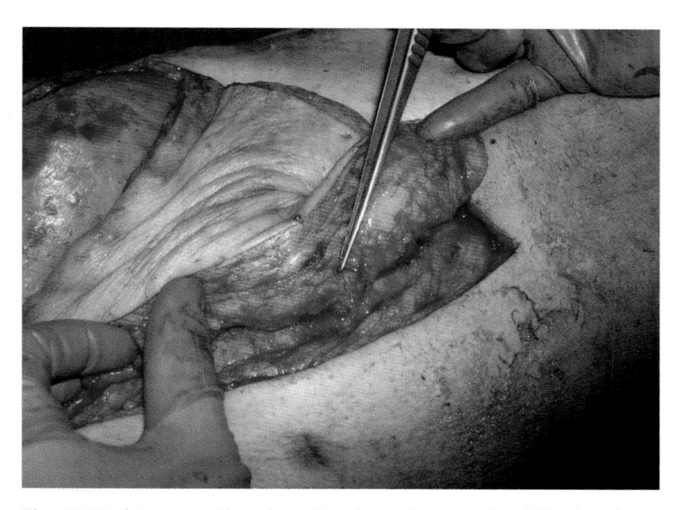

• **Fig. 27.13** Intraoperative view showing a large periumbilical perforator on which the flap would be based.

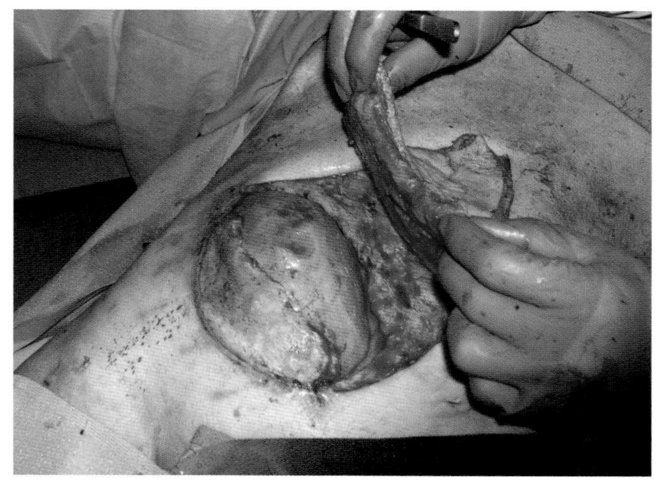

• **Fig. 27.14** Intraoperative view showing the flap that could easily be advanced to the dehisced wound and approximated to the muscle flap without tension.

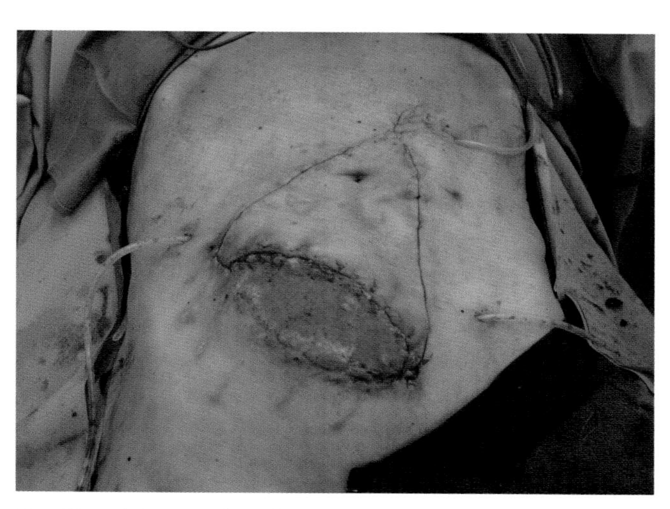

• **Fig. 27.15** Intraoperative view showing closure of the large V-to-Y periumbilical perforator- based cutaneous advancement flap.

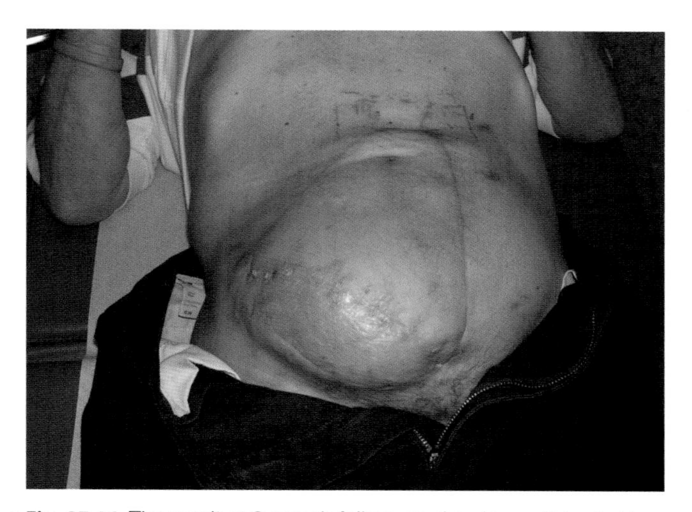

• **Fig. 27.16** The result at 2-month follow-up showing well-healed lower abdominal flap reconstruction site.

dehiscent wound over his flap reconstruction site with minimal scarring and has had stable renal allograft function since post-transplantation (Fig. 27.17). He has resumed his normal activities and has been followed by the transplant surgery service for routine follow-up.

Pearls for Success

With respect to wound healing, renal transplant recipients have long been recognized as disadvantaged for multiple reasons. There is no standardized approach to managing soft tissue wounds in posttransplant patients. Simple skin grafting to the transplanted kidney can be an option for temporary wound closure. However, a skin graft itself cannot provide stable wound coverage, thus allowing the possibility of further wound breakdown. Simple local tissue rearrangement as primary closure would also not be feasible in this large lower abdominal wound, complicated by an exposed renal allograft. Because of the large size of the wound, a rectus femoris muscle flap was selected in this case. It is well documented in the literature that a muscle flap can provide not only more

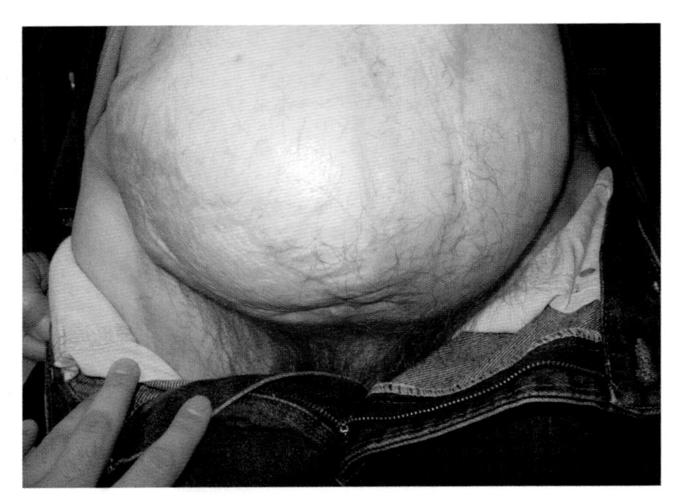

• **Fig. 27.17** The result at 2-year follow-up showing good and stable lower abdominal flap reconstruction site with good contour and minimal scarring.

stable wound coverage because of its bulkiness but also a better bacteria-killing environment because of its rich blood supply.

If the flap closure becomes dehiscent, attempted local tissue rearrangement can be performed. However, the wound may become dehiscent again, most probably because of impaired wound healing. In this case, it became obvious that additional flap reconstruction would be required for optimal wound closure. Based on the knowledge of periumbilical perforators used in breast reconstruction, a perforator-based cutaneous V-to-Y advancement flap can be designed during the operation for definitive wound closure because it can provide a more tension-free closure and can ensure healing of the lower abdominal wound. For this patient, encouragingly, the renal allograft, with stable soft-tissue coverage, has always maintained a good renal function.

Recommended Readings

Jeon H, McHugh PP, Ranjan D, Johnston TD, Gedaly R, Pu LLQ. Successful management of eviscerated renal allograft with preservation of function. *Am J Transplant.* 2008;8:1067–1070.

Landim FM, Tavares JM, Costa MLV, Landim RM, Feitosa RGF. Complex abdominal wall reconstruction after radiation therapy. *Am J Obstet Gynecol.* 2009;116:e1–e3.

Mericli AF, Baumann DP, Butler CE. Reconstruction of the abdominal wall after oncologic resection: defect classification and management strategies. *Plast Reconst Surg.* 2018;142:187S–196S.

Sumiya R, Tsukuura R, Mihara F, Yamamoto T. Free superficial circumflex iliac artery perforator fascial flap for reconstruction of upper abdominal wall with extensive infected herniation: a case report. *Microsurgery.* 2021;41:270–275.

Tamai M, Nagasao T, Miki T, Hamamoto Y, Kogure T, Tanaka Y. Rotation arc of pedicled anterolateral thigh flap for abdominal wall reconstruction: how far can it reach? *J Plast Reconstr Aesthet Surg.* 2015;68:1417–1424.

28 Upper Back Reconstruction

Clinical Presentation

A 63-year-old White male underwent a wide local excision of his upper back soft tissue sarcoma by the surgical oncology service, which left a 12 × 12 cm large soft tissue defect down to the deep muscle. The plastic surgery service was asked to help to close this wound after the wide local excision had been made for the primary sarcoma resection leaving an adequate margin. Thus, the definitive soft tissue reconstruction would be performed in the same setting immediately after oncological resection of the primary tumor (Fig. 28.1).

Operative Plan and Special Considerations

Because the location of this soft tissue defect was primarily in the upper back and the trapezius muscle in the adjacent area remained intact after the wide local excision, bilateral trapezius myocutaneous advancement flaps could be used to close this soft tissue defect. The flap receives blood supply from the transverse cervical artery and can be approximated in the midline of the upper back. Its attachment to the thoracic vertebrae could be released. Such a reconstruction could eventually provide a durable soft tissue coverage, best possible cosmetic outcome, and almost no donor site healing issues.

Operative Procedures

Under general anesthesia, the patient was placed in the prone position. Once the wide local excision had been completed by the surgical oncology service, the soft tissue defect was inspected. The paraspinal muscles were exposed at the base of the wound. Within the upper back wound, each side of the medial trapezius muscle edge was identified. The extent of the flap dissection was outlined for each side (Fig. 28.2). The flap elevation was started by detaching its muscle attachment to the thoracic vertebrae. Once such a surgical dissection had been performed adequately, submuscular dissection was performed so that the muscle and its overlying subcutaneous tissue and skin were elevated as a single unit. Such a dissection could be easily performed with the aid of a mammary light retractor and electrical cautery. During the dissection, the main pedicle vessels was visualized under the muscle and should be protected.

Once each side of the flap elevation had been advanced beyond the midline, hemostasis was carefully accomplished. A drain was placed under each flap. The final closure was done in three layers. Both muscle layers were approximated with interrupted 2-0 PDS sutures. Both subcutaneous tissue layers were approximated with interrupted 3-0 Monocryl sutures and the skin edges with interrupted 3-0 nylon sutures (Fig. 28.3).

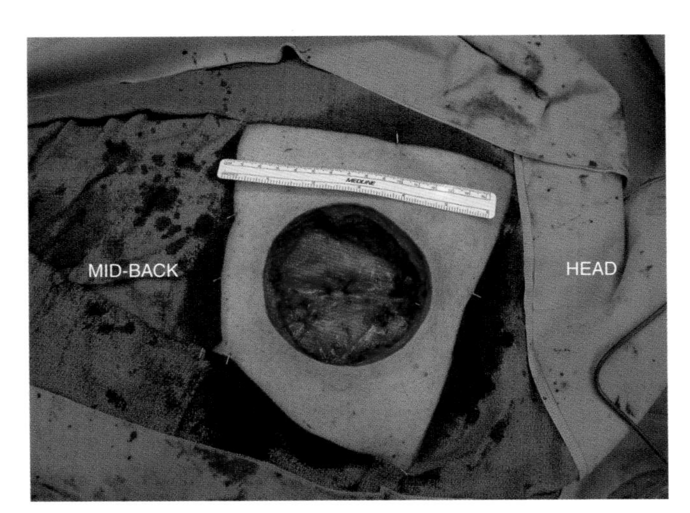

• **Fig. 28.1** Preoperative view showing a large soft tissue defect, measuring 12 × 12 cm, in the midline of the upper back down to the deep muscle after a wide local excision for soft tissue sarcoma.

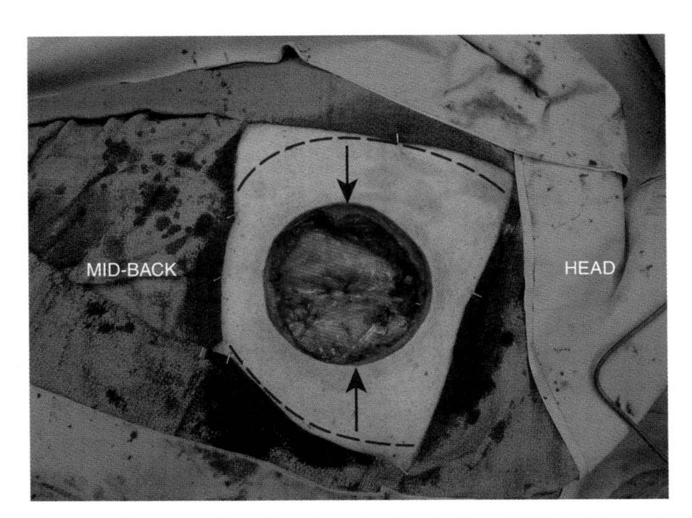

• **Fig. 28.2** Intraoperative view showing the design of bilateral trapezius myocutaneous advancement flaps and an extent of the submuscular flap dissection on each side.

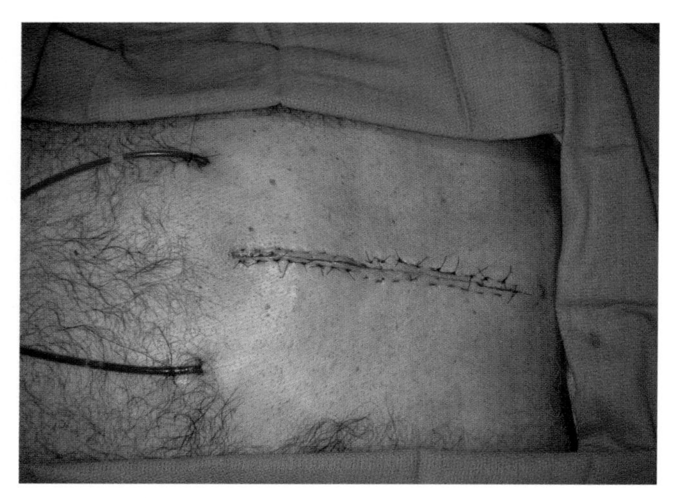

• **Fig. 28.3** Intraoperative view showing completion of bilateral trapezius myocutaneous advancement flaps for closure of this large upper back soft tissue defect.

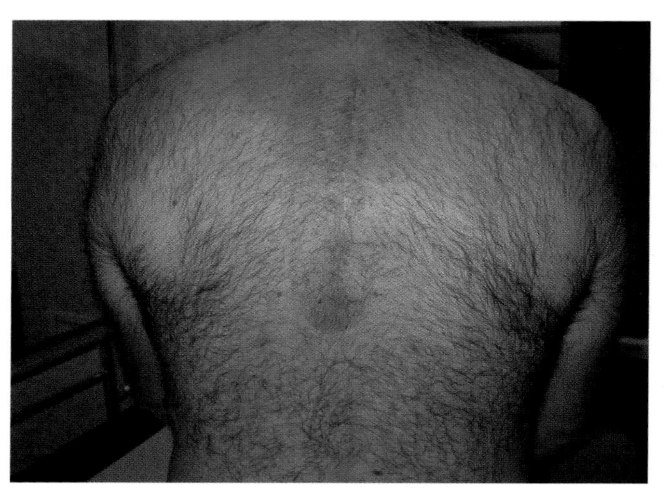

• **Fig. 28.4** The result at 2-month follow-up showing stable and well-healed upper back midline wound with good contour and minimal scarring.

Follow-Up Results

The patient did well postoperatively without any complications related to his bilateral trapezius myocutaneous advancement flaps for the wound closure. He was discharged from hospital on postoperative day 5. The drain was removed during subsequent follow-up visits. The upper back wound healed well and there was no seroma or contour issue in the flap site.

Final Outcome

The upper back wound after bilateral trapezius myocutaneous advancement flaps for soft tissue reconstruction healed well. Most importantly, there was durable soft tissue coverage with minimal scarring and no contour issue in the flap reconstruction site (Fig. 28.4). The patient has resumed his normal activities and is followed by the surgical oncology service for routine follow-up.

Pearls for Success

A large upper back midline soft tissue defect can successfully be reconstructed with bilateral trapezius myocutaneous advancement flaps. Such a flap reconstruction is similar to a sternal wound reconstruction where bilateral pectoral major myocutaneous advancement flaps are selected with an excellent outcome and good cosmetic result. In this case, the trapezium muscle was only partially detached medially based on the vertical length of the soft tissue defect. The extent of the horizontal flap elevation to the midline also depends on the degree of each flap's advancement toward the midline's soft tissue defect. Care should be taken not to injure the main pedicle vessels of each flap. A moderate amount of tension for the midline approximation may be tolerable for young and healthy patients but should be avoided for older patients or smokers. If performed correctly, such a flap reconstruction can be an excellent choice for the upper back midline soft tissue defect and the reconstructive outcome can be quite good as demonstrated in this case.

Recommended Readings

Baghaki S, Yalcin CE, Khankishiyev R, et al. Propeller and pre-expanded propeller use of a transversely oriented upper trapezius perforator flap in head and neck reconstruction: clinical experience and review of vascular anatomy of the supraspinal trapezius muscle. *J Plast Reconstr Aesthet Surg*. 2021;74:1534–1543.

Can A, Orgill DP, Ulrich JOD, Mureau MAM. The myocutaneous trapezius flap revisited: a treatment algorithm for optimal surgical outcomes based on 43 flap reconstructions. *J Plast Reconstr Aesthet Surg*. 2014;67:1669–1679.

Hallock GG. Reconstruction of posterior trunk defects. *Semin Plast Surg*. 2011;26:78–85.

Mathes DW, Thornton JF, Rohrich RJ. Management of posterior trunk defects. *Plast Reconst Surg*. 2006;118:73e–83e.

29 Middle Back Reconstruction

CASE 1

Clinical Presentation

A 45-year-old White female sustained a chronic radiation wound, measuring 10 × 9 cm, over her upper lumbar area with exposed spinal processes (Fig. 29.1). This wound was a complication of radiation to the area for treatment of a soft tissue sarcoma. She was referred by a surgical oncologist from outside hospital to our plastic surgery service for definitive soft tissue reconstruction. This patient also had a longstanding history of smoking. Therefore, her smoking history along with the location of this back wound would make this soft tissue reconstruction difficult and challenging (Fig. 29.2).

Operative Plan and Special Considerations

There are only a few reconstructive options for such a large soft tissue defect in the middle back after adequate debridement. Although a free flap transfer with recipient vessels based on the superior gluteal vessels can be a valid option, a revised latissimus dorsi muscle flap was considered for this case. The flap, based on two or three large lower thoracic and upper lumber perforators, could be turned over, in a revised fashion, to cover such a large soft tissue defect in this location. Depending on the presence, size, and number of those perforators, the revised latissimus dorsi muscle flap can be used to provide a durable soft tissue coverage for a sizable middle or upper lower back wound.

Operative Procedures

Under general anesthesia with the patient in a prone position, the wound was debrided by the neurosurgery service. The wound was located from T12 to L4 and measured 10 × 9 cm (Fig. 29.2). There were necrotic tissues on the surface with fibrotic tissues along all the edges of the wound. The wound was sharply debrided and all the visible necrotic or colonized tissues were removed. The wound was then irrigated thoroughly with Pulsavac.

Several major perforators for each side of the latissimus muscle flap were identified by a duplex scan. This flap could be based on the 3–5 major perforators along the same side of the thoracic spine. Two larger perforators were identified on the left side and the left latissimus muscle was selected for the flap reconstruction (Fig. 29.3). An oblique incision was made to explore the pedicle vessels of the left latissimus muscle. The skin flap was raised on either side of the latissimus muscle. Once the medial and the lateral border of the latissimus muscle had been identified, the dissection was performed toward the left axilla. The thoracodorsal vessels were identified and divided with hemoclips. The muscle was divided from its proximal insertion and elevated along with the submuscular tissue plane. By further dissection around those perforators, the latissimus dorsi muscle flap was turned over to cover the wound without too much tension (Fig. 29.4).

The flap was temporarily inset into the defect and secured temporarily with several small towel clips (Fig. 29.5). At this point, fluorescein (500 mg) was injected intravenously and the fluorescein test was performed to assess the circulation to the flap based on the three perforators but in a turnover fashion. The intraoperative fluorescein test showed that most of the flap appeared to be well perfused. Therefore, the intraoperative decision was made to proceed with the final flap inset and a skin graft to the muscle flap.

The flap was inset into the wound defect. Two drains were placed in the left latissimus dorsi muscle flap donor site. One additional drain was inserted under the muscle flap. The flap was inset into the adjacent rest of the normal-looking skin with several interrupted 3-0 Monocryl sutures in horizontal mattress fashion. The left back latissimus dorsi muscle flap donor site was approximated with several interrupted 2-0 PDS sutures for deep dermal closure and the skin was closed with skin staples (Fig. 29.6).

A split-thickness skin graft was harvested from the left upper thigh with a Zimmer dermatome. The skin graft was meshed to 1:1.5 ratio and placed on the muscle flap and secured with multiple skin staples. Several chromic sutures were used as a quilting suture to secure the skin graft (Fig. 29.7).

Follow-Up Results

The patient did well postoperatively without any complications related to the latissimus dorsi muscle turnover flap reconstruction for coverage of the lower middle and upper lower back wound. She was discharged from hospital on postoperative day 5. All drains were removed during subsequent follow-up visits. The lower middle back and upper lower back wound healed well and there was no recurrent infection or wound breakdown (Fig. 29.8).

Final Outcome

The lower middle and upper lower back wound after a reversed latissimus dorsi muscle turnover flap reconstruction healed well.

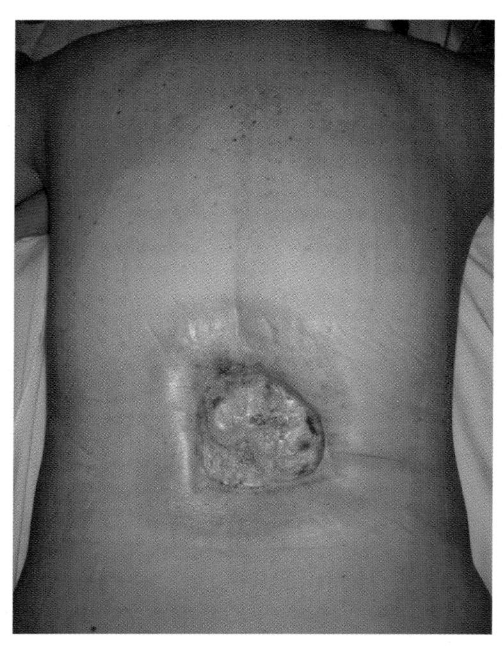

• **Fig. 29.1** Preoperative view showing a large radiation wound, measuring 10 × 9 cm, located in the lower middle and upper lower back.

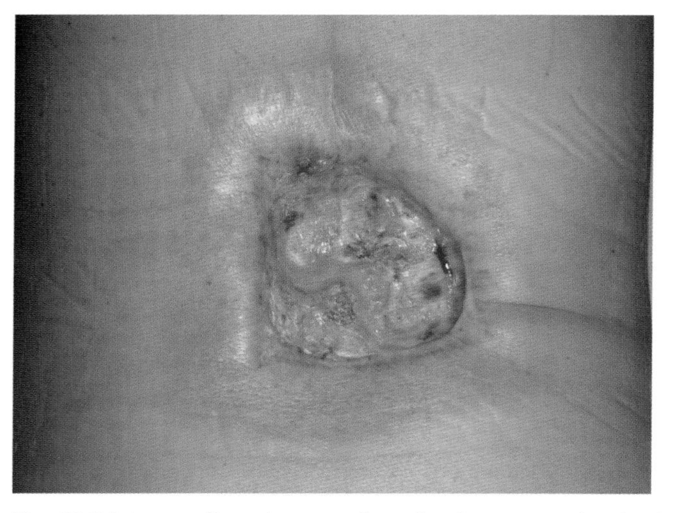

• **Fig. 29.2** Intraoperative close-up view showing a complex back wound with fibrotic and necrotic tissues and exposed spinal processes.

Most importantly, the patient has had no recurrent infection or wound breakdown during long-term follow-up. She has resumed her normal activities and been followed by the plastic surgery service as needed.

Pearls for Success

Soft tissue reconstruction for a lower middle back and/or upper lower back wound remains challenging because there is no adjacent soft tissue available for such a large back wound reconstruction. A reverse latissimus dorsi muscle flap can be an option for such a reconstruction. The flap is based on several large perforators from the lower thoracic and upper lumber areas. According to a previous published work (see Reference 6), the flap

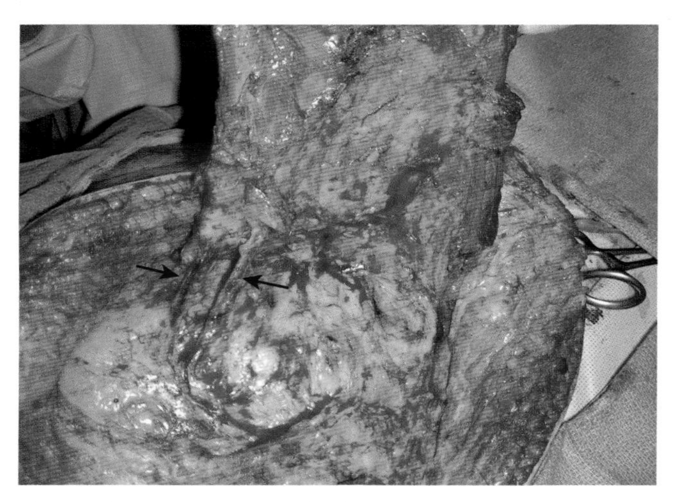

• **Fig. 29.3** Intraoperative view showing two large lower thoracic perforators of the reverse latissimus dorsi muscle flap.

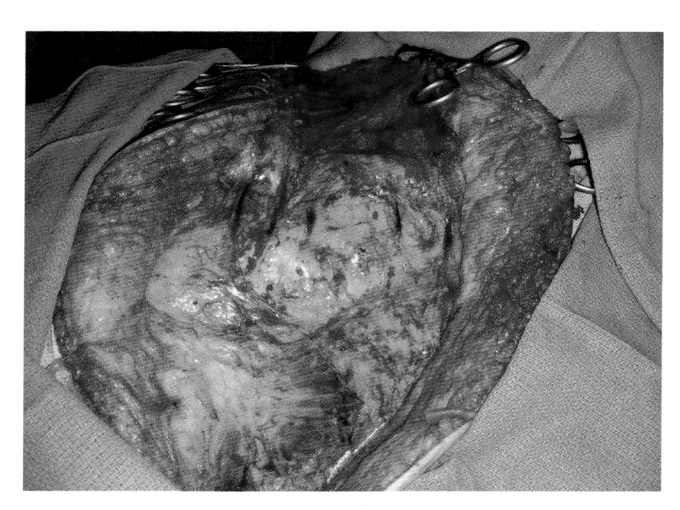

• **Fig. 29.4** Intraoperative view showing the reverse latissimus dorsi muscle flap after its turnover to cover this complex back wound temporarily. The flap was based on two larger lower thoracic perforators and three other relatively small thoracic and lumber perforators.

can be based on T10–T12 perforators. However, actual intraoperative dissection is encouraged to identify the presence of those large perforators as well as the status of their blood flow. Furthermore, an intraoperative perfusion study could be performed to assess adequate blood supply to the flap based on those perforators. In this case, several lumber artery perforators were included in the flap as long as they did not limit the degrees of the flap turnover. Although T10–T12 perforators might be adequate as a turnover flap for most patients, more perforators were included to the flap in this case because the patient was a long-term smoker.

CASE 2

Clinical Presentation

A 30-year-old White female with significant congenital spine problem had an infection after previous spine surgery. She was

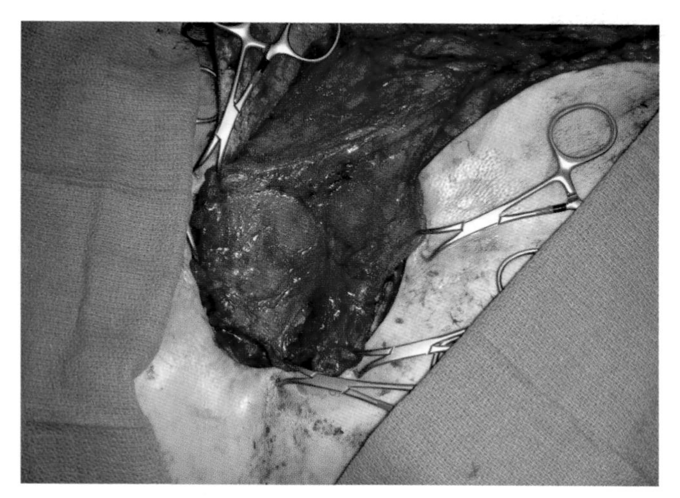

• **Fig. 29.5** Intraoperative view showing temporary inset of the flap to this complex back wound. The distal portion of the muscle appeared to be well perfused.

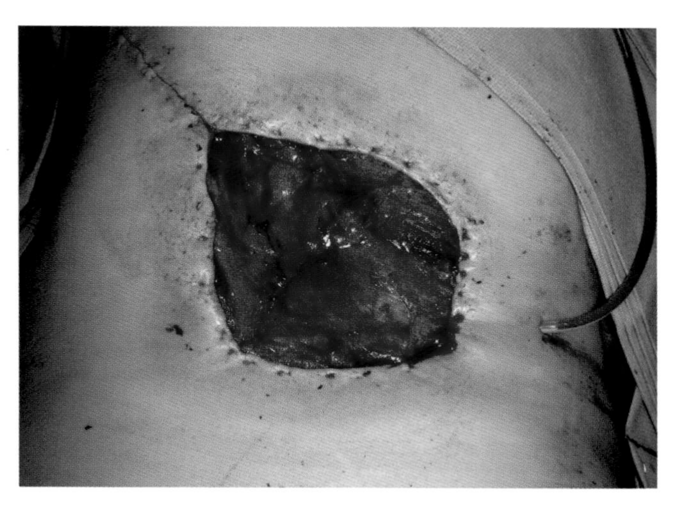

• **Fig. 29.6** Intraoperative view showing completion of the flap inset before placement of the skin graft.

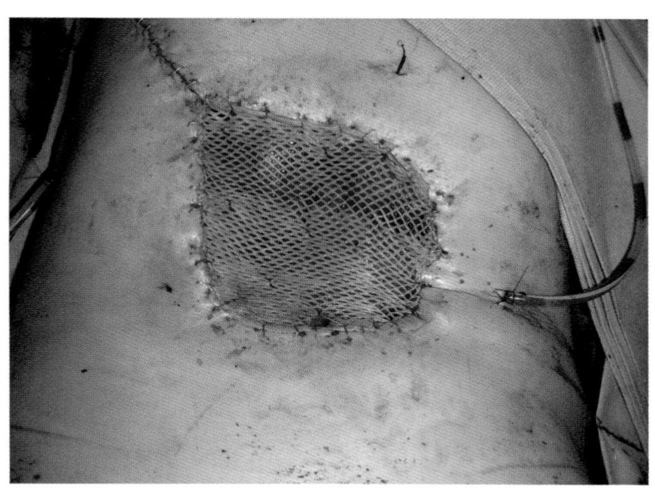

• **Fig. 29.7** Intraoperative view showing completion of the skin graft placement to the muscle flap and final appearance of the reconstruction.

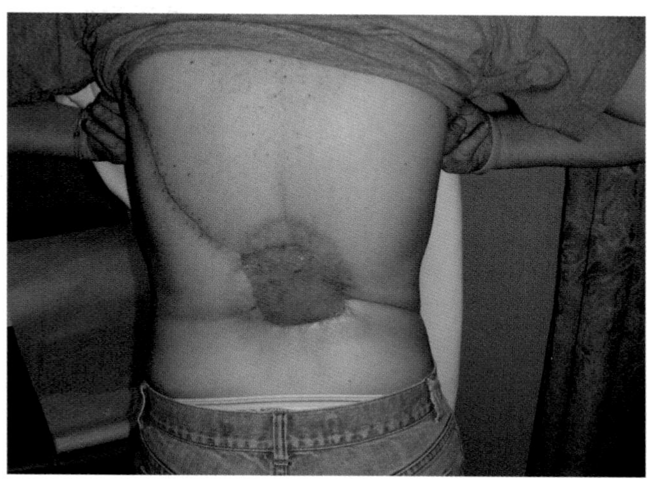

• **Fig. 29.8** The result at 7-week follow-up showing well-healed lower middle and upper lumber back wound. The flap provided a stable wound coverage and good contour.

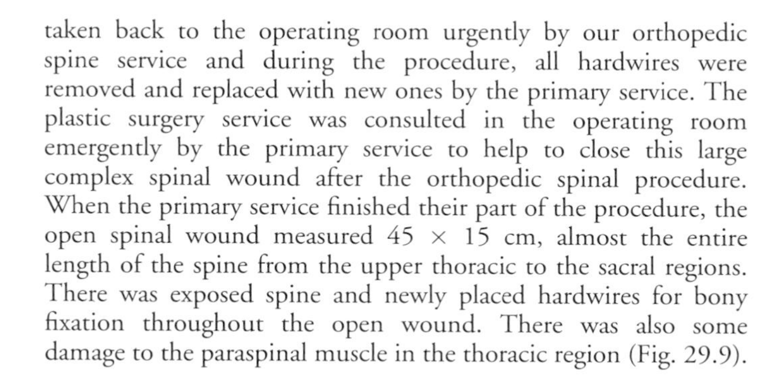

taken back to the operating room urgently by our orthopedic spine service and during the procedure, all hardwires were removed and replaced with new ones by the primary service. The plastic surgery service was consulted in the operating room emergently by the primary service to help to close this large complex spinal wound after the orthopedic spinal procedure. When the primary service finished their part of the procedure, the open spinal wound measured 45 × 15 cm, almost the entire length of the spine from the upper thoracic to the sacral regions. There was exposed spine and newly placed hardwires for bony fixation throughout the open wound. There was also some damage to the paraspinal muscle in the thoracic region (Fig. 29.9).

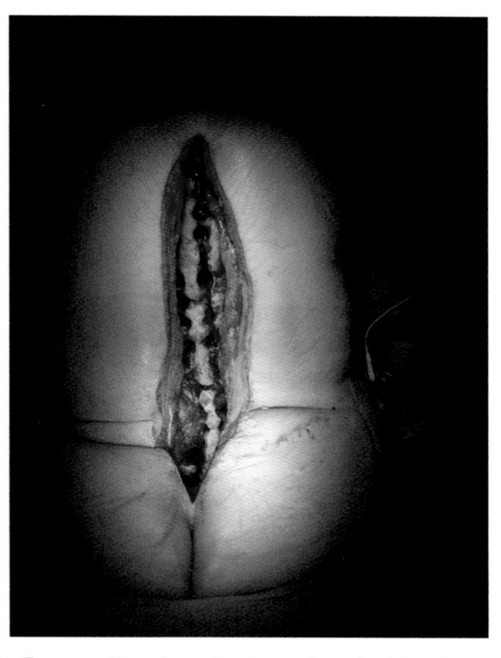

• **Fig. 29.9** Preoperative view showing a long incisional spine wound, measuring 45 × 15 cm, with exposed spine and hardware.

Operative Plan and Special Considerations

This spinal wound, although it was primarily located in the middle back, involved a portion of the upper back and most of the lower back. For such a long spinal wound, adjacent muscles from both sides of the wound edge could be used to cover the exposed spine and hardware. The latissimus dorsi muscle could be mobilized from each side to cover most of the middle back wound because the paraspinal muscles in the area were traumatized during the spine surgery. The untraumatized paraspinal muscle from each side could be used to cover the upper part of the lower back. The lower part of the lower back wound could be covered with the gluteal muscle from each side after approximation. Once the exposed spine and hardware had been covered with multiple muscle flaps that were approximated in the midline, the entire adjacent skin from each side could also be mobilized from each side and approximated to the midline for final skin closure.

Operative Procedures

Under general anesthesia with the patient in the prone position, the plastic surgery part of the procedure started after the spinal wound had been thoroughly debrided and the new hardware was replaced for spine stabilization by the orthopedic spine service. Once again, this was a 45 × 15 cm wound with the exposed spine and hardware. Two Blake drains were placed on the surface of the spine by the primary service (Fig. 29.10). There was also significant scarring and fibrosis in the muscle layers. The procedure was started by performing extensive undermining in the suprafascial tissue plane along the entire wound. The extensive undermining of the skin from each side was performed and each side of the skin flap could be advanced to the midline without too much tension. In this way, the edges of the latissimus dorsi muscle, paraspinal muscle, and gluteal muscle could be clearly visualized and elevated under direct vision. Both sides of the multiple muscles were elevated adequately and could be advanced to the midline and approximated with 0-PDS sutures in an interrupted fashion.

After multiple muscles were approximated in the midline, there was a 12 × 5 cm gap that could not be approximated because of the poor muscle condition in the gluteal area. Therefore, the

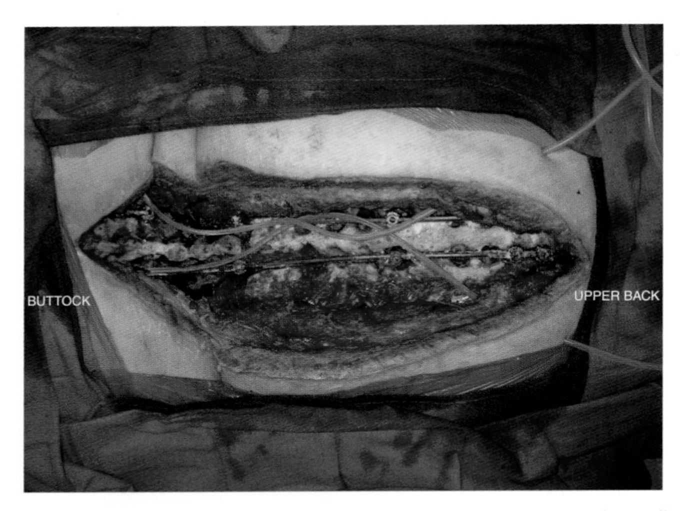

• **Fig. 29.10** Intraoperative view showing completion of the orthopedic spine surgery with new hardware and deep drain placements. The upper portion of the paraspinal muscle was traumatized and the gluteal muscle was scarred and in poor quality.

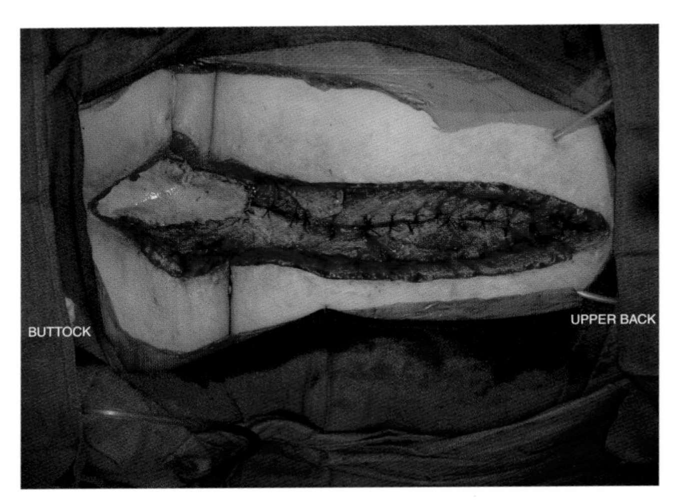

• **Fig. 29.11** Intraoperative view showing completion of the latissimus dorsi, paraspinal, and gluteal muscle closure in the midline with the placement of an acellular dermal matrix for the first-layer closure over the exposed spine and hardware.

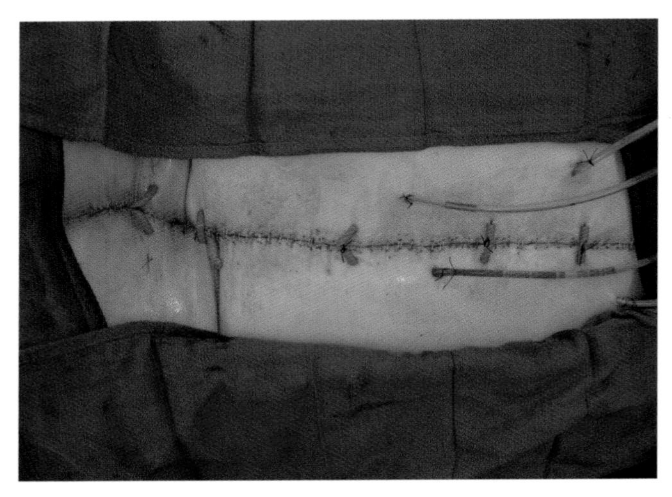

• **Fig. 29.12** Intraoperative view showing completion of the skin closure at the end of the operation. Several retention sutures were placed to release tension on the skin closure.

intraoperative decision was made to close this defect with an acellular dermal matrix as a biological mesh in this potentially infected wound.

A 12 × 5 cm ultra-thick AlloDerm tissue was selected and trimmed to an appropriate size and shape. It was then sutured to the adjacent muscle edge to cover this open area with interrupted 2-0 PDS sutures (Fig. 29.11). The final skin closure was performed in two layers. The deep dermal closure was approximated with several interrupted 2-0 PDS sutures. The skin was closed with skin staples and five retention sutures were placed for the final skin closure (Fig. 29.12).

Follow-Up Results

The patient did well postoperatively without problems related to the spinal wound closure. She was discharged from hospital on postoperative day 10. The drain was removed during subsequent follow-up visits by the primary service. The entire spinal wound

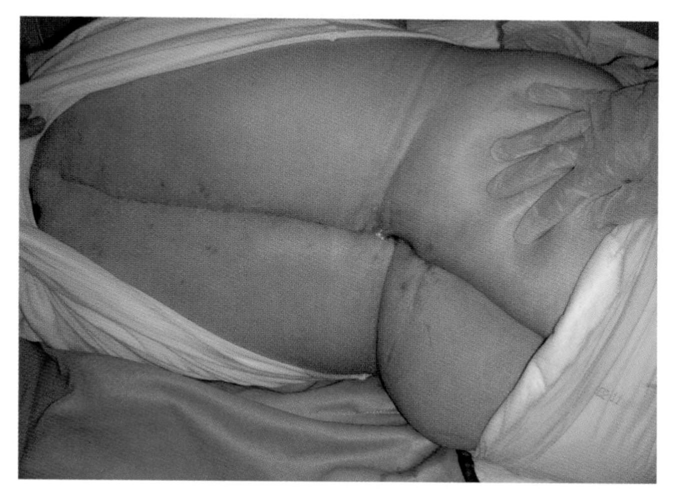

• **Fig. 29.13** The result at 2-month follow-up showing stable and well-healed spine wound with minimal scarring.

healed well without wound infection or any issues related to the new hardware placement.

Final Outcome

The spinal wound after adjacent bilateral latissimus dorsi, paraspinal, and gluteal muscle flap closure healed well with minimal scarring and no wound breakdown, infection, or seroma (Fig. 29.13). She has resumed her normal activities and is followed by the orthopedic spine surgery service for routine follow-up.

Pearls for Success

The spinal incisional wound after previous spine surgery can be challenging to manage because of poor adjacent tissue condition including muscle. Bilateral skin advancement flap closure may not be reliable on its own and additional muscle layer closure over the exposed spine and hardware is desirable. Paraspinal muscle along the spine can be a good choice to provide a good muscular layer coverage but multiple previous spine surgeries may make such an option less feasible. The latissimus dorsi muscle is usually away from the spinal wound (so undamaged) and can be used to cover most of the middle back wound. If any portion of the paraspinal muscle remains healthy and less scarred, it can be used to cover the midline back wound as shown in this case. If any adjacent muscles cannot be mobilized, a thicker acellular dermal matrix can be used as a biologic mesh to cover the exposed spine or hardware. Good quality of the skin closure over the muscle closure, that is, good approximation and tension-free deep dermal closure and placement of some retention sutures, may ensure proper healing of the skin closure.

Recommended Readings

Dumanian GA, Ondra SL, Liu J, Schafer MF, Chao JD. Muscle flap salvage of spine wounds with soft tissue defects or infection. *Spine.* 2003;28:1203–1211.

Hallock GG. Reconstruction of posterior trunk defects. *Semin Plast Surg.* 2011;25:78–85.

Inglesby DC, Young ZT, Alshareef M, et al. Paraspinous muscle flaps for the treatment of complex spinal wounds. *Spine.* 2020;45:599–604.

Mathes DW, Thornton JF, Rohrich RJ. Management of posterior truck defects. *Plast Reconstr Surg.* 2006;118:75e–83e.

Miyamoto S, Kayano S, Umezawa H, Fujiki M, Nakao J, Sakuraa M. Efficient design of a latissimus dorsi musculocutaneous flap to repair large skin defects of the upper back. *Microsurgery.* 2014;34:20–22.

Stevenson TR, Rohrich RJ, Pollock RA, Dingman RO, Bostwick J, III. More experience with the "Reverse" latissimus dorsi musculocutaneous flap: precise location of blood supply. *Plast Reconstr Surg.* 1984;74:237–243.

30 Lower Back Reconstruction

CASE 1

Clinical Presentation

A 14-year-old Black American morbidly obese female underwent hemipelvectomy for a pelvis osteosarcoma. She subsequently underwent pelvic reconstruction with a free fibular vascularized bone graft and a reconstruction plate by the orthopedic oncology and hand surgery services. Unfortunately, she developed complex and pending lower back, gluteal, and sacral wounds with potential exposure of the fibular bone graft and hardware. The plastic surgery service was asked to provide better soft tissue wound closure to improve the chance of primary healing of the surgical incision sites (Fig. 30.1).

Operative Plan and Special Considerations

All incision sites were reopened and all necrotic skin and subcutaneous tissue were debrided. There was a significant amount of hematoma under the skin incisions and the hardware used for reconstruction could potentially be exposed (Fig. 30.2). In this location, there are no local muscle or myocutaneous flaps available for soft tissue reconstruction. Because this patient was quite large with thick subcutaneous tissue even though she was only 14 years old, a large perforator-plus fasciocutaneous rotation/advancement flap was planned. One or two large perforators were identified by a handheld Doppler and should be included within the flap design. With a suprafascial dissection, all identified perforator(s) might be visualized and should be preserved during the flap dissection. The back cut could safely be performed as long as those perforator(s) were preserved. The flap could also be readvanced with even more back cut.

Operative Procedures

Under general anesthesia with the patient in the prone position, the entire lower back, sacral and gluteal incisions were reopened. There was a fair amount of necrotic skin and subcutaneous tissue along all previous incisions. All necrotic tissues were sharply debrided. Hematoma within the pelvic cavity was removed manually. The wound was then irrigated thoroughly with antibiotic solution.

A good gluteal perforator was mapped with a handheld Doppler. A 30 × 15 cm large skin rotation flap was designed based on the location of the perforator and soft tissue defect (Fig. 30.3). The proposed incision of the flap was infiltrated with 1% lidocaine with 1:100,000 epinephrine.

The flap elevation was started by making an incision through the skin, subcutaneous tissue, down to the subfascial plane. The subfascial dissection was performed to raise the flap (Fig. 30.4). During the dissection, the perforator was identified and the flap elevation was performed based on this single large perforator. The flap was easily rotated and advanced into the defect (Fig. 30.5). The flap donor site, measuring 30 × 10 cm, was approximated after the skin advancement from the nonflap side. A drain was inserted into the left pelvic cavity. Another drain was inserted under the flap. Six retention sutures were used to insure the wound approximation without too much tension. The entire flap closure was performed with interrupted 2-0 PDS sutures for the deep tissue closure and the subcutaneous tissue was closed with several interrupted 3-0 Monocryl sutures. The skin was closed with skin staples (Fig. 30.6).

Management of Complications

The patient developed partial wound dehiscence with potentially exposed hardware at postoperative 3 weeks (Fig. 30.7). She was taken back to the operating room and all necrotic tissues were debrided (Fig. 30.8). The large skin flap was re-elevated (Fig. 30.9) and rotated and advanced into the defect without any difficulties (Fig. 30.10). The flap site was closed again with the same sutures as the previous flap closure and retention sutures were again used (Fig. 30.11).

She unfortunately developed additional skin edge necrosis during the following month and was taken back to the operating room for more debridement (Fig. 30.12). The open wound was reclosed after some undermining and tissue rearrangement and retention sutures were again used (Fig. 30.13).

Several days later, she developed more skin edge necrosis probably from a direct compression (Fig. 30.14). She underwent another wound debridement and wound closure was performed again in the operating room (Fig. 30.15).

Follow-Up Results

After all surgeries and more than 2 months in-patient care, the lower back, pelvis, and gluteal wounds finally healed. The primary service was able to discharge her home. Unfortunately, she had a residual infection of the hardware and was taken back by the orthopedic oncology service for hardware removal and replacement (Fig. 30.16). The plastic surgery service was asked to reopen the previous flap site and to re-elevate the flap for access to the left pelvis (Fig. 30.17). During this procedure, the hardware inside the

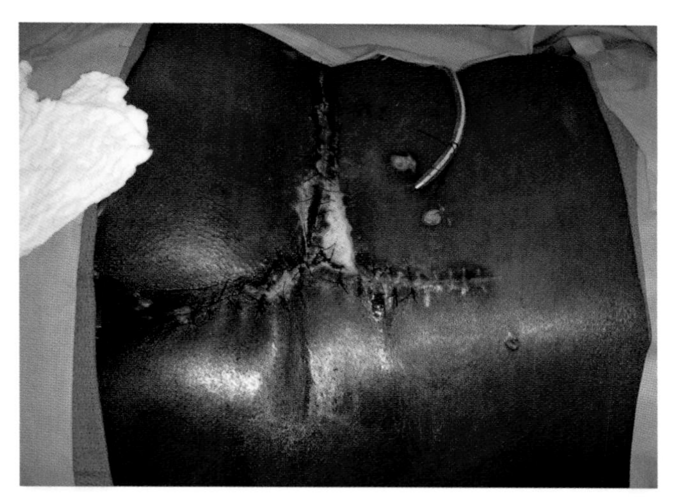

• **Fig. 30.1** Preoperative view showing a pending tissue necrosis of the primary incision closure sites for pelvic tumor resection and bony reconstruction.

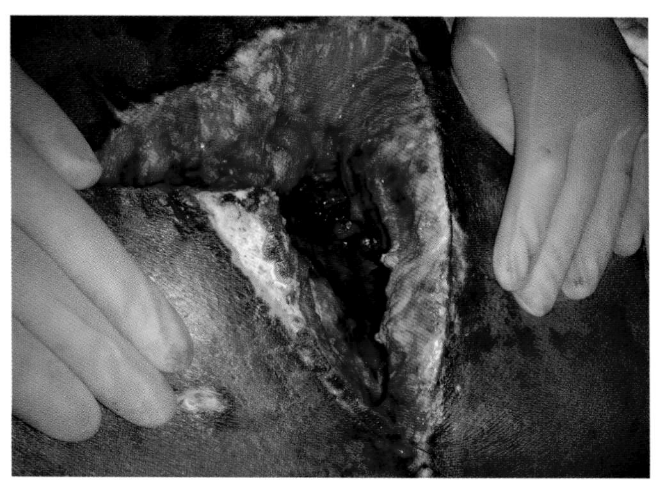

• **Fig. 30.2** Intraoperative view showing hematoma and potentially exposed hardware if wound dehiscence would occur.

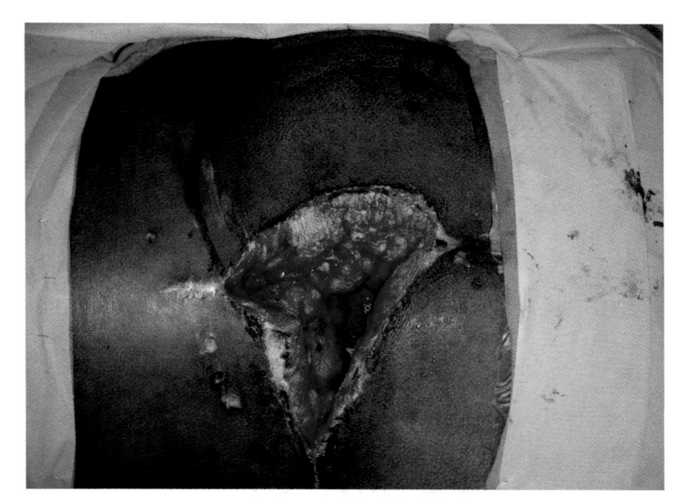

• **Fig. 30.3** Intraoperative view showing the design of a large perforator-plus skin rotation and advancement flap. Without proper wound closure, the hardware used for pelvic bony reconstruction would be exposed.

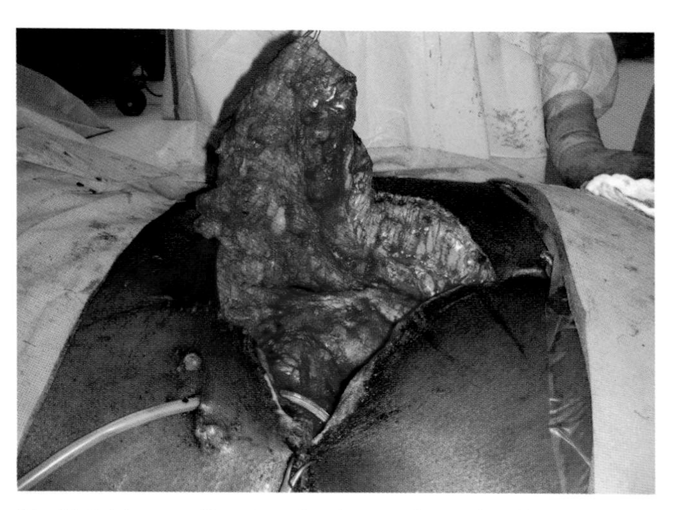

• **Fig. 30.4** Intraoperative view showing an elevated perforator-plus skin rotation and advancement flap.

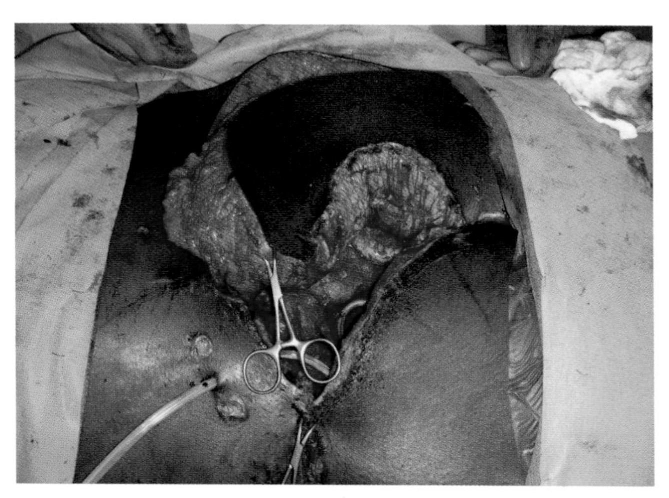

• **Fig. 30.5** Intraoperative view showing preliminary inset of the perforator-plus skin rotation and advancement flap for wound closure.

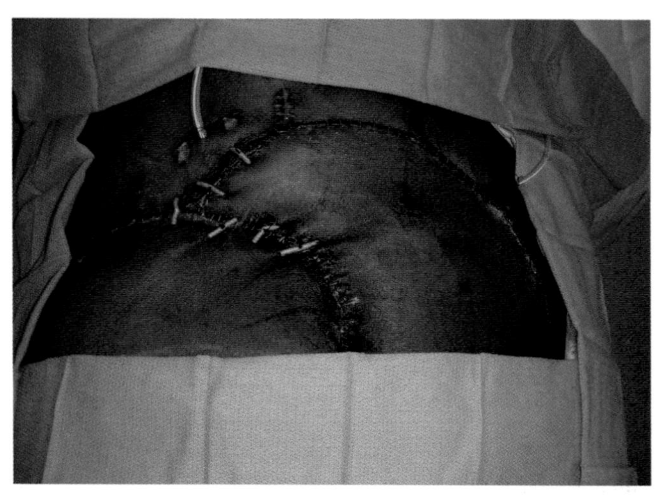

• **Fig. 30.6** Intraoperative view showing completion of the wound closure from the perforator-plus skin rotation and advancement flap.

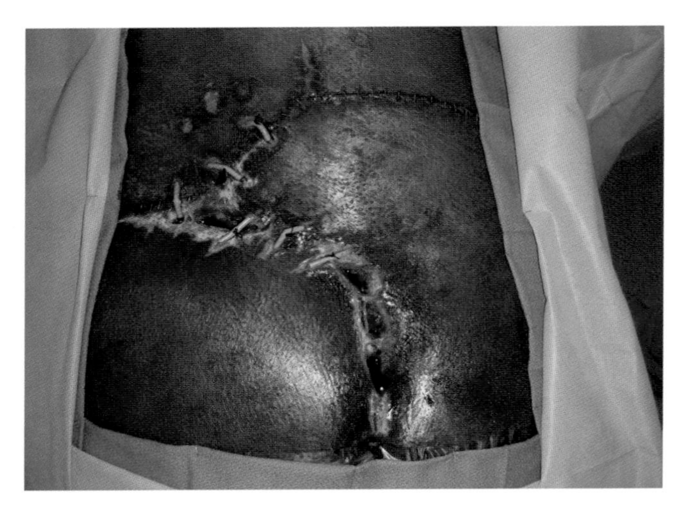

• **Fig. 30.7** Preoperative view showing several areas of wound dehiscence after the wound closure with perforator-plus skin rotation and advancement flap.

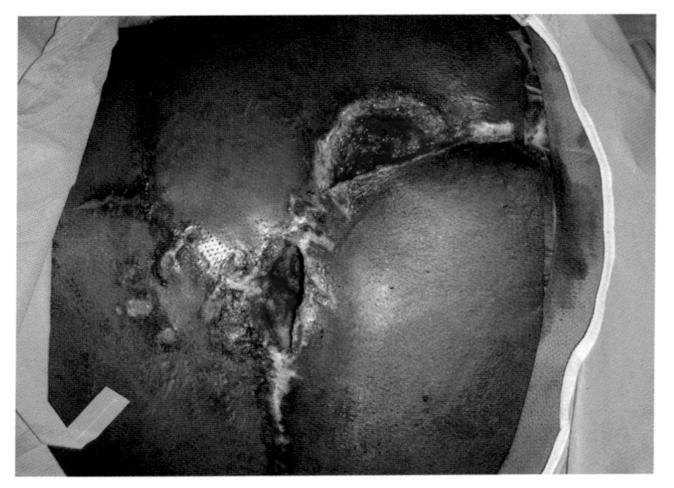

• **Fig. 30.8** Intraoperative view showing completion of the wound debridement after the perforator-plus skin rotation and advancement flap for wound closure.

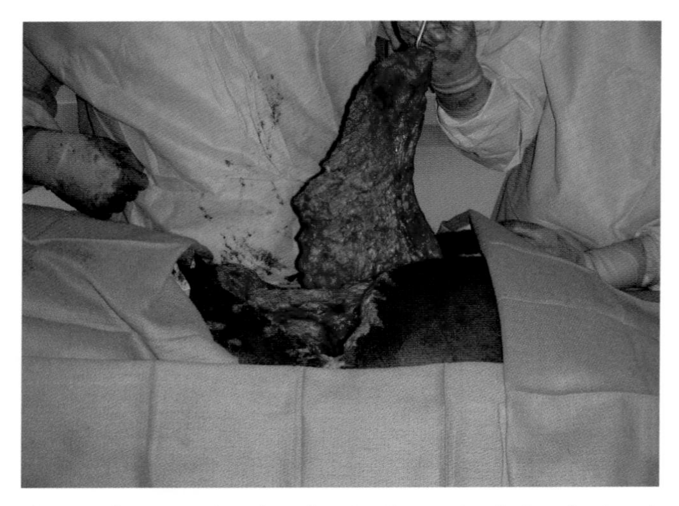

• **Fig. 30.9** Intraoperative view showing the re-elevated perforator-plus skin rotation and advancement flap.

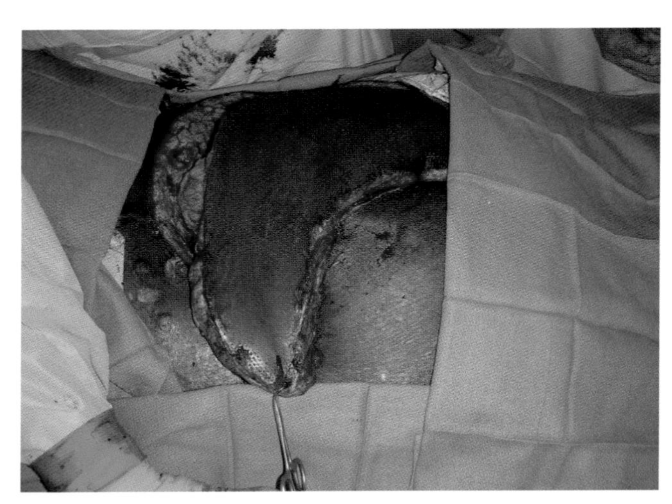

• **Fig. 30.10** Intraoperative view showing preliminary inset of the re-elevated perforator-plus skin rotation and advancement flap for wound closure.

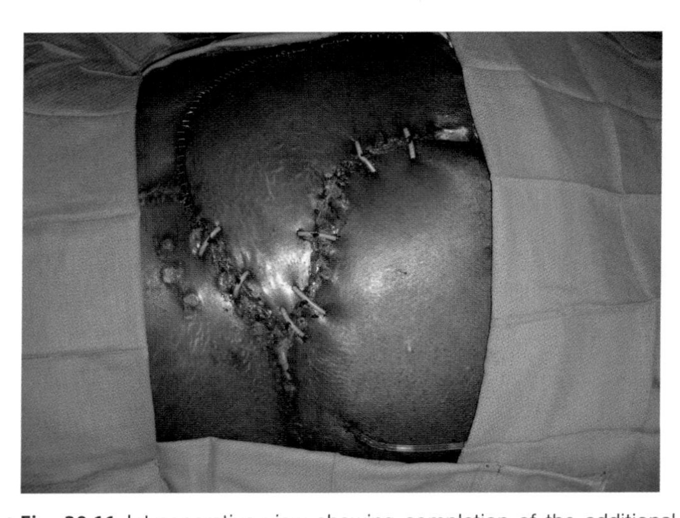

• **Fig. 30.11** Intraoperative view showing completion of the additional wound closure from the re-elevated perforator-plus skin rotation and advancement flap.

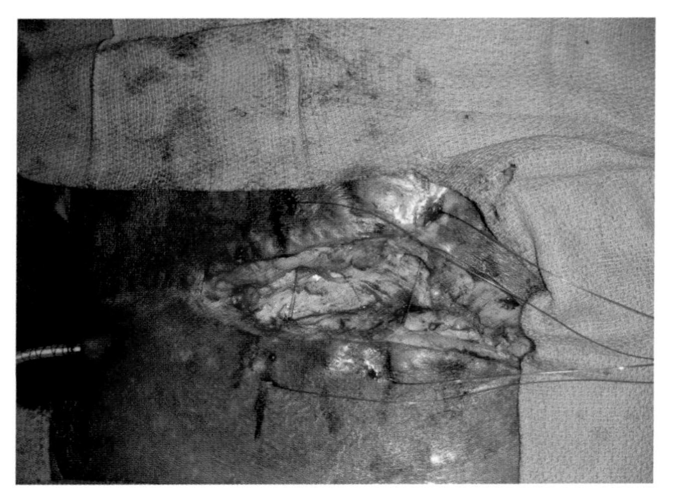

• **Fig. 30.12** Preoperative view showing the fresh open wound after debridement of newly developed skin edge necrosis in the operating room.

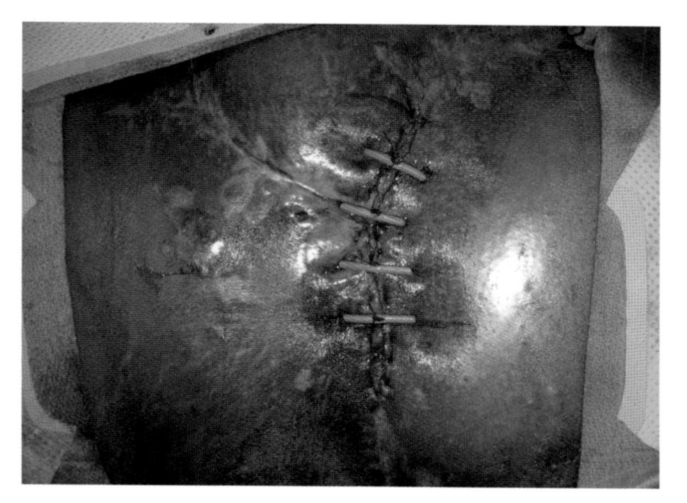

• **Fig. 30.13** Intraoperative view showing completion of the wound closure with complex closure and local tissue rearrangement. New retention sutures were placed.

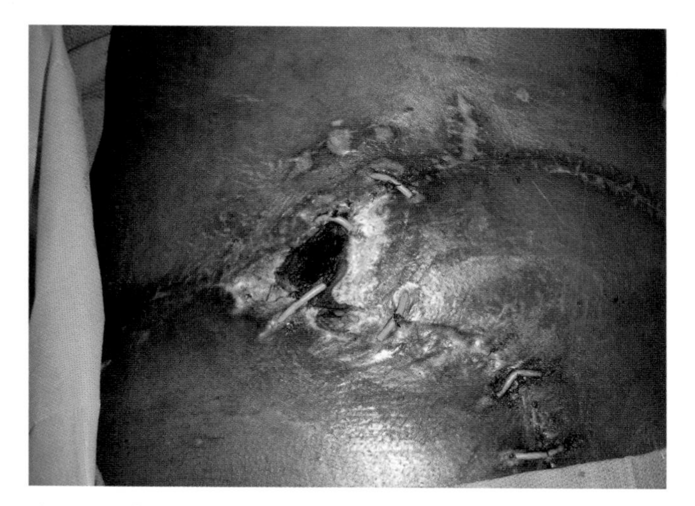

• **Fig. 30.14** Preoperative view showing newly developed distal skin flap necrosis that would need surgical debrided in the operating room.

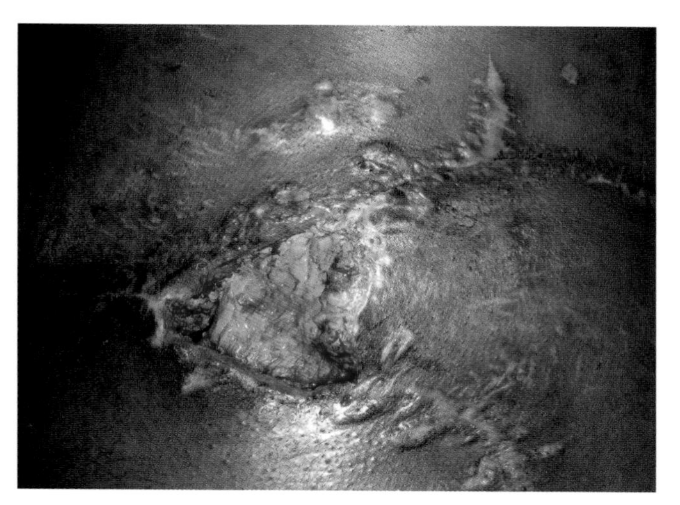

• **Fig. 30.15** Intraoperative view showing completion of the wound debridement. This wound could be closure with complex closure and local tissue rearrangement.

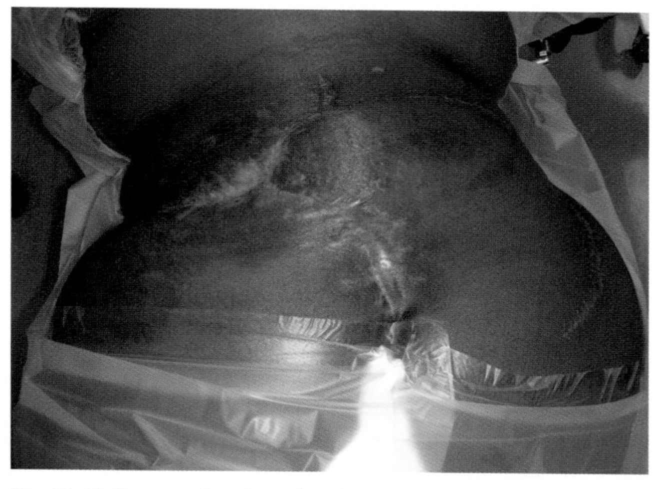

• **Fig. 30.16** Preoperative view showing well-healed flap wound closure sites with advanced perforator-plus skin rotation and advancement flap.

left pelvis was replaced. Some scar tissue over the previous flap site was excised and the open wound was closed again with the flap advancement and placement of retention sutures (Fig. 30.18).

Final Outcome

After multiple operative procedures including the flap re-elevation for new hardware replacement, the lower back, pelvic, and sacral wounds finally healed (Fig. 30.19). During the subsequent follow-up visits, there was no evidence of recurrent infection and the flap reconstruction site healed well with minimal scarring and good contour (Fig. 30.20). The patient has resumed her normal

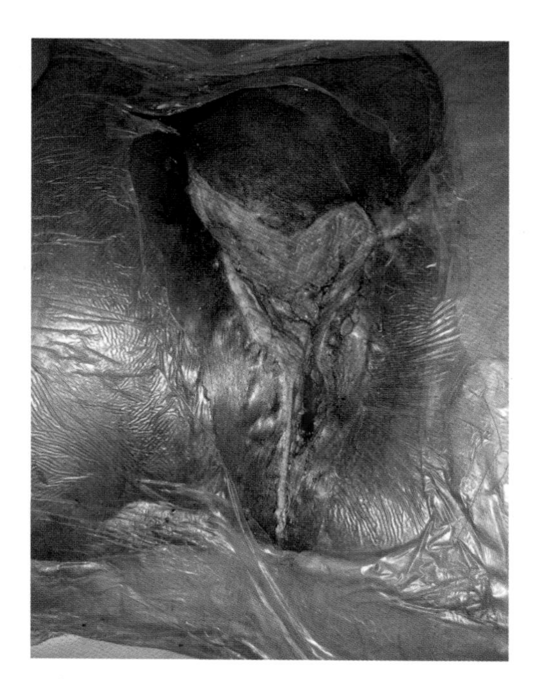

• **Fig. 30.17** Intraoperative view showing completion of the wound debridement. This wound could be closed with complex closure and local tissue rearrangement.

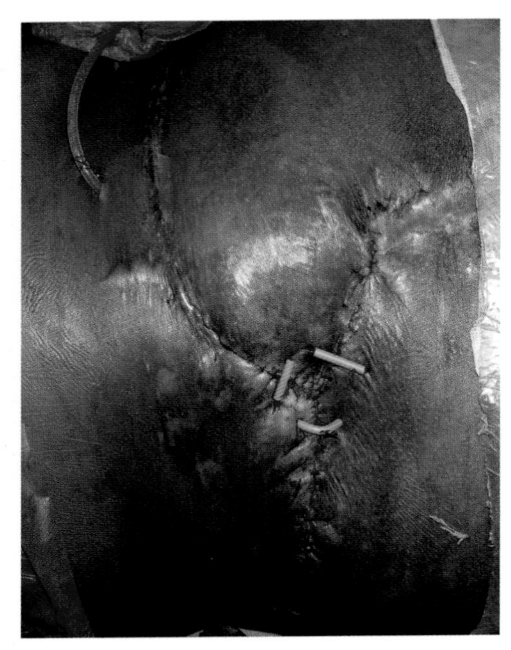

• **Fig. 30.18** Intraoperative view showing completion of another wound closure after local tissue rearrangement. New retention sutures were placed.

activities and been followed by the primary service for routine follow-up.

Pearls for Success

Reconstruction for a lower back wound can be challenging. This is especially true for an obese patient. However, as demonstrated in this patient, a large skin perforator-plus rotation and advancement flap can be a good option for reconstruction of a lower back wound because these patients may have some redundant skin over their lower back. It is worthwhile to include a large perforator in the flap design so that the venous outflow of the flap can be improved. Such a perforator can be identified with a handheld Doppler. During the flap elevation, the perforator and a skin bridge should be preserved. If needed, the flap can be re-elevated and advanced for subsequent soft tissue reconstruction. Skin edge necrosis can be an issue for these patients and more wound debridement may be needed. A small skin defect can be closed with complex closure or local tissue rearrangement. Retention sutures can also be added to ensure tension-free wound closure and prevent wound dehiscence.

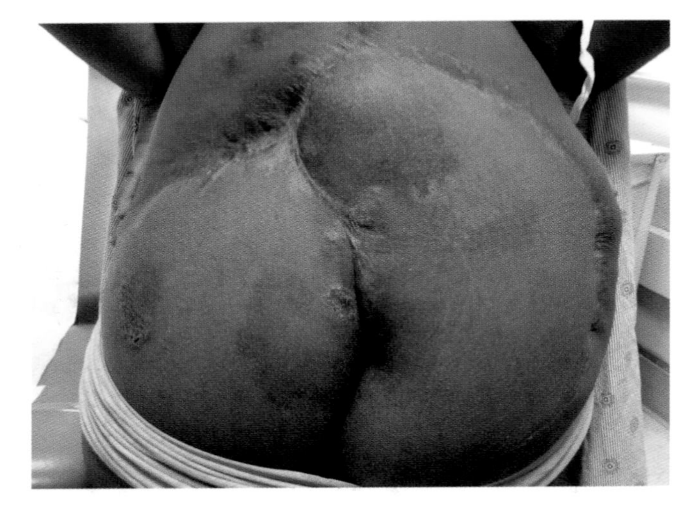

• **Fig. 30.19** The result at 3-year follow-up after final surgery for hardware replacement. The lower back, pelvic, and sacral wounds healed well.

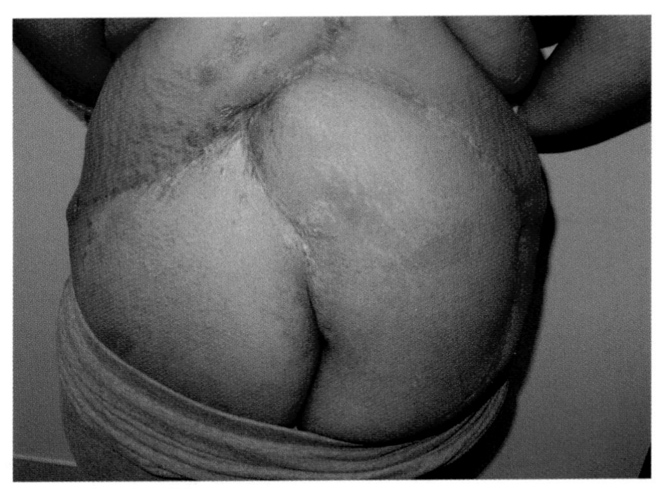

• **Fig. 30.20** The result at 3.5-year follow-up showing well-healed lower back, pelvic, and sacral wounds with good contour.

CASE 2

Clinical Presentation

A 53-year-old White male with metastatic lung cancer developed a complex spinal wound between L2 and L5 secondary to an urgent depression and stabilization of a pathologic L4 burst fracture. He also had postoperative radiation to the area and chemotherapy as part of his cancer treatment, which left a 7 × 5 cm open spinal wound with the exposed spine and hardware (Fig. 30.21). He was referred by an outside neurosurgeon to the plastic surgery service for wound reconstruction with a major flap.

Operative Plan and Special Considerations

Once adequate debridement within this wound had been completed, an extended, pedicled latissimus dorsi myocutaneous flap could be planned for the reconstruction. For this patient, an extended portion of the fasciocutaneous flap from the muscle could be designed and used to provide adequate soft tissue coverage for the wound closure. The pedicle length can be 15 cm and is usually accompanied by a single vena comitans. The flap can be harvested up to 20 × 35 cm. The long pedicle and large size make this a workhorse flap for soft tissue reconstruction of the lower back.

The extended latissimus dorsi flap is a modification that elongates the skin island inferiorly and medially. Dissection to include the muscle and subcutaneous tissue is performed with careful preservation of the descending branch of the thoracodorsal artery. This is vital to the survival of the flap. The insertion of the

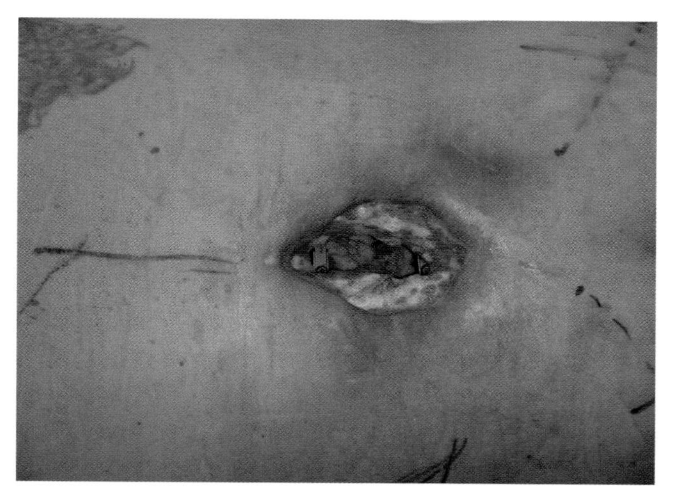

• **Fig. 30.21** Preoperative view showing a large lower back wound with exposed spine and hardware from previous radiation and spine surgery.

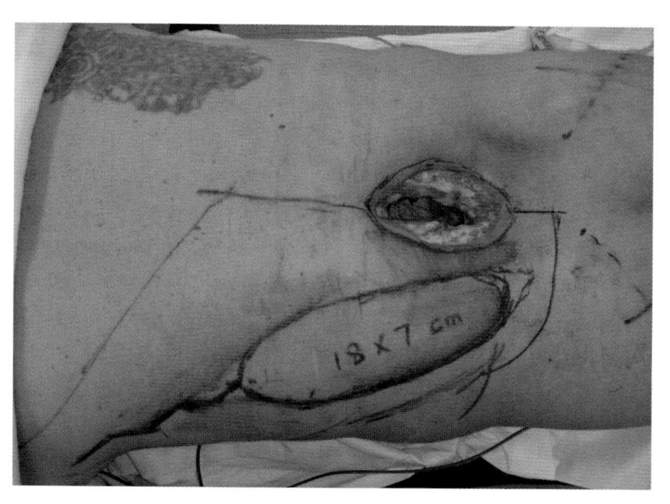

• **Fig. 30.23** Intraoperative view showing the design of this pedicled, extended latissimus dorsi myocutaneous flap for potential lower back wound coverage.

latissimus dorsi to the humerus can be divided to provide more freedom to reach further. Thus, it can be used to cover even the lower back soft tissue defect with an extension of the flap.

Operative Procedures

Under general anesthesia with the patient in the prone position, the procedure started with adequate debridement of the open spinal wound. Intraoperative neurosurgery consultation was obtained to ensure the debridement would be adequate but without injury to the spinal cord (Fig. 30.22). The wound area was gently curetted to remove all necrotic tissues including necrotic spinal tissue and the skin edge was freshened with a blade. After surgical debridement, the wound was irrigated thoroughly with Pulsavac (Fig. 30.23).

An extended latissimus dorsi myocutaneous flap was designed. The skin paddle was marked to 18 × 7 cm and designed as low as possible to catch some of the fasciocutaneous tissue from the extended portion of the muscle (Fig. 30.24). Once the incision had been made around the skin paddle down to the deep fascia, the muscle could be identified. The extended flap measured about 45 cm from the pedicle to the distal portion. The distal portion of the flap was elevated with cutaneous extention of the flap. The flap was then dissected free from the medial and lateral borders and extended toward the axilla. During the dissection, the pedicle was identified and the branch to the serratus muscle was divided. The pedicle dissection was further done toward the axillary vessels. The insertion of the latissimus dorsi muscle to the humerus was divided under direct vision. Further dissection was done to free the pedicle, so that the extended latissimus dorsi myocutaneous flap could be used as a pedicle and rotated to cover the midline lower back wound.

The flap was rotated and inset into the defect temporarily and the defect could be covered by the flap without any problems (Fig. 30.25). The distal excess portion of the flap was excised except for the fascia, which was folded and placed inside the wound (Fig. 30.26). The muscle layer was sutured to the adjacent subcutaneous tissue of the wound with 3-0 Monocryl sutures in two layers. The skin paddle of the flap was approximated to the

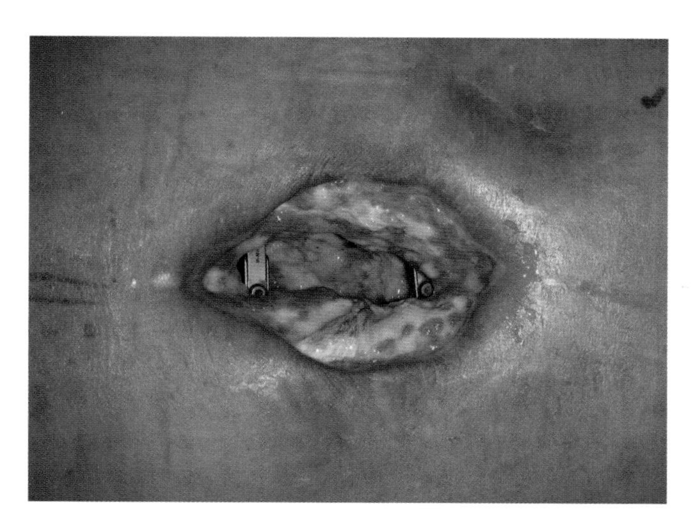

• **Fig. 30.22** Intraoperative close-up view showing this large lower back wound with exposed spine and hardware.

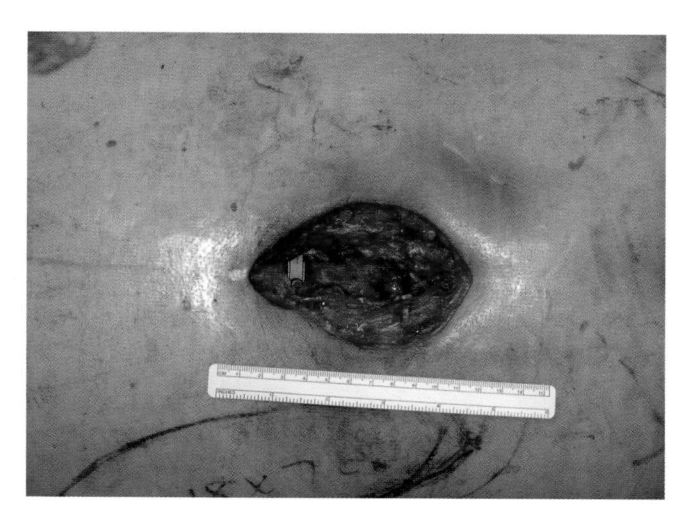

• **Fig. 30.24** Intraoperative view showing the appearance of the wound after careful surgical debridement.

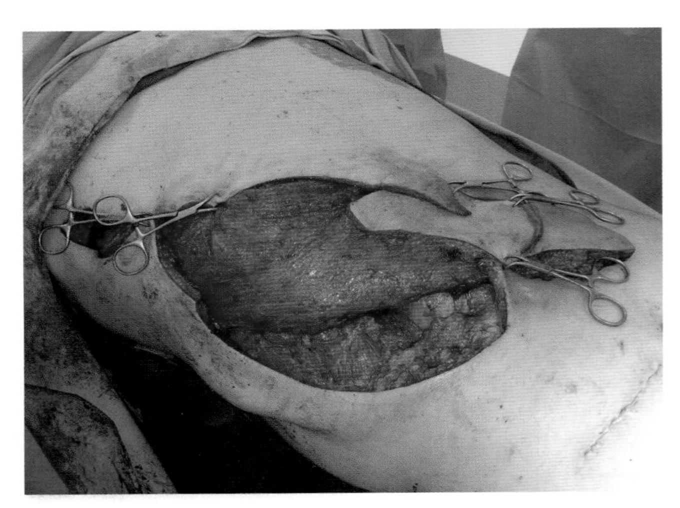

• **Fig. 30.25** Intraoperative view showing completion of the flap dissection. The lower back defect was completely covered by the extended portion of the flap.

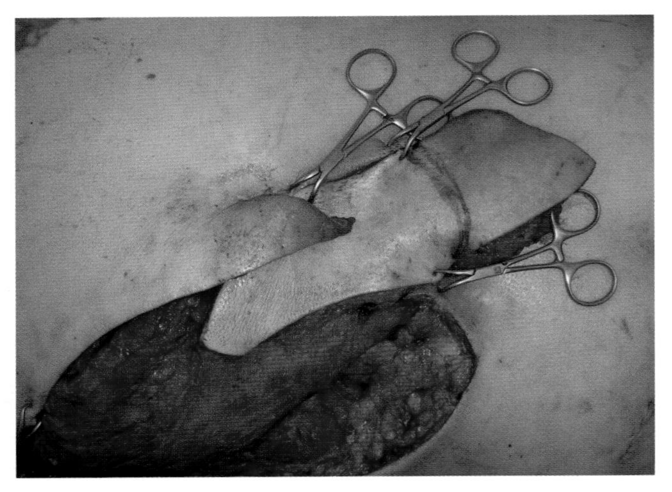

• **Fig. 30.26** Intraoperative view showing completion of the temporary flap inset into the lower back wound that was completely covered by the extended portion of the flap. The excess skin portion of the flap was discarded, but the fascial portion with adequate perfusion was preserved.

adjacent skin with interrupted 3-0 Monocryl half-buried horizontal sutures. Two drains were placed within the flap's donor site and one drain was placed under the flap.

The flap's donor site was closed in two layers. The rest of the skin defect in the flap donor site was closed with a split-thickness skin graft. The split-thickness skin graft was harvested from the left upper lateral thigh and meshed to 1:1.5 ratio. The skin graft was placed and secured with multiple skin staples (Fig. 30.27).

Follow-Up Results

The patient did well postoperatively without any complications related to the extended latissimus dorsi myocutaneous flap reconstruction. He was discharged from hospital on postoperative day 5. Drains were removed during subsequent follow-up visits. His lower back wound healed well and skin graft was successful (Fig. 30.28).

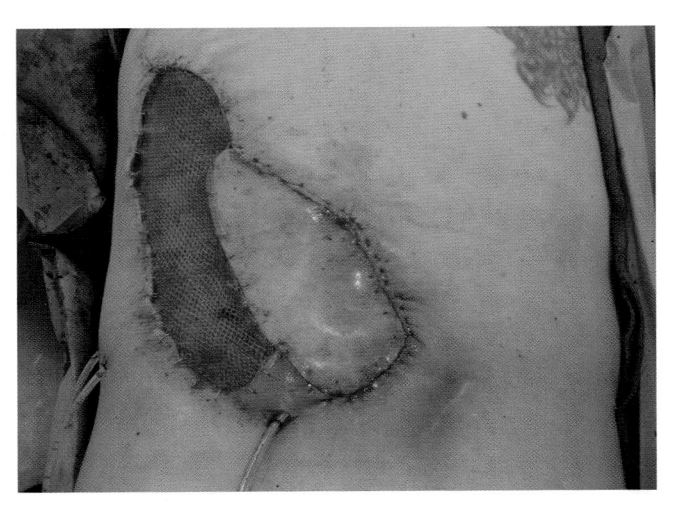

• **Fig. 30.27** Intraoperative view showing completion of the flap inset and skin graft placement as well as closure of the flap's donor site.

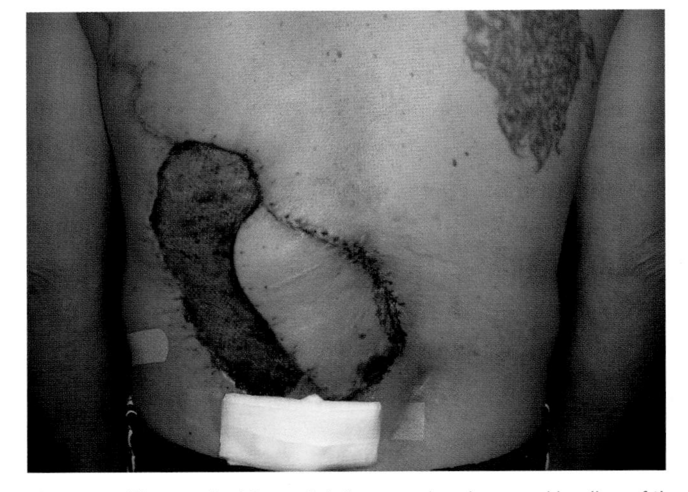

• **Fig. 30.28** The result at 3-week follow-up showing good healing of the lower back wound after the flap reconstruction.

Final Outcome

The lower back wound after the extended pedicled latissimus dorsi myocutaneous flap reconstruction healed well with minimal scarring (Fig. 30.29). The patient has had no recurrent infection, seroma, or wound breakdown. He remains cancer-free and has resumed his normal activities. He has been followed by the outside referring neurosurgeon for routine follow-up.

Pearls for Success

A pedicled, extended latissimus dorsi myocutaneous flap can be a reasonably good option for soft tissue coverage of the lower back wound, commonly secondary to complicated spine surgery. The flap can be designed with an extended skin paddle that receives blood supply via perforators from the very distal portion of the muscle flap. This part of the muscle can be reliably elevated with adequate blood supply if the design of the flap follows the course of the descending branch of the thoracodorsal artery. Division of the latissimus dorsi muscle's insertion in the humerus may add

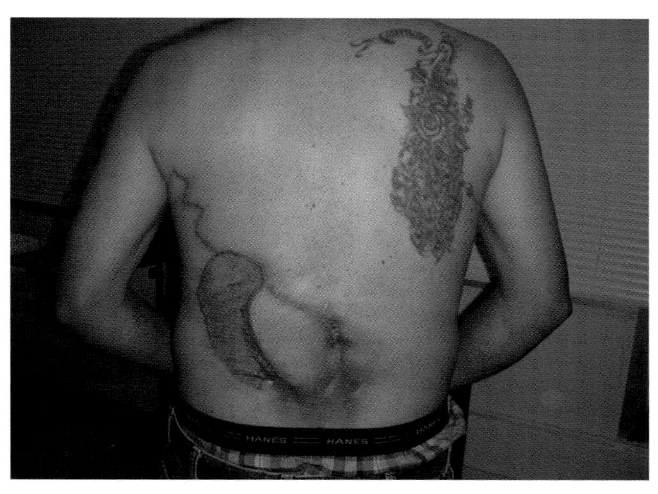

• **Fig. 30.29** The result at 5-month follow-up showing well-healed lower back wound with good contour and minimal scarring after the flap reconstruction.

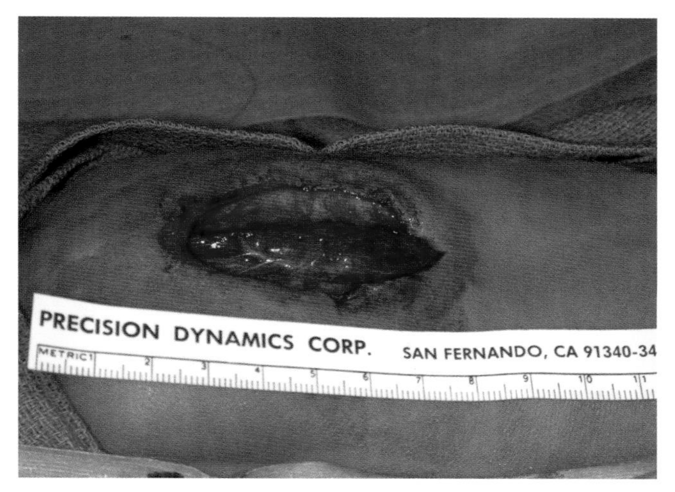

• **Fig. 30.30** Preoperative view showing a large lumbosacral myelomeningocele after the dural repair by the pediatric neurosurgery service.

more length of the flap rotation or advancement. Further dissection around the pedicle as for a free latissimus dorsi flap may also add more length for the flap rotation or advancement. The donor site's skin defect can be skin grafted for closure. Attention should also be paid to ensure that the pedicle vessels are not stretched when the flap is inset into the lower back wound.

CASE 3

Clinical Presentation

A 1-day-old baby boy had a large lumbosacral myelomeningocele at birth. His exposed spinal cord was covered with clean and moist dressing. Pediatric neurosurgery was asked to manage this complex and urgent neurosurgical condition. He was urgently taken to the operating room where the dura repair was performed. The plastic surgery service was asked by the pediatric neurosurgery service to perform soft tissue reconstruction for coverage of the large lumbosacral wound, measuring 6 × 3 cm (Fig. 30.30).

Operative Plan and Special Considerations

Once the dura had been repaired by the pediatric neurosurgery service, the next important step was to provide good soft tissue coverage with various local flaps for reconstruction. For a large lumbosacral wound, each side of the latissimus dorsi and gluteus maximus myocutaneous flaps can be elevated as one unit and advanced medially and approximated in the midline. Each flap unit is based on the thoracodorsal and superior gluteal vessels and the intervening thoracolumbar fascia, providing relatively tension-free and durable soft-tissue coverage over the dural repair site in a single procedure. No lateral relaxing incisions or skin grafts are needed.

Operative Procedures

Under general anesthesia with the patient in the prone position, the dural repair was completed by the pediatric neurosurgery service and no cerebrospinal fluid (CSF) leak was found. The edge of the latissimus dorsi and gluteus maximus muscles were identified after simple surgical excision of the excess skin and additional dissection. The latissimus dorsi muscle was freed from its attachments to the external oblique and serratus muscles. The gluteus maximus muscle was detached from the iliac crest and sacrum and dissection carried in the plane between the gluteus maximus and medius. Both latissimus dorsi and gluteus maximum myocutaneous flaps were elevated as a single unit and submuscular dissection was done toward the posterior axillary line. Once each side of the flap unit had been advanced medially across the midline, each flap dissection was completed.

The final soft tissue closure was performed in three layers over the repaired dura. The muscle layer was approximated with interrupted 3-0 PDS sutures. The subcutaneous tissue layer was approximated with interrupted 3-0 Monocryl sutures and the skin was closed with 3-0 nylon in an interrupted fashion with eversion of both skin edges (Fig. 30.31). Blood loss for this procedure was less than 5 cc.

Follow-Up Results

The baby boy did well postoperatively without any complications related to the flap reconstruction. He was observed at the pediatric ICU for the first two days and then transferred to the pediatric floor. His lumbosacral myelomeningocele reconstruction site showed good healing and there was no evidence of CSF leak. He was discharged from hospital on postoperative day 7 (Fig. 30.32). During subsequent follow-up visits, the lower back reconstruction site was noted to have healed well with minimal scarring (Fig. 30.33).

Final Outcome

The lumbosacral myelomeningocele reconstruction site healed well with no evidence of CSF leak and wound breakdown (Fig. 30.34). The patient showed no residual neurological deficit and has grown appropriately for his age. He has been followed by the pediatric neurosurgical service for routine follow-up.

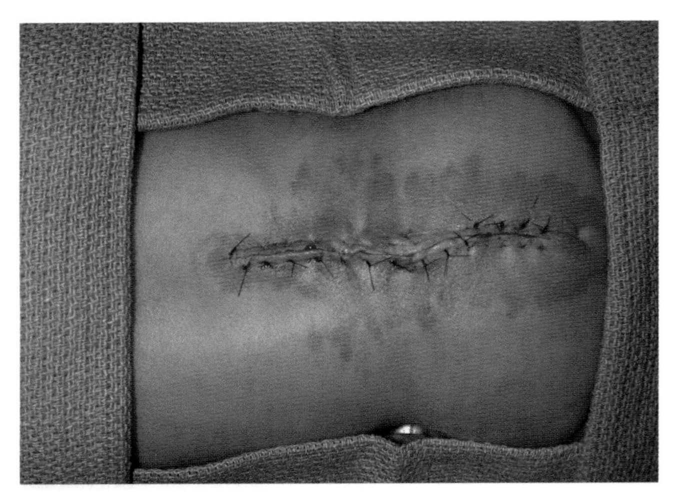

• **Fig. 30.31** Intraoperative view showing completion of bilateral latissimus dorsi and gluteus maximus myocutaneous advancement flaps for primary wound closure.

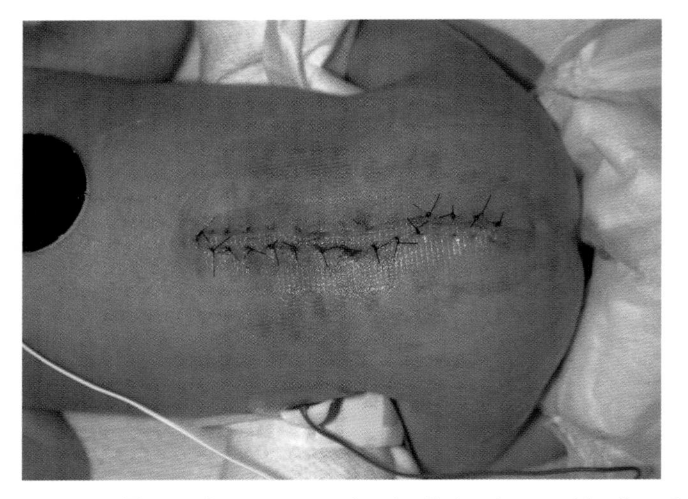

• **Fig. 30.32** The result at postoperative day 7 showing good healing of the lumbosacral wound.

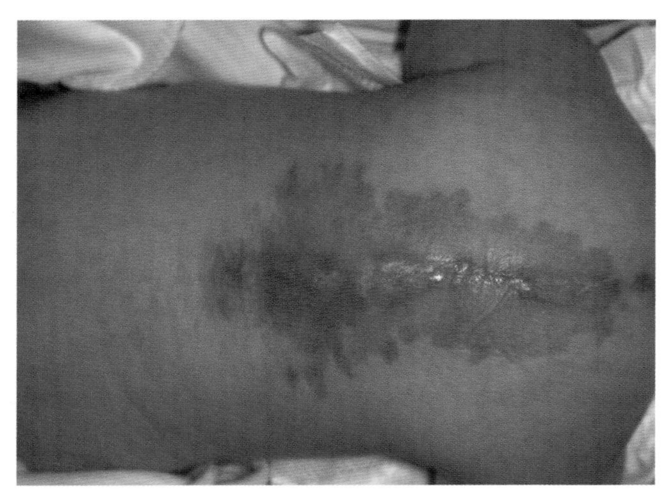

• **Fig. 30.33** The result at 4-week follow-up showing stable and well-healed lumbosacral wound with no evidence of cerebrospinal fluid leak.

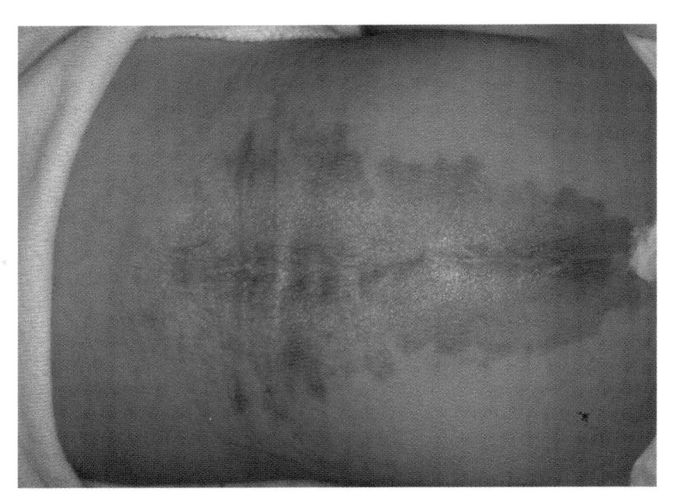

• **Fig. 30.34** The result at 6.5-month follow-up showing stable and well-healed lumbosacral wound with minimal scarring.

Pearls for Success

A large lumbosacral myelomeningocele is a pediatric neurosurgery emergency and a durable soft tissue reconstruction is required after dural repair by the primary service. The latissimus dorsi muscle and gluteus maximus muscle each receive blood supply from the independent pedicle but there is a rich anastomosis between the two muscles. Therefore, both muscles can be elevated as a single unit from each side and both flaps can be approximated in the midline after proper submuscular dissection as an advancement flap and provide a three-layer closure over the repaired dura. Such a reconstruction can be done in one stage and unlike other fasciocutaneous flaps described elsewhere, there will be no additional scar apart from the midline one. With more precise surgical dissection following submuscular tissue plane, blood loss can be minimized except bleeding from the skin edge.

Recommended Readings

Casella D, Nanni J, Lo Torto F, et al. Extended Latissimus Dorsi Kite Flap (ELD-K Flap): revisiting an old place for a total autologous breast reconstruction in patients with medium to large breasts. *Aesthetic Plast Surg*. 2021;45:390–391.

Eom JS, Hong JP. Lower back defect coverage using a free-style gluteal perforator flap. *Ann Plast Surg*. 2011;67:516–519.

Hifny MA, Hamdan AR. The keystone island perforator flap in reconstruction of large myelomeningocele defects. *Ann Plast Surg*. 2020;84:575–579.

Holoyda KA, Kim EN, Tuncer FB, et al. Layered closure of lumbosacral myelomeningocele defects with bilateral paraspinous muscle and composite fasciocutaneous flaps. *PRS Global Open*. 2020;8:e2884.

Mehrotra S. Perforator-plus flaps: a new concept in traditional flap design. *Plast Reconstr Surg*. 2007;119:590–598.

Mirmanesh M, Mazzaferro D, Borab Z, Pu LLQ. Posterior, extended, pedicled latissimus dorsi flap for the reconstruction of a large complicated lower back wound. *Eplasty*. 2016;16:ic32.

Ramirez OM, Ramasastry SS, Granick MS, Pang D, Futrell JW. A new surgical approach to closure of large lumbosacral meningomyelocele defects. *Plast Reconstr Surg*. 1987;80:799–807.

SECTION 4

Pelvis, Groin, Sacrum, Buttock, Perineum and Genitals

31

Hip Reconstruction

CASE 1

Clinical Presentation

A 68-year-old White male had a complicated postoperative course after an osteocutaneous flap harvest from his right hip by another surgical service. He had a significantly large open wound over the right hip, measuring 25 × 10 cm, with exposed pelvic structures (Fig. 31.1). This patient had previous wound debridement and a wound vacuum-assisted closure (VAC) by the primary service. Some granulation tissue had developed within the wound. The primary service used acellular dermal matrix that appeared to be incorporated with the wound bed (Fig. 31.2). The plastic surgery service was asked by our ENT microvascular team to carry out a definitive wound closure.

Operative Plan and Special Considerations for Reconstruction

For this large soft tissue wound with exposed pelvic structures in the lateral hip and pelvis, a distant muscle flap with a relatively large amount of well-vascularized tissue, such as a rectus femoris muscle flap, can be selected to provide a one-stage soft tissue coverage and obliterate the potential space. The flap, which receives a blood supply primarily from the descending branch of the lateral circumflex femoral artery, is a type II muscle flap but is fairly reliable if the patient is free of peripheral vascular disease in the profound artery. It is a large muscle flap that can be used to cover lower abdominal wall or pelvic soft tissue defect. Approximation of the vastus lateralis and vastus medialis after the rectus femoris muscle flap harvest may possibly reduce weakness of the knee extension. An adjacent abdominal skin rotation flap can be added to facilitate the entire wound closure in addition to a skin graft to the muscle flap in this case.

Operative Procedures

Under general anesthesia with the patient in a supine position, the right hip wound was debrided first. All floating acellular dermal matrix was also excised but incorporated acellular dermal matrix was left in place.

The design for the right rectus femoris muscle flap harvest was marked. The skin incision was made from the anterior iliac spine to the central part of the patella after infiltration with 1% lidocaine with 1:100,000 epinephrine. The skin, subcutaneous tissue, and fascia were incised and the rectus abdominis muscle was identified. The muscle was elevated and a Penrose drain was used to wrap around the muscle. The dissection was done to free its attachment to the vastus lateralis and vastus medialis muscles. The muscle flap was then divided more distally close to the patella. The muscle was elevated and the pedicle vessels were identified. One minor pedicle vessel was temporally clamped first and then divided with hemoclips. Further dissection was made around the major pedicle. (Fig. 31.3). The proximal end of the muscle was divided and the flap was then tunneled to the right hip wound and secured using interrupted 3-0 Monocryl sutures.

Because of the area with the exposed acellular dermal matrix, an adjacent skin rotation flap was also elevated. This flap, measuring 12 × 3 cm, was rotated into the area to cover the exposed acellular dermal matrix. The skin flap donor site was approximated with several interrupted 3-0 Vicryl sutures and the skin closure was done with skin staples. A 10 flat JP was inserted under the muscle flap. The flap was inserted into the right hip wound and secured with multiple 3-0 Monocryl sutures to create a better contour and soft tissue coverage (Fig. 31.4).

A split-thickness skin graft was harvested with a dermatome from the right lateral thigh. It was meshed to 1:1/2 ratio. The skin graft was placed over the muscle and the rest of the granulation wound and secured with multiple skin staples (Fig. 31.5). A VAC dressing was placed over the skin grafted muscle flap and connected to a VAC machine (Fig. 31.6).

The rectus femoris muscle flap donor site was closed after irrigation. A 10 flat JP was inserted into the donor site. Both vastus lateralis and vastus medialis muscles were approximated with interrupted 2-0 Prolene sutures. The deep dermal closure was performed with interrupted 3-0 Monocryl sutures and the skin was closed with skin staples.

Follow-Up Results

The patient did well postoperatively without any issues related to flap reconstruction and donor wound closure. He was discharged from the hospital on postoperative day 7. His right hip and pelvic wound healed uneventfully (Fig. 31.7). He was followed by both the primary service and the plastic surgery service for subsequent care.

Final Outcome

The patient was routinely followed by the primary service for his postsurgical visits. His right hip flap reconstruction site has healed well with no wound breakdown or any other long-term issues related to the soft tissue reconstruction (Fig. 31.8).

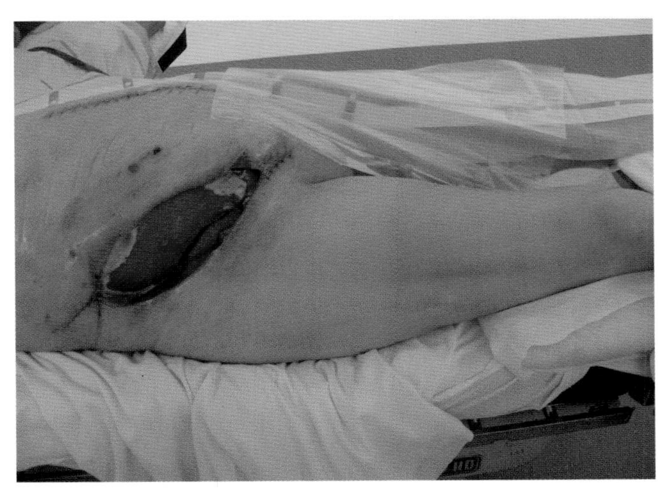

• **Fig. 31.1** A preoperative view showing a large and complex hip and pelvic wound with exposed deep pelvic structures.

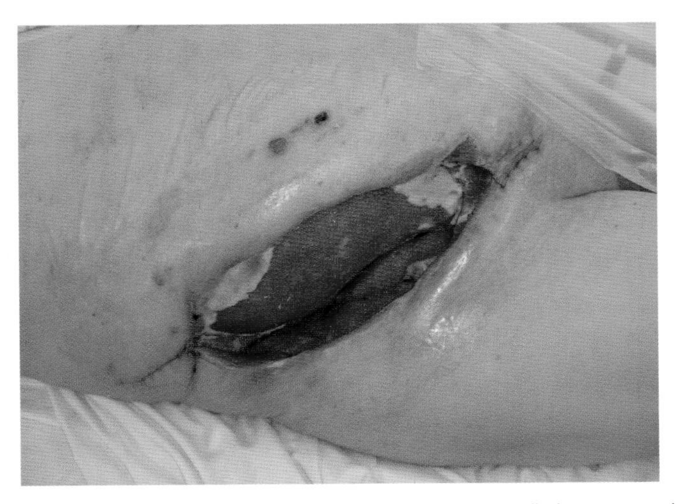

• **Fig. 31.2** A preoperative close-up view showing partially incorporated acellular dermal matrix and exposed deep pelvic structures.

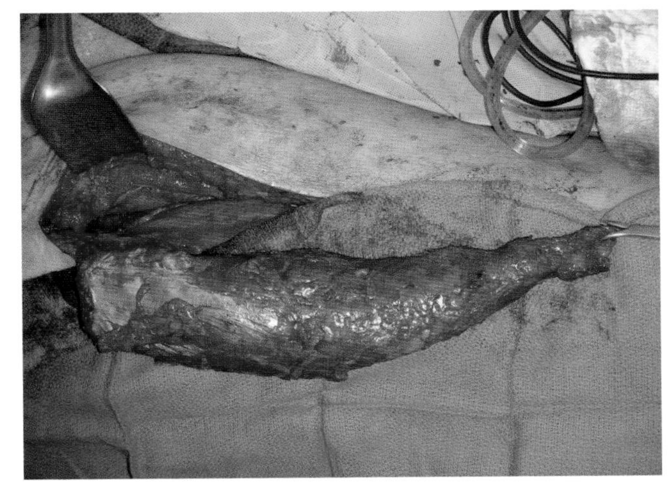

• **Fig. 31.3** An intraoperative view showing completion of the rectus femoris muscle flap dissection. The flap appeared to be quite large and well vascularized.

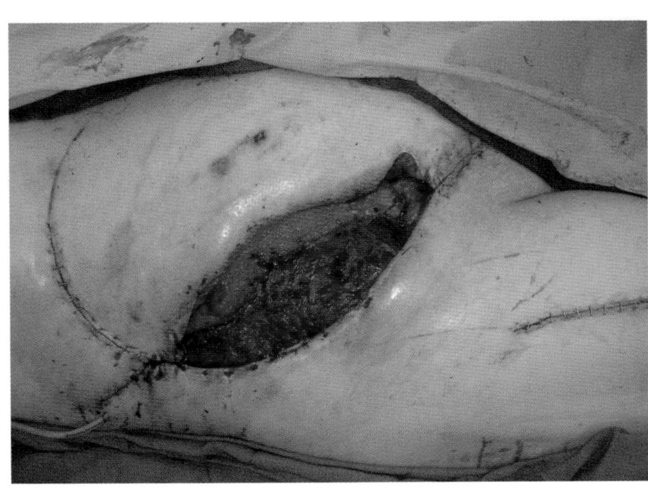

• **Fig. 31.4** An intraoperative view showing completion of the rectus femoris muscle flap inset and closure of the adjacent skin rotation flap.

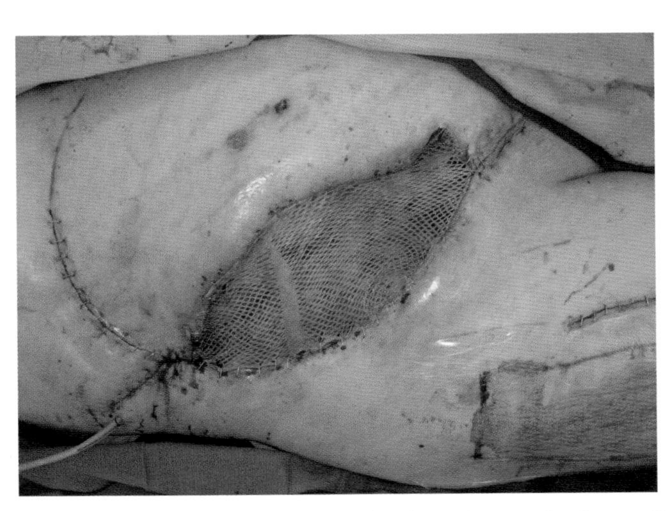

• **Fig. 31.5** An intraoperative view showing placement of a split-thickness skin graft to the rectus femoris muscle flap.

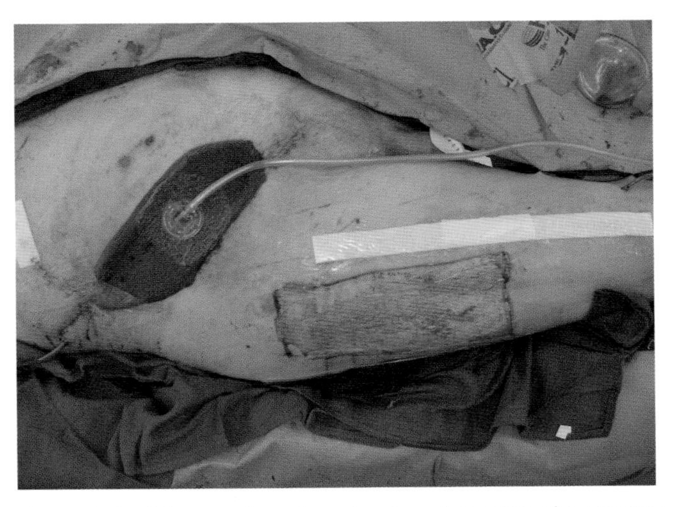

• **Fig. 31.6** An intraoperative view showing placement of a vacuum-assisted closure dressing over the skin-grafted rectus femoris muscle flap at the end of the procedure.

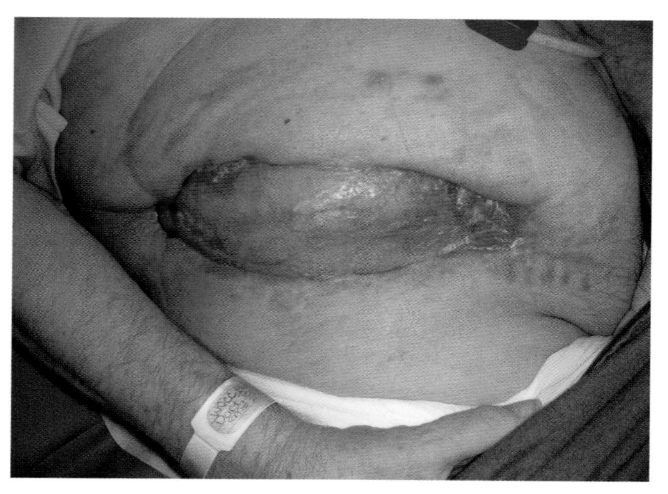

• **Fig. 31.7** Result at 2-month follow-up showing nearly complete healed right hip and pelvic wound after reconstruction.

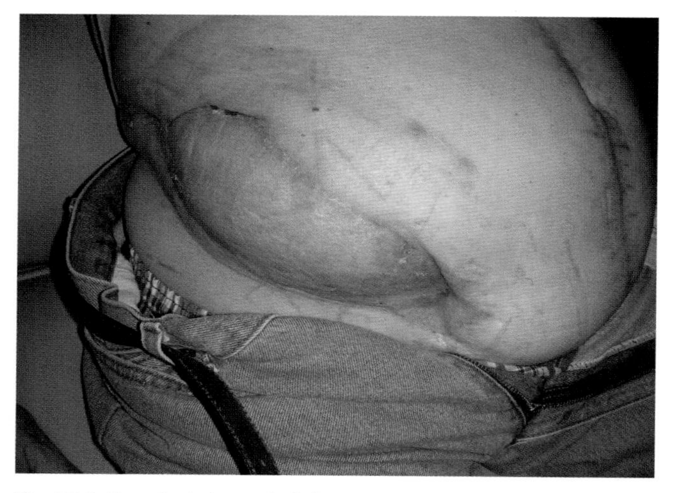

• **Fig. 31.8** Result at 4-month follow-up showing well-healed right hip and pelvic wound after reconstruction.

Pearls for Success

A large distant muscle flap, such as a rectus femoris muscle flap, can be selected to cover a large soft tissue wound in the hip and pelvic regions. The flap is fairly reliable and its flap dissection can be quickly performed. It can provide adequate vascularized tissue for an optimal wound closure because of its rich blood supply and the size of the muscle. It can also be used to obliterate a deep space in the pelvis as a pedicle flap. Both proximal and distal insertions can be divided to improve the flap's arch of rotation and filling the potential dead space. If necessary, a sizable skin paddle can be included although the muscle flap alone is used more often because it is large enough. A proper vascular evaluation for the femoral vessels and/or profunda vessels may be necessary if the patient sustains peripheral vascular disease. A split-thickness skin graft is commonly used to place over the muscle flap and the healing can be enhanced with a 5-day VAC therapy. Approximation of the vastus lateralis and vastus medialis muscles may minimize the weakness of the knee extension after the rectus femoris muscle harvest.

CASE 2

Clinical Presentation

A 26-year-old White male was involved in a motor vehicle accident and sustained multiple traumas including a left hip soft tissue avulsion with pelvic ring fracture. The fracture was fixed by the orthopedic trauma service, but a 33 × 15 cm large soft tissue wound was left with the exposed pelvic rim, which clearly required soft tissue coverage (Fig. 31.9). The patient also underwent pelvic vessel embolization to control pelvic bleeding by interventional radiology when he was admitted to the hospital after trauma. The plastic surgery service was asked to provide a soft tissue reconstruction with a major flap so that his left hip open pelvic fracture site could be covered. With this complex wound in this location, a free tissue transfer would obviously be required to cover this large soft tissue wound.

Operative Plan and Special Considerations for Reconstruction

A free latissimus dorsi flap with skin graft could be offered to this patient for soft tissue reconstruction. The flap has a long pedicle and can provide a large and well-vascularized tissue for soft tissue reconstruction of the hip and pelvic open fracture wound. Unfortunately, the recipient vessels for the free tissue transfer from a branch of the left femoral vessel might not be reliable because of previous embolization and also within the zone of the injury. Obviously, proper selection of the recipient vessels for free tissue transfer would be critical. In addition, the flap reconstruction should be done with the patient in a lateral decubitus position making access to a branch of the femoral vessel difficult for microvascular anastomoses. However, based on the author's previous experience and an innovative technique, the descending branch of the lateral circumflex femoral vessel could be selected after surgical dissection and turnover to create a recipient vessel from the distant area. In this way, microvascular anastomoses could be performed adjacent to the hip soft tissue defect.

Operative Procedures

Under general anesthesia with the patient in a right lateral decubitus position, the procedure was started by debriding and preparation of the left hip and pelvic wound. All the colonized tissues were removed and skin edge of the wound was freshened with a blade. The wound was then irrigated with antibiotic solution.

The descending branch of the lateral circumflex femoral vessels was first dissected out through a skin incision over the anterolateral thigh region. The branch was exposed between the rectus femoris and vastus lateralis muscles. The entire course of the descending branch was dissected free and additional dissection was performed toward the profunda. Once its distal end had been divided, the descending branch including both artery and two veins was turned over and placed into the left hip soft tissue wound. The artery had a good pulsation even grossly and one of the veins appeared to be a good size (Fig. 31.10).

The left latissimus dorsi myocutaneous flap was dissected out next. Once the skin paddle was incised down to the muscle, the dissection was performed to free the entire latissimus muscle

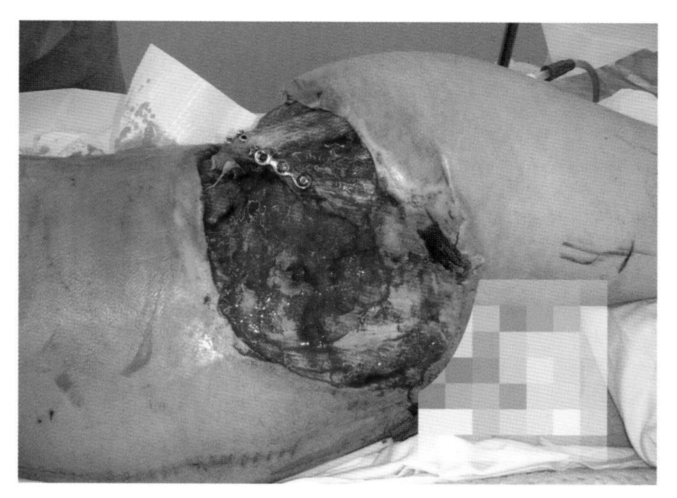

• **Fig. 31.9** A preoperative view showing a large soft tissue defect, measuring 33 × 15 cm, in the left hip, pelvic, and groin regions with exposed pelvic fracture site and hardware.

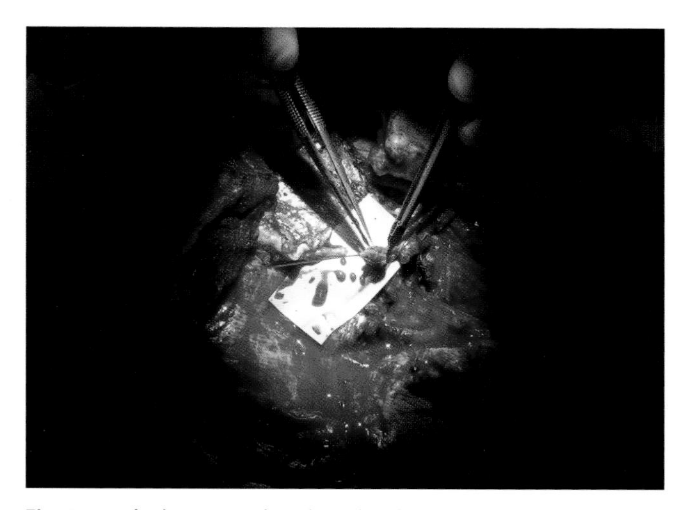

• **Fig. 31.10** An intraoperative view showing a good arterial flow of the descending branch of the femoral circumflex vessels after its dissection and turnover.

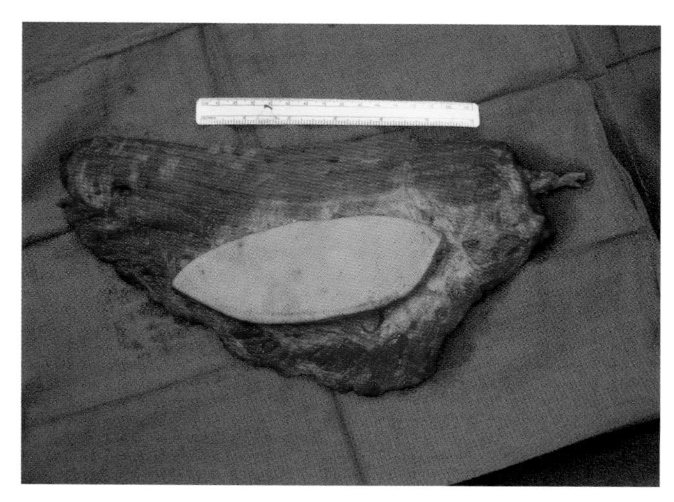

• **Fig. 31.11** An intraoperative view showing completion of a free left latissimus dorsi muscle flap dissection with a skin paddle.

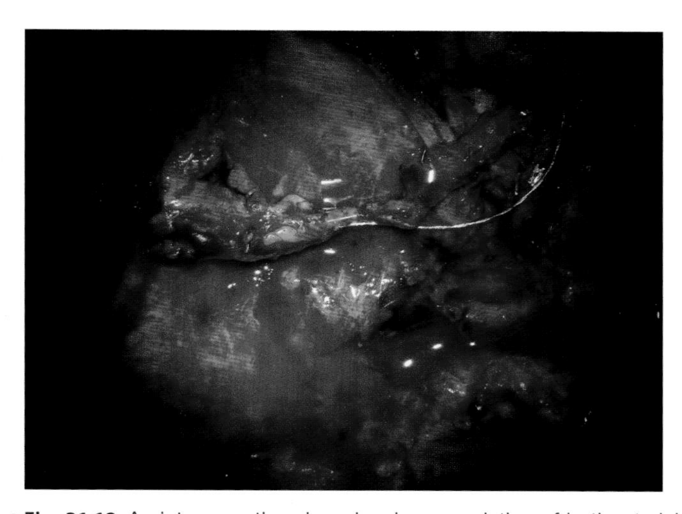

• **Fig. 31.12** An intraoperative view showing completion of both arterial and venous microvascular anastomoses under an operating microscope. The Cook Doppler probe was wrapped around the pedicle artery just distal to the anastomosis.

laterally, inferiorly, and medially. Distally the muscle was divided from the posterior iliac spine. Both medial and lateral borders of the muscle were dissected free. During dissection, the serratus muscle was identified and was left down to the chest wall. By further dissection toward the axilla, the serratus branch of the thoracodorsal vessel to the serratus muscle was divided and the latissimus dorsi muscle attachment to the humerus was also divided under direct vision. The pedicle dissection was then performed toward the axilla. The thoracodorsal nerve was divided and the pedicle dissection was completed near the axillary vessel. Both artery and vein were divided individually with hemoclips (Fig. 31.11).

Both the pedicle artery and the vein were prepared under loupe magnification. The artery was flushed with heparinized saline solution. The flap was then placed to the left hip defect and microanastomosis was performed under microscope. An end-to-end arterial anastomosis was performed with 8-0 nylon suture in an interrupted fashion. For venous anastomosis, a 2-mm coupler device was used. Once all clamps were released, there was a good signal within the flap and the flap appeared well perfused. A Cook Doppler probe was used to monitor the blood flow of the arterial anastomosis (Fig. 31.12).

The flap was inset with a 3-0 Monocryl suture in half-buried horizontal mattress fashion. Two drains were placed into the left hip wound under the flap. The entire left hip soft tissue defect was covered with the free latissimus dorsi myocutaneous flap (Fig. 31.13). The rest of the muscle flap and the rest of the wound were covered with a split-thickness skin graft, harvested from the left thigh with a dermatome. The skin graft was approximated to the wound skin edges with staples and in between with 5-0 chromic sutures (Fig. 31.14).

Two drains were placed within the latissimus dorsi flap donor site. The incision was closed in three layers. The scape's fascia was closed with 2-0 interrupted PDS sutures. The deep dermal layer was closed with 3-0 interrupted Monocryl sutures. The skin was closed with 3-0 V-loc suture in a running intradermal fashion.

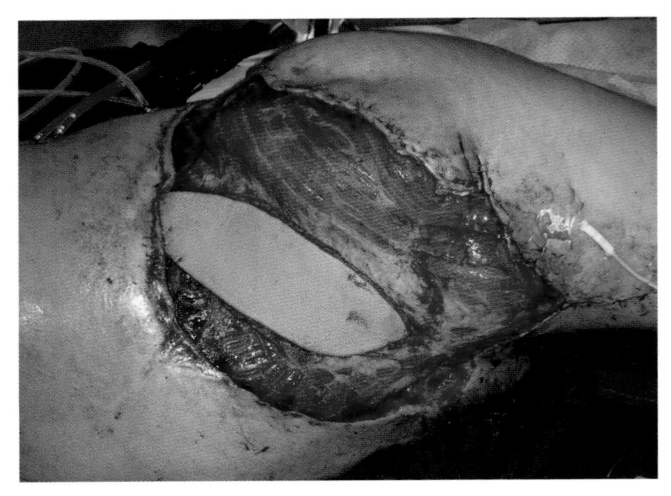

• **Fig. 31.13** An intraoperative view showing completion of initial inset of the free latissimus dorsi flap for the wound coverage.

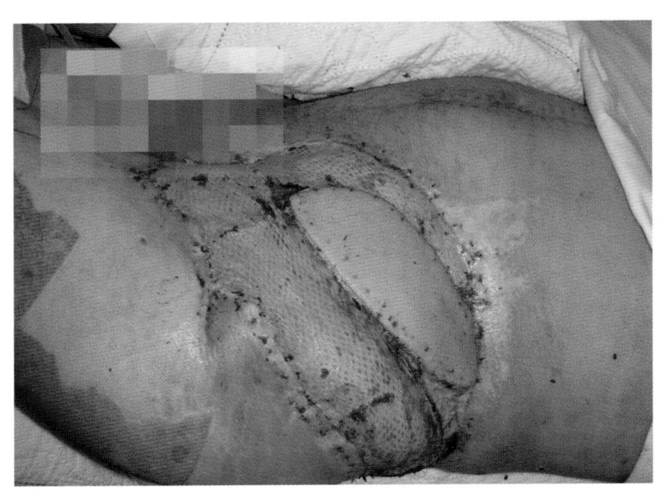

• **Fig. 31.15** Early result at 2-week follow-up showing initial healing of the left hip, pelvic, and groin wound.

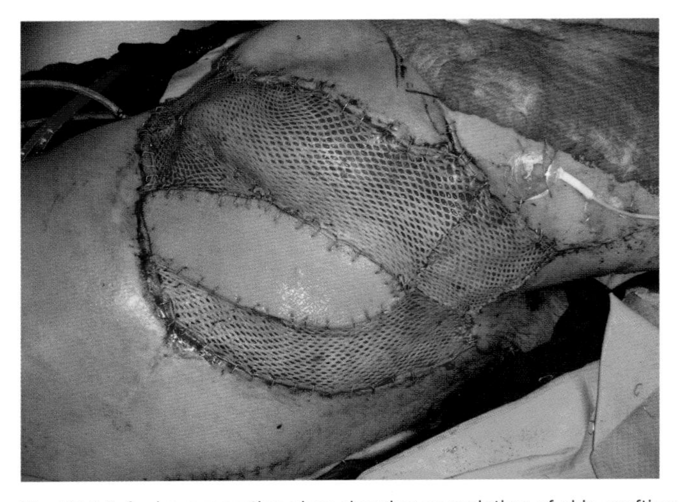

• **Fig. 31.14** An intraoperative view showing completion of skin grafting over the rest of the latissimus dorsi muscle flap for the wound closure.

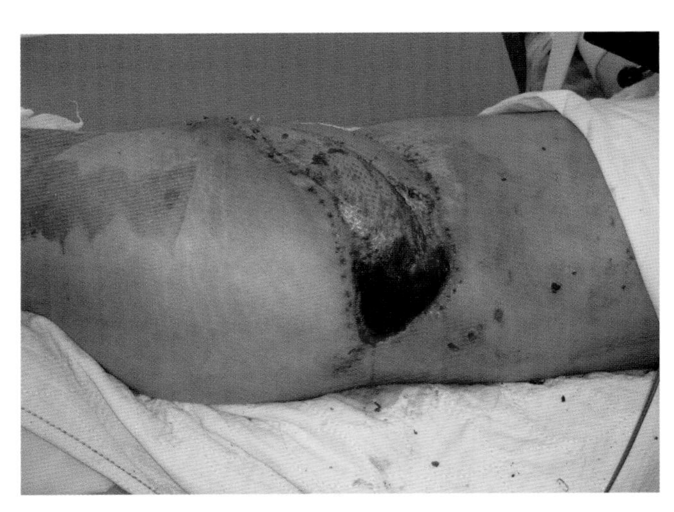

• **Fig. 31.16** Postoperative after 3 weeks showing the distal flap necrosis caused by direct compression of the brace.

Follow-Up Results

The patient did well postoperatively without any complications related to the free latissimus dorsi flap transfer. The flap site and the skin graft over the muscle flap also healed well (Fig. 31.15). He had a normal postoperative course and started physical therapy as instructed by the rehabilitation service. About 3 weeks later, he developed a distal flap necrosis and the cause of this condition was thought to be direct compression from a brace used to immobilize his nonoperative lumbar spine fracture (Fig. 31.16).

Management of Complications

The patient was brought back to the operating room for debridement of the necrotic portion of the flap and subsequent soft tissue reconstruction with a skin graft. During the procedure, the necrotic portion of the flap was debrided to the healthy bleeding flap tissue and a split-thickness skin graft, measuring 8 × 5 cm and harvested from the left thigh, was placed for wound closure. VAC was used over the skin graft site for possible enhancement of the graft healing (Fig. 31.17). Unfortunately, his skin graft procedure was not successful and an open wound remained that was treated with prolonged VAC for 2 months.

He was brought back to the operating room for another operation. At this time, the left hip wound measured 12 × 7 cm with a potential dead space (Fig. 31.18). A large lumbar perforator-based free-style skin rotation flap, with a skin island measuring 17 × 9 cm, was designed for definitive soft tissue reconstruction. Intraoperatively, several perforators were identified with a handheld Doppler but only a large perforator with a strong Doppler signal was used for the flap design (Fig. 31.19). The flap was raised and completely based on this single large perforator. At least 4 cm of intramuscular dissection of the perforator was performed until the perforator was reasonably free (Fig. 31.20). The entire skin island was easily rotated into the defect with no tension on the perforator (Fig. 31.21). The entire soft tissue wound was covered by the flap and the significant dead space of the wound was obliterated by the de-epithelialized portion of the flap. Several retention sutures were used to secure the wound closure. A skin graft was also used to close the flap donor site defect (Fig. 31.22).

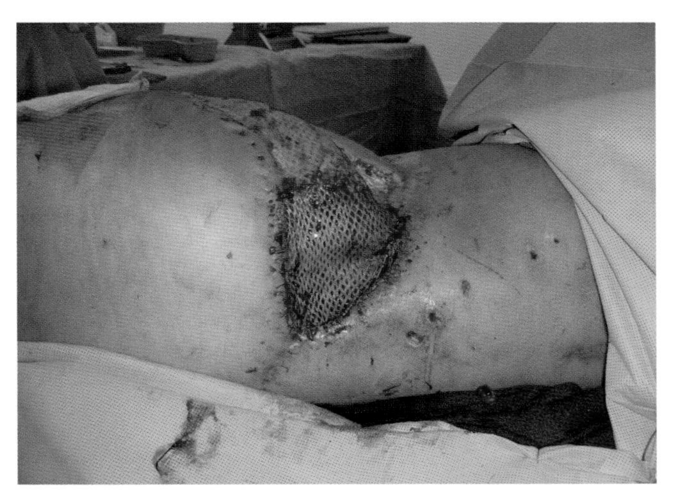

• **Fig. 31.17** An intraoperative view showing completion of the flap debridement and a skin graft placement after reoperation.

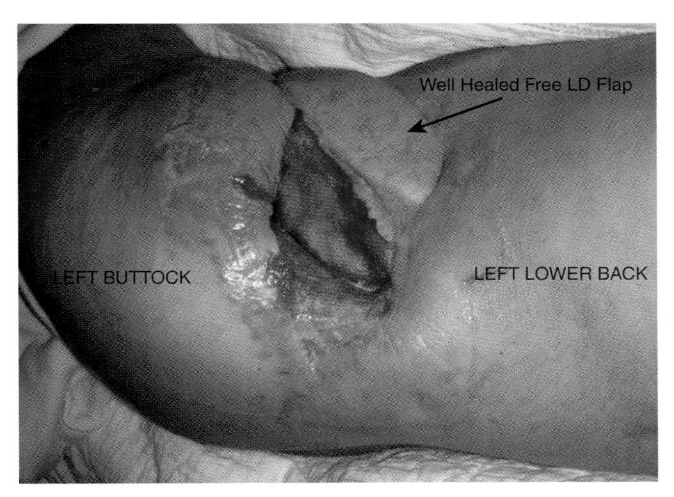

• **Fig. 31.18** A preoperative view showing a resulting 12 × 7 cm complex hip wound following a debridement of the distal necrotic free latissimus dorsi flap and a loss of the subsequent skin graft.

Final Outcome

The patient had an uneventful postoperative course and there were no postoperative issues related to the final operative flap reconstruction (Fig. 31.23). He was eventually discharged home. During follow-up, the left hip wound healed well with stable and durable soft tissue coverage and the patient has been fully ambulating without any problems (Fig. 31.24).

Pearls for Success

A large muscle flap, such as a free latissimus dorsi flap, can be selected to cover a large soft tissue wound in the hip and pelvic regions. The flap can be fairly reliable, if successfully transferred after microvascular anastomoses, and used to reconstruct this hip and pelvic wound and obliterate its dead space after the flap inset. Proper selection of recipient vessels for stress-free microvascular anastomoses would be key for success. As demonstrated in this case, the descending branch of the lateral circumflex femoral

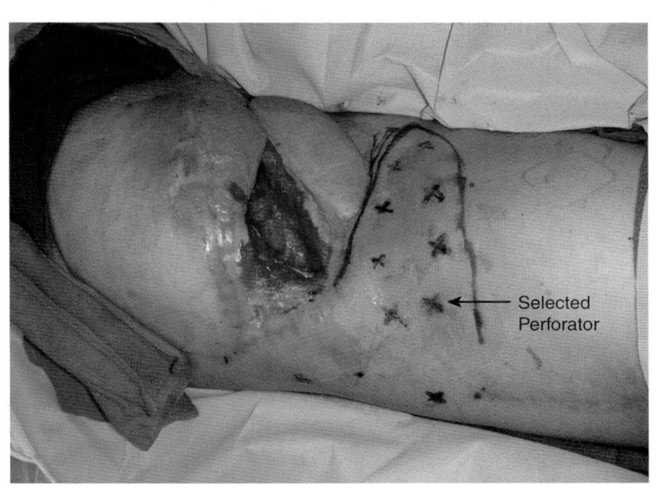

• **Fig. 31.19** An intraoperative view showing the design of an adjacent freestyle pedicled perforator rotation flap for the wound closure. Several perforators were identified (see the *marks*) preoperatively with a hand-held Doppler, but the flap would be successfully elevated based on one large perforator.

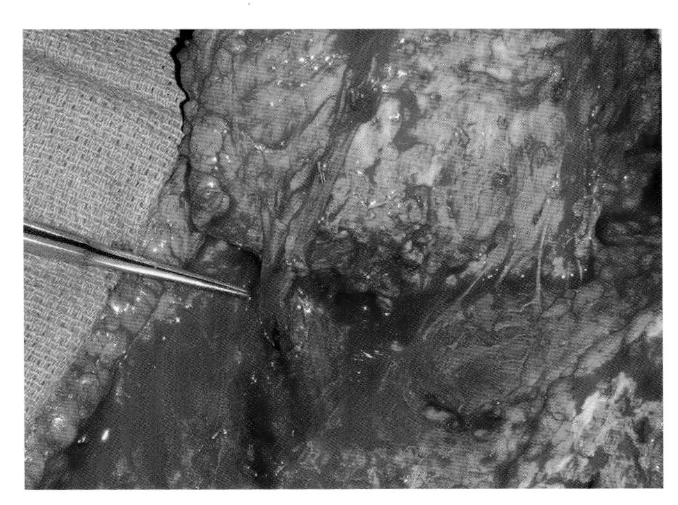

• **Fig. 31.20** An intraoperative view showing the selected perforator (indicated by *forceps*) that was dissected further intramuscularly to ensure adequate length for the flap rotation.

vessels could be used, after surgical dissection, to create a reliable recipient vessel from the distant area. Thus, microvascular anastomoses could be performed in a relatively straightforward fashion without any difficulties. adjacent to the hip and pelvic soft tissue defect. The descending branch of the femoral circumflex vessels is located in the deep layer of the thigh and is usually free of trauma. It can be dissected free and turned over to the area close to the hip and pelvis region.

In this case, a freestyle local perforator flap was successfully elevated and used to cover the subsequent defect in the hip region. Once perforators have been located perioperatively, the flap can be custom designed around the perforator with a skin island tailored to the shape of the soft tissue defect. These flaps can be successfully performed everywhere in the body if an appropriate perforator and an adequate amount of local tissue are present. When elevating a freestyle local perforator flap, once the perforator has

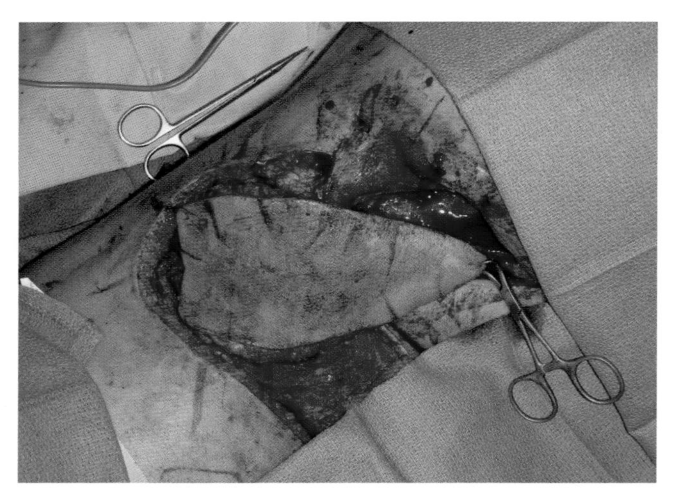

• **Fig. 31.21** An intraoperative view showing the free-style pedicled perforator flap that was elevated as an island and easily rotated into the wound for good soft tissue coverage.

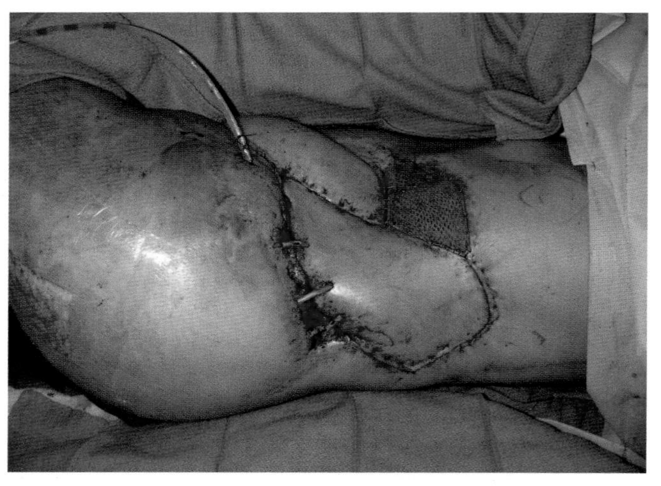

• **Fig. 31.22** An intraoperative view showing the completion of the flap inset and the donor site closure with a skin graft.

been identified and the size is thought suitable for the flap, intramuscular dissection of the perforator may be needed after the fascia is opened so that the length of the dissected perforator is long enough for the flap rotation and advancement. Care should be taken to avoid any tension or twisting placed on the perforator. With appropriate planning and execution, any freestyle cutaneous perforator flaps can be elevated successfully and can be a good alternative to conventional pedicled or free flap.

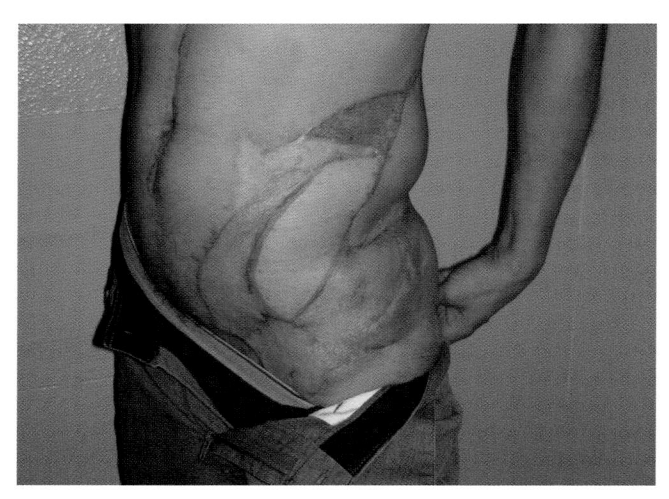

• **Fig. 31.23** Result at 7-week follow-up showing well-healed left hip, pelvic, and groin wounds.

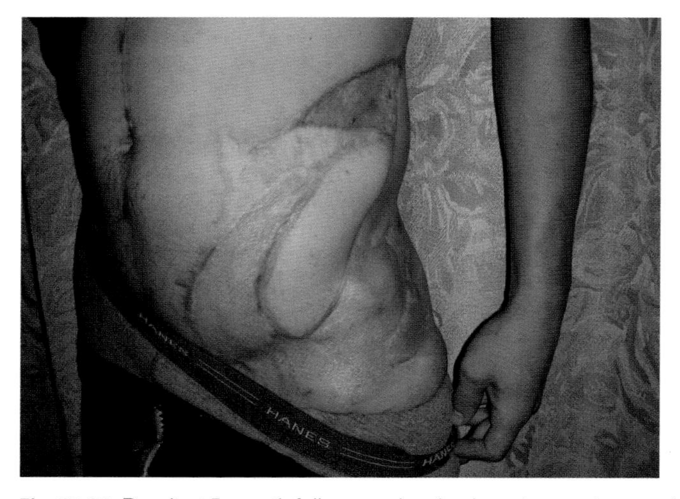

• **Fig. 31.24** Result at 5-month follow-up showing long-term outcome of the well-healed left hip, pelvic, and groin wounds after reconstructive procedures.

Recommended Readings

Alkon JD, Smith A, Losee JE, Illig KA, Green RM, Serletti JM. Management of complex groin wounds: preferred use of the rectus femoris muscle flap. *Plast Reconstr Surg*. 2005;115:776–783.

Diageler A, Dodic T, Awiszus F, Schneider W, Fansa H. Donor-Site Morbidity of the pedicled rectus femoris muscle flap. *Plast Reconstr Surg*. 2005;115:786–792.

Kapur SK, Liu J, Baumann DP, Butler CE. Surgical outcomes in lateral abdominal wall reconstruction: a comparative analysis of surgical techniques. *J Am Coll Surg*. 2019;229:267–276.

Kludt N, Pu LLQ. The clinical application of free-style cutaneous perforator flaps. *Eur J Plast Surg*. 2015;38:71–76.

Mathes SJ, Steinwald PM, Foster RD, Hoffman WY, Anthony JP. Complex abdominal wall reconstruction: a comparison of flap and mesh closure. *Ann Plast Surg*. 2000;232:586–596.

Sacks JM, Broyles JM, Baumann DP. Considerations in abdominal wall reconstruction. *Semin Plast Surg*. 2012;26:5–7.

Tashiro K, Arikawa M, Fukanaga Y, et al. Free latissimus dorsi musculocutaneous flap for external hemipelvectomy reconstruction. *Microsurgery*. 2019;39:138–143.

32
Groin Reconstruction

CASE 1

Clinical Presentation

A 64-year-old White male with a history of hypertension and two previous coronary artery bypass grafting surgeries underwent uneventful heart transplantation for severe congestive heart failure. During his cardiac transplant surgery, the left femoral artery and vein were cannulated for cardiopulmonary bypass. He was placed on routine immunosuppression protocol for postoperative heart transplant care. Three months after the successful heart transplantation, the patient presented with a large seroma secondary to lymphorrhea in the left groin cannulation site and underwent an incision and drainage of the seroma and placement of a closed drain by the cardiothoracic surgery service. Unfortunately, the patient developed persistent and uncontrollable drainage of lymphatic fluid (300–400 mL/day) from the left groin over the course of the next 2 weeks with no signs of improvement. The bacterial culture from the drain showed *Pseudomonas* and the patient was given appropriate antibiotics. The plastic surgery service was asked to manage recalcitrant groin lymphorrhea (Fig. 32.1).

Operative Plan and Special Considerations for Reconstruction

Intraoperative lymphatic mapping technique with intradermal injection of blue dye was selected to identify all lymphatic leak sites so that lymphorrhea could be controlled by ligating those afferent lymphatic vessels. A selected local muscle flap, such as sartorius muscle flap, was selected to provide reliable soft tissue coverage to the femoral vessels, eliminate dead space within the groin wound, seal lymphatic leak sites, and eradicate infection by increasing vascularity. In addition, it might act as a conduit for lymphatic drainage in the groin.

Operative Procedures

Eight weeks after the initial presentation of the groin seroma, 3 cc of isosulfan blue dye (Lymphazurin) was injected intradermally just proximal to the left ankle under general anesthesia. The injection was done circumferentially in order to incorporate all lymphatic drainage of the lower extremity (Fig. 32.2). The injected area was gently massaged and the leg was elevated to speed migration of the blue dye. The blue dye can usually be seen emerging from the damaged lymphatic vessels after 15 minutes. The previous left groin incision was reopened. Within the left groin wound, several blue-stained lymphatic vessels were identified and directly ligated with metallic surgical clips or PDS sutures (Fig. 32.3). A large sentinel lymph node and its afferent lymphatic vessel were also identified and directly ligated (Fig. 32.4). During gentle surgical dissection of the femoral vessels, more blue-stained lymphatic vessels were identified and they were directly ligated with suture-ligatures or metallic clips. A sizable well-formed capsule was found lateral and superior to the femoral vessels. The capsule was only partially removed because of the amount of dense adhesion to the femoral vessels. After a thorough irrigation and adequate hemostasis, the sartorius muscle was identified and elevated. Once the insertion of the sartorius was divided from the anterior superior iliac spine, the flap was easily transposed medially to cover the femoral vessels after the first perforator to the muscle was divided (Fig. 32.5). A drain was placed within the groin wound. The subcutaneous tissue and deep dermal layers of the incision were closed with interrupted absorbable sutures and the skin incision was closed with skin staples.

Follow-Up Results

The patient did well without any postoperative complications. He was discharged from hospital on postoperative day 5. The left groin incision healed uneventfully and the drain was removed once the drain's output became minimal. The left groin lymphorrhea subsided and was eventually resolved within 3 weeks after the surgery.

Final Outcome

The patient returned to his active normal lifestyle and has been followed by the cardiothoracic surgery service since then for routine post heart transplant office visits. No local lymphorrhea or wound breakdown of the left groin recurred during the following 2 years (Fig. 32.6).

Pearls for Success

The combination of intraoperative lymphatic mapping and sartorius muscle flap may be more effective than either method used alone for treating recalcitrant groin lymphorrhea in high-risk patients. Such a combination may not only identify disrupted lymphatic vessels directly in the groin but also obliterate a dead space within the groin wound. Some small lymphatic leaks, not

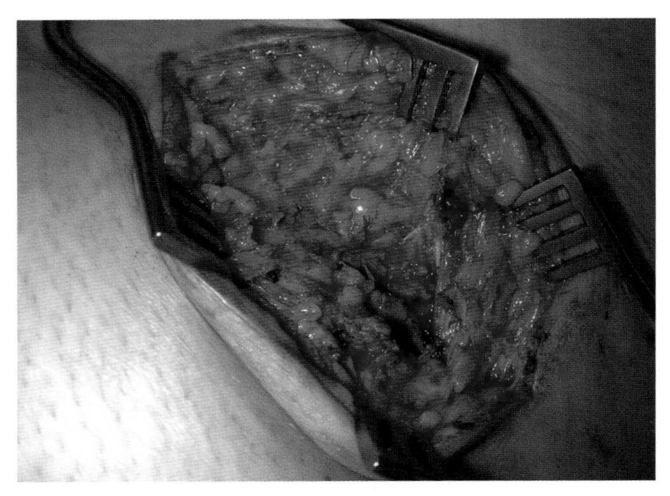

• **Fig. 32.1** An intraoperative view showing the patient's left groin lymphorrhea wound after surgical debridement.

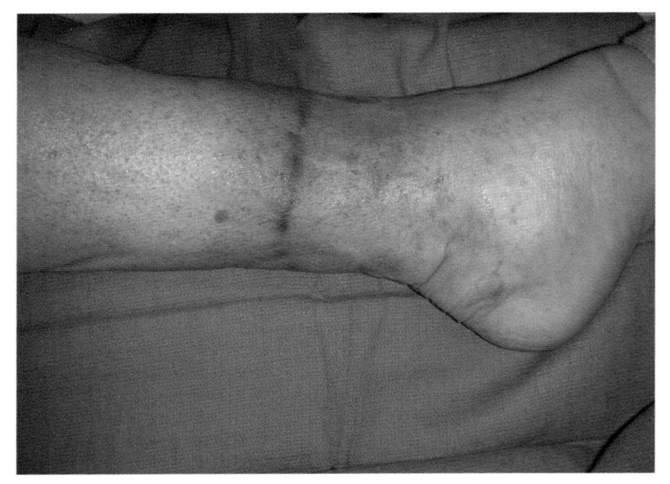

• **Fig. 32.2** An intraoperative view showing intradermal injection of blue dye (Lymphazurin) circumferentially just proximal to the left ankle.

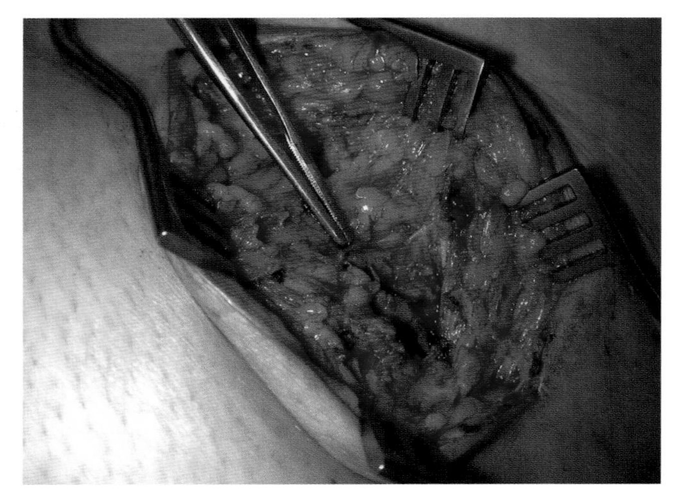

• **Fig. 32.3** Intraoperative view showing a disrupted, blue-stained lymphatic vessel within the left groin wound (indicated by a *forceps*).

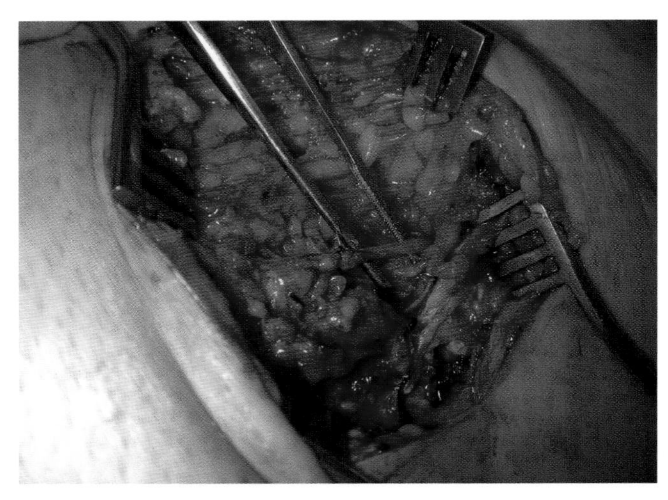

• **Fig. 32.4** Intraoperative view showing a blue-stained sentinel lymph node and its afferent lymphatic vessel (ligated with a PDS suture) within the left groin wound. Several small lymphatic vessels (occluded with surgical clips) surrounding the lymph node were also noted.

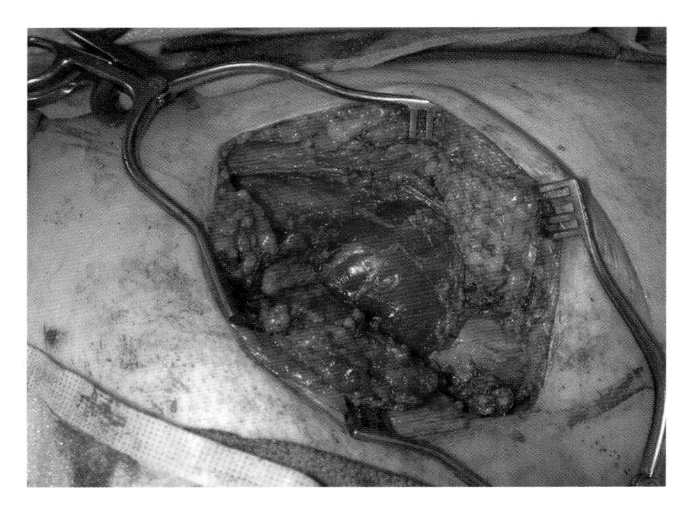

• **Fig. 32.5** Intraoperative view showing the femoral vessels of the left groin were completely covered by the sartorius muscle flap. Additional dead space within the groin wound would also be filled by the flap.

identified by intraoperative lymphatic mapping, can also be controlled with the sartorius muscle flap.

Two local muscle flaps, primarily sartorius and rectus femoris flaps, are used for treating vascular bypass graft infection or lymphorrhea in the groin. The sartorius muscle is a readily available muscle flap adjacent to the femoral vessels and causes minimal functional loss to the thigh when it is scarified and should be the local muscle flap of choice for small soft tissue defect of the groin, for coverage of femoral vessels when there is pending soft tissue necrosis over the femoral triangle, or for "filling" the space within the groin wound complicated with lymphorrhea. Because of its segmental blood supply from the superficial femoral artery (SFA), only the first branch of the SFA can be divided to allow adequate rotation of the muscle flap to cover the femoral triangle and to ensure adequate blood supply to the muscle flap. Division of more than two branches from the SFA should be avoided.

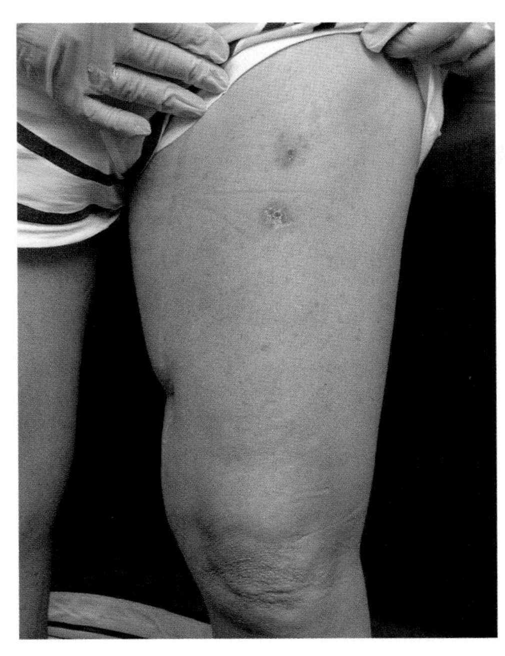

• **Fig. 32.6** Well-healed left groin wound with no evidence of recurrent lymphorrhea at 7-month follow-up.

CASE 2

Clinical Presentation

A 33-year-old, Black American male with a history of right testicular cancer presented with an advanced testicular cancer over the right groin. He had developed a large metastatic and fungating mass in the right groin involving the adjacent vital structures. Both urology and surgical oncology services had planned to perform the tumor resection to achieve a surgical control of the locally advanced metastatic disease (Fig. 32.7). The plastic surgery service was asked to perform a critical soft tissue reconstruction with a major flap so that the right groin wound with exposed femoral vessels could be closed and all vital structures could be protected after extensive tumor resection (Fig. 32.8). The retroperineal and paraaortic lymph node dissection was also performed via a midline laparotomy approach (Figs. 32.9A and B).

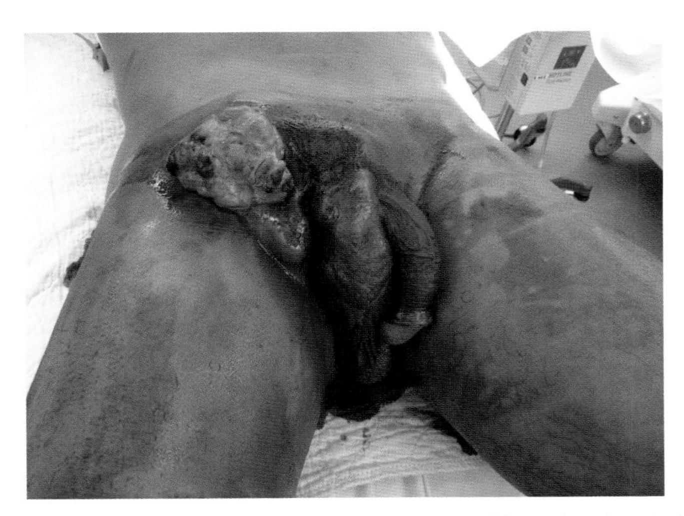

• **Fig. 32.7** A preoperative view showing a large and fungating ulcerated mass over the right groin.

Operative Plan and Special Considerations for Reconstruction

For this potential large soft tissue defect with the exposed femoral vessels and nerve and possible development of lymphatic leak in the groin, a reliable distant flap with a large skin paddle should be selected to provide a one-stage soft tissue coverage and obliterate the potential space.

Contralateral vertical rectus abdominis musculocutaneous (VRAM) flap could be a good option if the pedicle vessels are found to be intact. The flap can be harvested with a large and reliable skin paddle and can easily reach the contralateral groin area for a durable soft tissue reconstruction.

Operative Procedures

The defect after extensive tumor resection was assessed first. There was a large skin defect down to the femoral vessels. The inguinal ligament was completely excised. There was also significant scrotal defect on the right side. The VRAM flap was designed through both midline laparotomy incision and left lateral longitudinal abdominal incision. Three perforators of the rectus abdominis muscle were identified with a handheld Doppler. A 10 × 7 cm skin paddle was designed and both superior and inferior excess skin was incorporated into the flap skin paddle (Fig. 32.10).

Once the laparotomy incision had been temporarily closed with staples, the left lateral abdominal incision was made longitudinally and a suprafascial dissection was performed so that more anterior rectus sheath could be preserved. Once the anterior rectus

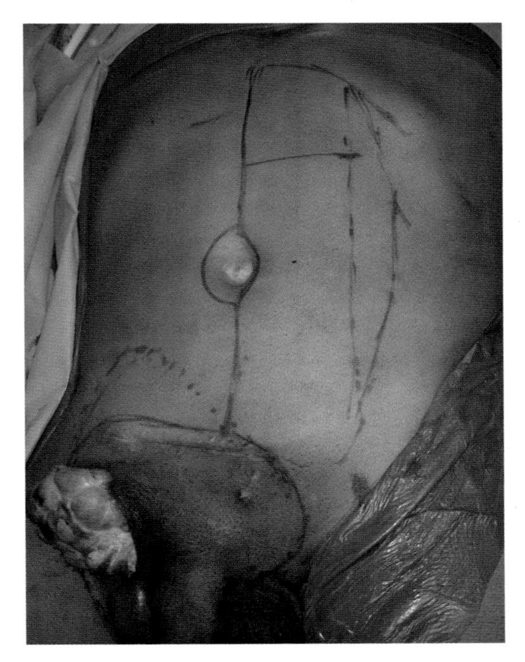

• **Fig. 32.8** An intraoperative view showing the extent of the surgical resection in the right groin and preliminary design of a contralateral VRAM flap for reconstruction.

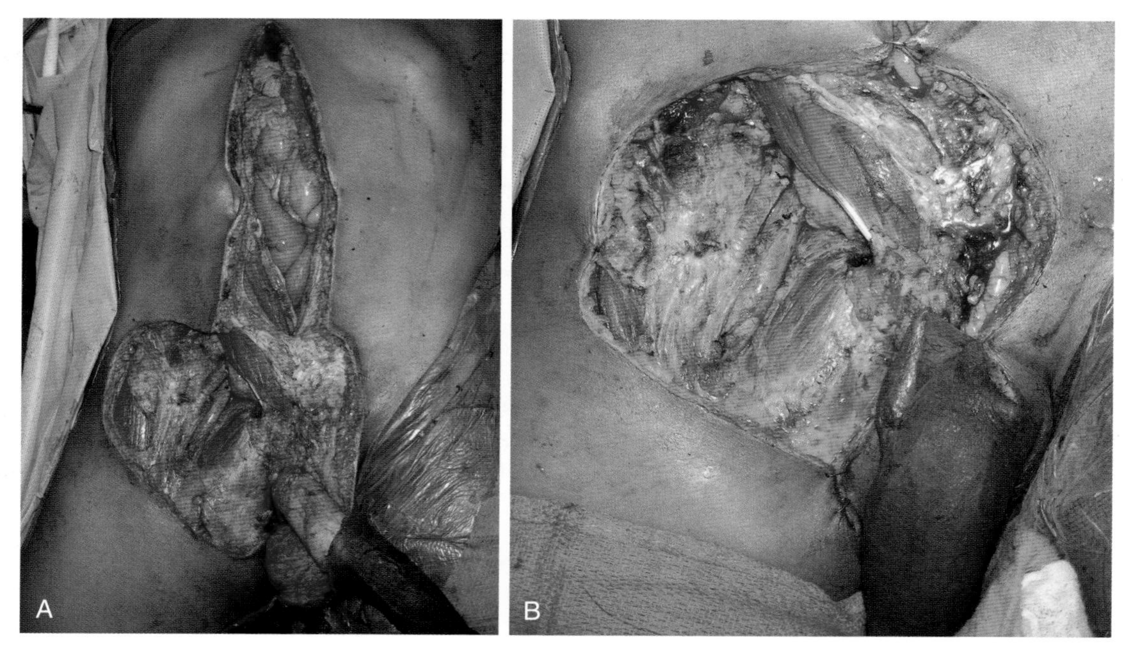

• **Fig. 32.9** (A) An intraoperative view showing completion of the right groin tumor resection and retroperitoneal and paraaortic lymph node dissection. (B) The exposed femoral vessels and the complete removal of the inguinal ligament and the portion of the anterior rectus sheath are shown.

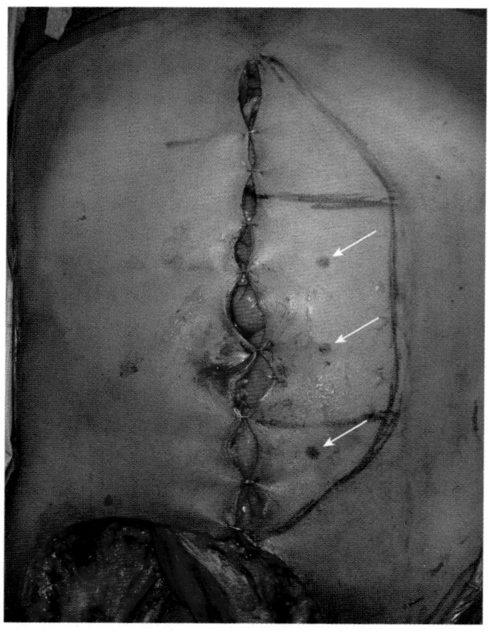

• **Fig. 32.10** An intraoperative view showing the design of the skin paddle for the contralateral VRAM flap. Three perforators were identified and marked by *arrows*. The excess portion of the skin was also marked proximally and distally and was elevated with the skin paddle of the flap.

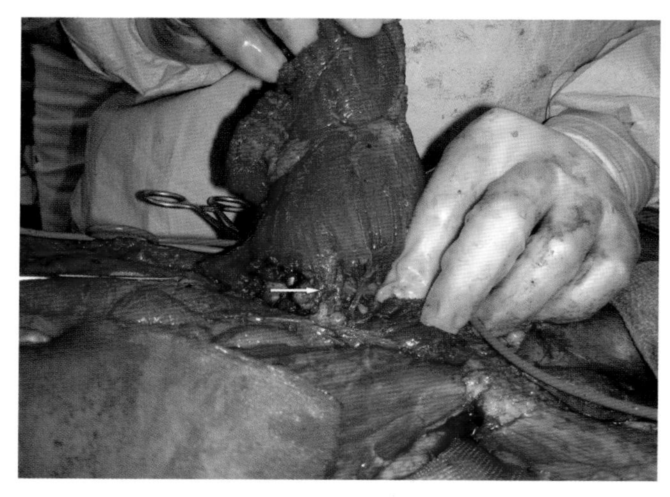

• **Fig. 32.11** An intraoperative view showing a completely dissected muscle portion of the vertical rectus abdominis musculocutaneous flap. The pedicle vessels of the flap were clearly visualized *(arrow)* and protected.

sheath had been incised down to the muscle, muscle dissection was performed to free the lateral and medial border of the muscle. Close to the costal margin, the rectus muscle was divided. During dissection, the inferior epigastric vessels were identified and were well protected. The inferior attachment of the muscle was also divided. The VRAM flap was elevated with its skin paddle (Fig. 32.11). The flap could be easily transposed to the right groin without difficulty. The abdominal incision was closed accordingly. The anterior rectus sheath was approximated with PDS sutures in simple running fashion. The skin incision was then approximated with skin staples.

The inguinal ligament was reconstructed with Prolene mesh (Fig. 32.12). The final inset of the VRAM flap was then performed. The muscle covered the exposed femoral vessels and the reconstructed inguinal ligament. The flap was inset into the right groin defect and secured to the adjacent subcutaneous tissues with Monocryl sutures and the skin paddle was approximated to the adjacent skin with the skin staples. The scrotal wound was closed

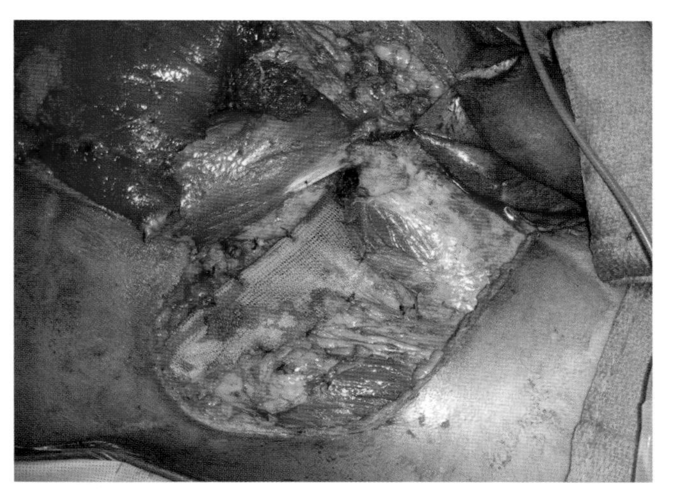

• **Fig. 32.12** An intraoperative view showing completion of the reconstructed inguinal ligament with Prolene mesh over the exposed femoral vessels.

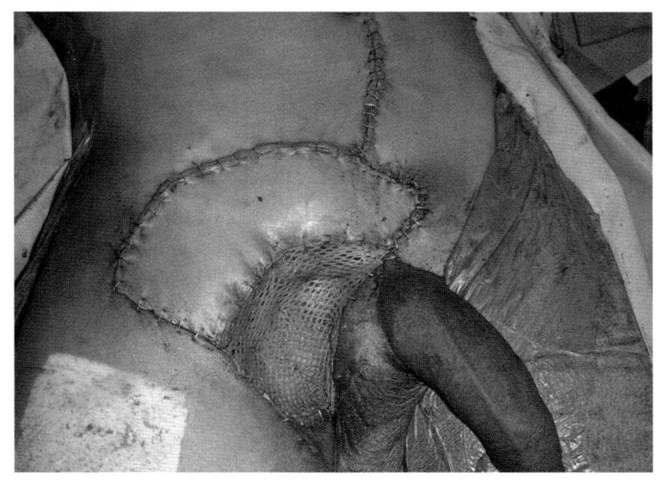

• **Fig. 32.13** An intraoperative view showing immediate result after the vertical rectus abdominis musculocutaneous flap reconstruction for the groin wound and local tissue rearrangement and a split-thickness skin graft for the scrotal wound coverage.

with local tissue rearrangement and a split-thickness skin graft (Fig. 32.13).

Follow-Up Results

The patient did well postoperatively without any complications related to the extensive tumor resection and VRAM flap reconstruction for the right groin wound. He was discharged from hospital on postoperative day 4. The right groin flap site healed uneventfully (Fig. 32.14) and the patient was followed by his primary service for testicular cancer care and medical oncology service for additional chemotherapy.

Final Outcome

The patient was routinely followed by the urology service for his postsurgical visits. The right groin flap reconstruction site had no wound breakdown and no long-term postoperative complications related to the extensive tumor resection (Fig. 32.15).

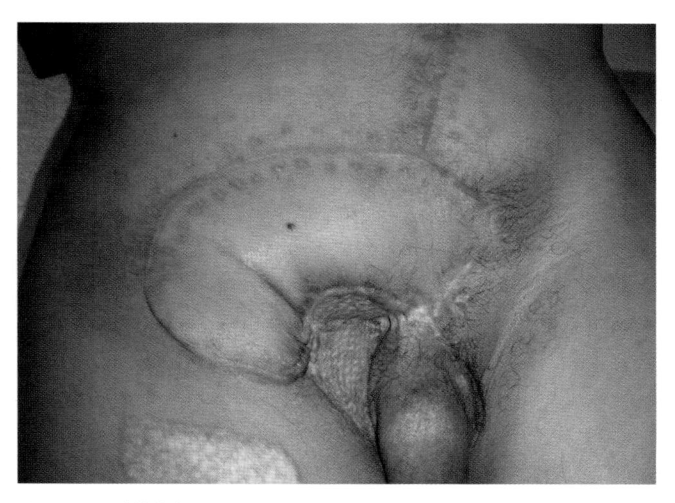

• **Fig. 32.14** Well-healed right groin wound after the vertical rectus abdominis musculocutaneous flap reconstruction and right scrotal wound after local tissue rearrangement and a skin graft at 5-month follow-up.

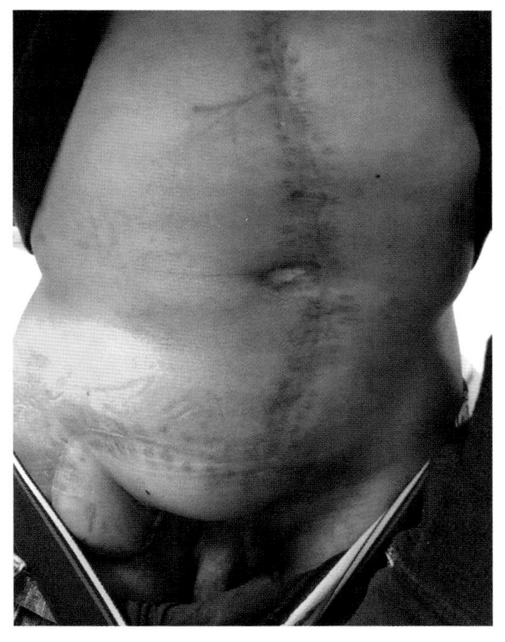

• **Fig. 32.15** Result at 11-month follow-up showing well-healed stable right groin and scrotal wounds.

Pearls for Success

A large distant myocutaneous flap, such as a VRAM flap, can be selected to cover such a large soft tissue wound in the groin with the exposed femoral vessels and nerve. The flap is fairly reliable and has a large skin paddle from the contralateral abdomen. Its pedicle vessels are usually intact and not within "the zone of injury." It can provide well-vascularized tissues to cover such a large groin wound with the exposed vital structures after surgical resection for a locally advanced metastatic tumor.

A few good perforators can be identified over the contralateral rectus abdominis muscle by a handheld Doppler and the skin paddle of the VRAM flap would be more reliable because one or two perforators can be incorporated within the flap design. Because the location of perforator(s) is(are) marked in the skin paddle, more anterior rectus sheath can be preserved after suprafascial dissection from both medial and lateral directions. In this way, less anterior rectus sheath (usually about only 2 cm wide) is taken during the VRAM flap dissection and thus the defect of the anterior rectus sheath after the flap dissection can be closed primarily. The proximal insertion of the rectus abdominis muscle may be divided carefully to allow the entire flap's rotation and advancement but can also partially be divided to prevent tension on the pedicle vessels during the flap rotation and advancement.

Recommended Readings

Combs PD, Sousa JD, Louie O, Said H, Neligan PC, Mathes DW. Comparison of vertical and oblique rectus abdominis myocutaneous flaps for pelvic, perineal, and groin reconstruction. *Plast Recontr Surg.* 2014;134:315–323.

Fisher JP, Mizabeigi MN, Sieber BA, et al. Outcome analysis of 244 consecutive flaps for managing complex groin wounds. *J Plast Reconstr Aesthet Surg.* 2013;66:1396–1404.

Graham RC, Omotoso O, Hudson DA. The effectiveness of muscle flaps for the treatment of prosthetic graft sepsis. *Plast Reconstr Surg.* 2002;109:108–113.

Pu LLQ, Jahania MS, Mentzer RM. Successful management of recalcitrant groin lymphorrhoea with the combination of intraoperative lymphatic mapping and muscle flap. *J Plast Reconstr Aesthet Surg.* 2006;59:1363–1366.

Reiffel AJ, Handerson PW, Karwowski JK, Spector JA. An interdisciplinary approach to the prevention and treatment of groin wound complications after lower extremity revascularization. *Ann Vasc Surg.* 2012;26:365–372.

Stadelmann WK, Tobin GR. Successful treatment of 19 consecutive groin lymphoceles with the assistance of intraoperative lymphatic mapping. *Plast Reconst Surg.* 2002;109:1274–1280.

33 Sacral Reconstruction

CASE 1

Clinical Presentation

A 35-year-old Hispanic paraplegic female developed a sacral pressure sore when she was in hospital to give birth (Fig. 33.1). This was the first time she had a pressure sore since she became paraplegic as a result of an accident. She was offered a flap reconstruction to close the sacral pressure sore after excision of the entire wound because she was a highly motivated individual with good social support from her husband. She fully understood the potential risks and benefits of the procedure and was willing to follow our postoperative instructions for an optimal flap healing.

Operative Plan and Special Considerations

Adequate surgical debridement for this sacral pressure wound should be performed first. With advance knowledge of perforator flap surgery, a gluteal perforator flap could be planned for the reconstruction. The flap itself can be based on one or two large perforators identified by an intraoperative Doppler finding. It can be raised as a V-to-Y fasciocutaneous advancement flap and the sacral soft tissue defect can be closed without tension. After the perforator has been identified, flap dissection can be done aggressively to elevate the entire skin paddle as an island flap. Such a flap's advancement can be done freely to close a large sacral wound and the bulkiness of the flap can easily be advanced to fill any dead space of the sacral wound. Obviously, for any paraplegic patient, postoperative care is critical to ensure no tension or sheer force for the flap reconstruction site.

Operative Procedures

Under general anesthesia with the patient in a prone position, methylene blue was used to stain the entire bursa of the sacral pressure sore. Surgical debridement was first performed to excise the entire pressure sore including the bursa. This was achieved first by using a blade and including some normal skin and then by using electrocautery to remove the entire bursa of the sacral pressure sore. During the procedure, this patient had a significant amount of bleeding from several sizable vessels around the bursa of the pressure sore. All bleeding was controlled with hemoclips, electrocautery, surgicel, and pressure dressing. The wound was then irrigated with antibiotic solution

A 15 × 9 cm triangular, superior gluteal artery perforator flap was designed. Based on a preoperative duplex scan finding, there was a sizable perforator that measured about 2 mm in diameter with an excellent flow. Therefore, this perforator was included for the design of the superior gluteal artery perforator flap (Fig. 33.2).

The skin incision was made along the planned triangular fasciocutaneous flap and was followed by subfascial dissection of the flap. Several small perforators were encountered but were divided. The flap's attachment to the underlying superior gluteus muscle was then dissected freely and the superior gluteal artery perforator was identified (Fig. 33.3). Precise dissection was performed around the perforator so that the flap could be advanced freely.

This single perforator-based superior gluteal artery perforator flap was then advanced into the midline sacral defect in a V-Y fashion without any tension (Fig. 33.4). Some excess of the flap skin was trimmed and the flap was approximated to the contralateral midline without any tension. A 10-mm flat JP was inserted into the wound. The deep layer closure was approximated with several interrupted 2-0 PDS sutures. The deep dermal closure was made with several interrupted 3-0 Monocryl sutures. The skin closure was approximated first with four 3-0 nylons in half-buried horizontal mattress fashion. The rest of the skin closure was made with multiple skin staples (Fig. 33.5).

Follow-Up Results

The patient was placed on a special bed in a prone position postoperatively on the floor. She had no immediate complications related to the flap closure. She was doing well during her hospital care and was discharged from hospital on postoperative day 14. The drain was removed during the subsequent follow-up visit. Her sacral pressure sore flap closure site healed well during the early postoperative follow-up (Fig. 33.6).

Final Outcome

The sacral pressure sore wound after the superior gluteal artery perforator flap reconstruction healed well with minimal scarring (Fig. 33.7). There has been no recurrent infection, seroma, or wound breakdown. The patient remains wound-free and has resumed her activities. She has been followed by the plastic surgery service as needed.

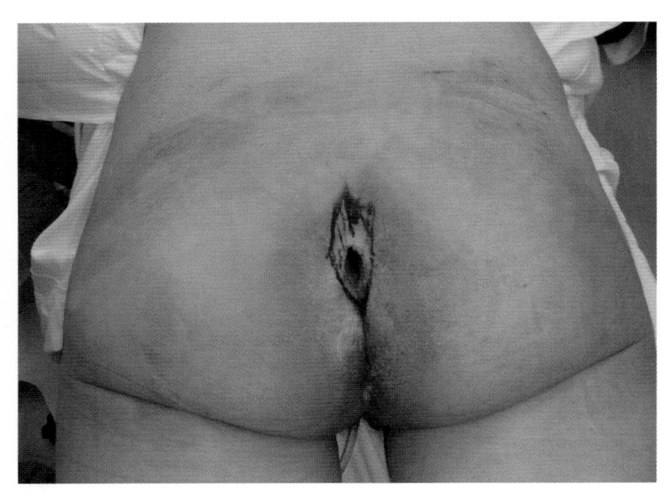

• **Fig. 33.1** Preoperative view showing a sacral pressure sore wound with the outlined scar tissue around it.

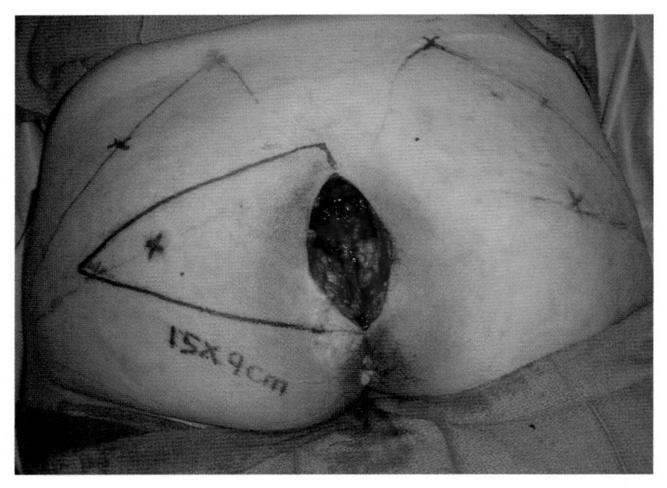

• **Fig. 33.2** Intraoperative view showing the design of the superior gluteal artery perforator V- to-Y fasciocutaneous advancement flap. The perforator was clearly mapped and marked.

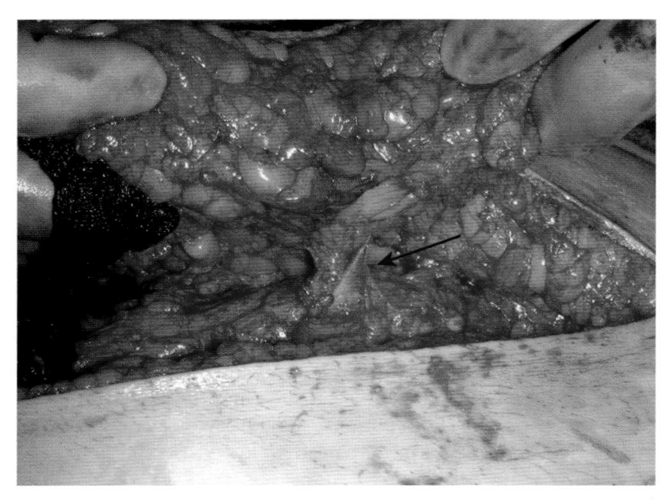

• **Fig. 33.3** Intraoperative view showing the perforator that was identified during the flap dissection.

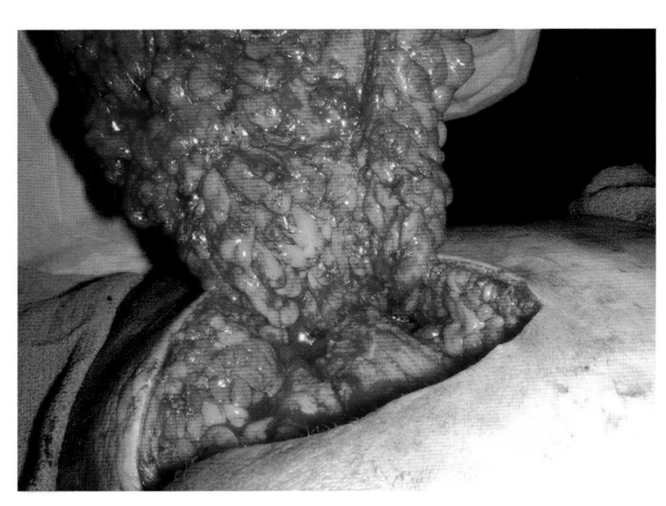

• **Fig. 33.4** Intraoperative view showing completion of the flap dissection for this perforator-bassed flap. The flap could be advanced freely to the sacral defect.

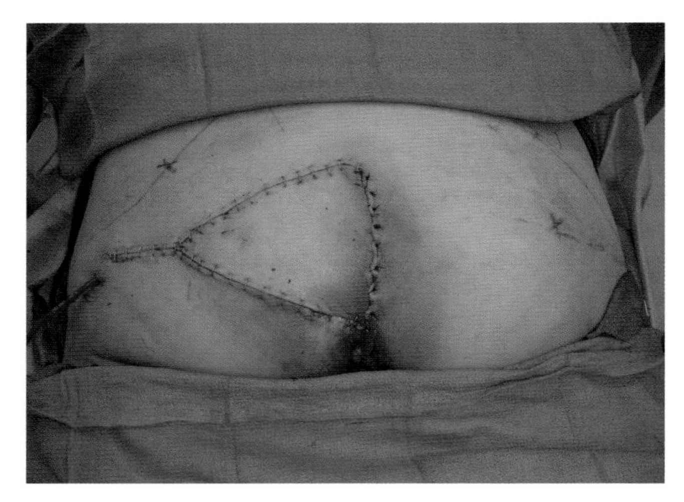

• **Fig. 33.5** Intraoperative view showing completion of the flap inset and closure as well as closure of the flap's donor site.

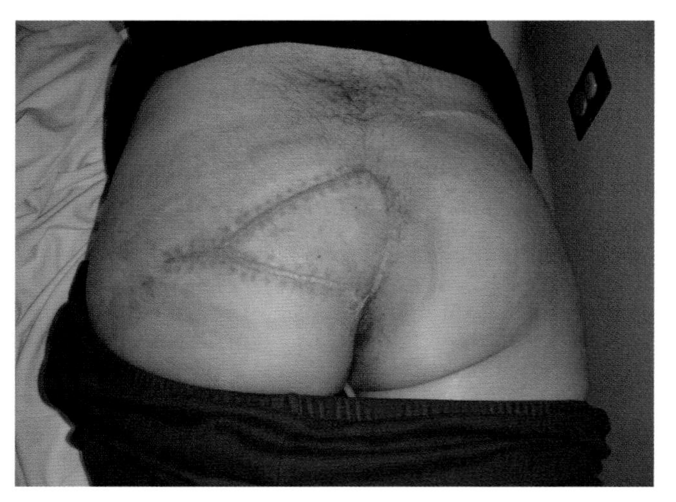

• **Fig. 33.6** The result at 2-month follow-up showing good healing of the sacral pressure sore wound after the flap reconstruction.

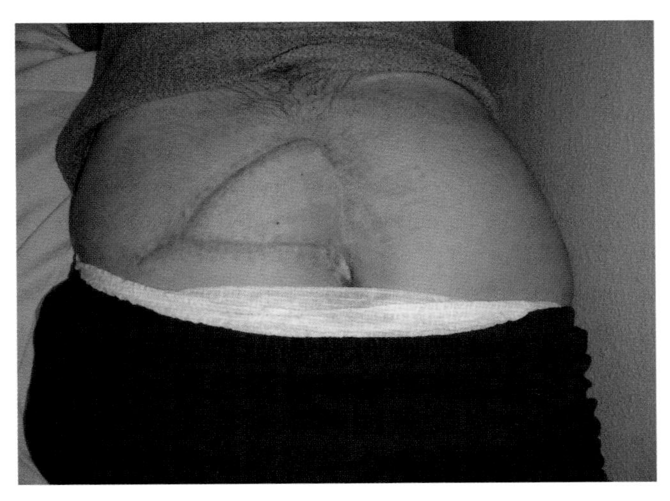

• **Fig. 33.7** The result at 6-month follow-up showing well-healed sacral pressure sore wound with minimal scarring and good contour after the flap reconstruction.

Pearls for Success

A superior gluteal artery perforator flap, elevated and advanced in a V-to-Y fashion, can be an excellent option for soft tissue reconstruction of a sacral pressure sore wound after adequate surgical debridement. The flap can be elevated based on one or two large perforators with a large skin paddle. The flap can be raised as an island flap and with further perforator dissection including intramuscular dissection, it can be easily advanced to the midline sacral soft tissue wound. In addition, the proximal portion of the flap can be de-epithelized and fill the dead space of the wound without difficulty. The final closure for a V-to-Y fashion may minimize scarring of the flap donor site and also facilitate the flap's advancement. Compared with a conventional gluteal fasciocutaneous V-to-Y advancement flap, the perforator flap has more advantages in terms of the freedom for the flap's advancement and flap inset. Further intramuscular dissection around the perforator can be performed so that the flap can be advanced beyond the midline sacral wound. Attention should be paid not to stretch or twist the perforator during the flap's advancement or inset. Venous congestion may occur after the flap closure and this condition can be resolved by leech therapy or adjustment of the flap inset.

CASE 2

Clinical Presentation

A 60-year-old White male developed a sacral pressure sore from his prolonged trauma care in the surgical ICU after a motor vehicle accident. Although he recovered from his traumatic injuries, he developed a 5.5 × 4.5 cm sacral pressure sore down to the subcutaneous tissue (Fig. 33.8). He was referred by the trauma service for wound closure with a flap. A local fasciocutaneous rotation flap was offered to this patient. Because he had been fully ambulating, good reconstructive outcome should be anticipated.

Operative Plan and Special Considerations

After adequate debridement within the wound, an adjacent fasciocutaneous rotation flap can be planned for reconstruction. For this patient, a large fasciocutaneous rotation flap could be designed and used to provide adequate soft tissue coverage for the sacral wound closure. The arc arch rotation of the flap could be designed large enough with potential "back cut" to ensure tension-free closure and can be readvanced if wound dehiscence occurs near the primary defect. The flap donor site can usually be closed primarily without a skin graft.

Operative Procedures

Under general anesthesia with the patient in a prone position, the procedure started with adequate debridement of the sacral wound. The wound area was gently curetted to remove all necrotic tissues and the skin edge was freshened with a blade. After such surgical preparation, the wound was irrigated thoroughly with Pulsavac.

The design of an adjacent gluteal fasciocutaneous rotation flap was then marked. The arc rotation of the flap was designed large

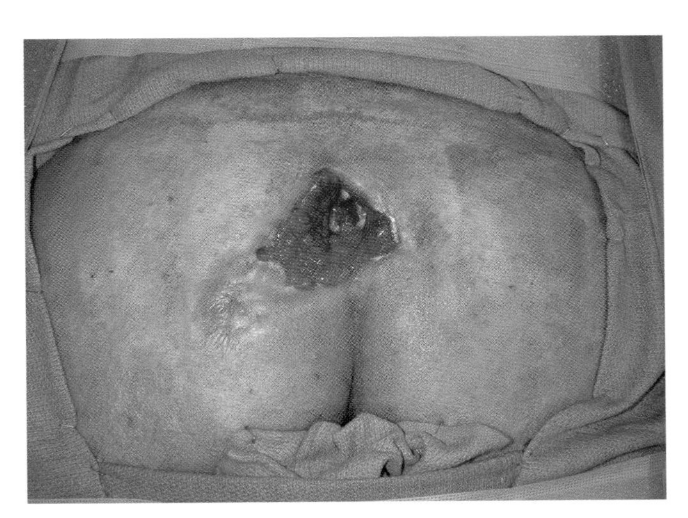

• **Fig. 33.8** Preoperative view showing a 5.5 × 4.5 cm sacral pressure sore wound down to the subcutaneous tissue.

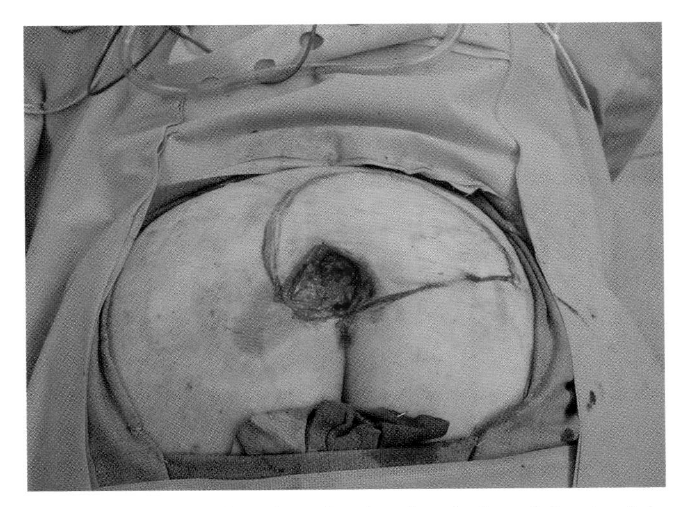

• **Fig. 33.9** Intraoperative view showing the design of the local fasciocutaneous rotation flap with longer arc of rotation and possible back cut.

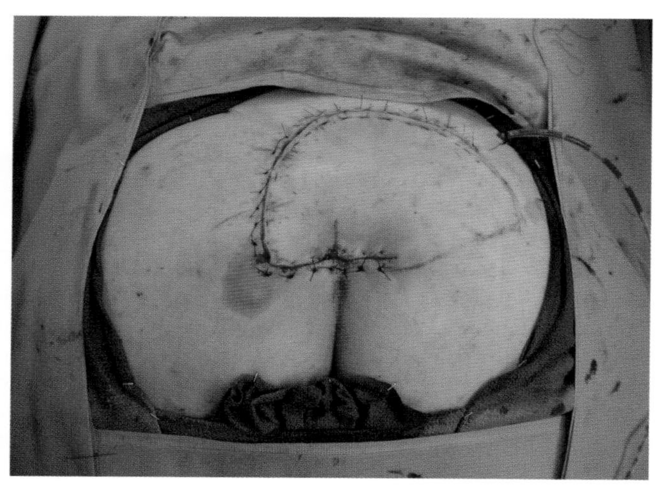

• **Fig. 33.10** Intraoperative view showing completion of the flap inset for sacral pressure sore wound closure.

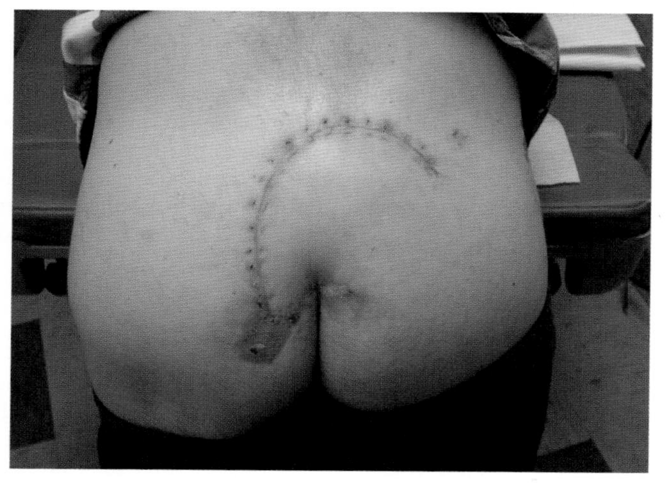

• **Fig. 33.11** The result at 4-week follow-up showing good healing of the sacral pressure sore wound closure after the flap reconstruction.

enough for easy flap rotation and a back cut could be added if necessary to facilitate the flap rotation (Fig. 33.9). Once the incision was made through the skin, subcutaneous tissue, and fascia down to the gluteal muscle, the flap was elevated as a single unit. The extend of the flap's rotation was made only necessary while allowing adequate attachment of the skin to the muscle as a fasciocutaneous flap. The flap was then rotated into the sacral wound and inset into the soft tissue defect and no back cut was needed in this case. The flap closure was done in two layers. The deep dermal layer was closed with interrupted 3-0 Monocryl sutures and the skin was closed with interrupted 3-0 nylon in half-buried horizontal mattress fashion. One drain was placed under the flap (Fig. 33.10).

Follow-Up Results

The patient did well postoperatively without any issues related to the flap reconstruction. He was discharged from hospital on postoperative day 5. The drain was removed during subsequent follow-up visits. The sacral wound closure remained intact and healed well (Fig. 33.11). He started fully ambulating at 6 weeks postoperatively.

Final Outcome

The sacral pressure sore wound after an adjacent fasciocutaneous rotation flap closure healed well without any complications. There is no recurrent infection, seroma, or wound breakdown. The patient has resumed his normal activities and has been followed by the plastic surgery service as needed.

Pearls for Success

For a less extensive sacral wound, a local fasciocutaneous rotation flap can be a reasonably good option for soft tissue reconstruction. The flap can be designed with a relatively large arc of the rotation to achieve an optimal wound closure. A back cut can also be incorporated into the flap design and be used to facilitate the flap rotation. A relatively large arc of the flap rotation is designed so that the flap can be rotated with a back cut in case a further operation is needed for wound dehiscence. A half-buried horizontal mattress suture can be used for flap closure to minimize skin edge ischemia and to ensure a better contour. With advanced knowledge of a skin perforator flap, a gluteal perforator-based flap can also be designed and used to reconstruct the same kind of sacral wound for a durable soft tissue coverage.

Recommended Readings

Acarturk TO, Seyhan T, Bengur FB, Erbas VE. A single superior gluteal artery perforator flap in reconstruction of large midline sacral defects: a method for practical harvest and safe closure. *Ann Plast Surg.* 2022;88:313–318.

Cheon YW, Lee MC, Kim YS, Rah DK, Lee WJ. Gluteal artery perforator flap: a viable alternative for sacral radiation ulcer and osteoradionecrosis. *J Plast Reconstr Aesthet Surg.* 2010;63:642–647.

Kimura H, Nasu W, Kashiwa K, Kobayashi S. Reconstruction of the sacral region using the lumbo-gluteal sensory flap. *J Plast Reconstr Aesthet Surg.* 2013;66:239–242.

Lin CT, Chang SC, Chen SG, Tzeng YS. Modification of the superior gluteal artery perforator flap for reconstruction of sacral sores. *J Plast Reconstr Aesthet Surg.* 2014;67:526–532.

Lin PY, Kuo YR, Tsai YT. A reusable perforator-preserving gluteal artery-based rotation fasciocutaneous flap for pressure sore reconstruction. *Microsurgery.* 2012;32:189–195.

Miles WK, Chang DW, Kroll SS, et al. Reconstruction of large sacral defects following total sacrectomy. *Plast Reconstr Surg.* 2000;105:2388–2394.

34
Buttock Reconstruction

CASE 1

Clinical Presentation

A 63-year-old White female had chronic recurrent drainage from her right buttock for the past 2 years. She had a resection of malignant fibrohistiocytoma and postoperative irradiation in the region approximately 20 years ago. She was evaluated by the surgical oncology service and multiple biopsy specimens from the region were negative for recurrent sarcoma (Fig. 34.1). Wide local resection was performed by the surgical oncologist and all irradiated tissues and a chronic drainage tract were excised. A 20 × 15 cm gluteal soft tissue defect with an exposed small area of the sacrum was left after resection. The gluteus maximus muscle appeared to be fibrotic (Fig. 34.2).

Operative Plan and Special Considerations

For a large gluteal soft tissue defect, reconstruction with local flaps is usually possible because there are some redundant tissues in the adjacent areas. Double-opposing V-Y fasciocutaneous advancement flaps could be designed based on the size of the defect with mobilization of the excess adjacent gluteal tissue in both superior and inferior directions. Each fasciocutaneous flap would be designed as a V-to-Y advancement flap and both flaps could be approximated in an opposing fashion for the final wound closure. A single large fasciocutaneous rotation flap may also be an option, but it would create more surgical incision and dissection for the same wound closure. In terms of blood supply to these flaps, it is possible that the superior flap receives its blood supply from the superior gluteal artery perforators and the inferior flap receives its blood supply from the inferior gluteal artery perforators.

Operative Procedures

Under general anesthesia with the patient in the prone position, the gluteal soft tissue defect was assessed for size and dimensions. Each V-Y fasciocutaneous flap was designed superiorly or inferiorly to the defect and opposing to each other. The length of each flap measured 1.5 or 2 times the longitudinal diameter of the defect. The maximal width of the flap was equal to the width of the defect (Fig. 34.3).

The incision was made on the arms of the V and the subcutaneous tissue was incised and beveled away from the flap, possibly catching more direct cutaneous blood supply to the flap, down to the deep fascia. The deep fascial layer was incised in a V fashion according to the flap design to aid advancement of the flap. Both flaps were approximated to each other temporarily and additional flap dissections were performed if necessary. Any fibrous connections that might restrict the advancement of the flap were divided between the flap and the adjacent tissues.

Once sufficient advancement of the flap had been accomplished, the flap donor site was closed over a suction drain in two layers (deep dermis with interrupted 3-0 Monocryl sutures and skin with skin staples) primarily in V-Y fashion. The approximation of two opposing V-Y fasciocutaneous advancement flaps was performed in three layers over one suction drain. The deep subcutaneous was approximated with interrupted 2-0 PDS sutures and the deep dermal closure was done with interrupted 3-0 Monocryl sutures. The skin was closed with interrupted 3-0 nylon sutures (Fig. 34.4). Postoperatively, the patient was placed in the lateral decubital position with the operated side of the buttock up for the first several days. Patients would be allowed slow ambulation afterward but should avoid sitting or flexing their hips for approximately 6 weeks.

Follow-Up Results

Moderate venous congestion of the superior flap developed at the end of the procedure but was resolved with application of nitroglycerin ointment during the first 2 postoperative days. The postoperative course was also unremarkable and the patient was discharged from the hospital on postoperative day 6. During subsequent follow-up visits, she had well-healed flap sites in the gluteal region and all drains were removed. She was able to ambulate without problems (Fig. 34.5).

Final Outcome

The gluteal reconstruction site healed well with minimal scarring and acceptable contour (Fig. 34.6). The patient has had no infection, seroma, or wound breakdown. She remains cancer-free and has resumed her normal activities. She has been followed by the surgical oncology team for routine follow-up.

Pearls for Success

An effective reconstruction for a large gluteal soft tissue defect has not been established. The double-opposing V-Y fasciocutaneous advancement flaps are designed and used successfully to cover a large gluteal soft tissue defect. The flap design and dissection are relatively straightforward considering the size and contour of the

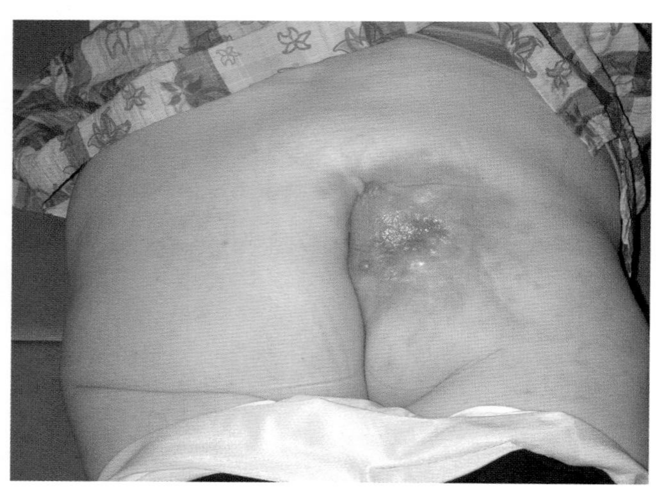

• **Fig. 34.1** Preoperative view showing a chronic irradiated wound with extensive fibrosis and induration within the right gluteal region.

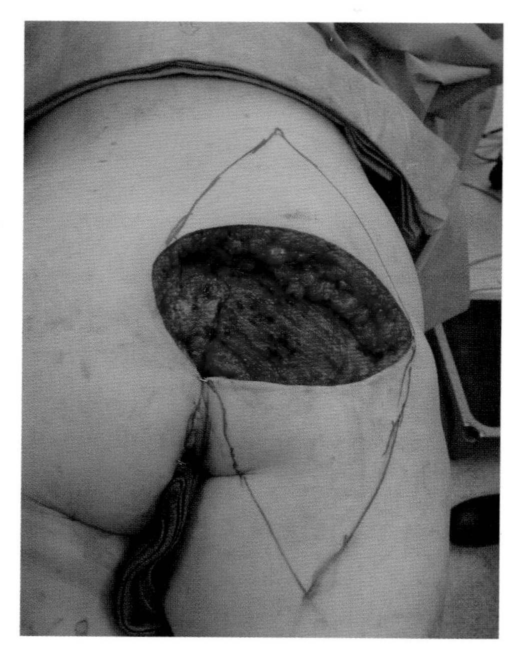

• **Fig. 34.3** Intraoperative view showing the design of the double-opposing V-Y fasciocutaneous advancement flaps.

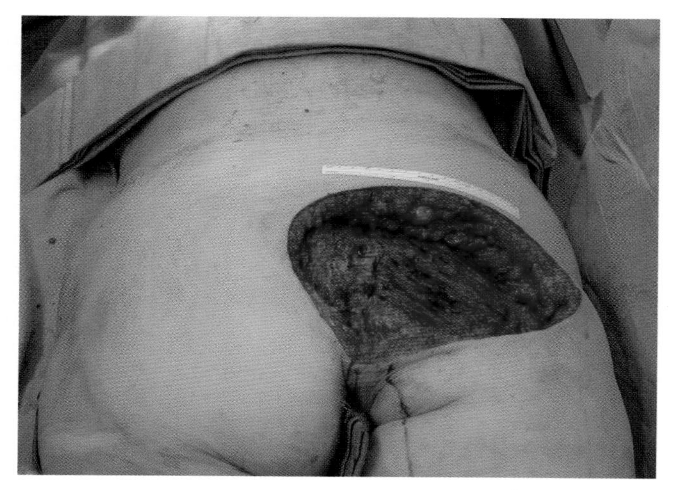

• **Fig. 34.2** Intraoperative view showing a 20 × 15-cm gluteal soft tissue defect after wide local resection of the chronic irradiated wound. A small area of the sacrum was also exposed.

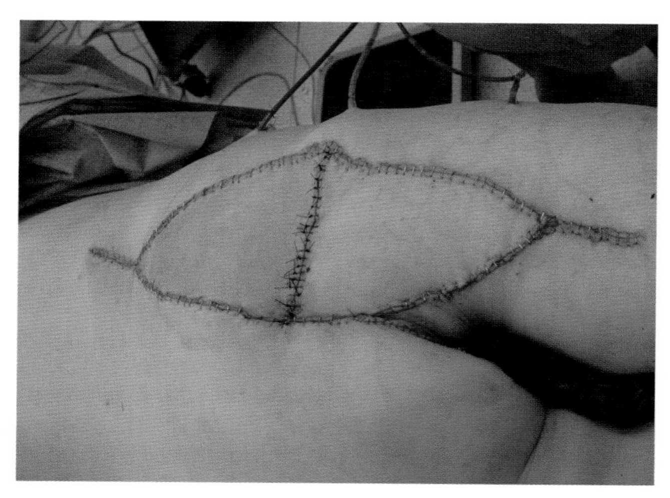

• **Fig. 34.4** Intraoperative view showing completion of the flap closure for the large gluteal soft tissue defect. Moderate venous congestion of the superior flap was noticed and treated successfully with nitroglycerin ointment.

defect. However, some degree of contour deformity may occur in the reconstructed gluteal region. For flap dissection, some degree of the difference in flap movement between the superior and inferior flaps can exist because the inferior flap usually moves well after flap elevation, but the superior flap may be tethered by the iliac wing. This might have been responsible for the transient venous congestion of the superior flap seen in this case. Therefore, complete release of the fibrous connection of the superior flap to the iliac wing should be performed to ease flap movement.

CASE 2

Clinical Presentation

A 33-year-old paraplegic White male had a long-standing history of left ischial pressure sore (Fig. 34.7). After assessing all risk factors for a flap reconstruction, he was offered an excision of the pressure sore and a flap reconstruction for the ischial wound closure. This patient also had osteomyelitis of the ischium and required bony debridement by the orthopedic surgery service (Fig. 34.8). He had specifically been informed about the high likelihood of wound dehiscence after the pressure sore wound closure. He fully understood the risk and the potential benefit of the procedure and was willing to accept the high risks of wound healing complications.

Operative Plan and Special Considerations

Adequate debridement of the ischial pressure sore wound with removal of all scarred and fibrotic tissues including a bursa would

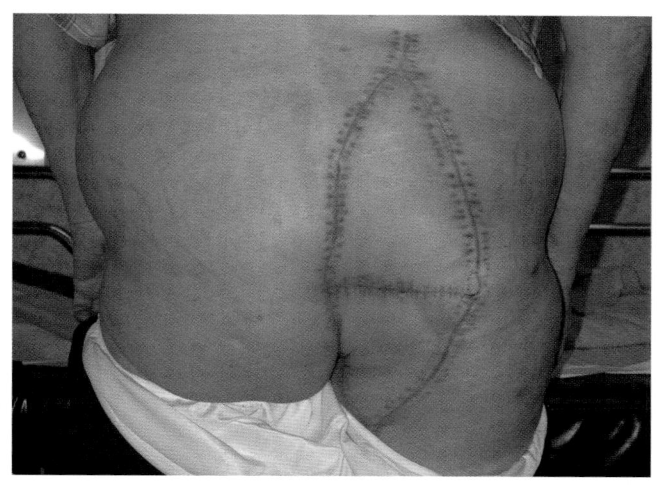

• **Fig. 34.5** The result at 5-week follow-up showing good healing of the gluteal wound after the flap reconstruction.

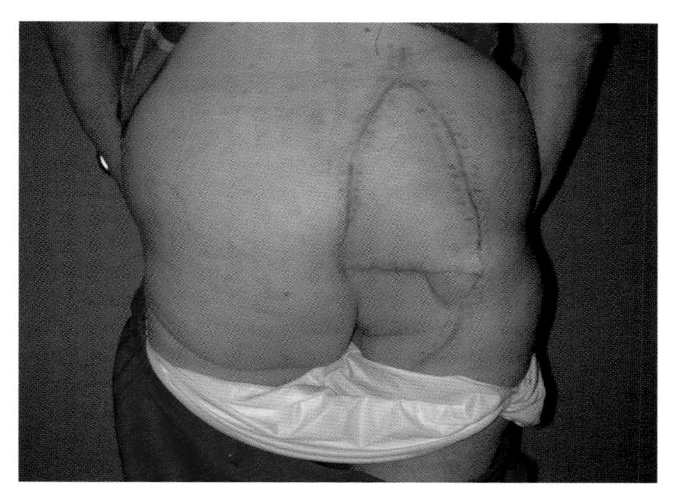

• **Fig. 34.6** The result at 4-month follow-up showing well-healed gluteal wound with minimal scarring and good contour after the flap reconstruction.

be a critical step toward the success of the wound closure. If indicated, adequate bony debridement should also be performed to remove all infected bones. A large posterior thigh fasciocutaneous rotation flap could be designed to close an ischial pressure wound. The flap should be designed long enough for it to be used again to rotate into the ischial defect if wound dehiscence occurs. In addition, a back cut can be done to facilitate the flap's rotation if perforators in the posterior thigh are identified. The proximal portion of the flap can be de-epithelialized and rotated into the wound to fill the dead space. Several retention sutures can be added to prevent sheer force of the flap closure.

Operative Procedures

Under general anesthesia with the patient in the prone position, the procedure started by excising the left ischial pressure sore. All visible or palpable fibrotic scar tissues and the bursa were excised down to normal-looking tissues at the base of the pressure sore

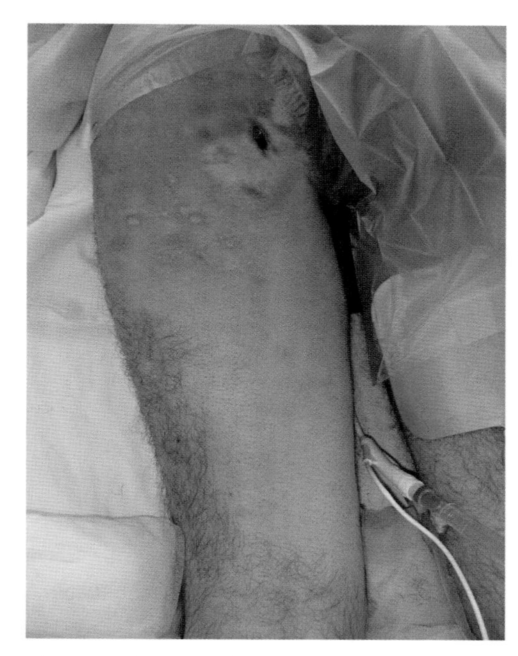

• **Fig. 34.7** Preoperative view showing a typical ischial pressure sore wound.

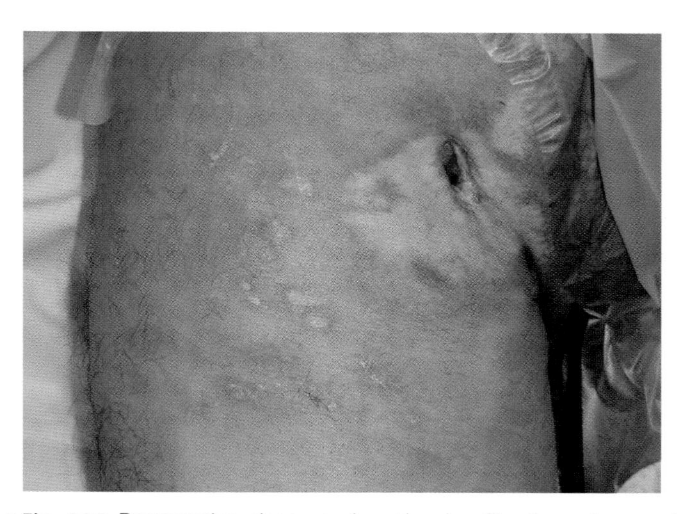

• **Fig. 34.8** Preoperative close-up view showing fibrotic and scarred tissues including a bursa around the open pressure sore wound.

wound. The curette was used to remove all residual bursa and colonized tissues. At this point, the orthopedic service was involved to complete all necessary bony debridement of the ischium. The wound was irrigated with Pulsavac and hemostasis was carefully controlled with placement of several 2-0 PDS sutures (Fig. 34.9).

A large posterior thigh fasciocutaneous rotation flap was designed and marked (Fig. 34.10). Two perforators were mapped by a Doppler. All proposed incisions were infiltrated with local anesthetic with epinephrine. The flap was elevated along the subfascial plane and inferiorly to the mid and lower third of the thigh. The fasciocutaneous flap was elevated off the gluteal muscle first and then off the posterior thigh muscles. Adequate elevation was accomplished and all two perforators in the posterior thigh

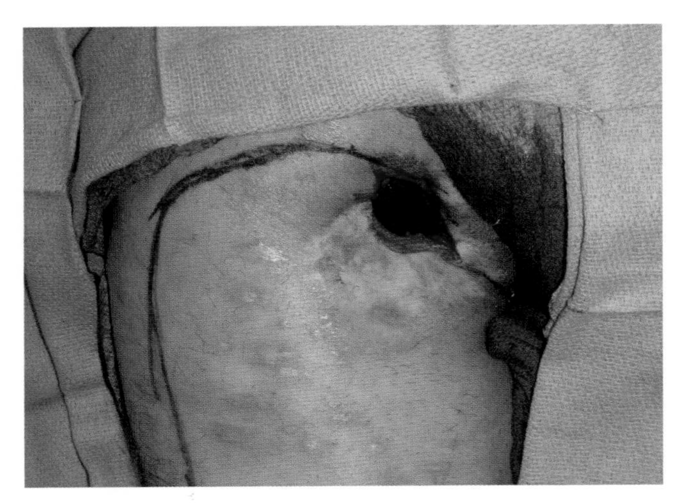

• **Fig. 34.9** Intraoperative view showing the appearance of the fresh pressure sore wound after adequate debridement.

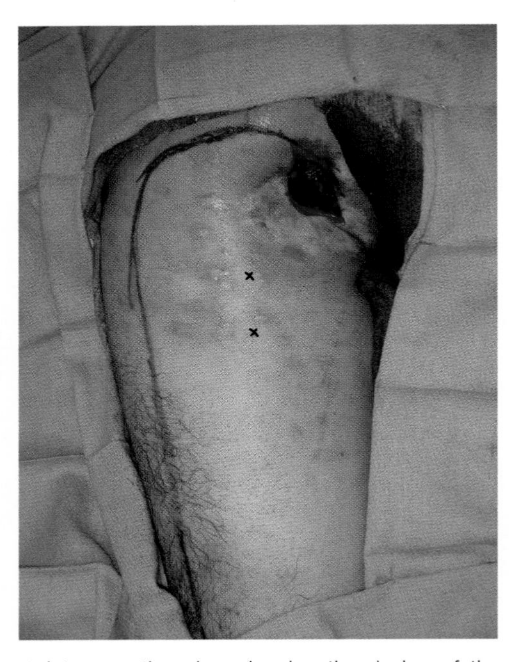

• **Fig. 34.10** Intraoperative view showing the design of the posterior thigh fasciocutaneous rotation flap for potential ischial pressure sore wound coverage. Two perforators were identified and marked.

were preserved. The flap could easily be rotated into the ischial wound without any tension.

The proximal portion of the flap was de-epithelialized. The part of the flap could be folded into the ischial pressure sore wound to fill the entire dead space and secured with several interrupted 2-0 PDS sutures (Fig. 34.11). The rest of the flap closure was performed in three layers. The deep tissue closure was approximated with several 2-0 PDS sutures in an interrupted fashion. The deep dermal closure was approximated with several interrupted 3-0 Monocryl sutures. Prior to the completion of the flap closure, two 10-mm JP drains were inserted (one from the ischial area and one from the flap donor site).

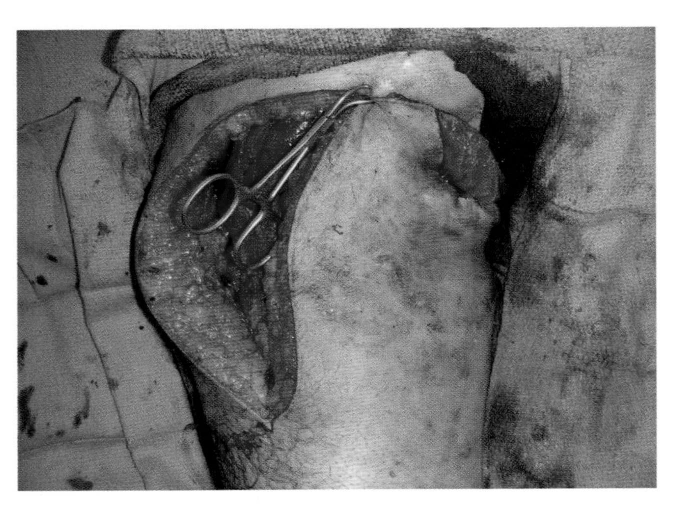

• **Fig. 34.11** Intraoperative view showing completion of the flap dissection. The proximal portion of the flap was de-epithelialized and easily rotated into the wound without tension. The posterior thigh non-flap tissue was undermined for closure of the flap's donor site.

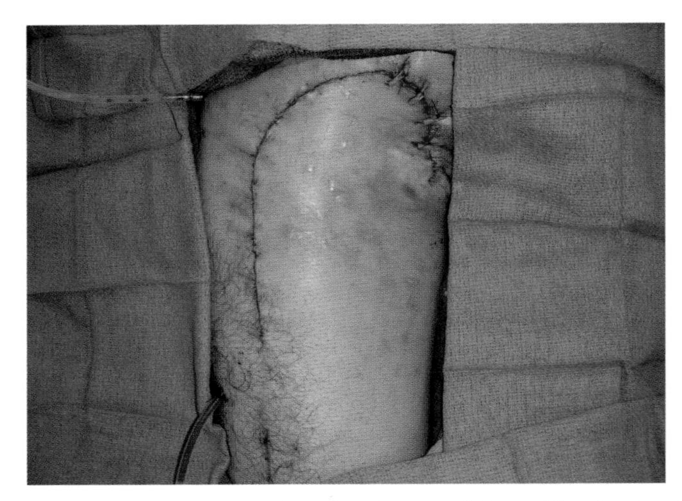

• **Fig. 34.12** Intraoperative view showing completion of the flap inset and closure including the flap's donor site closure.

Four retention sutures were placed at the critical part of the flap closure. The final closure of the rest of the flap was performed. The flap's donor site was closed primarily after some undermining of the posterior thigh nonflap tissue. The deep dermal closure was approximated with several interrupted 3-0 Monocryl sutures. The final skin closure was performed with a 3-0 V-Loc suture intradermally in a running fashion (Fig. 34.12).

Follow-Up Results

Postoperatively, the patient was placed in a special bed in the right lateral decubitus position. The patient did well without any issues related to the posterior thigh fasciocutaneous rotation flap surgery. He was discharged from hospital on postoperative day 14. Drains and retention sutures were removed during subsequent follow-up visits. The ischial pressure sore wound healed well.

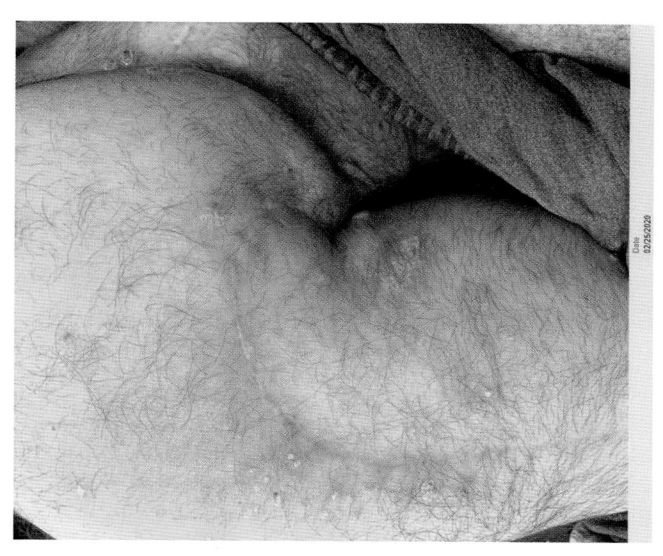

• **Fig. 34.13** The result at 6-month follow-up showing well-healed ischial pressure sore wound with good contour and minimal scarring after the flap reconstruction.

Final Outcome

The ischial pressure sore wound after debridement and the posterior thigh fasciocutaneous rotation flap reconstruction healed well with minimal scarring (Fig. 34.13). The patient has had no recurrent infection, seroma, or wound breakdown. He remains free from pressure sores and has resumed his normal activities. He has been followed by the plastic surgery service as needed.

Pearls for Success

A posterior thigh fasciocutaneous rotation flap is a workhorse for soft tissue reconstruction of an ischial pressure sore after adequate soft tissue and bony debridements. The flap can be designed, based on mapped posterior thigh perforators, as a large rotation flap with a possible back cut to facilitate wound closure. In addition, the flap can be elevated and used again to cover an ischial wound if the initial flap closure is failed. If necessary, the flap can be elevated even more as long as the perforator is preserved during the flap dissection. It should be elevated as a fasciocutaneous flap because the inclusion of the fascia may enhance blood supply of the flap. The flap can be reliable and the final contour after flap reconstruction can be quite good. It has replaced all other myocutaneous flaps in the area to become the first choice for soft tissue coverage in the ischial region, especially a pressure sore wound. The flap donor site can usually be closed primarily without the need for a skin graft.

Recommended Readings

Djedovic G, Morandi EM, Metzler J, et al. The posterior thigh flap for defect coverage of ischial pressure sores—a critical single-centre analysis. *Int Wound J*. 2017;14:1154–1159.

Friedman JD, Reece GR, Eldor L. The utility of the posterior thigh flap for complex pelvic and perineal reconstruction. *Plast Reconstr Surg*. 2010;126:146–155.

Legemate CM, Van der Kwaak M, Gobets D, Huikeshoven M, Van Zuijlen PPM. The pedicled internal pudendal artery perforator (PIPAP) flap for ischial pressure sore reconstruction: technique and long-term outcome of a cohort study. *J Plast Reconstr Aesthet Surg*. 2018;71:889–894.

Ordenana C, Pozza ED, Rampazzo A, et al. Wide posterior gluteal-thigh propeller flap for reconstruction of perineal defects. *Microsurgery*. 2021;41:146–156.

Pu LLQ. Reconstruction of a large gluteal soft-tissue defect with the double opposing V-Y fasciocutaneous advancement flap. *Plast Reconstr Surg*. 2007;119:599–603.

Sinnott CJ, Stavrides S, Boutros C, Kuruvilla A, Glickman LT. Dual-plane gluteal myocutaneous flap for reconstruction of ischial tuberosity pressure wounds. *Ann Plast Reconstr Surg*. 2020;85(S1 Suppl 1):S23–S27.

Yang CH, Kuo YR, Jeng SF, Lin PY. An ideal method for pressure sore reconstruction. *Ann Plast Surg*. 2011;66:179–184.

35 Perineal Reconstruction

Clinical Presentation

A 34-year-old White male was diagnosed with advanced rectal cancer and had been scheduled for an abdominoperineal resection (APR) by the colorectal service. Because his perineal resection could be extensive with a potential dead space within the pelvic cavity, the plastic surgery service was asked to perform a perineal reconstruction with a filling of the flap tissue into the pelvic cavity after an APR. In the operating room, an APR was completed by the colorectal service, which left a 10 × 6 cm perineal defect (Fig. 35.1).

Operative Plan and Special Considerations

A vertical rectus abdominis myocutaneous (VRAM) flap can be a classic option for a patient's perineal soft tissue reconstruction with the soft tissue filling of the dead space within the pelvic cavity. With proper design, the flap can carry a large skin paddle but only sacrifice a small amount of the anterior rectus sheath if perforators can be identified and incorporated within the skin paddle. The flap can be completely elevated and tunneled through the pelvis to fill the dead space within the pelvic cavity and be brought out for perineal soft tissue reconstruction. If only a small amount of the anterior rectus sheath is harvested with the flap, the actual fascial defect can be closed primarily and no mesh is needed for the abdominal donor site closure.

Operative Procedures

Under general anesthesia with the patient in the lithotomy position, the perineal wound was assessed after an APR procedure was completed by the colorectal service. It measured 10 × 6 cm and communicated with the pelvic cavity. A 12 × 6 cm skin paddle was designed and two perforators within the skin paddle were confirmed by a handheld Doppler (Fig. 35.2). The maximum width of the skin paddle could be estimated by a skin pinch test. The proposed incision was infiltrated with 1% lidocaine with 1:100,000 epinephrine.

The procedure was started by making a skin incision of the skin paddle down to the anterior rectus sheath. By further dissection toward the midline, the anterior rectus sheath was incised. The rectus abdominus muscle was identified. The dissection was performed to free the lateral boarder of the left rectus abdominus muscle and each tendinous intersection was also dissected free. Several tacking sutures were used to attach the muscle to the skin paddle. At this point, the muscle close to the xiphoid was divided with electrocautery and care was taken to control the superior epigastric vessels completely. The muscle and its skin paddle was elevated from the posterior rectus sheath and the dissection was done toward the pedicle. During dissection, the inferior epigastric vessels were identified and dissected free toward to the inguinal area. The inferior insertion of the muscle was completely divided while the pedicle vessels were well protected. The entire flap was tunneled through the pelvis and brought out to the perineal area. The proximal portion of the flap was de-epithelialized after it was placed back on the abdomen (Fig. 35.3). The flap was again tunneled through the pelvis and inset into the perineal area without any tension.

The final closure of the perineal wound was performed next. A large drain was placed within the pelvic cavity. The deep tissue closure was approximated with several interrupted 2-0 PDS sutures. The skin was closed with 3-0 Monocryl in an interrupted half-buried horizontal mattress fashion. Four retention sutures were placed (two on each side) (Fig. 35.4). At the end of the procedure, the skin paddle appeared to be well perfused with a good Doppler signal. The patient remained in the operating room for a colostomy and abdominal incision closure by the colorectal service.

Follow-Up Results

The patient did well postoperatively without any complications related to the VRAM flap for the perineal reconstruction. He was discharged from hospital on postoperative day 7. Drains were removed during subsequent follow-up visits. All retention sutures were removed 3 weeks postoperatively. His perineal wound healed well (Fig. 35.5).

Final Outcome

The perineal wound after the VRAM flap reconstruction healed well with minimal scarring (Fig. 35.6). The patient underwent postoperative radiation to his perineal area. There has been no evidence of seroma or wound breakdown. The abdominal flap

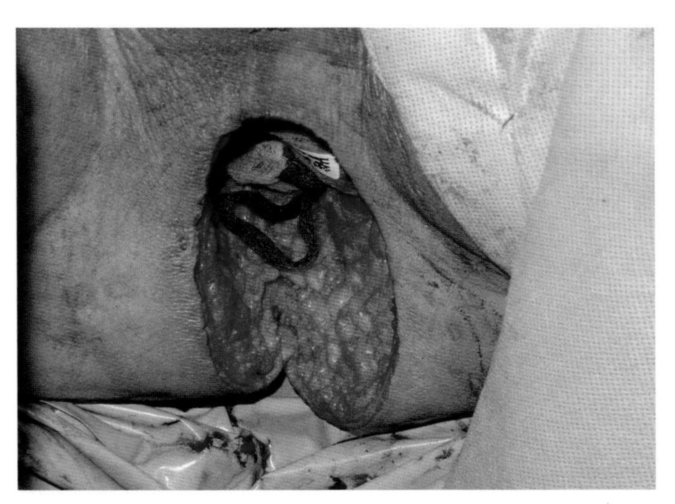

• **Fig. 35.1** Preoperative view showing a large, 10 × 6 cm, perineal soft tissue defect after an abdominoperineal resection procedure with direct communication to the pelvic cavity.

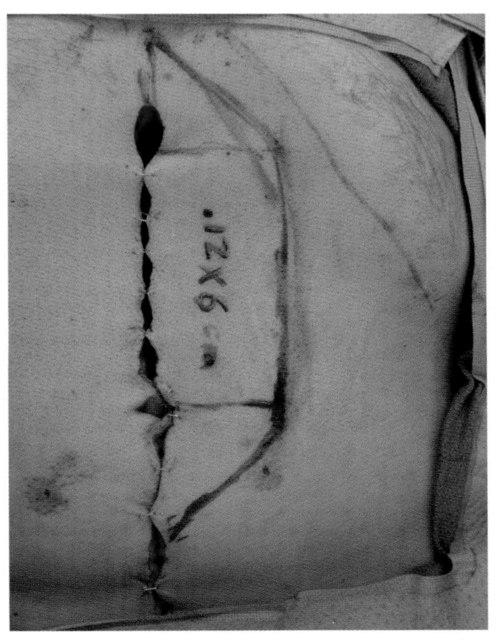

• **Fig. 35.2** Intraoperative view showing the design of the left vertical rectus abdominus myocutaneous flap for perineal wound coverage.

donor site also healed well and there was no evidence of a ventral hernia (Fig. 35.7). The patient remains cancer-free and has resumed his normal activities (Fig. 35.8). He has been routinely followed by the colorectal service for .

Pearls for Success

A VRAM flap is a classic choice for a large perineal wound reconstruction. The flap is usually harvested from the left abdomen if a colostomy can be placed on the right abdomen. The design of the skin paddle can be determined by the size of the perineal defect but should usually be slightly large. The maximum width of the skin paddle can be estimated by a skin pinch test. If

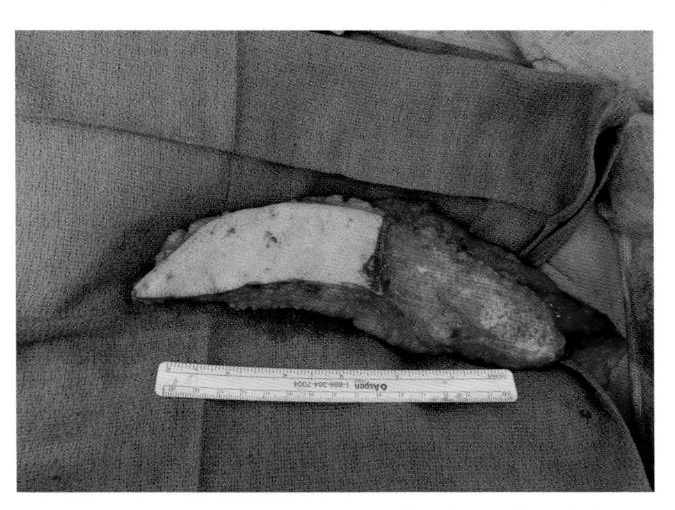

• **Fig. 35.3** Intraoperative view showing the elevated vertical rectus abdominus myocutaneous flap based on the inferior epigastric vessels. The proximal portion of the flap was de-epithelialized.

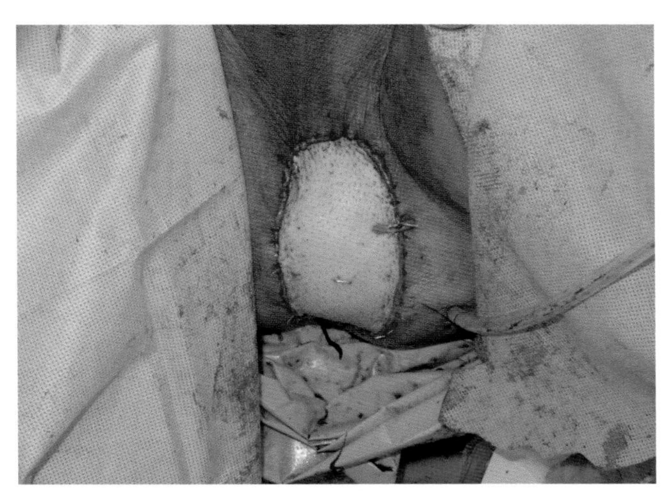

• **Fig. 35.4** Intraoperative view showing completion of the flap inset. The perineal wound was closed using the skin paddle of the vertical rectus abdominus myocutaneous flap.

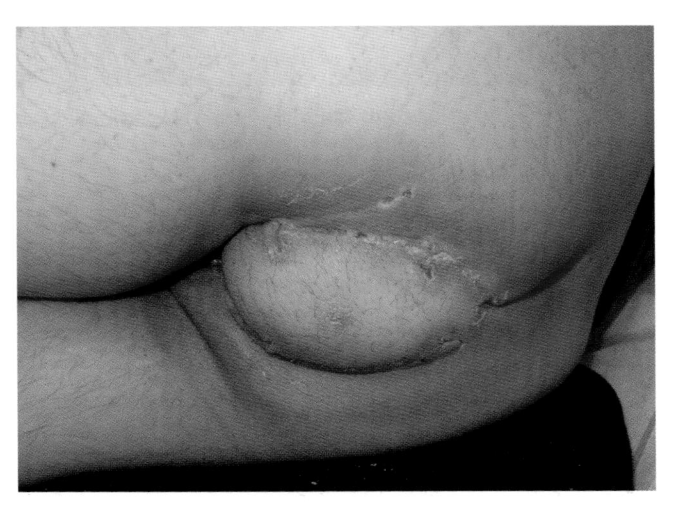

• **Fig. 35.5** The result at 4-week follow-up showing good healing of the vertical rectus abdominus myocutaneous flap for the perineal wound closure.

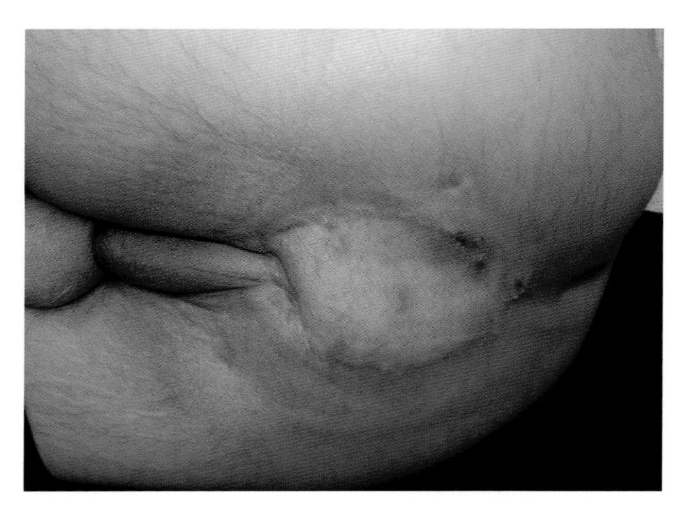

• **Fig. 35.6** The result at 3-month follow-up showing well-healed perineal wound after the vertical rectus abdominus myocutaneous flap reconstruction.

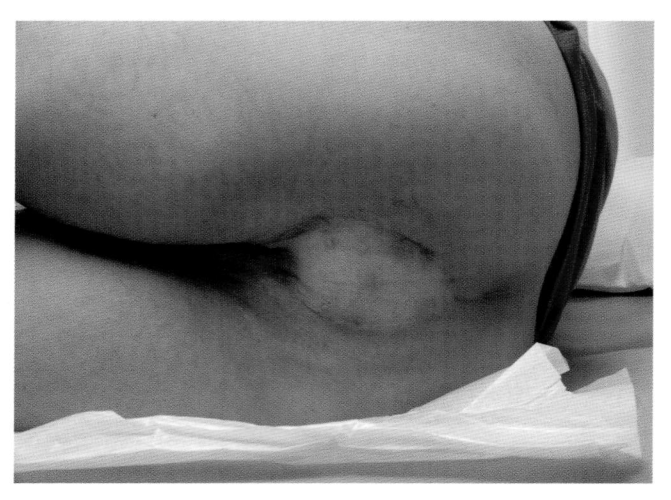

• **Fig. 35.8** The result at 6-month follow-up showing well-healed perineal wound after the vertical rectus abdominus myocutaneous flap reconstruction with minimal scarring and good contour.

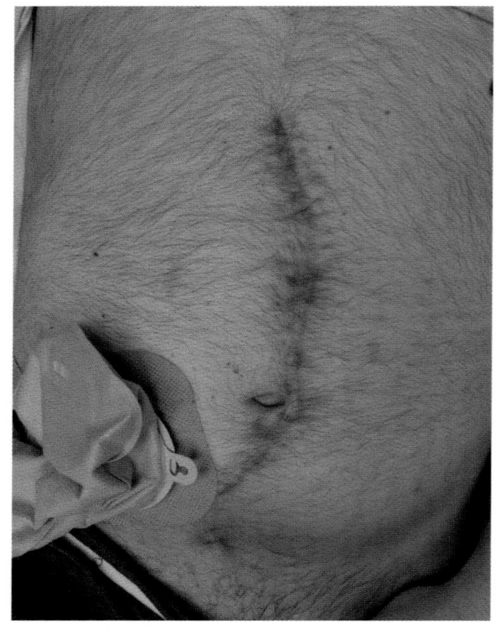

• **Fig. 35.7** The result at 3-month follow-up showing well-healed abdominal flap donor site after the vertical rectus abdominus myocutaneous flap reconstruction.

one or two perforators, especially periumbilical ones, can be identified and mapped, the actual need of the fascial defect can be reduced significantly so that the primary approximation of the fascial defect can be achieved without difficulty. No mash is ever needed for the fascial closure. When dividing the origin of the rectus abdominis muscle near the suprapubic area, a small portion of the muscle attachment can be preserved so that the trauma to the pedicle vessels during the flap tunnel can be minimized. Retention sutures should be added to the final flap closure because the wound dehiscence in the perineal area is extremely common due to sheer force. If wound dehiscence occurs, delayed primary closure should be attempted as long as the tissue condition permits.

Recommended Readings

Butler CE, Gündeslioglu AO, Rodriguez-Bigas MA. Outcomes of immediate vertical rectus abdominis myocutaneous flap reconstruction for irradiated abdominoperineal resection defects. *J Am Coll Surg*. 2008;206:694–703.

Myers PL, Krasniak PJ, Day SJ, Bossert RP. Gluteal flaps revisited: technical modifications for perineal wound reconstruction. *Ann Plast Surg*. 2019;82:667–670.

Özkaya Ö, Ergan Şahin A, Üsçetin İ, Güven H, Sağlam F. Immediate perineal reconstruction after extralevatory abdominoperineal excision: buried desepidermised fasciocutaneous V-Y advancement flap. *Ann Plast Surg*. 2018;80:154–158.

Sinna R, Qassemyar Q, Benhaim T, et al. Perforator flaps: a new option in perineal reconstruction. *J Plast Reconstr Aesthet Surg*. 2010;63:e766–e774.

Weichman KE, Matros E, Disa JJ. Reconstruction of peripelvic oncologic defects. *Plast Reconstr Surg*. 2017;140:601e–612e.

36 Vulvar Reconstruction

Clinical Presentation

An 86-year-old White female underwent a wide local excision (WLE) for a vulvar squamous cell cancer (SCC) by the gynecologic oncology service. A 15 × 8-cm large soft tissue defect remained over the vulva down to the deep muscles and tissues. The plastic surgery service was asked to help to close this large vulvar wound once the WLE was confirmed to be adequate for a vulvar cancer surgical excision. Therefore, the definitive soft tissue reconstruction could be performed in the same setting immediately after oncological WLE of the vulvar SCC cancer (Fig. 36.1).

Operative Plan and Special Considerations

The shape and size of this vulvar soft tissue defect and availability of the adjacent normal perineal and thigh skin determine that bilateral V-to-Y skin advancement flaps could be designed to close the defect after complex closure for direct approximation for both superior and inferior aspects of the defect based on an intraoperative decision. The closure with such bilateral V-to-Y advancement flaps may provide a relatively simple reconstruction with almost no donor site problems. It would be a better option than a skin graft procedure for durable vulvar soft tissue reconstruction. Wound separation after any flap reconstruction is common in this location and the patient should be well informed about such a complication.

Operative Procedures

Under general anesthesia, the patient was placed in the lithotomy position and the vulva soft tissue defect was assessed. A Folly catheter was placed prior to surgical excision. The superior and inferior areas of the defect could be closed after simple skin undermining. Bilateral skin V-to-Y advancement flaps were designed and the skin marking was extended to the proximal thigh. The extent of the flap dissection was outlined for each side (Fig. 36.2).

Each side of the skin flap was incised and elevated toward the midline and approximated temporarily in a V-to-Y fashion. Care should be taken to maintain adequate attachment of the skin flap to the deep tissue. Once a surgical dissection for each skin V-to-Y advancement flap had been completed, both flaps could be sutured together in the midline for final wound closure.

For deep tissue closure in the midline, such an approximation was performed with interrupted 3-0 PDS sutures. The rest of the deep dermal closure for the entire V-to-Y flaps was performed with interrupted 3-0 Monocryl sutures. All skin closure was done with running 3-0 chromic sutures except around the urethra and vagina, where interrupted 3-0 Vicryl sutures were used (Fig. 36.3).

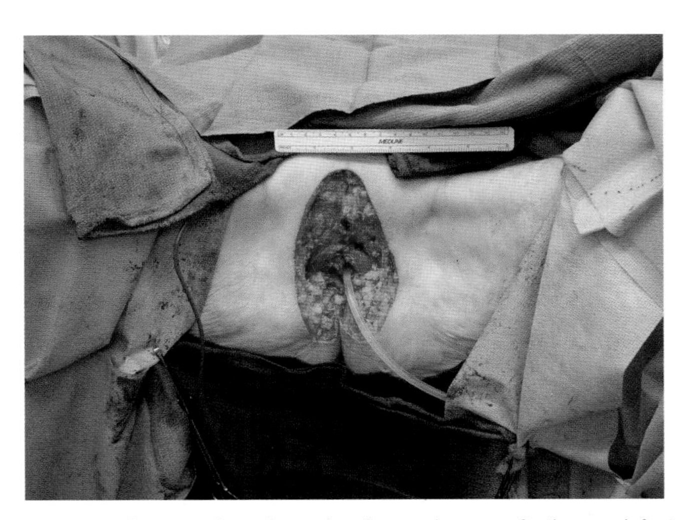

• **Fig. 36.1** Preoperative view showing a large soft tissue defect, measuring 15 × 8 cm, in the midline vulva down to the deep muscles and tissues after a wide local excision for squamous cell cancer.

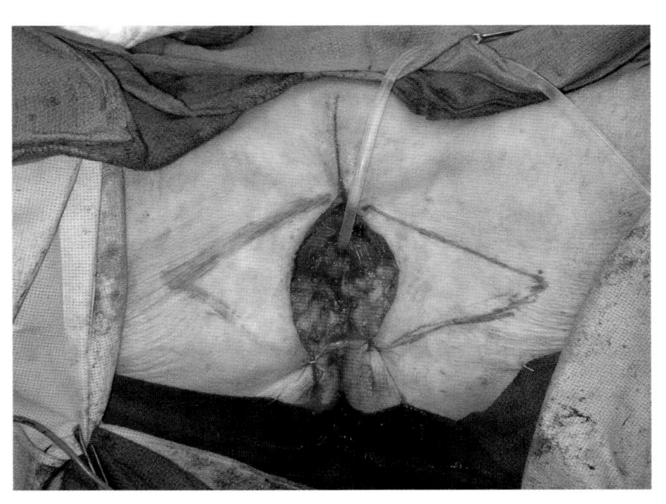

• **Fig. 36.2** Intraoperative view showing the design of bilateral V-to-Y skin advancement flaps after approximation of the upper and lower aspects of the wound.

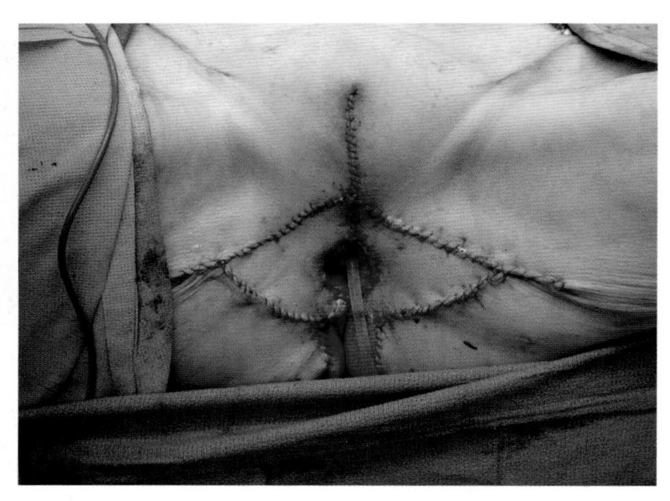

• **Fig. 36.3** Intraoperative view showing completion of bilateral V-to-Y skin advancement flaps for closure of this large vulvar soft tissue defect. The superior and inferior aspects of the wound were closed after undermining.

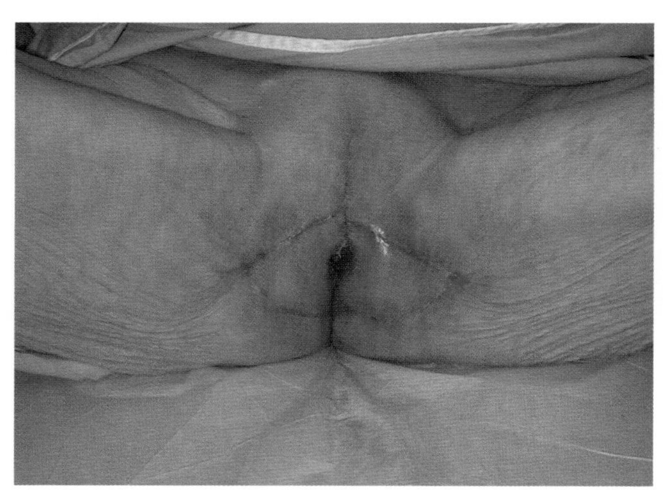

• **Fig. 36.4** The result at 4-week follow-up showing stable and well-healed vulvar wound with good contour and minimal scarring.

Follow-Up Results

The patient did well postoperatively without any complications related to the bilateral skin V-Y advancement flaps for the vulvar wound closure. She was discharged from hospital on postoperative day 5. The Folly catheter was removed postoperatively during the 2-week follow-up visit. The vulvar wound healed well and there was no wound dehiscence or necrosis of the flap (Fig. 36.4).

Final Outcome

After bilateral V-to-Y skin advancement flaps for soft tissue reconstruction the vulvar wound healed well. Most importantly, the patient has had durable soft tissue coverage with minimal scarring and no contour issues in either flap site. She has resumed her normal activities and has routinely been followed by the gynecological oncology service.

Pearls for Success

A large vulvar soft tissue defect after vulvectomy for cancer would need a skin flap rather than a skin graft for more durable soft tissue reconstruction. As demonstrated in this case, bilateral V-to-Y skin advancement flaps can be designed and used to close such a large defect. Some of the areas in this large soft tissue defect can be closed after simple skin undermining. The excess thigh skin can be incorporated into the V-shaped skin flap design. Adequate release of the skin flap to the base of the flap should be done to enable adequate advancement of the flap. With advanced knowledge for a free-style local perforator flap, the V-shaped skin flap can be dissected freely based on the location of the perforator. The moderate amount of tension for the midline approximation in this location may be tolerable for young and healthy patients but should be avoided for older patients or smokers. If performed correctly, bilateral V-to-Y skin advancement flaps can be a relatively straightforward operation for a large vulvar soft tissue reconstruction.

Recommended Readings

Gentileschi S, Servillo M, Garganese G, et al. Surgical therapy of vulvar cancer: how to choose the correct reconstruction? *J Gynecol Oncol.* 2016;27:e60.

Huang JJ, Chang NJ, Chou HH, et al. Pedicle perforator flaps for vulvar reconstruction—new generation of less invasive vulvar reconstruction with favorable results. *Gynecol Oncol.* 2015;137:66–72.

Lazzaro L, Guarneri GF, Rampino Cordaro E, et al. Vulvar reconstruction using a "V-Y" fascio-cutaneous gluteal flap: a valid reconstructive alternative in post-oncological loss of substance. *Arch Gynecol Obstet.* 2010;282:521–527.

O'Dey DM, Bozkurt A, Pallua N. The anterior obturator artery perforator (aOAP) flap: surgical anatomy and application of a method for vulvar reconstruction. *Gynecol Oncol.* 2010;119:526–530.

Salgarello M, Farallo E, Barone-Adesi L, et al. Flap algorithm in vulvar reconstruction after radical, extensive vulvectomy. *Ann Plast Surg.* 2005;54:184–190.

Zeng A, Qiao Q, Zhao R, Song K, Long X. Anterolateral thigh flap-based reconstruction for oncologic vulvar defects. *Plast Reconstr Surg.* 2011; 127:1939–1945.

37 Vaginal Reconstruction

Clinical Presentation

A 68-year-old Asian woman had radiation therapy for early-stage cervical cancer about 40 years ago in Asia and remained cancer free for a long time but unfortunately developed recurrent cervical cancer. She was offered an anterior pelvic exenteration by the gynecological oncology service and an ileal conduit by the urology service. The plastic surgery service was asked to perform a vaginal reconstruction after anterior pelvic exenteration and ileal conduit. She was prepared for multiple surgical procedures in the same setting by three surgical services, each performing a specialty procedure for an optimal outcome (Fig. 37.1).

Operative Plan and Special Considerations

A vertical rectus abdominis myocutaneous (VRAM) flap is a classic option for vaginal reconstruction and soft tissue filling of the dead space within the pelvic cavity. With an appropriate design, the flap can carry a sizable skin paddle for the vaginal reconstruction but only sacrifice a small amount of the anterior rectus sheath if perforators can be identified and incorporated within the skin paddle. The flap can be completely elevated and tunneled through the pelvis to fill the dead space within the pelvic cavity and a reconstructed vagina, formed by folding the skin paddle of the flap into a tube, can be brought out for closure of the perineal wound at the same time. If a smaller amount of the anterior rectus sheath is harvested with the flap, the actual fascial defect can be closed and no mesh is needed for the abdominal donor site closure.

Operative Procedures

Under general anesthesia with the patient in the lithotomy position, anterior pelvic exenteration was completed by the gynecological oncology service through a midline laparotomy. After careful assessment of the left abdominal wall including the left inferior epigastric vessels, a left VRAM flap was performed as planned. Two perforators were identified with a hand-held Doppler and marked and incorporated within the skin paddle design of the flap. A 10 × 10 cm skin paddle was designed from the midline based on the pinch test and potential excess skin for the closure of the abdomenal skin defect was incorporated with the skin paddle design (Fig. 37.2). The skin paddle was incised down to the anterior rectus sheath. The suprafascial dissection was performed to identify the perforators. In this way, only a small portion of the anterior rectus sheath was sacrificed during the flap elevation.

Further dissection was performed to free the muscle more proximally and the superior rectus abdominis muscle was divided with electrocautery. The muscle flap was elevated from the posterior rectus sheath. During dissection, several intercostal nerves were identified and divided with hemoclips. Inferiorly, the muscle was dissected free toward its insertion. The muscle flap was then completely elevated based on the inferior epigastric vessels (Fig. 37.3A). The anterior rectus sheath was tacked to the subcutaneous tissue with 3-0 Vicryl sutures to prevent shear force (Fig. 37.3B). The pedicle dissection was performed within the pelvis under direct vision. The entire flap was easily turned over and tunneled through the pelvic cavity and brought out in the perineal opening without any tension.

The new vagina was then created using the skin paddle of the flap. With a 3-cm diameter stand, a spiral type of closure was performed to form a new vaginal canal (Fig. 37.4). This was done in two layers. The deep tissue layer was approximated with several interrupted 2-0 Vicryl sutures in figure-of-eight fashion and the skin was approximated with several interrupted 2-0 Vicryl sutures (Fig. 37.5). The proximal end of the reconstructed vagina was approximated with 2-0 Vicryl sutures, once again in two layers (Fig. 37.6). The entire flap was tunneled through the pelvis and brought out in the perineal opening (Fig. 37.7). Two 15-Fr Blake drains were inserted in the pelvis and brought out in the buttock area. At this point, the urology service started the ileal conduit procedure through the right abdomen.

Once the urology service had finished their part of the procedure, the final abdominal incision closure and the inset of the new vagina were performed. The opening of the new vagina was defatted under direct vision to reduce the bulk and maintain a good size of the new vaginal lumen. After adequate defatting, the final closure of the perineal opening was done with 2-0 Vicryl sutures in interrupted half-buried horizontal mattress fashion. The closure was completed and a nearly watertight closure was performed from the skin edge of the flap within the perineal opening. Several additional layers of the closure were placed with 2-0 Vicryl sutures in simple interrupted fashion (Fig. 37.8). A Xeroform gauze was inserted into the new vagina and served as a stent (Fig. 37.9).

The abdominal midline incision closure was performed next. The omentum was used to cover the intestine evenly. In the midline lower abdomen, the posterior rectus sheath was approximated with a 0-Metzenbaum suture in simple running fashion. The anterior rectus sheath was also approximated to the midline anterior rectus sheath with a 0-Metzenbaum suture in a simple running fashion. In the upper abdomen where the skin paddle was harvested, significant undermining was performed laterally along

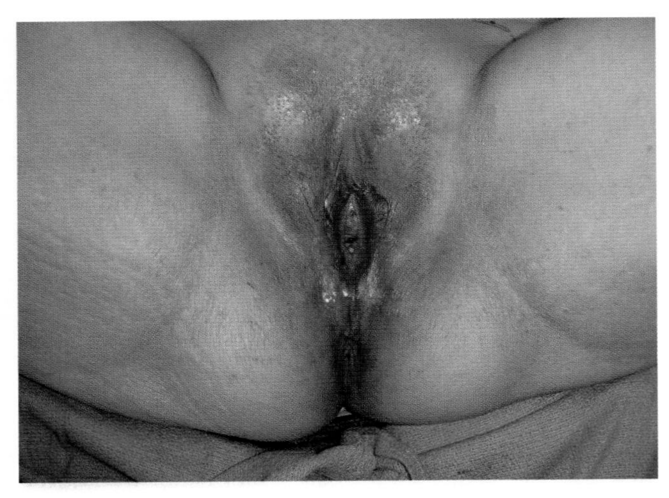

• **Fig. 37.1** Preoperative view showing a recurrent cervical cancer from a lithotomy position.

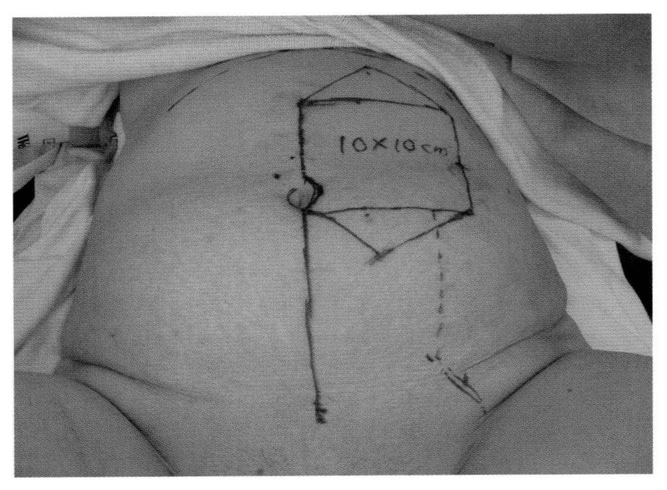

• **Fig. 37.2** Intraoperative view showing the design of the left vertical rectus abdominus myocutaneous flap for the vaginal reconstruction.

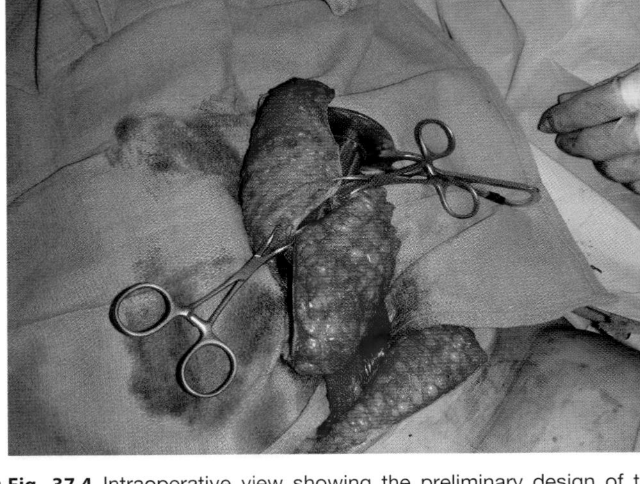

• **Fig. 37.4** Intraoperative view showing the preliminary design of the flap's skin paddle closure in a spiral fashion for the vaginal reconstruction.

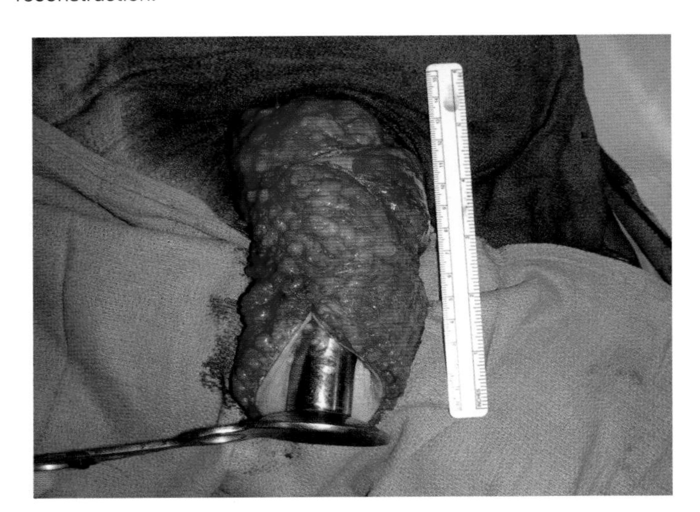

• **Fig. 37.5** Intraoperative view showing the approximation of the flap's skin paddle in a spiral fashion for the vaginal reconstruction.

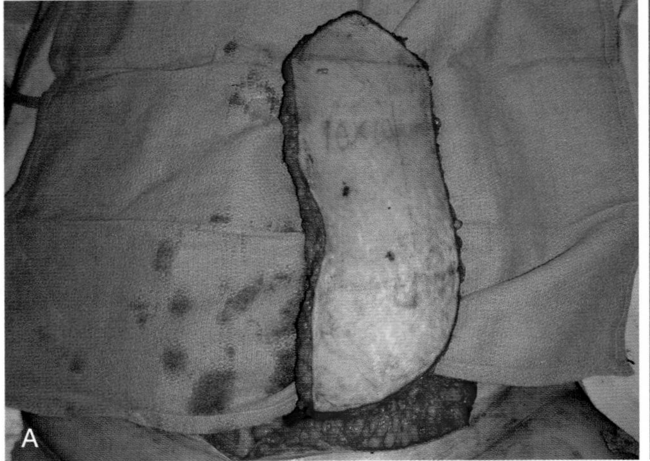

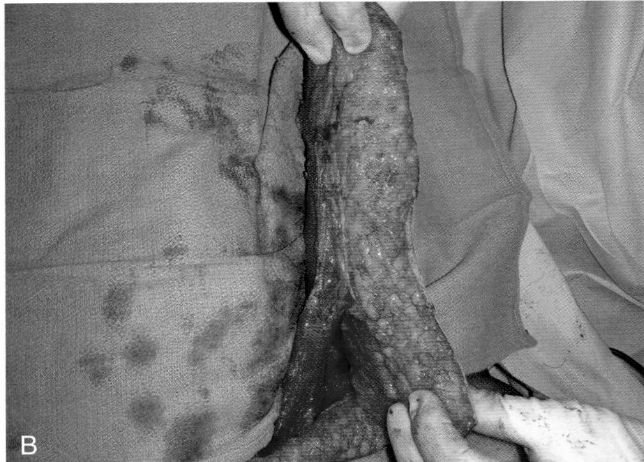

• **Fig. 37.3** (A) Intraoperative view showing the elevated vertical rectus abdominis myocutaneous (VRAM) flap based on the inferior epigastric vessels. Based on the location of the perforators, minimal anterior rectus sheath could be harvested so that the fascial defect would not be significant. (B) Intraoperative view showing the elevated VRAM flap in a lateral view. The fascia was sutured to the subcutaneous tissue to prevent a shear force between the muscle and the skin paddle.

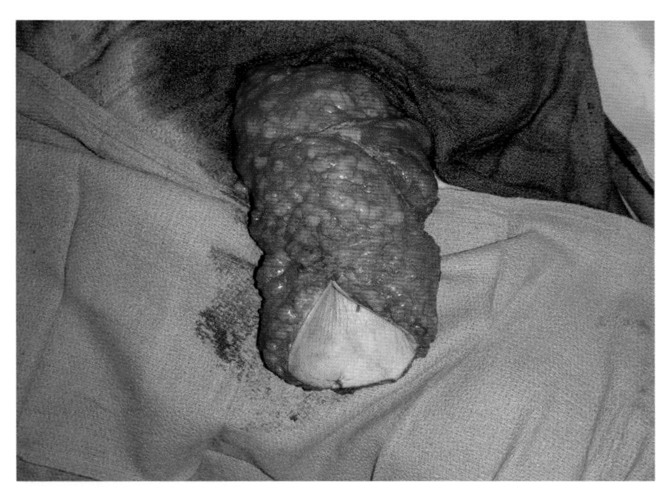

• **Fig. 37.6** Intraoperative view showing the completion of the vaginal closure from the flap's skin paddle for the vaginal reconstruction.

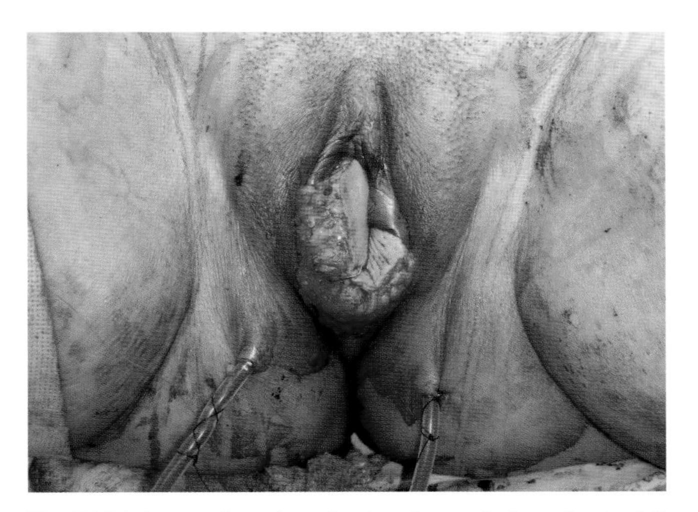

• **Fig. 37.7** Intraoperative view showing the preliminary inset of the reconstructed vagina in the perineal region.

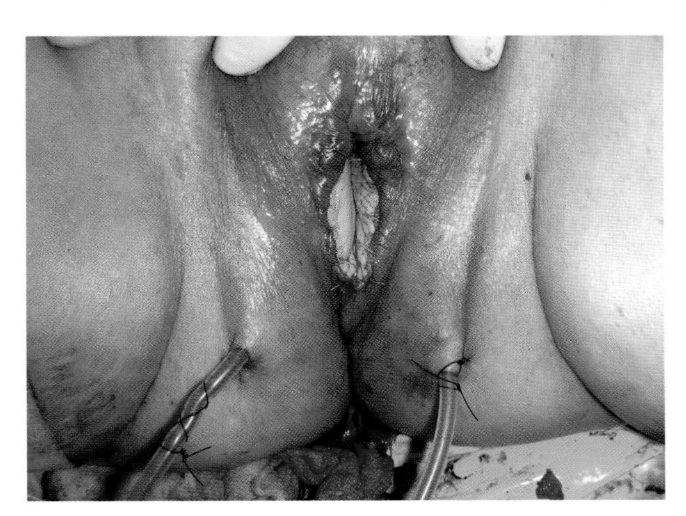

• **Fig. 37.8** Intraoperative view showing completion of the closure for the reconstructed vagina in the perineal region.

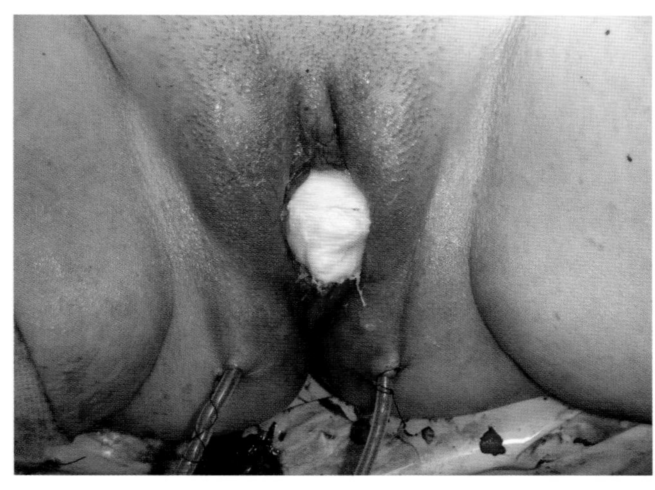

• **Fig. 37.9** Intraoperative view showing the placement of Xeroform as a stent inside the reconstructed vagina at the end of the procedure.

the suprafascial plane. The deep dermal closure was approximated with several interrupted 3-0 Monocryl sutures. A 10-mm flat JP was placed in the subcutaneous tissue pocket. The skin closure was approximated with skin staples.

Follow-Up Results

The patient did well postoperatively without any complications related to the VRAM flap for the vaginal reconstruction. She was discharged from hospital on postoperative day 5. Drains were removed during subsequent follow-up visits. The perineal wound and reconstructed vagina healed well. She also dilated the reconstructed vagina under the guidance of the gynecological oncology service (Fig. 37.10). During longer follow-up, the newly reconstructed vagina looked quite good and all surgical services and the patient were satisfied with the outcome (Fig. 37.11).

In the subsequent long-term follow-up, the adequate size of the reconstructed vagina was maintained (Fig. 37.12). However, the patient complained about some protruding flap tissue from

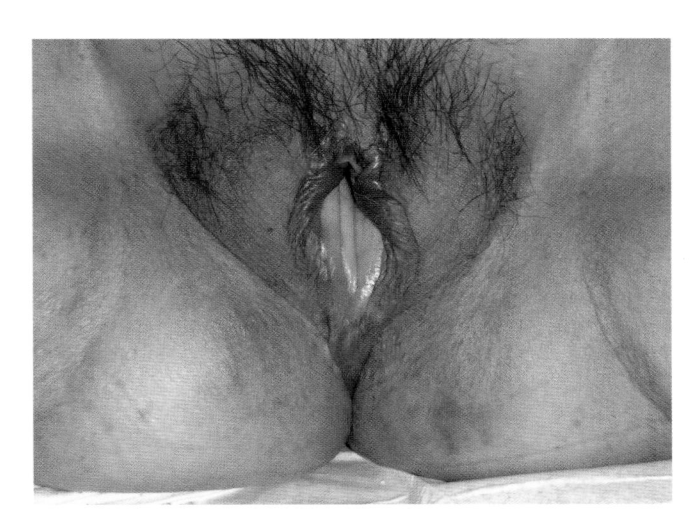

• **Fig. 37.10** The result at 2-month follow-up showing good healing of the vertical rectus abdominis myocutaneous flap for the vaginal reconstruction.

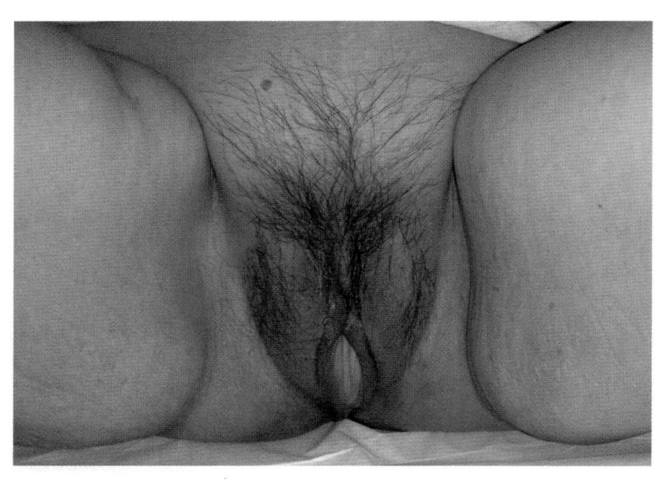

• **Fig. 37.11** The result at 11-month follow-up showing well-healed vertical rectus abdominis myocutaneous flap for the vaginal reconstruction.

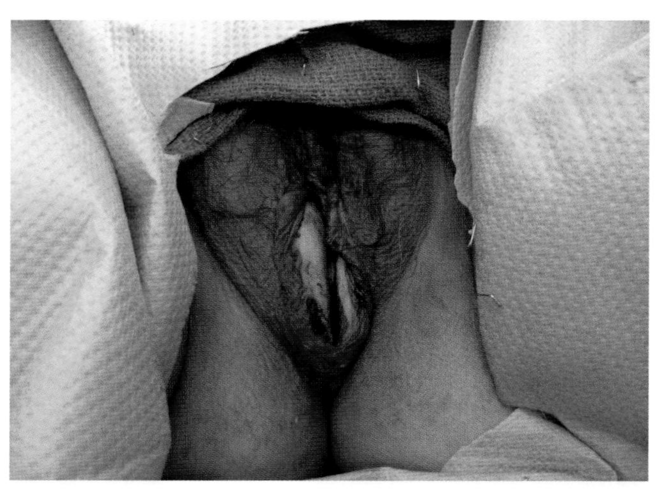

• **Fig. 37.13** Preoperative view at 18-month before revisional surgery showing excess tissues *(marked)* from the skin paddle of the flap.

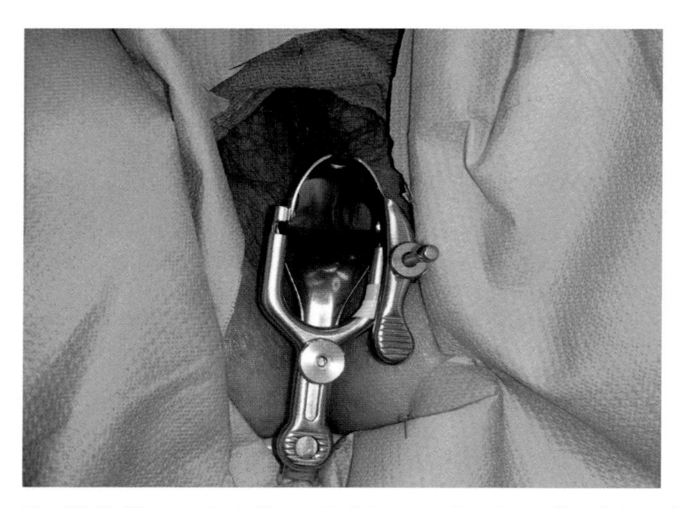

• **Fig. 37.12** The result at 18-month follow-up showing well-maintained size of the reconstructed vagina after the vertical rectus abdominis myocutaneous flap reconstruction.

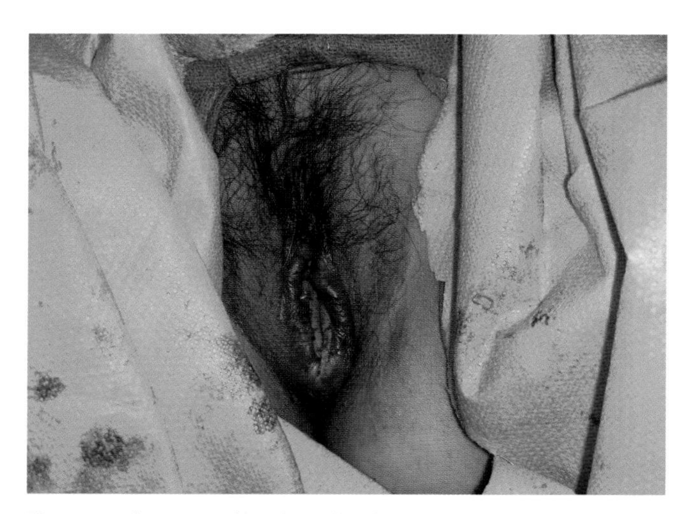

• **Fig. 37.14** Intraoperative view showing completion of the revisional surgery by excising excess tissues from the flap's skin paddle and closing with local tissue rearrangement.

the flap's skin paddle in the opening of the reconstructed vagina (Fig. 37.13). She was taken to the operating room and under general anesthesia, all excess tissues from the skin paddle were excised and the opening of the reconstructed vagina was closed with local tissue rearrangement (Fig. 37.14).

Final Outcome

The vaginal reconstruction with the VRAM flap healed well and the size of the new vagina has been maintained after revisional surgery to excise excess tissues from the flap's skin paddle. The patient has had minimal scarring in the perineal area and no evidence of wound breakdown or hypertrophic scar. The abdominal flap donor site also healed well and there is no evidence of the ventral hernia. She remains cancer-free and has resumed her normal activities including sexual intercourse. She has been routinely followed by the gynecological oncology service.

Pearls for Success

A VRAM flap is a classic choice for the vaginal reconstruction. The dead space in the pelvic cavity after anterior pelvic exenteration can be filled by the flap tissue but the skin paddle of the flap can be folded as a tube as a simultaneous vaginal reconstruction if the patient desires so. Therefore, the perineal defect can be closed after the flap's inset. The flap is usually harvested from the left abdomen if an ileostomy and/or colostomy are selected on the right abdomen. The design of the skin paddle can be determined by the size of required reconstructed vagina. The maximum width of the skin paddle can be estimated by a skin pinch test. However, the approximation of the flap's skin paddle in a spiral way as demonstrated in this case could limit the width of the skin paddle needed for a vaginal reconstruction so that the flap's donor site closure may be performed with less difficulty. If one or two perforators, especially periumbilical ones, can be identified and mapped, the actual size of the anterior fascial defect can be reduced significantly so that the primary approximation of the fascial defect can be accomplished without difficulty. If the actual fascial defect is not significant, no mash is needed for the fascial closure. When dividing the origin of the rectus abdominis muscle near the suprapubic area, a small portion of the muscle attachment can be preserved so that the trauma to the pedicle vessels during the flap tunneling can be minimized. Further revision after initial vaginal reconstruction may be needed for an optimal reconstructive outcome.

Recommended Readings

Pusic AL, Mehrara BJ. Vaginal reconstruction: an algorithm approach to defect classification and flap reconstruction. *J Surg Oncol.* 2006;94: 515–521.
Pusic AL, Mehrara BJ. Vaginal reconstruction: an algorithm approach to defect classification and flap reconstruction. *J Surg Oncol.* 2006;94: 515–521.
Rietjens M, Maggioni A, Bocciolone L, Sideri M, Youssef O, Petit JY. Vaginal reconstruction after extended radical pelvic surgery for cancer: comparison of two techniques. *Plast Reconstr Surg.* 2002;109:1592–1597.

Tobin GR, Day TG. Vaginal and pelvic reconstruction with distally based rectus abdominis myocutaneous flaps. *Plast Reconstr Surg.* 1988; 81:62–73.

Wang X, Qiao Q, Burd A, et al. A new technique of vaginal reconstruction with the deep inferior epigastric perforator flap: a preliminary report. *Plast Reconstr Surg.* 2007;119:1785–1790.

Yang B, Wang N, Zhang S, Wang M. Vaginal reconstruction with sigmoid colon in patients with congenital absence of vagina and menses retention: a report of treatment experience in 22 young women. *Int Urogynecol J.* 2013;24:155–160.

38 Penile Reconstruction

Clinical Presentation

A 14-year-old intersex White person had been born with ambiguous genitalia. The patient decided to be a male but unfortunately all male genital organs had been removed at a young age. The patient now strongly desired a transformation from female to male and was seen by the pediatric urology service for a total penile reconstruction (Fig. 38.1). The plastic surgery service was asked to perform a microvascular penile reconstruction in conjunction with the patient's entire surgical care for penile reconstruction.

Operative Plan and Special Considerations

There are several options with a microvascular flap for total penile reconstruction. Among them, free radial forearm flap or free fibular osteocutaneous flap is the common option. However, free fibular osteocutaneous flap can provide a total penile reconstruction without the need for a penile implant. In addition, urethral reconstruction can also be done within the flap to provide a more functional reconstructed penis. In this case, a two-stage reconstruction was planned. During the first stage, a prefabricated urethroplasty was designed and performed in the proposed free fibular osteocutaneous flap donor site so that urethral reconstruction could be accomplished first. The formal penile reconstruction was performed during the second stage and a free fibular osteocutaneous flap was dissected out and a reconstructed penis could be created. This type of penile reconstruction may prevent future implant extrusion that might be experienced after a free radial forearm flap for a total penile reconstruction. Preoperative arterial angiogram would be needed to make sure there was normal vascular anatomy of the selected lower leg for a free fibular osteocutaneous flap donor site.

Operative Procedures

For this patient, the total penile reconstruction was performed in two stages. During the first-stage procedure, a prefabricated urethroplasty was performed. Under general anesthesia with the patient in the supine position, a free fibular osteocutaneous flap was designed and marked in the left leg. Two perforators were identified by a handheld Doppler and marked. A 10 × 11 cm skin paddle was marked based on the location of the fibula and the two identified perforators. The location of the proposed new urethra was also marked (Fig. 38.2). A 15 × 2 cm full thickness skin graft was designed in the left groin and then harvested (Fig. 38.3). This full-thickness skin graft was sutured to form a tube over a rubber catheter with 3-0 Vicryl suture in a running fashion. This newly created urethra was buried under the skin within the skin paddle of the planned free fibular osteocutaneous flap (Fig. 38.4). The catheter remained in place and acted as a stent for the prefabricated urethral reconstruction.

Eleven months later, the patient underwent the second-stage procedure where the total penile reconstruction was performed. A suprapubic catheter was placed for urinary drainage. Under general anesthesia with the patient in the supine position, the free fibular osteocutaneous flap was marked including two septocutaneous perforators that were confirmed by a handheld Doppler scan. A catheter was easily passed through the prefabricated and reconstructed new urethra with the flap. A 10 × 11 cm of the skin paddle was again designed (Fig. 38.5).

The left free fibular osteocutaneous flap was harvested. Under tourniquet control, the skin paddle was incised down to the fascia. The suprafascial dissection was performed toward the posterior intermuscular septum. Two septocutaneous perforators were identified within the septum and carefully preserved. The dissection was performed to release the muscle attachment to the fibula from the soleus muscle. Once the peroneal vessels had been identified, the distal osteotomy was performed at a level of 6 cm proximal to the lateral malleolus. By further dissection of the hallucis longus muscle's attachment, the peroneal vessels and the fibula were dissected free. A longitudinal skin incision was extended further toward the fibular head and the proximal osteotomy was performed (Fig. 38.6). Following more dissection around the pedicle, the peroneal vessels were dissected free toward the bifurcation of the tibioperoneal trunk (Fig. 38.7).

At this point, the skin paddle was wrapped around the fibula and sutured in two layers with the appropriate amount of tension. The deep dermal closure was approximated with interrupted 3-0 Vicryl sutures and the skin was closed with 3-0 Vicryl suture in a simple running fashion (Fig. 38.8). Once the bifurcation was visualized, the pedicle was divided. A 12-cm segment of the fibula was obtained after additional proximal osteotomy and the flap's dissection was completed. The distal end of the flap was also approximated in two layers as for the other skin closure (Fig. 38.9).

The fibular osteocutaneous flap was inserted into the perineal area. The periosteum of the proximal fibula was sutured to the corpus cavernosum with 2-0 Prolene sutures in an interrupted fashion (Fig. 38.10). Once the superficial femoral artery and the femoral vein had been exposed through a groin skin incision, the pedicle vessels were tunneled subcutaneously. An end-to-side

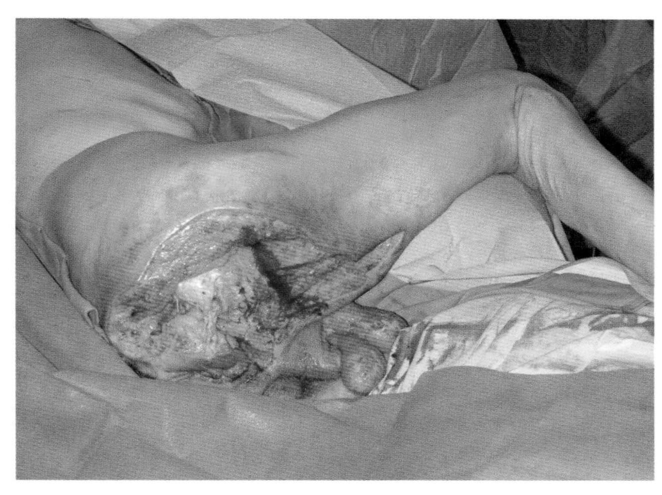

• **Fig. 39.1** A preoperative view showing large ischial, gluteal, and posterior thigh wounds as well as scrotal wounds after surgical debridement by the urology service.

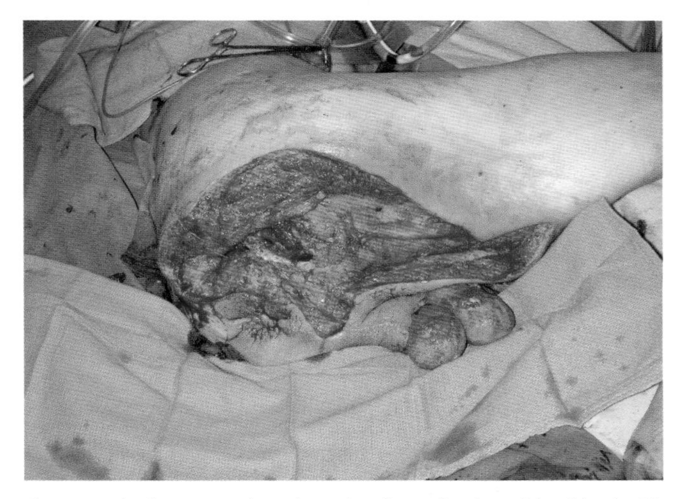

• **Fig. 39.2** An intraoperative view showing a fresh and healthy-looking wound after additional debridement by the plastic surgery service.

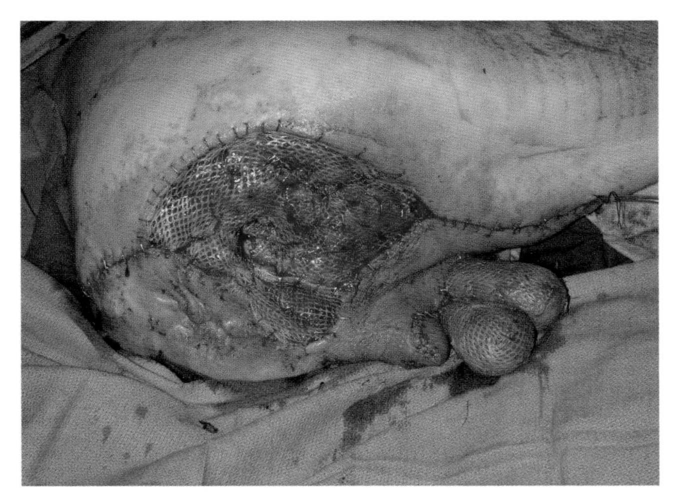

• **Fig. 39.3** Intraoperative view showing completion of the definitive soft tissue reconstruction of this extensive large wound with a combination of split-thickness skin graft and local tissue rearrangement for direct closure.

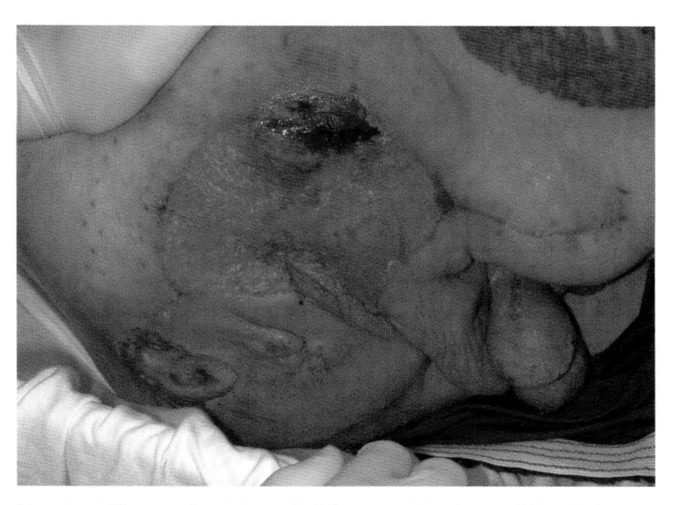

• **Fig. 39.4** The result at 4-week follow-up showing well-healed wound after definitive reconstruction with a combination of split-thickness skin graft and local tissue rearrangement for direct closure. The patient unfortunately developed a new pressure sore as shown.

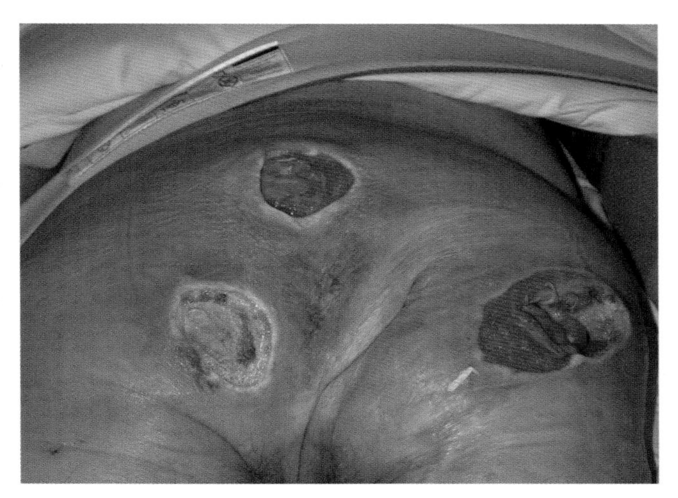

• **Fig. 39.5** The result at 4-month follow-up showing well-healed gluteal and posterior thigh wounds but newly developed pressure sores as an ongoing problem.

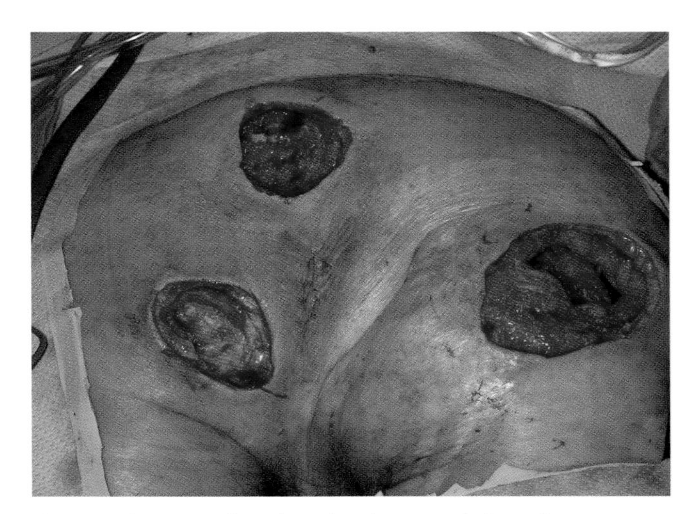

• **Fig. 39.6** Intraoperative view showing completion of new pressure sore debridement after further operation for this ongoing problem.

Recommended Readings

Chen SY, Fu JP, Chen TM, Chen SG. Reconstruction of scrotal and perineal defects in Fournier's gangrene. *J Plast Reconstr Aesthet Surg.* 2011;64:528–534.

Konofaos P, Hickerson WL. A technique for improving osmosis after primary scrotum reconstruction with skin grafts. *Ann Plast Surg.* 2015;75:205–207.

Mopuri N, O'Connor EF, Iwuagwu FC. Scrotal reconstruction with modified pudendal thigh flaps. *J Plast Reconstr Aesthet Surg.* 2016;69:278–283.

Salgado CJ, Monstrey S, Hoebeke P, Lumen N, Dwyer M, Mardini S. Reconstruction of the penis after surgery. *Urol Clin North Am.* 2010;37:379–401.

Tan BK, Rasheed MZ, Wu WT. Scrotal reconstruction by testicular apposition and wrap- around skin grafting. *J Plast Reconstr Aesthet Surg.* 2011;64:944–948.

SECTION 5

Lower Extremity

40

Upper Thigh Reconstruction

CASE 1

Clinical Presentation

A 40-year-old White male had a very complicated injury to his right hip and lateral thigh regions with a pelvic fracture and extensive muscle necrosis over his right hip region as a result of a motor vehicle accident. He unfortunately developed heterotopic ossification requiring resection of the head of the right femur. A definitive treatment plan, proposed by the orthopedic trauma service, was to perform right total hip replacement as soon as possible after additional bony debridement. However, because of lack of good soft tissue and the poor skin quality secondary to the heterotopic ossification and the frequent surgeries in the area (Fig. 40.1), the primary service felt that it would be critical to obtain better soft tissue coverage to the area immediately after the total hip replacement. The plastic surgery service was consulted to provide reliable soft tissue coverage for the potential right hip prosthesis. Because there was no reliable local option available, a free tissue transfer would be required for this kind of soft tissue coverage. However, the lack of recipient vessels for free tissue transfer presented a real challenge because all potential recipient arteries were occluded during initial embolization to control bleeding.

Operative Plan and Special Considerations

Because there was no reliable local option after total hip replacement, a free latissimus dorsi muscle flap could be selected to provide a good and reliable soft tissue coverage for potentially exposed hip prosthesis. The flap has a long pedicle and can provide large but well-vascularized soft tissue to obliterate the deep space for reliable soft tissue coverage. Because of the previous arterial embolization to the pelvic vessels to control bleeding, no suitable recipient vessel could be identified on preoperative angiogram to be used for free tissue transfer. The descending branch of the lateral circumflex femoral vessels in the thigh is well known because of increased experience by surgeons in harvesting an anterolateral thigh perforator flap. After a straightforward dissection between the rectus femoris and vastus lateralis muscles, the descending branch of the lateral circumflex femoral vessels in the thigh, when dissected with adequate length, can be placed in the lateral thigh to serve as an excellent recipient vessel for free tissue transfer to the thigh or hip.

Operative Procedures

Under general anesthesia, the patient was placed in the left lateral decubitus position. Prior to the procedure, the descending branch of the lateral circumflex femoral vessels was identified by duplex scan and marked (Fig. 40.2).

The previous right hip incision was reopened. There was a fair amount of blood clots as well as seroma. All were removed and the open wound was then irrigated. The entire potential wound measured 30 × 11 cm. Based on the duplex finding, the right lateral thigh incision was extended more medially and inferiorly and the space between the rectus femoris and the vastus lateralis was opened. The descending branch of the lateral circumflex vessels was identified and the vessel was divided with hemoclips at the most distal level near the knee. Retrograde dissection was then performed along the entire length and the many small branches from it were divided with microclips (Fig. 40.3A). The motor nerve was spared during dissection. The dissection again followed a retrograde fashion in the space between the rectus femoris and vastus lateralis toward the profunda. At least 12 cm of the pedicle was dissected free (Fig. 40.3B) and then tunneled under the vastus lateralis and brought out superficially to serve as extended recipient vessels with a good arterial flow (Fig. 40.4). Care was taken to ensure that the entire pedicle was not kinked or compressed.

The right latissimus dorsi muscle was harvested next. An oblique incision was made down to the latissimus dorsi muscle fascia. Once both medial and lateral borders of the latissimus muscle were identified, the muscle was divided with electrocautery medially, inferiorly, and laterally. Under direct vision, the latissimus dorsi muscle was elevated from the chest wall, but the serratus muscle was left intact. After division of the serratus branch of the artery, the latissimus dorsi muscle attachment to the humerus was divided with electrocautery. The pedicle dissection was performed under direct vision with proper retraction. The thoracodorsal nerve was divided first and both thoracodorsal artery and vein were then divided after further pedicle dissection (Fig. 40.5).

The muscle flap was prepared on a separate table. The pedicle artery and vein were irrigated with heparinized saline solution. The muscle flap was temporarily placed into the right hip wound. Under a microscope, an end-to-end arterial microanastomosis was performed with an interrupted 8-0 nylon suture. A 3.0-mm coupler device was used for an end-to-end venous microanastomosis (Fig. 40.6). After all the clamps had been removed, the flap was

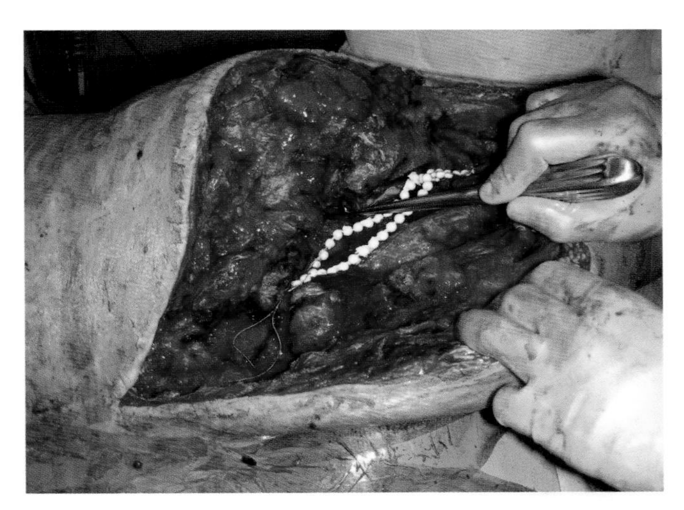

• **Fig. 40.1** An intraoperative view showing a 30 × 11 cm complex soft tissue wound in the right hip and upper thigh. The area of the hip joint space is indicated.

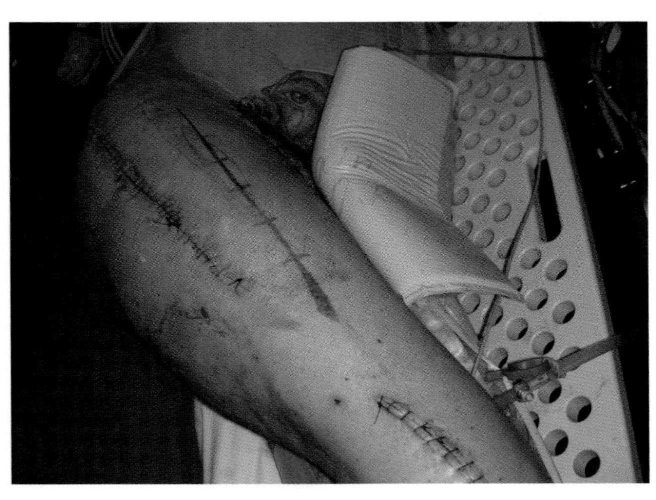

• **Fig. 40.2** An intraoperative view showing the course of the descending branch of the lateral circumflex femoral vessels that was mapped by intraoperative duplex scan.

instantly perfused with good Doppler signals throughout. The flap was placed over the hip region for 1 hour and it appeared to be stable with good arterial and venous flow (Fig. 40.7).

At this point, the orthopedic trauma service performed the right total hip replacement with prosthesis while the flap was temporarily placed near the area. The right total hip replacement was completed by the primary service. Because of the skin condition and the amount of swelling, it was initially impossible to close the right hip wound. Therefore, the intraoperative decision was made to place the muscle flap to cover the entire prosthesis and the hip wound (Fig. 40.8). The muscle flap was inserted into the entire wound with 2-0 PDS sutures in a figure-of-eight. The most proximal part of the hip wound and the distal part of the thigh wound were approximated temporarily with towel clips. The skin edge was sutured to the surface of the muscle flap (Fig. 40.9). The split-thickness skin graft was harvested from the right lateral thigh. The skin graft was meshed to 1:1.5 ratio and placed over almost the entire muscle flap and secured with skin staples. The muscle flap appeared to be well perfused and viable at the end of the procedure (Fig. 40.10). The rest of the skin incision was closed in two layers. The deep dermal layer was approximated with several interrupted 2-0 PDS sutures. The skin was closed with either skin staples or 3-0 nylon in a mattress fashion. A large vacuum-assisted closure sponge dressing was placed over the skin graft site and connected with a machine.

The right back flap donor site was closed last. Two 15-Fr Blake drains were inserted into the donor site and the incision was closed in two layers. The deep dermal layer was approximated with several interrupted 2-0 PDS sutures. The skin was closed with 3-0 Monocryl sutures in running subcuticular fashion.

Follow-Up Results

The patient did well postoperatively without any complications related to the free latissimus dorsi muscle flap reconstruction. Skin grafts over the muscle flap healed well. He was discharged from the hospital on postoperative day 10. All drains were removed during subsequent follow-up visits. The right hip and upper thigh reconstruction sites healed well.

Management of Complications

Apparently, this patient was also treated with Coumadin for anticoagulation as part of routine postoperative orthopedic management. Unfortunately, he developed some swelling over his right back latissimus flap donor site and presented to the clinic 2 days after discharge. Needle aspiration showed clear seroma fluid. A few days later, he had a spike in fever and went to a local hospital with diagnosis of fever. He was then admitted to our hospital and had an ultrasound-guided placement of a seroma catheter. However, he had persistent swelling around the right back donor site and was brought to the operating room for incision and drainage of a possibly infected seroma. Under general anesthesia with the patient in the left lateral decubitus position, a 5-cm incision was made through the previous well-healed incision. Some cloudy fluid was discovered and was evacuated. The wound was curetted thoroughly and irrigated with Pulsavac. After thorough debridement, the wound was packed with Kerlix. The donor site seroma was resolved after an open drainage.

At 5 weeks after the free tissue transfer, this patient unfortunately developed an infection of the total hip arthroplasty, which required open drainage. The plastic surgery service was asked by the primary service to elevate the free latissimus dorsi muscle flap for an open drainage of the right hip arthroplasty (Fig. 40.11). In the operating room with the patient in the left lateral decubitus position, the pedicle of the latissimus dorsi muscle flap was identified with a Doppler and marked. The skin incision was reopened with a knife, followed by the sharp dissection of the muscle flap beveled away from the muscle flap. The incision was opened carefully to avoid injury to the pedicle of the latissimus dorsi free flap. After the adequate elevation of the muscle flap had been completed, the orthopedic trauma service performed the open drainage of the left hip joint and closed the incision appropriately.

Final Outcome

The right hip and upper thigh free flap reconstruction site healed well with minimal scarring. There was no recurrent infection under

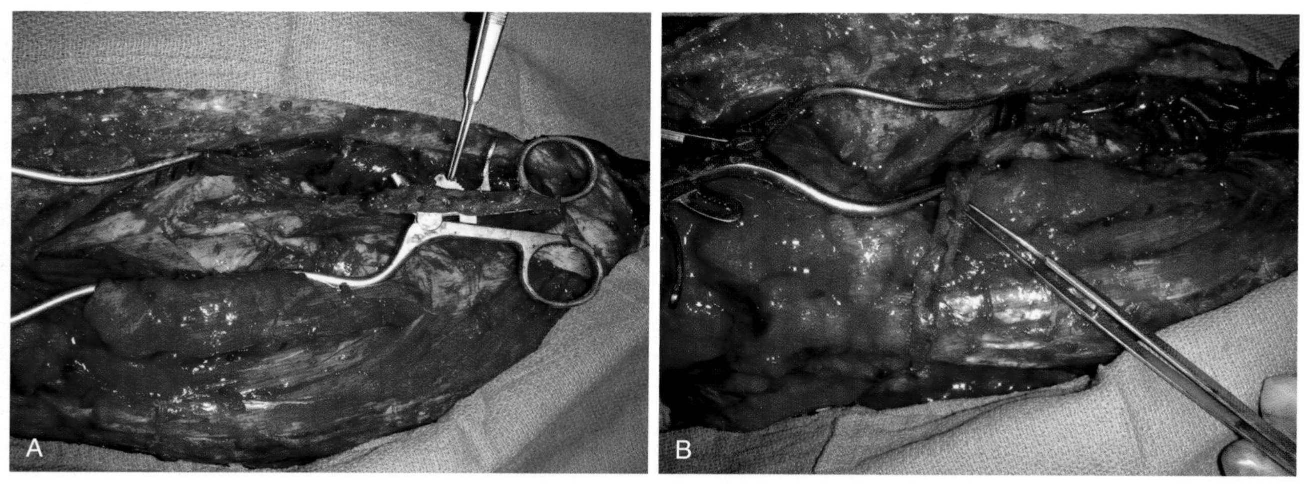

• **Fig. 40.3** (A) An intraoperative view showing the dissected and freed descending branch of the lateral circumflex femoral vessels (both artery and vein) between the rectus femoris and vastus lateralis muscles. (B) An intraoperative view showing the descending branch of the lateral circumflex femoral vessels rotated above the vastus lateralis muscle before it was tunneled.

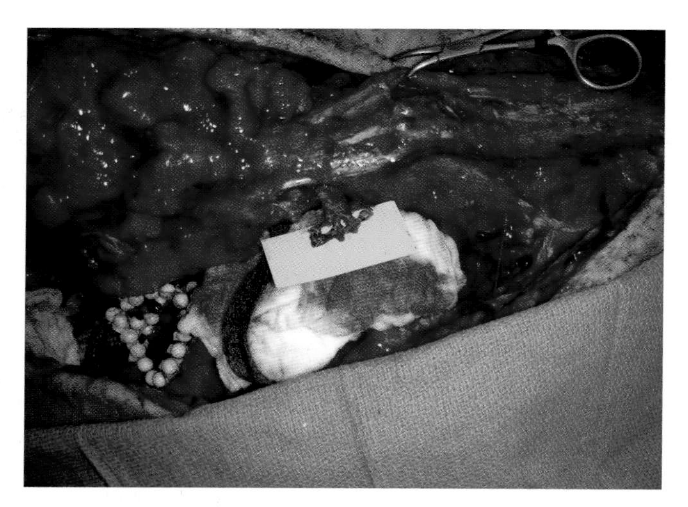

• **Fig. 40.4** An intraoperative view showing the descending branch of the lateral circumflex femoral vessels tunneled under the vastus lateralis muscle as a created recipient vessel for easy microvascular anastomosis.

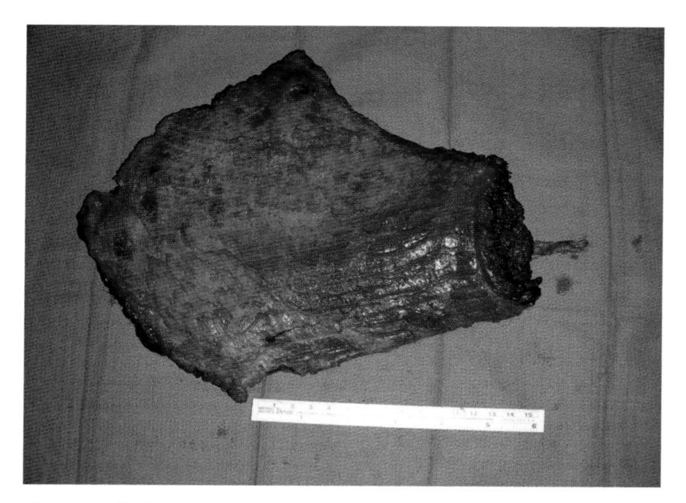

• **Fig. 40.5** An intraoperative view showing completion of a free latissimus dorsi muscle flap dissection.

the flap (Fig. 40.12). The patient has resumed his normal activities and is routinely followed by the orthopedic trauma service.

Pearls for Success

For a complex hip and upper thigh wound when critical soft tissue coverage is needed for the success of an orthopedic procedure, a free latissimus dorsi flap can be selected as a valid reconstructive option. The flap is large enough and can be harvested as a muscle flap to provide well-vascularized tissue for a reliable soft tissue coverage. However, there are issues on selection of a good recipient vessel for such a free tissue transfer in some cases. The descending branch of the lateral circumflex femoral vessels can be surgically dissected and placed near some difficult reconstructed areas of the lower extremity and serve as a recipient vessel for free tissue transfer such as in this case. Alternatively, the nearby recipient vessel might only be found in a deep or less convenient

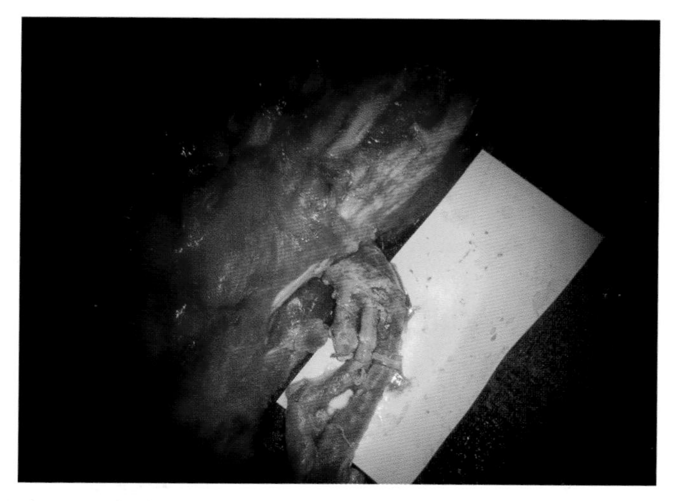

• **Fig. 40.6** An intraoperative view showing completion of easy microvascular anastomoses under an operating microscope.

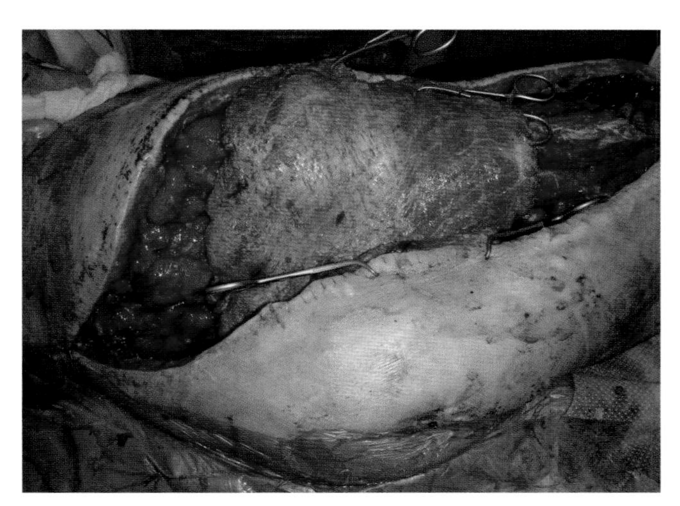

• **Fig. 40.7** An intraoperative view showing preliminary flap inset into the soft tissue wound.

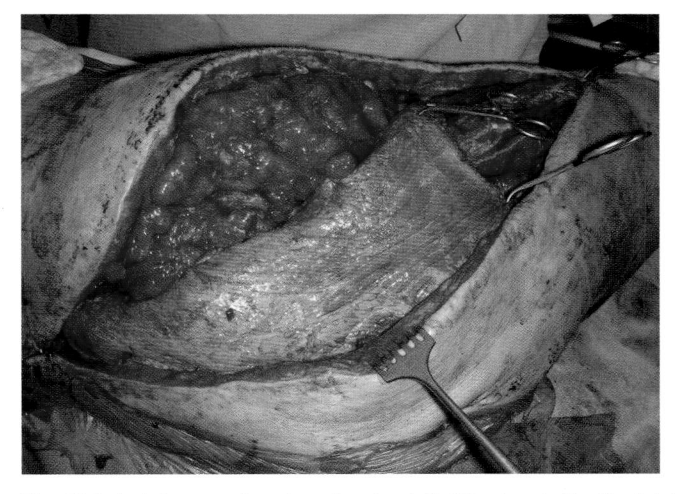

• **Fig. 40.8** An intraoperative view showing initial flap inset after the total hip replacement with a prosthesis.

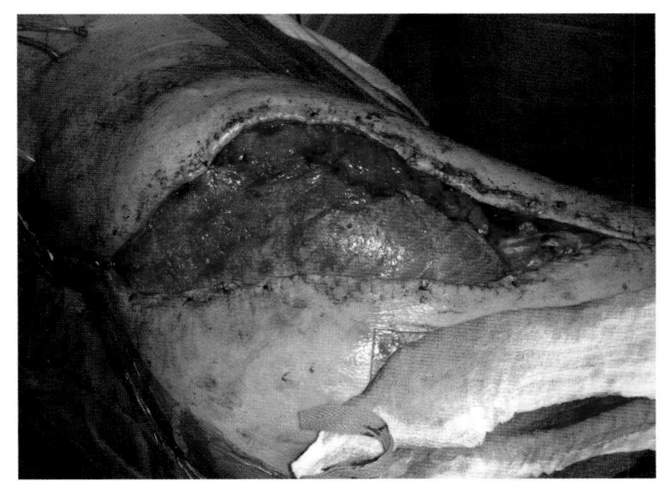

• **Fig. 40.9** An intraoperative view showing completion of the flap inset and the rest of the wound closure after the total hip replacement with a prosthesis.

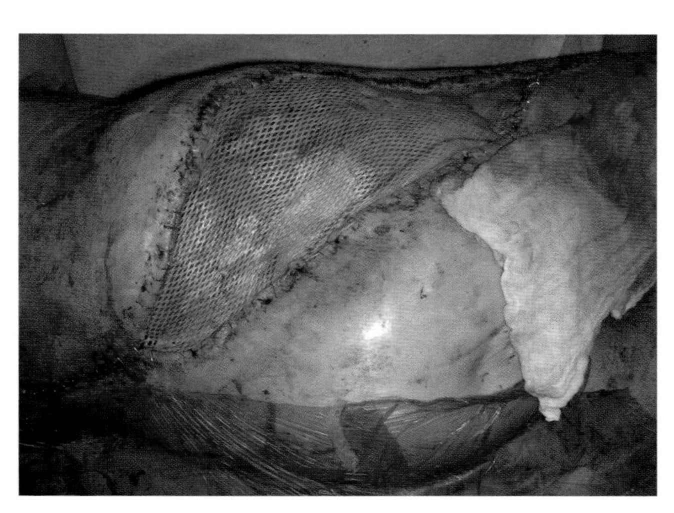

• **Fig. 40.10** An intraoperative view showing completion of the flap reconstruction after skin graft placement.

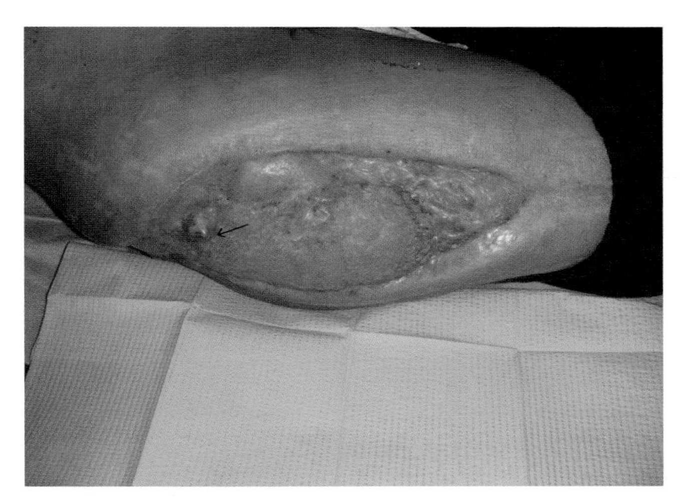

• **Fig. 40.11** The result at 5-week follow-up showing well-healed free flap reconstruction site and a chronic draining site through the flap *(arrow)*.

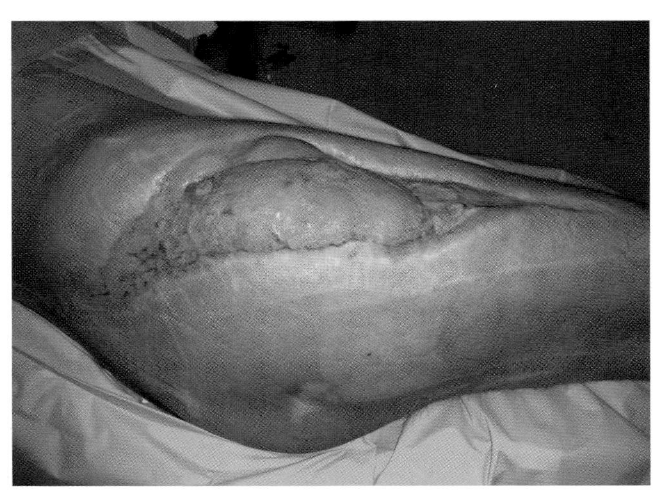

• **Fig. 40.12** The result at 2-month follow-up showing well-healed and stable right hip and upper thigh free flap site with good contour.

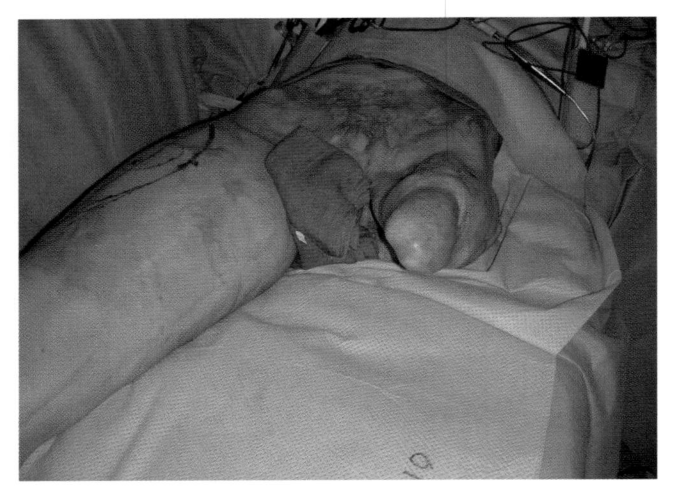

• **Fig. 40.13** A preoperative view showing a high above knee amputation stump with poor padding soft tissue over the bone and surrounding tissues.

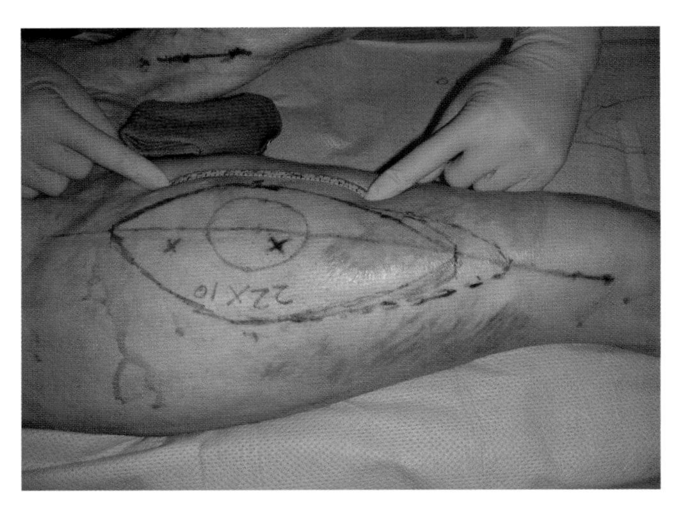

• **Fig. 40.14** An intraoperative view showing the design of the right anterolateral thigh perforator flap with a 22 × 11 cm skin paddle. Two perforators were identified with preoperative duplex scanning.

location for microvascular anastomosis. As demonstrated in this case, the descending branch of the lateral circumflex femoral vessels was mobilized and placed in a new location as a potential recipient vessel for easy microvascular anastomosis. This avoids the use of vein grafts and simplifies free flap reconstruction to those difficult areas with improved success. Creation of such a versatile and reliable recipient vessel for free tissue transfer to certain difficult areas of the lower extremity should be added to the armamentarium of the plastic surgeon when dealing with those complex reconstructive challenges.

CASE 2

Clinical Presentation

A 19-year-old White female sustained traumatic above knee amputation (AKA) of her left lower extremity. Although the left high AKA stump had healed, it had minimal soft tissue padding over the femur. This created many problems in terms of wearing a prosthesis that was a good fit. The patient had been managed by the burn reconstructive surgery service because of her associated burn injury. The plastic surgery service was asked to provide a better soft tissue coverage to her high AKA stump (Fig. 40.13). Because no available local soft tissue could be used to reconstruct her AKA stump, a free tissue transfer was proposed to the patient and the primary service.

Operative Plan and Special Considerations

In order to provide a better quality of soft tissue coverage for her high AKA stump and availability of the contralateral thigh tissue, a free anterolateral thigh (ALT) perforator flap was offered to this patient to cover such a relatively large AKA stump after initial reconstruction of the poor quality of the skin graft in the area. An ALT flap could provide a fasciocutaneous component of flap tissue that may be resistant to the sheer force over the stump. This may be more reliable than a skin-grafted muscle flap for the same reconstruction. The distal superficial femoral artery (SFA) could be explored and serve as a recipient vessel for arterial microanastomosis.

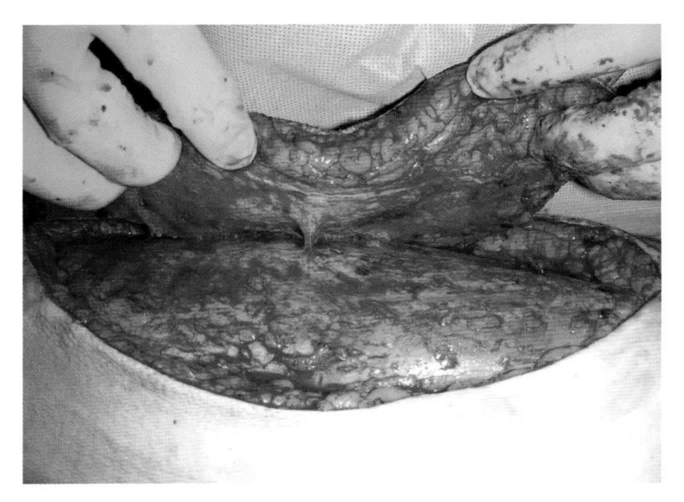

• **Fig. 40.15** An intraoperative view showing a single large perforator during the free anterolateral thigh perforator flap dissection.

Perforators in the right thigh could be mapped by duplex scan so that perforator dissection would potentially be less difficult.

Operative Procedures

Under general anesthesia, the left ALT perforator flap was designed based on the findings from preoperative duplex scan perforator mapping. The flap was based on two mapped perforators. A 22 × 10 cm skin paddle was designed and centered to one major perforator (Fig. 40.14). During elevation of the skin paddle, the fascia was incorporated as a fasciocutaneous flap. Several other less important perforators were divided and only one major perforator, close to the septum between the rectus femoris and the vastus lateralis muscle, was followed and dissected free to the descending branch of the lateral circumflex femoral vessels (Fig. 40.15). The pedicle dissection was performed to obtain more length of the pedicle. The descending branch was divided as proximal as possible from the profunda vessels. One artery and one vein were divided with hemoclips and the flap dissection was completed (Fig. 40.16).

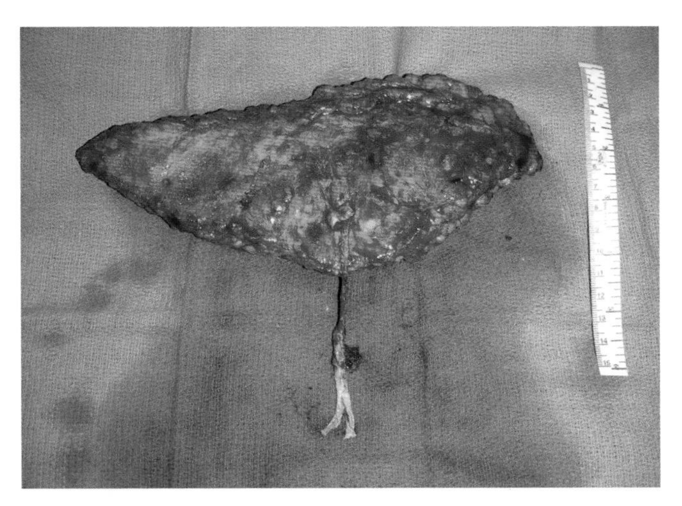

• **Fig. 40.16** An intraoperative view showing completion of a free anterolateral thigh perforator flap dissection.

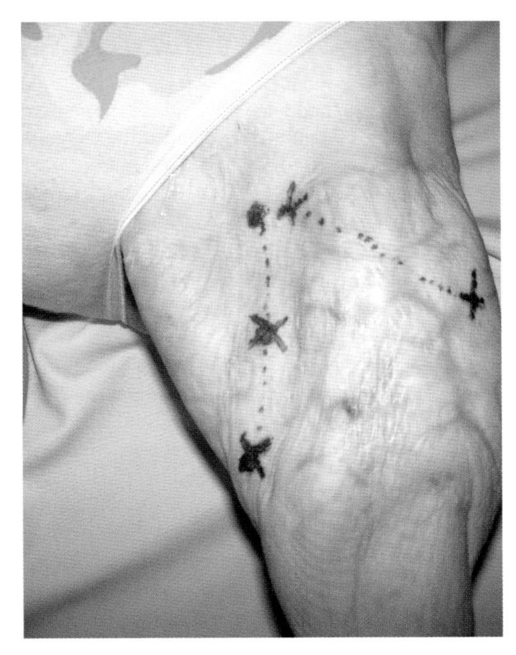

• **Fig. 40.17** An intraoperative view showing an outline of the surface anatomy for the superficial femoral artery and femoral vein in the thigh.

The AKA stump was opened and the distal SFA and femoral vein were explored as potential recipient vessels (Fig. 40.17). Under loupe magnification, the distal SFA and femoral vein were dissected free and prepared for arterial and venous microanastomoses.

The pedicle of the flap was also prepared under loupe magnification. With further preparation, one artery and one vein were ready for microvascular anastomoses. The artery was flushed with heparinized saline solution. The flap was temporarily placed over the AKA stump. The arterial microanastomosis was performed in an end-to-side fashion with interrupted 8-0 nylon sutures under a microscope. The venous microanastomosis was performed in an end-to-end fashion with a 3-mm Coupler Device. The flap appeared to be well perfused after all clamps had been removed (Fig. 40.18).

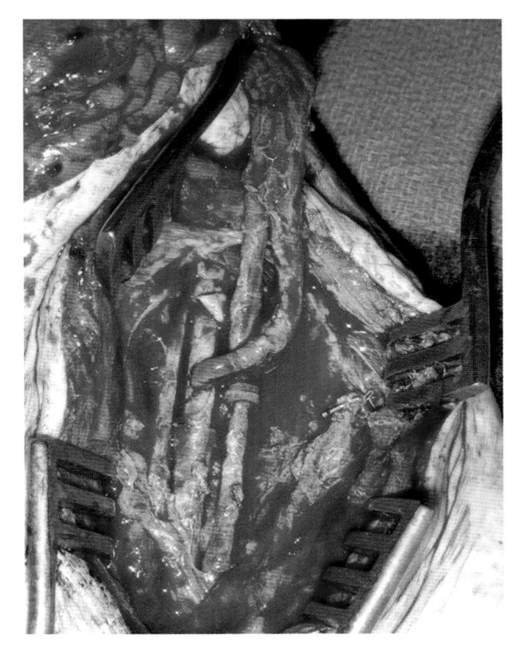

• **Fig. 40.18** An intraoperative view showing completion of the arterial microanastomosis (in an end-to-side fashion) and the venous microanastomosis (in an end-to-end fashion)

The final inset of the flap to the AKA stump was performed with interrupted, half-buried horizontal mattress 3-0 Monocryl sutures once excess flap tissues had been excised. A Penrose drain was placed under the flap and came out from the incision on each side. A Cook Doppler probe for monitored arterial flow was placed around the distal arterial anastomosis and connected with the machine. The right thigh flap donor site was closed in three layers after significant undermining.

Follow-Up Results

The patient did well postoperatively without any complications related to the free ALT flap reconstruction for the left high AKA stump. She was discharged from hospital on postoperative day 7. The drain was removed before discharge. The left thigh high AKA stump site healed well (Fig. 40.19). Adequate soft tissue padding to the left thigh AKA stump was accomplished after a free ALT flap reconstruction.

Final Outcome

The left high AKA stump reconstruction site healed well and the final contour has been good without any need for a debulking procedure (Fig. 40.20). The patient has resumed her normal life and now has a new prosthesis for the left AKA stump. No recurrent wound breakdown has occurred.

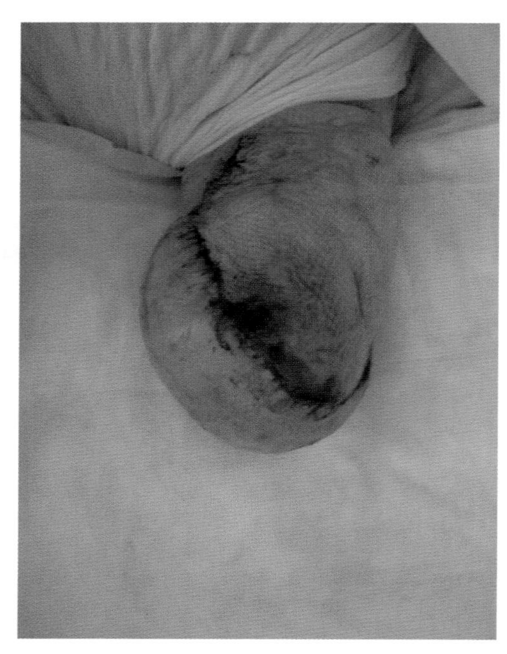

• **Fig. 40.19** The result at 2-week follow-up showing good healing of the knee amputation stump and good flap contour.

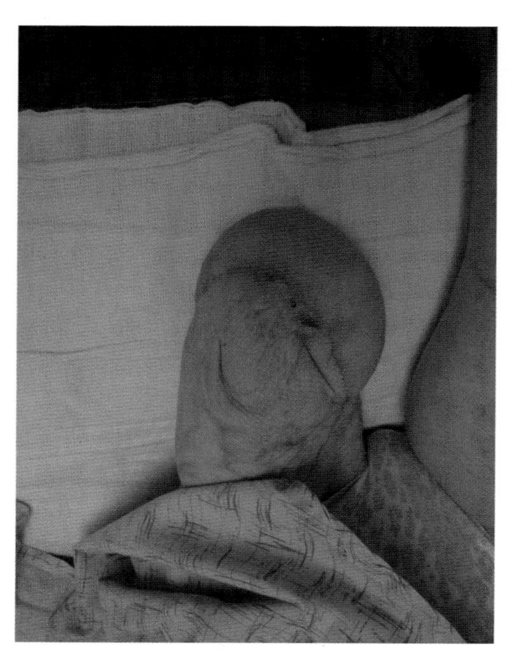

• **Fig. 40.20** The result at 2-month follow-up showing well-healed above knee amputation stump with good flap contour and minimal scarring. (The photo should be rotated 180 degree and oriented the same as Fig 40.19)

Pearls for Success

A free ALT perforator flap from the contralateral thigh can be a good option for reconstruction of an AKA stump as long as the patient has enough flap tissue and well-defined perforator(s) for the flap design. It has a long pedicle and can be harvested as a fasciocutaneous flap based on a single perforator for an AKA stump reconstruction. However, the flap dissection has a learning curve and can be time consuming. The distal SFA and femoral vein can be selected as recipient vessels. For arterial microanastomosis, an end-to-side anastomosis can be performed without difficulty. For venous microanastomosis, an end-to-end anastomosis can still be performed with a Coupler device. In addition, the perforator mapping with duplex scan can be helpful so that a reliable perforator for the flap design or dissection can be performed. Unlike a skin-grafted free muscle flap, a free ALT perforator flap may remain bulky even after 1 year. This would work well for an AKA stump reconstruction because such a reconstructed stump is more reliable and can tolerate shear force from a prosthesis. A flap debulking procedure is usually not necessary after this kind of reconstruction.

Recommended Readings

Dorfman DW, Pu LL. Using the descending branch of the lateral circumflex femoral artery and vein as recipient vessel for free tissue transfer to the difficult areas of the lower extremity. *Ann Plast Surg.* 2013;70:397–400.

Dorfman D, Pu LL. The value of color duplex imaging for planning and performing a free anterolateral thigh perforator flap. *Ann Plast Surg.* 2014;72(suppl 1):S6–S8.

Elswick SM, Wu P, Arkhavan AA, et al. A reconstructive algorithm after thigh soft tissue sarcoma resection including predictors of free flap reconstruction. *J Plast Reconstr Aesthet Surg.* 2019;72:1304–1315.

Hsu CC, Loh CYY, Wei FC. The anterolateral thigh perforator flap: its expanding role in lower extremity reconstruction. *Clin Plast Surg.* 2021;48:235–248.

Kim JT, Kim SW, Youn S, Kim YH. What is the ideal free flap for soft tissue reconstruction? A ten-year experience of microsurgical reconstruction using 334 latissimus dorsi flaps from a universal donor site. *Ann Plast Surg.* 2015;75:49–54.

Vijayasekaran A, Gibreel W, Carlsen BT, et al. Maximizing the utility of the pedicled anterolateral thigh flap for locoregional reconstruction: technical pearls and pitfalls. *Clin Plast Surg.* 2020;47:621–634.

41

Lower Thigh Reconstruction

CASE 1

Clinical Presentation

A 42-year-old White male had a complicated lateral thigh wound following an open distal femur fracture. He underwent an open reduction and internal fixation of the distal femur fracture by the orthopedic trauma service, which left a large open wound, measuring 12 × 8 cm, with the exposed fracture site and reconstructed plate (Figs. 41.1 and 41.2). The plastic surgery service was asked by the primary service to perform a soft tissue coverage and definitive wound closure.

Operative Plan and Special Considerations for Reconstruction

For this relatively large soft tissue wound with the exposed femur fracture site, hardware, and potential space, a local muscle flap with a relatively large size of well-vascularized tissue, such as the biceps femoris muscle, can be selected to provide a one-stage soft tissue coverage and also obliterate the potential space. The muscle, which received a blood supply from a few branches of the profunda femoris artery, is a type II muscle flap but is considered to be reliable if the patient is free of peripheral vascular disease in the profound artery. Its long head is a large muscle that can be used to cover lower lateral thigh soft tissue defect. A skin graft to the muscle flap would be needed for the final wound closure. Adjacent skin rearrangements can also be added to facilitate the entire wound closure in addition to a skin graft to the muscle flap.

Operative Procedures

Under general anesthesia with the patient in the supine position, the right distal lateral thigh wound was debrided. All colonized tissues were removed. The open wound appeared to be fresh and clean after a more definitive debridement by the plastic surgery service.

The design for the long head of the biceps femoris muscle flap was marked (Fig. 41.3). The skin incision was made through the skin, subcutaneous tissues, and fascia down to the hamstring muscles. Once the long head of the biceps femoris muscle had been identified, the flap dissection was carried out to explore its insertion to the head of the fibula. Once its attachment to the fibula had been divided, the muscle was gradually elevated from distal to proximal and its minor pedicles from the profunda artery were identified. The flap was then elevated so that it could be rotated to cover all exposed structures but only one minor pedicle was divided during the flap dissection (Fig. 41.4). The flap was temporarily inset into the wound to cover the entire fracture site and exposed hardware. One drain was placed under the flap (Fig. 41.5). The flap was inset into the wound with several interrupted 3-0 Monocryl sutures. Additional local tissue rearrangements were performed to facilitate a complete wound closure (Fig. 41.6).

A split-thickness skin graft was harvested with a dermatome from the right anteromedial thigh. It was meshed to 1:1.5 ratio. The skin graft was placed over the muscle and the rest of the granulation wound and secured with multiple skin staples (Fig. 41.7).

Follow-Up Results

The patient did well postoperatively without any issues related to the flap reconstruction and wound closure. He was discharged from hospital on postoperative day 7. The right distal lateral thigh wound healed uneventfully (Fig. 41.7). He was followed by both the primary service and the plastic surgery service for subsequent postoperative care.

Final Outcome

After acute care with the plastic surgery service, the patient was followed by the primary service for his routine postsurgical visits. The right lateral thigh flap reconstruction site has healed well and there has been no wound breakdown, recurrent infection, or any other long-term problems related to the flap reconstruction (Fig. 41.8).

Pearls for Success

A large local muscle flap, such as the long head of the biceps femoris muscle flap, can be used to cover a large soft tissue wound in the distal lateral thigh. The flap is reliable and its flap dissection is relatively straightforward. It can provide adequate vascularized tissue for an optimal wound closure because of its rich blood supply and convenient location. It can certainly be used to obliterate a deep space in the fracture site. During flap dissection, division of one or two minor pedicles may be needed so that the flap can be rotated to provide adequate soft tissue coverage and fill the potential dead space. A proper vascular evaluation for the femoral vessels and/or profunda vessels may be necessary if the patient has peripheral vascular disease. A split-thickness skin graft

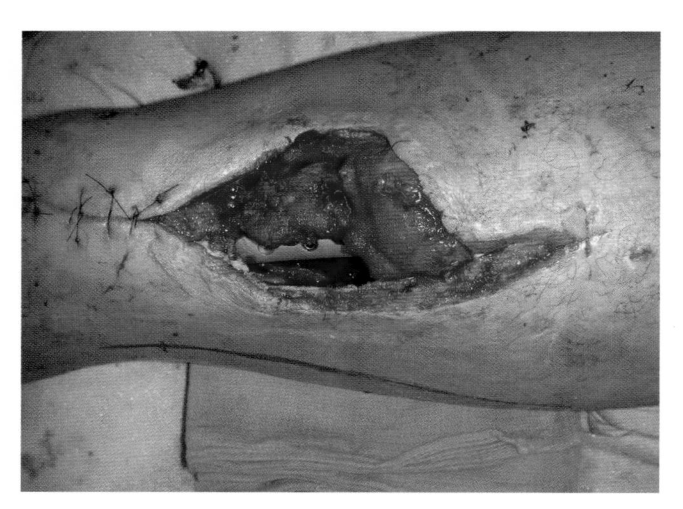

• **Fig. 41.1** A preoperative view showing a large and complex lateral thigh wound with the exposed fracture site and hardware.

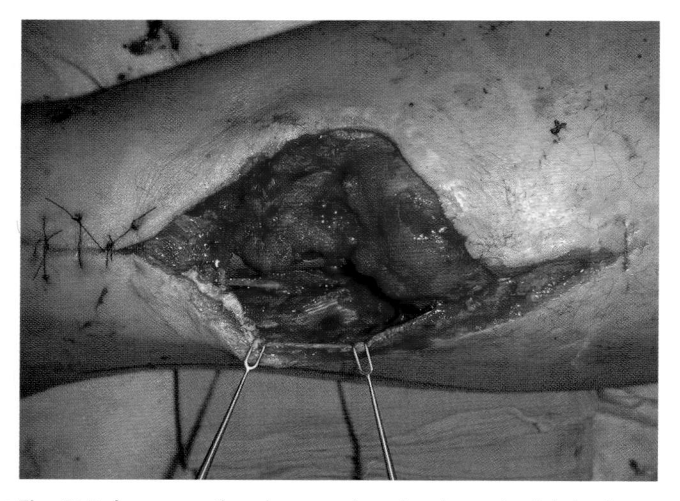

• **Fig. 41.2** A preoperative close-up view showing potential dead space around the fracture site after open reduction and internal fixation.

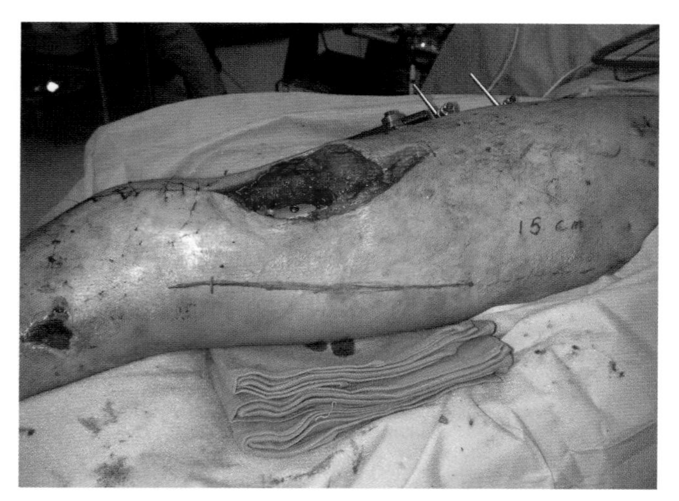

• **Fig. 41.3** An intraoperative view showing the planned incision for dissection of the long head of the biceps femoris muscle flap.

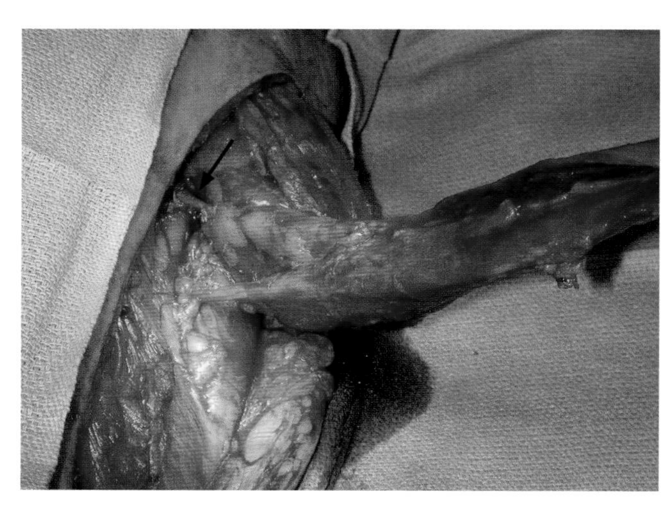

• **Fig. 41.4** An intraoperative view showing completion of the biceps femoris muscle flap (long head) dissection. Please note that only one minor pedicle *(see* hemoclip is visiable in the distal flap*)* was divided to facilitate the flap's rotation. One proximal pedicle from the profunda was preserved *(arrow)*.

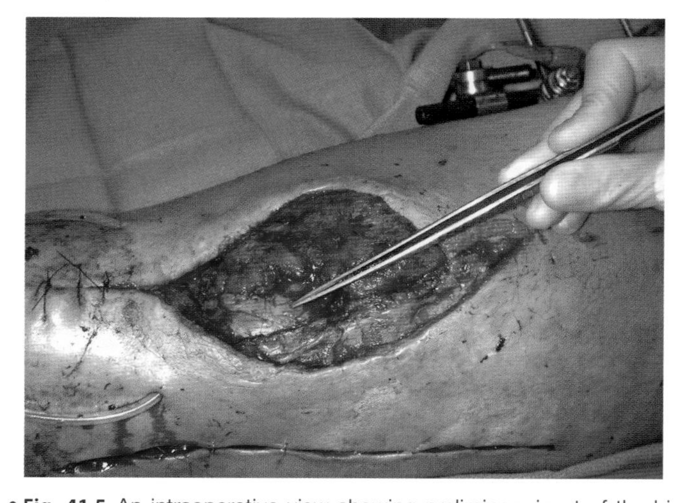

• **Fig. 41.5** An intraoperative view showing preliminary inset of the biceps femoris muscle flap (long head).

is commonly placed over the muscle flap for definitive wound closure.

CASE 2

Clinical Presentation

An 18-year-old White male sustained a significant orthopedic trauma to his right lower extremity. He had multiple complex wounds over his right lower extremity, the most critical of which was in the right lateral thigh and knee, measuring 30 × 12 cm, with the exposed sciatic nerve, femur, distal femur fracture site (Fig. 41.9). After open reduction and internal fixation (ORIF) of the distal femur fracture by the orthopedic trauma service, the plastic surgery service was consulted for soft tissue coverage of the lateral thigh and knee wounds (Fig. 41.10). The patient also had a complex wound over his right abdomen and right medial leg. He

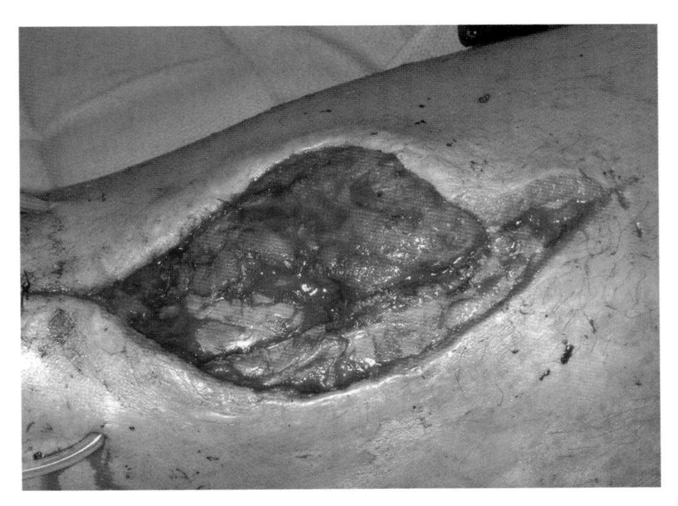

• **Fig. 41.6** An intraoperative close-up view showing completion of the flap's inset for the biceps femoris muscle flap (long head).

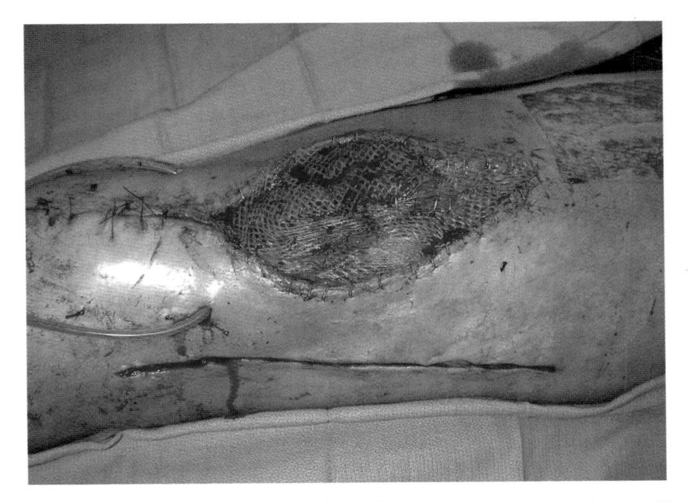

• **Fig. 41.7** An intraoperative view showing placement of a split-thickness skin graft to the biceps femoris muscle flap for definitive wound closure.

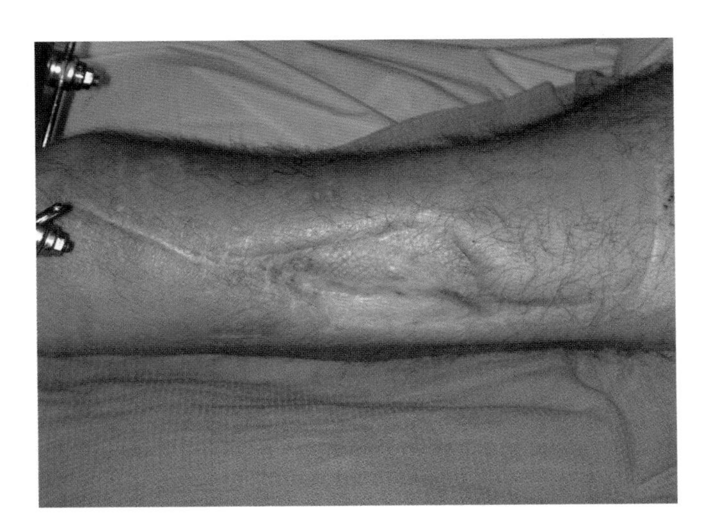

• **Fig. 41.8** Result at 4-month follow-up showing well-healed right distal lateral thigh wound after flap reconstruction.

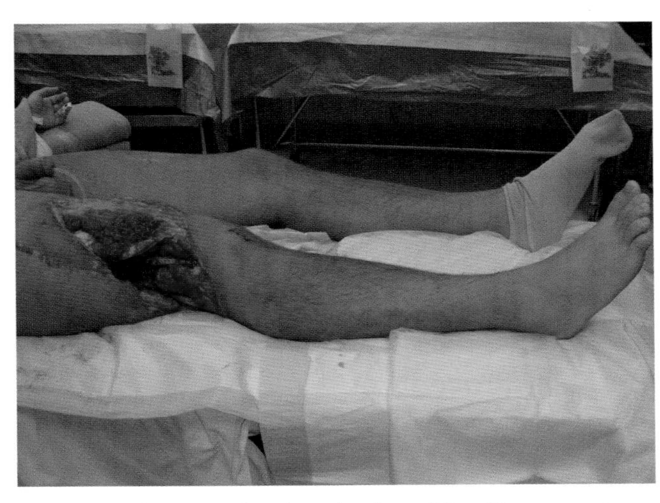

• **Fig. 41.9** An intraoperative view showing a 30 × 10 cm complex soft tissue wound in the distal lateral thigh and knee associated with comminuted femur fracture.

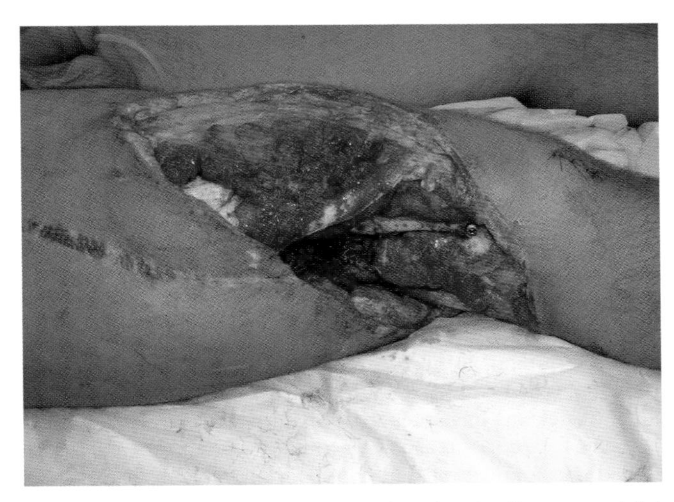

• **Fig. 41.10** An intraoperative close-up view showing the exposed distal femur fracture site and exposed hardware.

was brought to the operating room by our service for a free tissue transfer to cover the right lateral thigh and knee wounds, to close the right abdominal complex wound, and to apply a skin graft to the rest of the wounds.

Operative Plan and Special Considerations

The primary soft tissue wound over the right distal lateral thigh and knee was quite large and would require a free tissue transfer for wound coverage because there was no local option available to fulfil reconstructive need after ORIF of the distal femur fracture. In this case, a large anterolateral thigh (ALT) perforator flap from the contralateral thigh could be selected to provide a good and reliable soft tissue coverage for potentially exposed distal femur fracture site and hardware. The flap has a long pedicle and can provide a large amount of the fasciocutaneous soft tissue for reliable soft tissue coverage. However, it is always difficult, based on this author's experience, that a good and reliable recipient vessel may not be available for free tissue transfer. The descending branch of the lateral circumflex femoral vessels in the thigh is well known because of increased experience by surgeons harvesting the ALT perforator flap. The descending branch can be found between the rectus femoris and vastus lateralis muscles. Its distal portion can be dissected out in an adequate length and placed in the distal thigh close to the soft tissue wound. It can serve as an excellent recipient vessel for free tissue transfer to the distal thigh or knee. The surgeon should make sure that the descending branch is outside the zone of the injury, which can be confirmed during surgical exploration.

Operative Procedures

Under general anesthesia with the patient in supine position, the right lateral thigh and knee wounds were debrided. All colonized tissues were then removed and the wound was irrigated thoroughly with Pulsavac. After irrigation, the wound appeared to be fresh and clean.

The descending branch of the lateral circumflex femoral vessels in the right thigh was explored. A longitudinal skin incision over the right ALT was made through the skin and subcutaneous tissue. By incising the fascia over the muscle compartment, the descending branch of the lateral circumflex femoral vessels was identified within the space between the rectus femoris and the vastus lateralis muscles. Because of previous trauma, there appeared to be significant swelling around the descending branch. The dissection was carefully performed under loupe magnification toward the profunda vessels and multiple branches of the descending branch were divided with hemoclips. After the descending branch had been divided distally, both the artery and vein were identified and dissected free within the descending branch. It appeared to be small and further division was therefore done more proximally in order to obtain an adequate size of the artery and vein for microvascular anastomoses (Fig. 41.11). The pedicle vessel was then prepared for microvascular anastomosis.

An ALT perforator flap with a 30 × 10 cm skin paddle was mapped and marked on the left ALT (Fig. 41.12). The skin and subcutaneous tissue were incised down to the deep fascia. The fascia was included with the flap. During the flap dissection, two perforators were confirmed. One was within the circle; another was distal and appeared to have good pulsation. Therefore, the intraoperative decision was made to preserve this perforator. The perforator dissection was performed intramuscularly by dissecting the vastus lateralis muscle and by dissecting this descending branch of the lateral circumflex femoral vessel in a retrograde fashion. The most distal perforator was dissected intramuscularly and only a small portion of the vastus lateralis muscle was included. It was followed until it joined the descending branch. During the dissection, a motor nerve to the vastus muscle was spared. Once the distal descending branch had been divided, both perforators were incorporated into the descending branch. The entire skin paddle was supplied by these two perforators (Fig. 41.13). The descending branch was dissected from distal to proximal until it joined the profunda vessels (Fig. 41.14). The proximal descending branch was divided from the profunda with hemoclips and the flap dissection was completed (Fig. 41.15).

The pedicle of the flap was prepared under loupe magnification. Both artery and vein were dissected free and the artery was perfused with heparinized saline solution. Once the venous

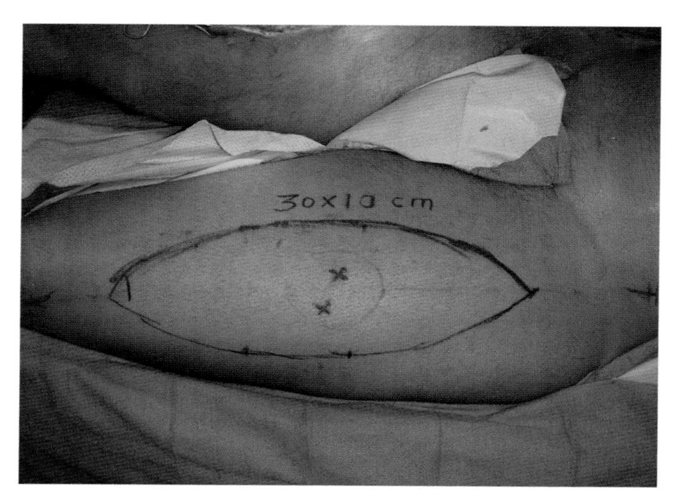

• **Fig. 41.12** An intraoperative view showing the design of the left anterolateral thigh perforator flap. Two perforators were marked.

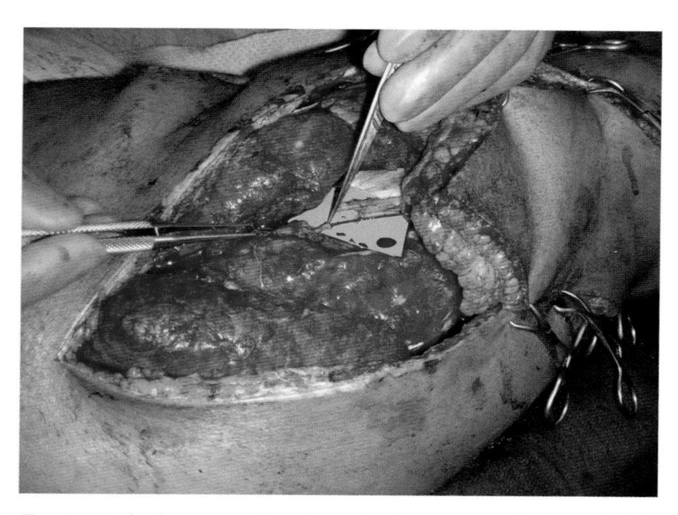

• **Fig. 41.11** An intraoperative view showing an excellent arterial flow from the descending branch of the right lateral circumflex femoral artery.

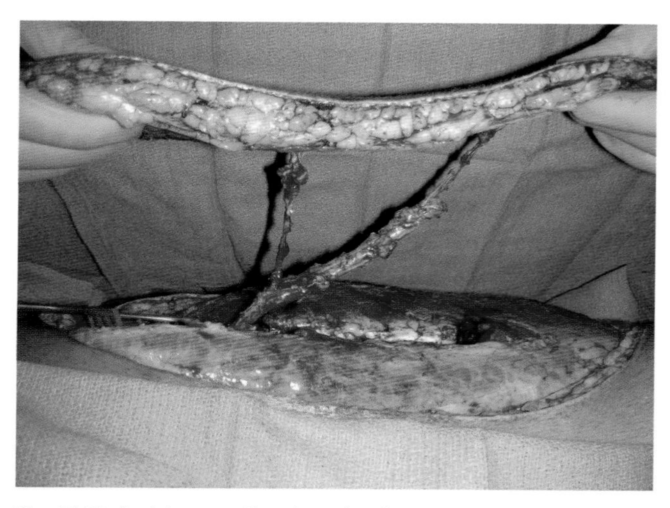

• **Fig. 41.13** An intraoperative view showing complete dissection of the anterolateral thigh flap's two perforators and portion of the left descending branch.

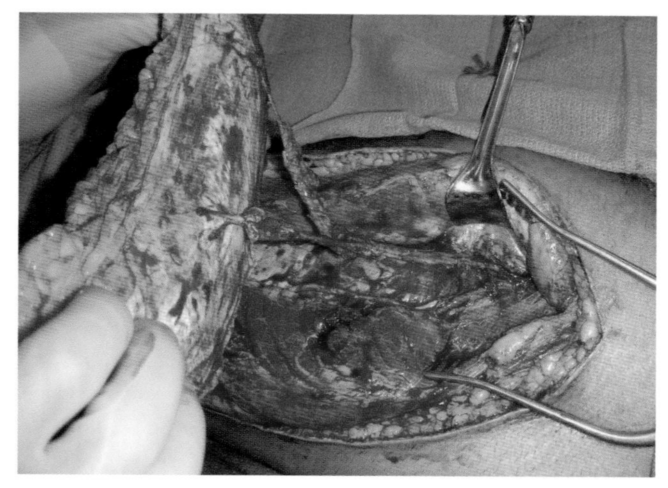

• **Fig. 41.14** An intraoperative view showing complete dissection of the anterolateral thigh flap with two perforators and the entire left descending branch.

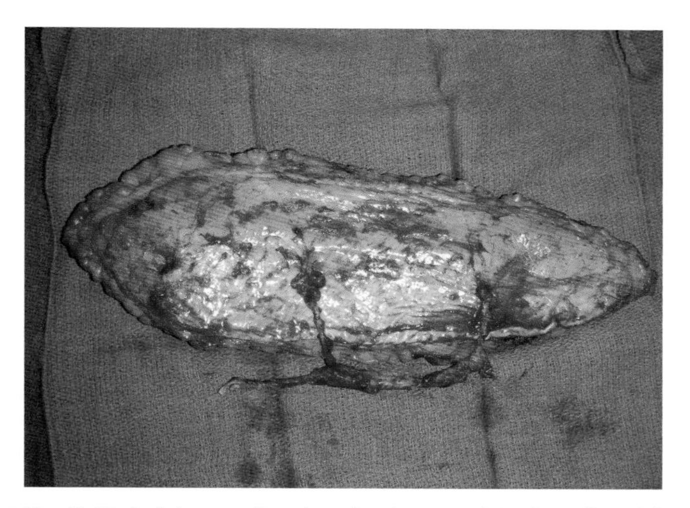

• **Fig. 41.15** An intraoperative view showing complete dissection of the left anterolateral thigh flap.

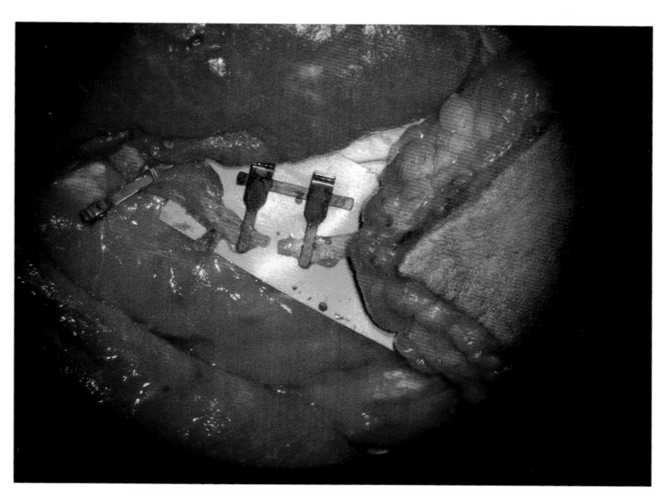

• **Fig. 41.16** An intraoperative view under an operating microscope showing an easy set-up for an end-to-end arterial microanastomosis.

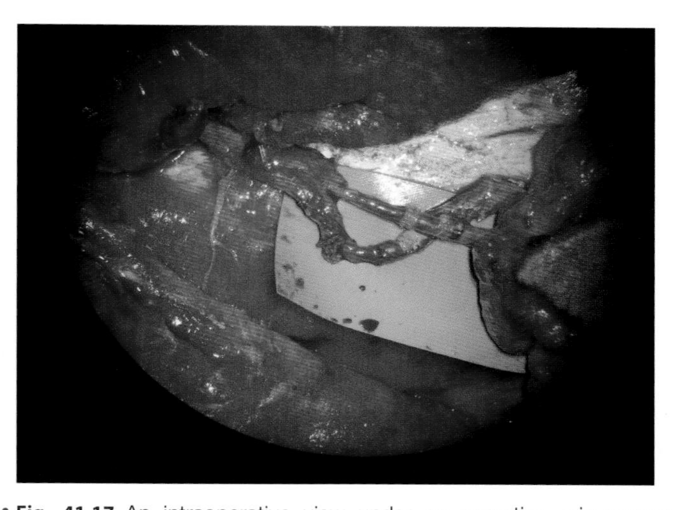

• **Fig. 41.17** An intraoperative view under an operating microscope showing completion of both arterial and venous microanastomoses.

outflow of the pedicle appeared to be clear, the flap was ready for microvascular anastomosis (Fig. 41.16).

The flap was temporarily inset into the defect. The recipient and pedicle vessels were placed next to each other and both microvascular anastomoses were performed under a microscope. The arterial microanastomosis was performed in an end-to-end fashion with interrupted 8-0 nylon sutures. The venous micro-anastomosis was performed with a 2-mm venous coupler, also in an end-to-end fashion. Once all clamps had been removed, the flap appeared to be well perfused with good arterial and venous Doppler signals (Fig. 41.17).

The flap inset was then performed. Prior to that, antibiotic beads were placed around the distal femur fracture site by the orthopedic trauma service. It was approximated to the adjacent skin edges with several interrupted 3-0 Monocryl sutures. Two drains were placed one under the flap and another with the descending branch dissection site. The rest of the deep dermal closure was approximated with interrupted 3-0 Monocryl sutures and all skin closure was done with skin staples.

The split-thickness skin graft was harvested from the right lateral thigh. The skin graft was meshed to 1:1.5 ratio and placed over the right anterior thigh, right posterior knee, and right medial leg wounds and secured with multiple skin staples. The skin graft site was covered with Xeroform, bacitracin ointment, and fluffs and secured with a vacuum-assisted closure sponge (Fig. 41.18).

The left ALT flap donor site was closed primarily after significant undermining and approximated in two layers.

Follow-Up Results

The patient did well postoperatively without any complications related to the free ALT flap reconstruction site. All skin graft sites also healed well. He was discharged from hospital on postoperative day 10. All drains were removed during subsequent follow-up office visits. The right lateral thigh and knee reconstruction site healed well (Fig. 41.19).

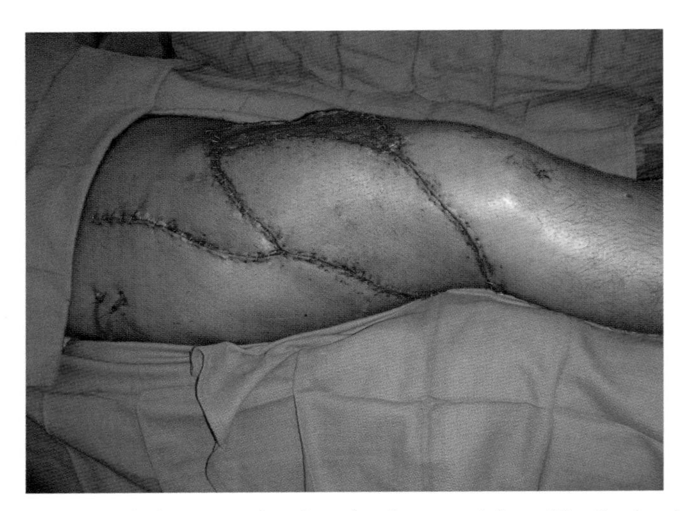

• **Fig. 41.18** An intraoperative view showing completion of the flap inset and the rest of the wound closure including a skin graft.

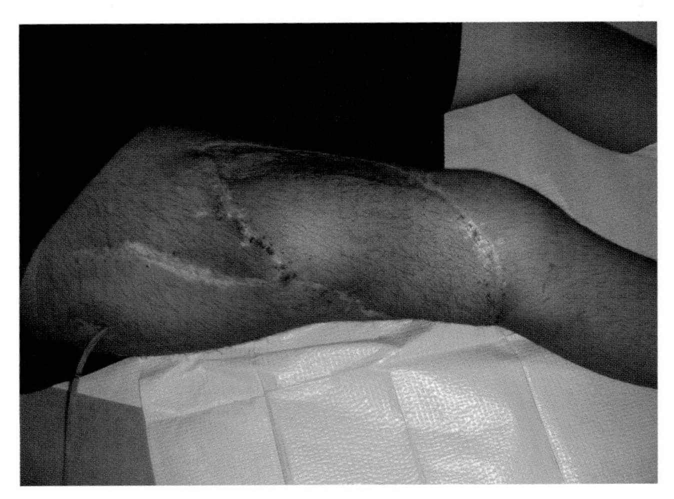

• **Fig. 41.19** The result at 4-week follow-up showing well-healed and stable right lateral thigh and knee free anterolateral thigh flap site with good contour and minimal scarring.

Final Outcome

The right lateral thigh and knee free flap reconstruction site healed well with minimal scarring. The distal femur fracture site also healed well. The patient has resumed his normal activities and been routinely followed by the orthopedic trauma service.

Pearls for Success

For a large complex wound in the lower lateral thigh when there is no good local reconstructive option available after an orthopedic procedure, a free ALT perforator flap can be selected as a valid reconstructive option. The flap is large enough and can be harvested as a fasciocutaneous flap for reliable soft tissue coverage. Microvascular free tissue transfer to the distal thigh can be challenging because good recipient vessels are lacking in the area. Although the distal superficial femoral artery can be selected because of its consistent anatomy, its location is quite deep and only end-to-side microvascular anastomosis could be performed. The descending branch of the lateral circumflex femoral vessels can be surgically dissected and placed near some difficult reconstructive areas of the lower extremity and serve as a recipient vessel for free tissue transfer. As demonstrated in this case, the descending branch of the lateral circumflex femoral vessels is dissected free and placed in a convenient location as a potential recipient vessel for easy microvascular anastomosis. It would avoid using vein grafts and simplify free flap reconstruction to some difficult areas of the lower extremity with improved success. Creation of such a versatile and reliable recipient vessel for free tissue transfer to some difficult areas of the lower extremity should be considered by the plastic surgeon when dealing with such complex reconstructive problems.

Recommended Readings

Demirseren ME, Ceran C, Aksam B, Demiralp CO. Clinical experience with the combination of a biceps femoris muscle turnover flap and a posterior thigh fasciocutaneous hatchet flap for the reconstruction of ischial pressure ulcers. *Ann Plast Surg.* 2016;77:93–96.

Dorfman DW, Pu LL. Using the descending branch of the lateral circumflex femoral artery and vein as recipient vessel for free tissue transfer to the difficult areas of the lower extremity. *Ann Plast Surg.* 2013;70:397–400.

Elswick SM, Wu P, Arkhavan AA, et al. A reconstructive algorithm after thigh soft tissue sarcoma resection including predictors of free flap reconstruction. *J Plast Reconstr Aesthet Surg.* 2019;72:1304–1315.

Hsu CC, Loh CYY, Wei FC. The anterolateral thigh perforator flap: its expanding role in lower extremity reconstruction. *Clin Plast Surg.* 2021;48:235–248.

Nazerali RS, Pu LL. Free tissue transfer to the lower extremity: a paradigm shift in flap selection for soft tissue reconstruction. *Ann Plast Surg.* 2013;70:419–422.

42

Knee Reconstruction

CASE 1

Clinical Presentation

A 29-year-old white male had significant left proximal tibia bone loss and open knee injury as a result of an explosive injury in a foreign country. The orthopedic injury was stabilized initially after debridement in an overseas military hospital. He was subsequently transferred to the orthopedic trauma service of our hospital for more definitive treatment. After admission, an aggressive orthopedic debridement was performed by our orthopedic trauma service. The open facture wound was temporally covered with a vacuum-assisted closure (VAC) dressing after an external fixator placement and patella reconstruction. The plastic surgery service was consulted for soft tissue coverage of this large upper tibial wound that extended to the knee (Fig. 42.1).

Operative Plan and Special Considerations

The potential definitive orthopedic management and soft tissue coverage was performed 8 months later after the initial injury. Because of the complexity of the composite injuries, the patient was taken to the operating room by the plastic surgery service for more definitive bony and soft tissue debridement. A plan for definitive soft tissue coverage along with the orthopedic reconstruction would be made at that time. Based on an intraoperative assessment, a successful soft tissue reconstruction could be performed after appropriate bony reconstructions for limb salvage. Because of the size of the upper tibial and knee wound and the long pedicle of the flap, a free latissimus dorsi muscle flap could be selected to provide adequate soft tissue coverage of the wound. However, good recipient vessels for a successful free flap reconstruction remained undetermined until direct intraoperative exploration would be carried out. If not feasible, the popliteal vessels could be explored as potential recipient vessels for free flap transfer and vein grafts could be avoided.

Operative Procedures

Under general anesthesia, the patient was placed in the supine position and the descending genicular vessels around the left knee were explored to see whether they could be used as recipient vessels. Unfortunately, these vessels appeared to be too small as recipient vessels for successful end-to-end microvascular anastomosis.

With the patient in a near prone position (not in a true prone position because of the external fixator), the popliteal vessels were explored as recipient vessels for microvascular anastomosis. A lazy S skin incision was made in the popliteal fossa. Once the dissection was through subcutaneous tissue, both the popliteal artery and vein were dissected free and prepared under a loupe magnification.

The left latissimus donor was harvested next. An oblique incision was made down to the fascia. After identifying both medial and lateral borders of the latissimus muscle, the muscle was divided using electrocautery medially, inferiorly, and laterally. Under direct vision, the latissimus dorsi muscle flap was elevated from the chest wall but the serratus muscle was left intact. Once the serratus branch of the artery had been divided, the latissimus dorsi muscle attachment to the humerus was also divided using electrocautery. The pedicle dissection was performed under direct vision with proper retraction. The thoracodorsal nerve was divided and the thoracodorsal artery and vein were both divided after further pedicle dissection from the axillary vessels.

The pedicle vessels of the muscle flap were prepared under loupe magnification. The pedicle artery and vein were irrigated with heparinized saline solution. The portion of the muscle flap including the pedicle was tunneled through the skin of the knee and the major portion of the muscle flap was temporarily placed into the knee and upper tibial wound. Both microvascular anastomoses to the popliteal vessles were performed under loupe magnification because of the unique position of the patient. End-to-side arterial and venous microanastomoses were performed with interrupted 8-0 nylon sutures. Once all the clamps had been removed, the flap was instantly perfused with good Doppler signals (Fig. 42.2). The major portion of the latissimus dorsi muscle flap was then inset into the upper tibial and knee wound with multiple interrupted horizontal mattress sutures over a closed suction drain. Split-thickness skin grafts were placed over the muscle flap and secured with multiple skin stapes (Fig. 42.3).

The left back flap donor site was closed after placing two drains into the donor site under the skin. The deep dermal layer was approximated with several interrupted 2-0 PDS sutures. The skin was then closed with 3-0 Monocryl in running subcuticular fashion.

Follow-Up Results

The patient did well postoperatively without any complications related to the free latissimus dorsi muscle flap reconstruction. Skin grafts over the muscle flap initially took. He was discharged from hospital on postoperative day 14. All drains were removed during subsequent follow-up visits. The left knee and upper tibial free flap reconstruction site healed well.

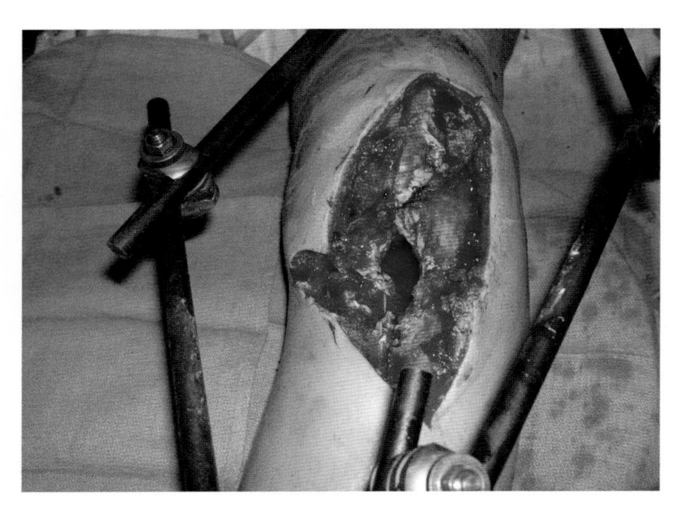

• **Fig. 42.1** A preoperative view showing a 22 × 10 cm upper tibial wound extending to the knee with the exposed tibial fracture and patella reconstruction sites.

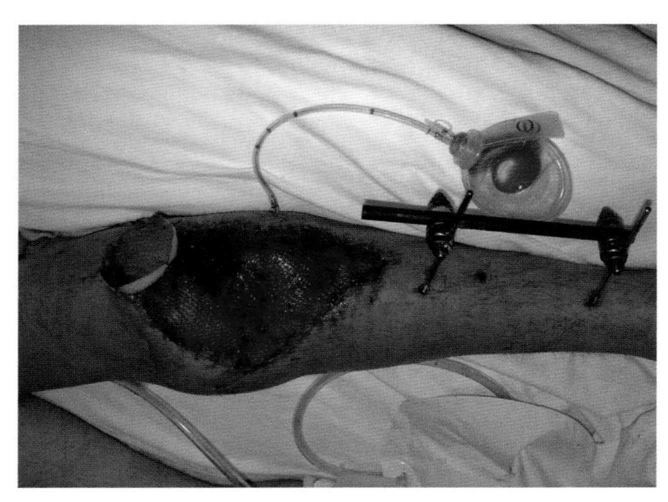

• **Fig. 42.3** One-week postoperative view showing a good soft tissue reconstruction to the wound after a successful free latissimus dorsi flap transfer.

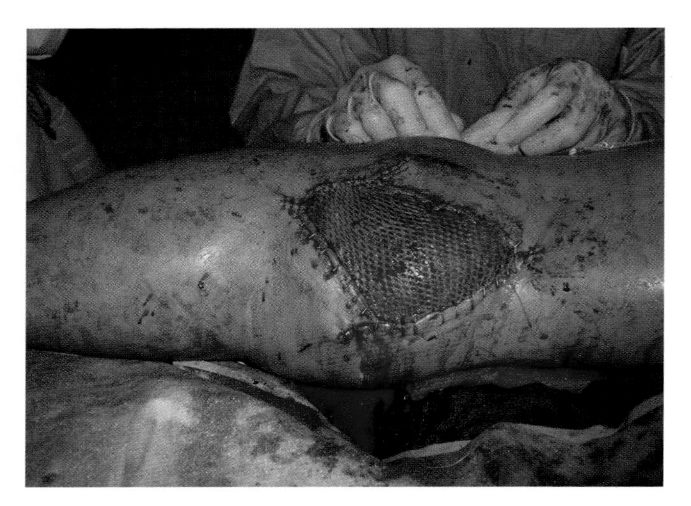

• **Fig. 42.2** An intraoperative view showing completion of the free latissimus dorsi muscle flap reconstruction. The popliteal wound used to explore both popliteal artery and vein were partially closed primarily and covered with the proximal portion of the skin-grafted muscle flap.

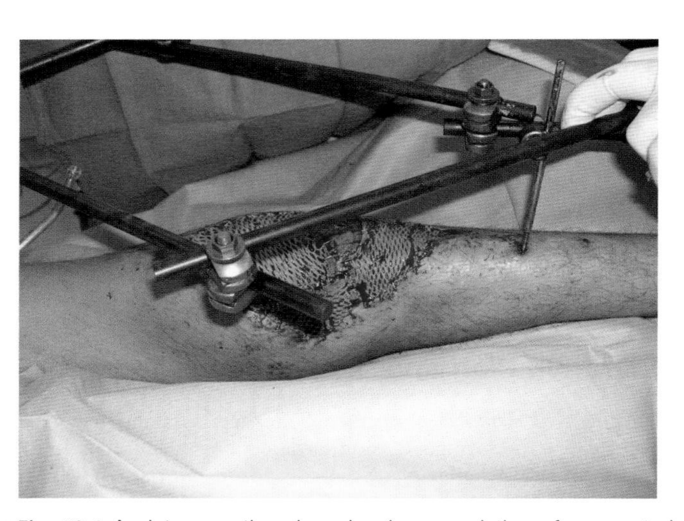

• **Fig. 42.4** An intraoperative view showing completion of a repeated skin graft procedure to the free latissimus dorsi muscle flap.

Management of Complications

The skin graft over the distal portion of the muscle flap had not healed well by postoperative 3 weeks. There were no issues related to the muscle flap. The patient was taken back to the operating room and underwent an additional skin graft procedure without difficulty (Fig. 42.4). The skin graft site over the muscle flap healed well after the subsequent operation (Fig. 42.5).

Final Outcome

Autologous bone grafting for the definitive fracture healing was performed 3 months later after the flap was elevated by the plastic surgery service (Figs. 42.6 and 42.7). The bone graft procedure went well and the fracture site healed. The knee and upper tibial free flap reconstruction site healed well with good contour and minimal scarring even after the second flap elevation. There was no recurrent infection under the flap. The patient has some stiffness in his left knee but he has resumed his normal activities and been routinely followed by the orthopedic trauma service (Fig. 42.8).

Pearls for Success

For a complex knee and upper tibial wound when a critical soft tissue reconstruction is necessary for the success of limb salvage, a free latissimus dorsi flap can be selected as a valid reconstructive option. The flap is large enough and can be harvested as a muscle flap to provide well-vascularized tissue for a reliable soft tissue coverage with skin graft. However, there are issues on selection of a good recipient vessel for such a free tissue transfer around the knee even though the muscle has a long pedicle. The popliteal vessels can be explored as a potential recipient vessel. However, both arterial and venous anastomoses should be performed end-to-side under loupe magnification. The proximal portion of the muscle flap could be used to close the popliteal incision. Because

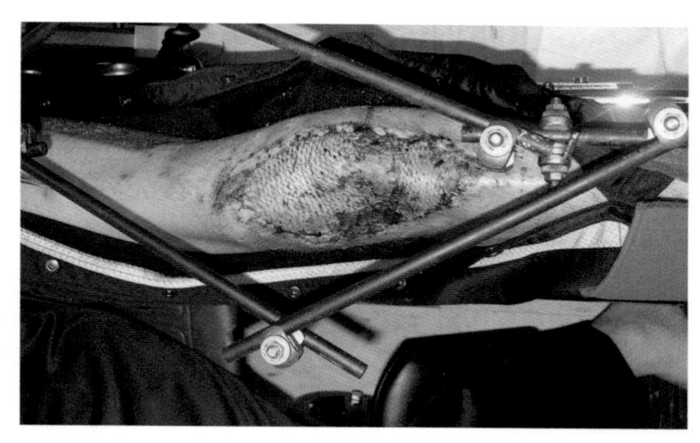

• **Fig. 42.5** A 10-day postoperative view after a repeated skin graft procedure showing almost complete adherence of skin grafts to the free latissimus dorsi muscle flap.

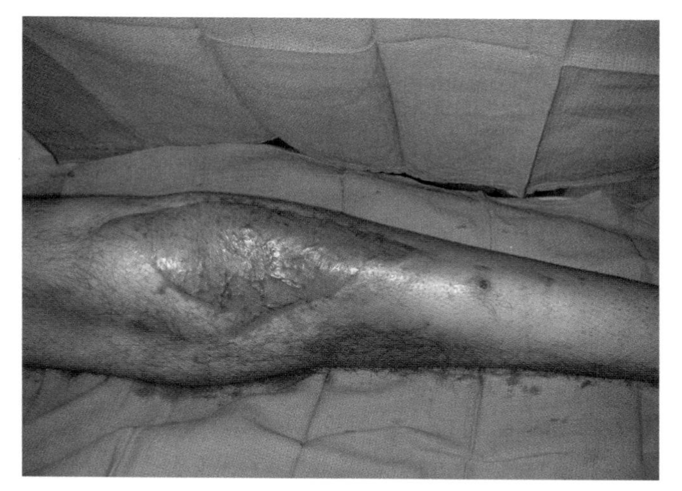

• **Fig. 42.6** A preoperative view 4 months after free latissimus dorsi muscle transfer showing well-healed flap reconstruction site.

of those external fixators, it might not be possible to place the patient in a true prone position. Thus, microvascular anastomoses of the flap reconstruction might be performed with some difficulty. The surgeon should routinely explore the descending genicular vessels. If those vessels can be determined as good recipient vessels, microvascular anastomoses for a free latissimus dorsi muscle flap can be performed while the patient is in the supine position. If not, the procedure can be done in the prone position where the popliteal vessels are selected as recipient vessels without the need for vein grafts. This unique vessel selection would avoid the use of a vein graft and yet still allow primary microvascular anastomoses. In addition, the size and shape of a latissimus muscle would naturally allow the muscle to fit well into a large knee and upper tibial wound after inset.

CASE 2

Clinical Presentation

A 36-year-old Asian male had a complex wound over the left lateral knee as a result of a gunshot wound. Apparently, part of the lateral femoral condyle was missing and there was a 13 × 9 cm soft tissue wound in the lateral knee. He was treated initially by our orthopedic trauma service with an external fixator and antibiotic spacer (Fig. 42.9). The plastic surgery service was consulted for soft tissue coverage to his lateral knee so that a future autologous bone graft could be performed for definitive bony reconstruction.

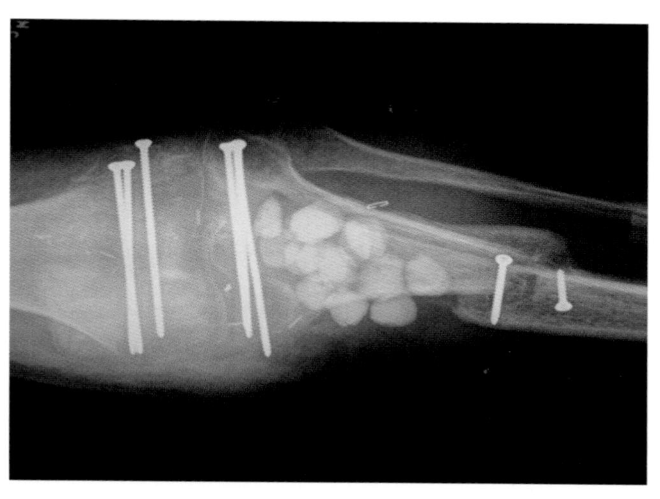

• **Fig. 42.7** An X-ray image before autologous bone graft procedure showing previously placed antibiotic beads in the fracture bony defect.

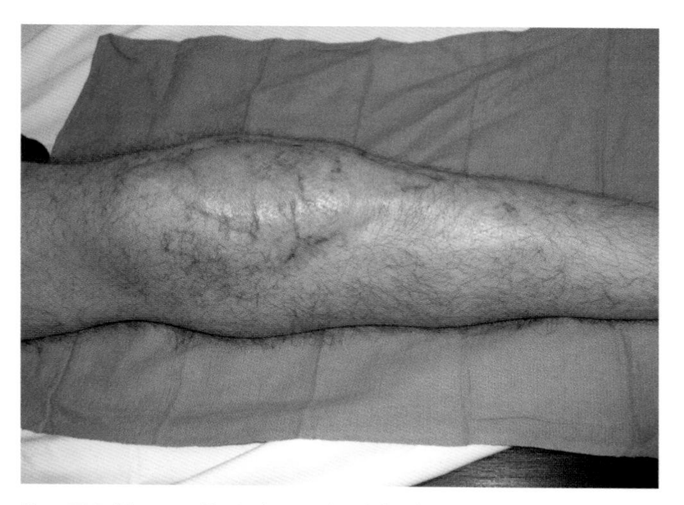

• **Fig. 42.8** The result at 4 months following autologous bone graft procedure and 8 months after free latissimus dorsi muscle transfer showing well-healed and stable left knee and upper tibial wound with good contour and minimal scarring.

Operative Plan and Special Considerations

For this complex lateral knee wound, a possible local fasciocutaneous flap, such as a reversed anterolateral thigh (ALT) perforator flap, was planned. The flap would provide adequate soft tissue for a reliable reconstruction. However, a free flap reconstruction should also be planned as a back-up option for the same reconstruction. A reverse ALT flap, based on the blood supply from perforators in the ALT region, is the same as a proximally based pedicle ALT flap. The flap, after adequate dissection, can be turned over to provide good soft tissue coverage in the knee. As

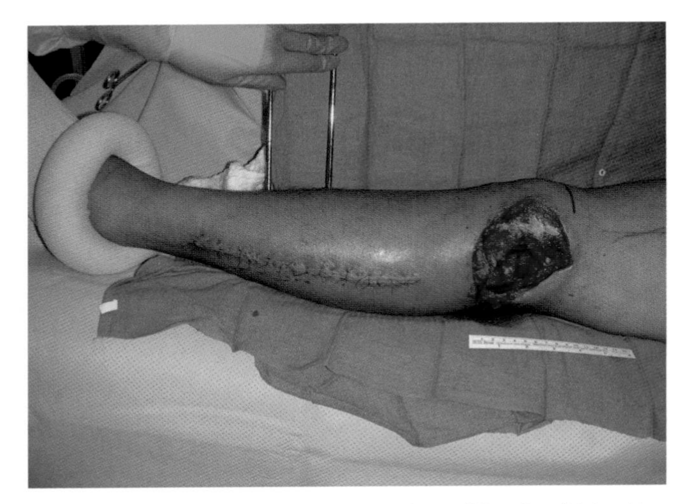

• **Fig. 42.9** A preoperative view showing a large (13 × 9 cm) lateral knee gunshot wound with the exposed underlying fracture and open knee joint.

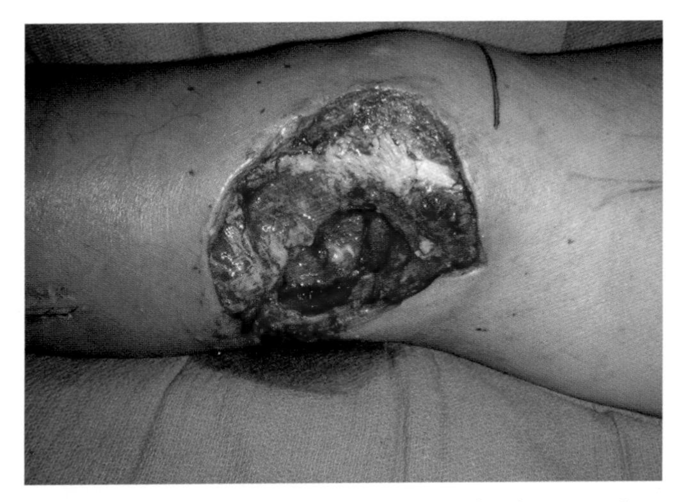

• **Fig. 42.10** An intraoperative close-up view showing the exposed open fracture site and open knee joint after debridemet.

with any ALT flap, the donor site can be closed primarily if the width of the flap is less than 8 to 9 cm. Otherwise, a skin graft would be needed to close the flap's donor site in the thigh. Preoperative mapping with a duplex scan would be helpful to identify proper perforators and the descending branch of the lateral circumflex femoral vessels.

Operative Procedures

Prior to the procedure, a duplex scan was performed by a vascular technician to map the perforators as well as the descending branch of the lateral circumflex femoral vessels. Under general anesthesia with the patient in the supine position, the left knee wound was debrided first and the skin edge was freshened with a blade. All colonized tissues were removed surgically. The wound was irrigated with Pulsavac and appeared to be clean and fresh (Fig. 42.10).

The left reversed ALT perforator flap with a 15 × 9 cm skin paddle was designed. Because of the location of the previous pin placement for an external fixator, the design of the skin paddle was shifted more laterally (Fig. 42.11). The skin and subcutaneous tissue were incised to the subfascial plane. The skin paddle of the flap was elevated along the subfascial plane. During dissection, several perforators were identified but only two major ones, which were much more medially located with reference to the skin paddle of the flap. By exploring the intramuscular space between the rectus femoris and vastus lateralis muscles, the descending branch of the lateral circumflex femoral vessels was identified. This could serve as a pedicle for the reversed ALT flap. However, by dissecting this branch further distally, it appeared that a segment of the branch had been damaged during the placement of the pin by orthopedic trauma service (Fig. 42.12). Therefore, the distally based reverse ALT flap was not possible because of the injury to the flap's pedicle.

However, the perforator dissection was carried out more proximally in the hope that this could be accomplished as a free

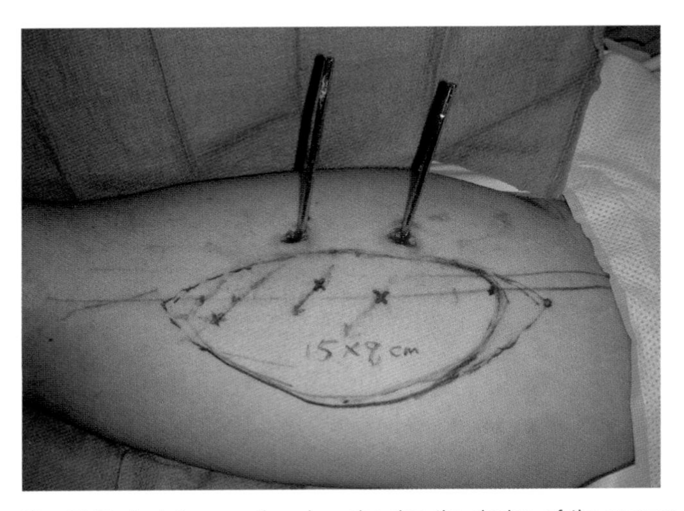

• **Fig. 42.11** An intraoperative view showing the design of the reverse anterolateral thigh flap with at least one confirmed sizable perforator within the skin paddle identified as a potential free-style free perforator flap.

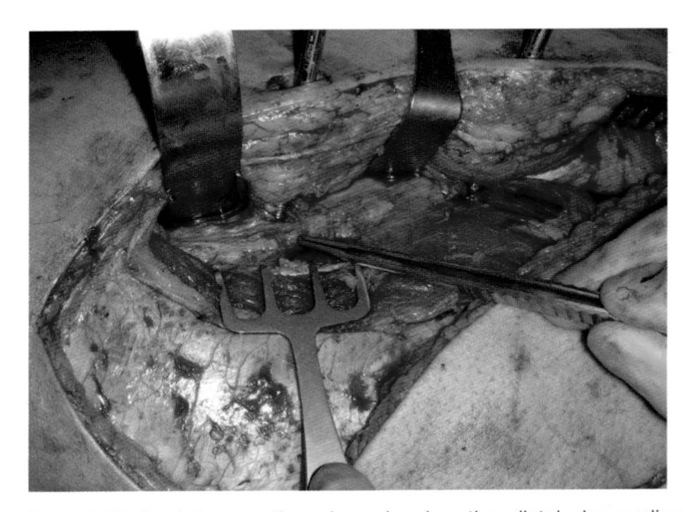

• **Fig. 42.12** An intraoperative view showing the distal descending branch of the lateral femoral circumflex vessels (the potential pedicle for the reversed anterolateral thigh flap) was injured by the pin placed for the external fixation.

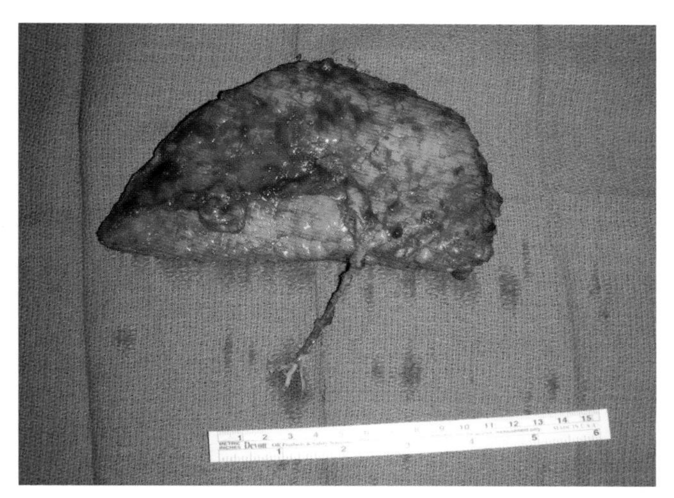

• **Fig. 42.13** An intraoperative view showing the free-style free thigh flap. In this case, after a tedious intramuscular dissection, an adequate length and diameter of the flap pedicle were obtained and the flap was elevated as a free-style free flap. The pedicle of this free-style free flap had one artery (approximately 1.2 mm) and two veins (one was approximately 1.5 mm).

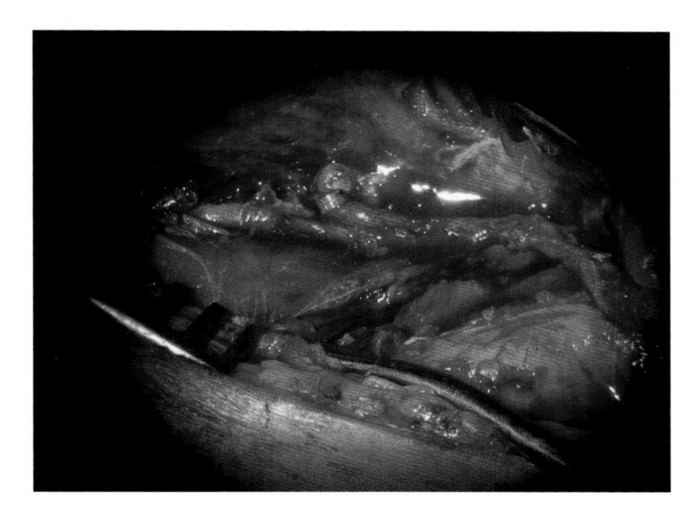

• **Fig. 42.14** An intraoperative view showing completion of both arterial (end-to-side) and venous (end-to-end) microanastomoses under an operating microscope.

ALT perforator flap. For a larger perforator, the fascia around it was opened longitudinal. A very tedious intramuscular dissection was performed under loupe magnification. With more intramuscular perforator dissection, many small branches were divided. It became obvious that the perforator dissection appeared to go quite deep inside the muscle and would not go to the proximal portion of the descending branch of the lateral circumflex femoral vessels. Therefore, an intraoperative decision was made to convert this flap to a free-style free thigh perforator flap. After intramuscular dissection of nearly 12 cm, the length (10–12 cm) and possible diameter (>1.2 mm) of the pedicle were thought to be adequate once it joined relatively large vessels. At this level, the pedicle could be divided as a free-style free skin perforator flap (Fig. 42.13).

Before dividing the pedicle, the anterior tibial vessels were explored based on a normal preoperative angiogram. The skin

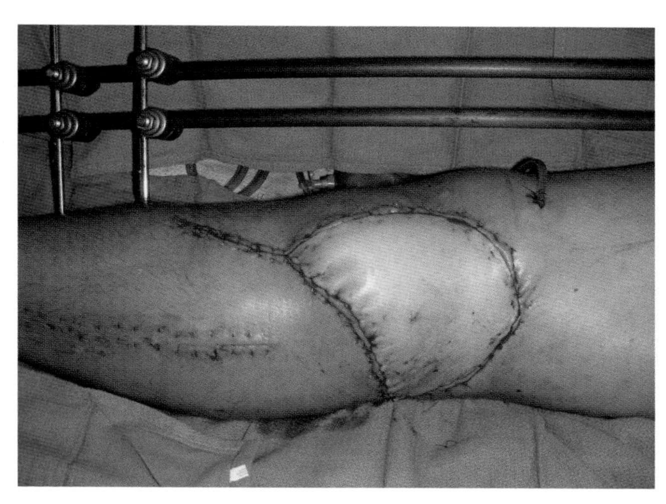

• **Fig. 42.15** An intraoperative view showing completion of the flap inset and closure of the incision used for exploration of the anterior tibial vessels.

incision was extended distally from the lateral knee wound and the anterior tibial vessels were identified in the space between the extensor digitorium longus and anterior tibialis muscles. The anterior tibial artery and vein were dissected free. Both vessels appeared to be a good size and could be used as recipient vessels for microvascular anastomosis.

The free-style free thigh perforator flap was prepared under loupe magnification. Both artery and vena comitans were prepared. One vein appeared to be bigger, measuring approximately 1.5 mm. The artery appeared to be quite small with a diameter of approximately 1.2 mm. The flap was flushed with heparinized saline (Fig. 42.13), placed temporarily into the wound, and secured with multiple towel clips.

Microvascular anastomosis was performed under an operating microscope. The end-to-side arterial microanastomosis was performed to the anterior tibial artery. A small arteriotomy was performed with an 11 blade and the arteriotomy opening was enlarged after trimming the wall of the artery. The pedicle artery was trimmed in an oblique fashion and in this way, there was a bigger opening for an end-to-side anastomosis. The anastomosis was done with interrupted 9-0 nylon sutures. The vena comitans was divided more distally. The venous microanastomosis was performed with a 1.5-mm coupler device in an end-to-end fashion. Once all clamps were removed, there was a good flow through the arterial anastomosis. After that, the flap appeared to be well perfused with a strong Doppler signal (Fig. 42.14).

The antibiotic spacer was placed back into the wound and a 10-flat JP was inserted under the flap. The incision for exposure of the anterior tibial vessel was approximated with multiple skin staples. The flap was then inset into the lateral knee wound and approximated to the adjacent skin with several interrupted 3-0 Monocryl sutures in half-buried horizontal mattress fashion (Fig. 42.15).

The left thigh donor site was closed next. The vastus lateralis muscle was approximated with several interrupted 3-0 Vicryl sutures. The fascial incision was closed with 3-0 Monocryl suture in a figure-of-eight. Much of the skin defect was closed with 2-0 PDS sutures. The remaining wound was closed with a split-thickness skin graft, which was harvested from the lateral thigh.

The skin graft was meshed to 1:1.5 ratio, placed on the wound, and secured with multiple skin staples to the wound edge. The skin graft site was covered with Xeroform, bacitracin ointment, some fluffs, and the vacuum-assisted closure sponge was secured with multiple skin staples. The skin graft donor site was covered with a Tegaderm dressing (Fig. 42.16).

Follow-Up Results

The patient did well postoperatively without any complications related to the free-style free thigh perforator flap for coverage of the left lateral knee wound. He was discharged from hospital on postoperative day 10. All drains were removed during subsequent follow-up visits. The left lateral knee reconstruction site healed well. The closure for the flap donor including a skin graft site also healed well (Fig. 42.17).

Final Outcome

The left lateral knee free flap reconstruction site healed well with good contour and minimal scarring (Fig. 42.18). The patient underwent an autologous bone grafting to the lateral femoral condyle about 4 months later at an outside hospital and had good bony union after the procedure. He has resumed his normal activities and been routinely followed by an outside orthopedic service.

Pearls for Success

For a large complex lateral knee wound, when there is no good local reconstructive option available including a reversed ALT flap, it can be converted to a free-style free thigh perforator flap if a sizable perforator can be identified, followed, and dissected safely. Such a surgical dissection can be very tedious and time-consuming. Thus, a free-style free flap requires much more sophisticated perforator dissection and microsurgical techniques, because the diameter of the pedicle vessels is smaller (<1.5 mm) and microvascular anastomosis can be challenging. As demonstrated in this case, an intraoperative decision can be made to convert to a free-style free flap if a sizable perforator is identified. A tedious intramuscular dissection can be performed successfully by following the perforator, if a pedicle longer than 10 cm can be dissected free, the diameter of the pedicle artery (>1.2 mm) is thought to be adequate to perform an end-to-side arterial microanastomosis, and the diameter of the pedicle vein (>1.5 mm) is thought to be adequate to perform an end-to-end venous microanastomosis. Proper amount of traction set up by the surgeon to the flap and staying relatively closer to the perforator during the perforator flap dissection may be the key for the success of a free-style free flap perforator dissection.

CASE 3

Clinical Presentation

A 64-year-old White female developed a complicated right popliteal wound secondary to previous radiation. Apparently, she had had a sarcoma in the area and underwent a surgical resection by the surgical oncology service. She then underwent post-operative radiation to the area. Unfortunately, the patient

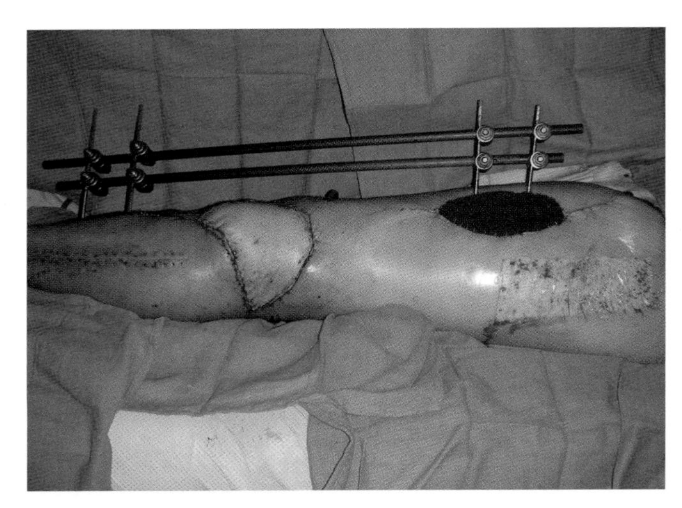

• **Fig. 42.16** An intraoperative view showing completion of the flap donor site closure with primary closure and skin grafting.

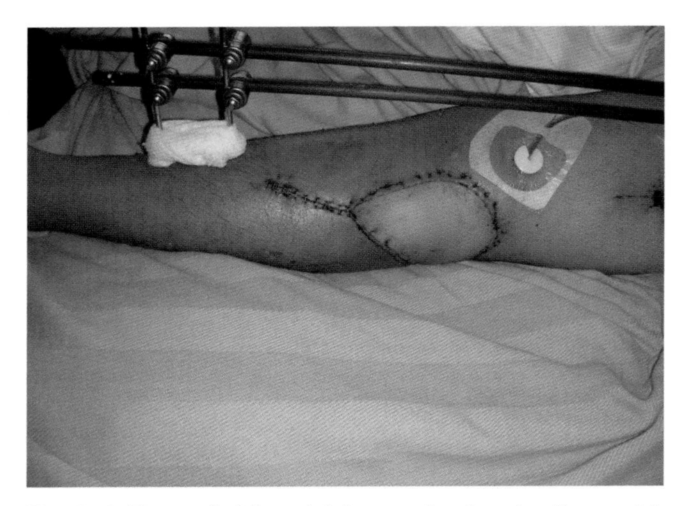

• **Fig. 42.17** The result at 2-week follow-up showing a healthy, surviving free-style free thigh perforator flap.

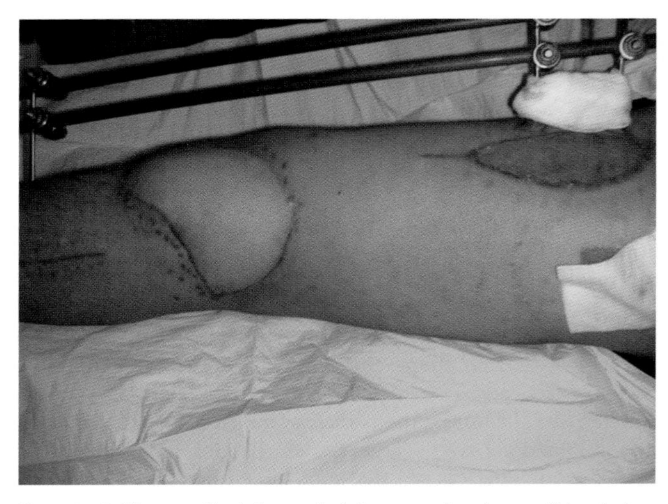

• **Fig. 42.18** The result at 4-month follow-up showing well-healed and stable left lateral knee free-style free thigh perforator flap site with good contour and minimal scarring. The flap donor site also healed well.

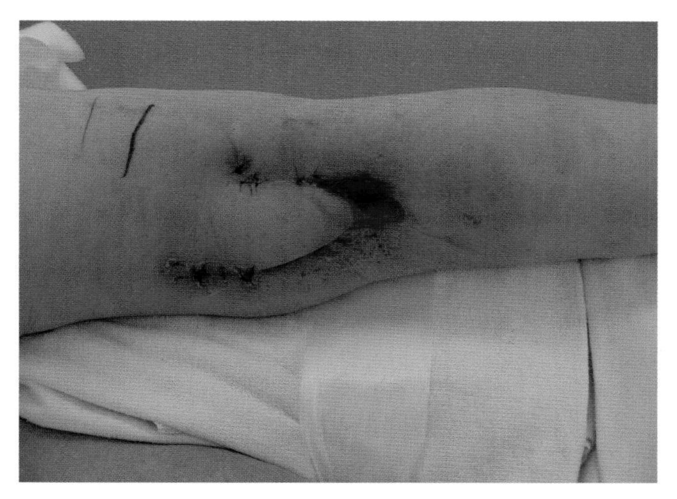

• **Fig. 42.19** An intraoperative view showing a 15 × 9 cm complex soft tissue radiation wound in the popliteal region.

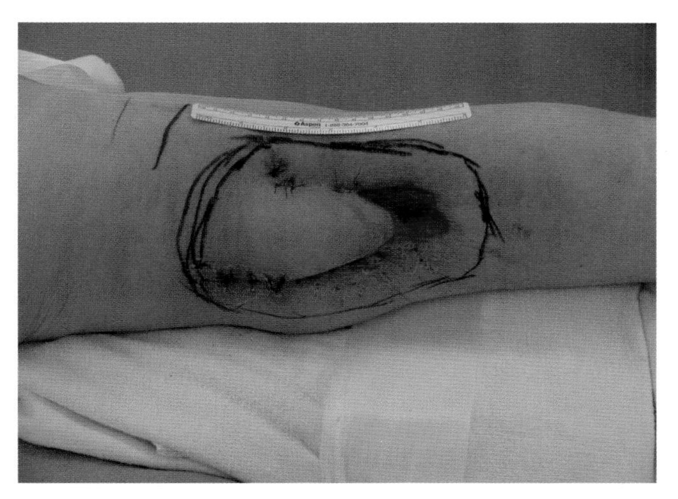

• **Fig. 42.20** An intraoperative close-up view showing the soft tissue radiation wound in the popliteal region. The zone of the radiation injury was marked.

developed a wound dehiscence after her oncological surgical resection. There was potential for exposure of the popliteal vessels at the base of the wound. The plastic surgery service was consulted to provide a soft tissue coverage for the popliteal wound. Two attempts at the local fasciocutaneous flap were performed. Although the local flap had completely survived, the patient developed a wound dehiscence between the flap and her native skin in the distal part of the wound with consistent drainage (Fig. 42.19). With consideration of limb salvage and prevention of a potential popliteal vessel blowout, a free flap reconstruction was offered to this patient in order to close this complex popliteal wound (Fig. 42.20).

Operative Plan and Special Considerations

The primary soft tissue wound over the popliteal area can be problematic because of potential exposure of the popliteal vessels. After failed local option for soft tissue coverage, a free flap should be considered to provide more reliable soft tissue reconstruction to

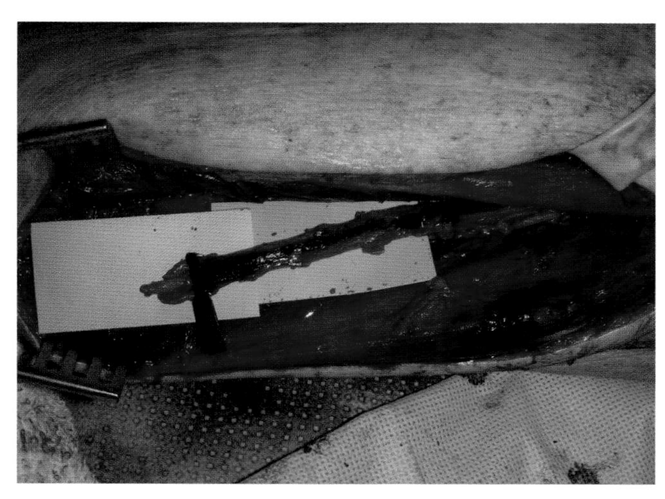

• **Fig. 42.21** An intraoperative view showing the anterior tibial vessels that were dissected free between the anterior tibialis and extensor digitorium longus muscles.

the popliteal region. In this case, a free latissimus dorsi muscle flap could be selected for such a reconstruction. The flap has a long pedicle and can provide a large amount of well-vascularized soft tissue for reliable soft tissue reconstruction in the popliteal region. However, based on this author's experience, it can be difficult because a good, reliable recipient vessel may not be readily available for the free tissue transfer to the poplieal area. When the patient has a normal vascular anatomy of the lower extremity, the anterior tibial vessels can be dissected free for an adequate length and act as a created recipient vessel once they are turned over to a superficial location near the popliteal region for two end-to-end microvascular anastomoses. In this way, both microvascular anastomoses can be performed without difficulty because the latissimus dorsi muscle also has a long pedicle and can be tunneled to a superficial location. A skin graft over the muscle flap would also be needed for the final wound closure.

Operative Techniques

Under general anesthesia with the patient in a left lateral decubitus position, the right popliteal wound, measuring 15 × 9 cm, was debrided. The large, radiated wound was then excised down to the fresh- and healthy-looking tissues. All colonized and scarred tissues within the wound were removed. The wound was irrigated with Pulsavac ready for definitive soft tissue coverage.

A longitudinal incision was made along the anterolateral leg. The incision was about 20 cm long and parallel to the lateral border of the tibia. The skin and subcutaneous tissue were incised and the fascia was opened. The anterior tibial neurovascular bundle was identified between the anterior tibialis muscle and extensor digitorum longus muscle and the deep peroneal nerve was dissected from the vessel. With the aid of loupe magnification, the dissection was performed along the entire anterior tibial vessels. Many small branches of the anterior tibial vessels were divided with hemoclips. A 20-cm section of anterior tibial vessels including the anterior tibial artery and its vena comitans were dissected free. The distal artery and its vena comitans were divided with hemoclips (Fig. 42.21). The subcutaneous tunnel was made between the wound and the anterolateral portion of the leg near the posterior knee (Fig. 42.22). The anterior tibial vessels were

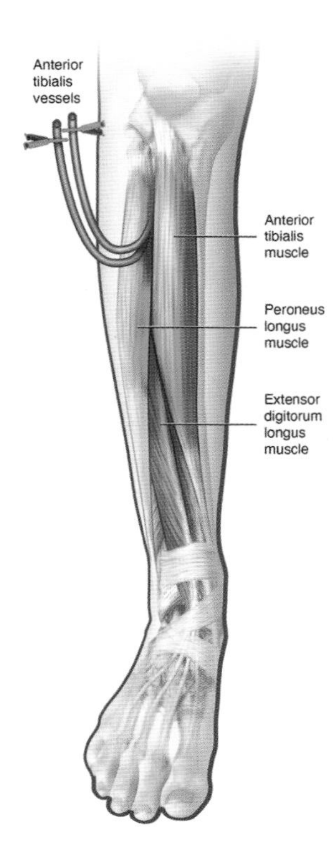

• **Fig. 42.22** The schematic diagram showing the anterior tibial vessels turnover as recipient vessels.

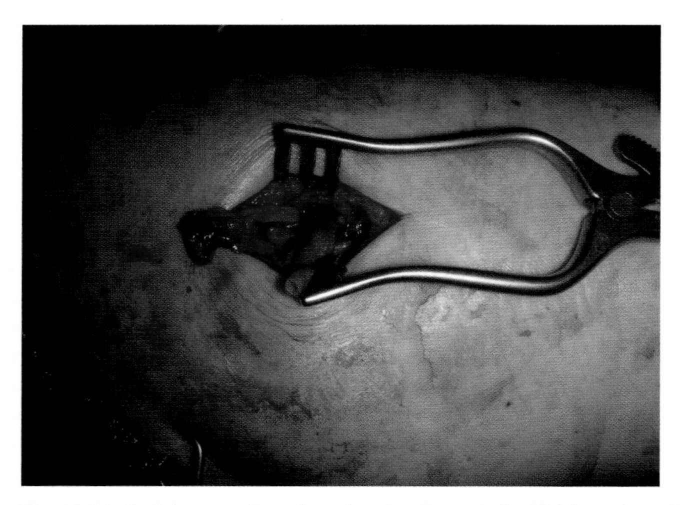

• **Fig. 42.23** An intraoperative view showing the anterior tibial artery and vein that were turned over, tunneled, and placed in a subcutaneous location near the popliteal wound.

turned over through the subcutaneous tunnel and the absence of kinking and twisting was confirmed. They were placed in a nearby superficial location for subsequent microvascular anastomoses (Fig. 42.23).

A right free latissimus dorsi free muscle flap was then harvested. With an oblique incision through the skin and subcutaneous tissue down to the fascia, the latissimus dorsi muscle was identified. The medial border was identified first and the muscle was then divided more distally close to the posterior iliac spine. Its lateral border was also dissected free. During dissection, the serratus muscle was

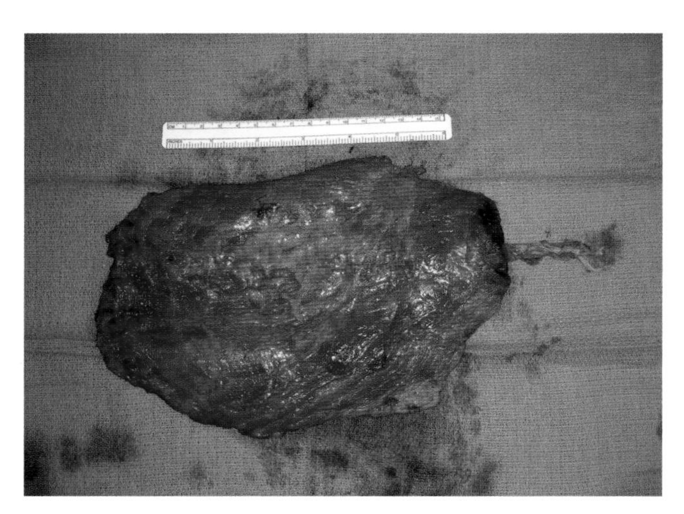

• **Fig. 42.24** An intraoperative view showing completion of temporarily free latissimus dorsi muscle flap inset and microvascular anastomoses for both artery and vein.

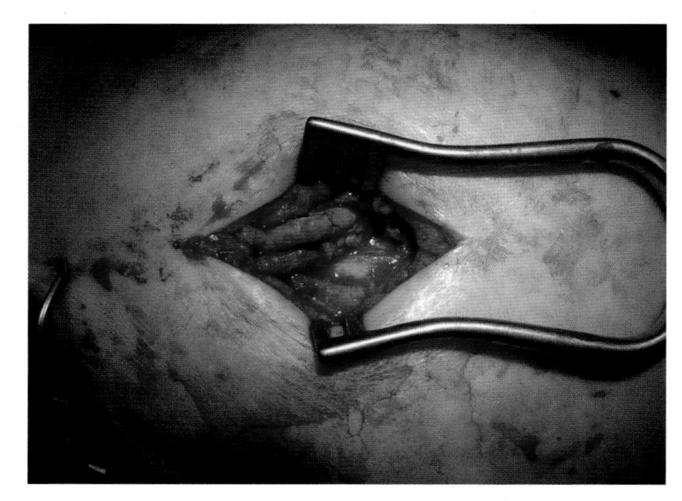

• **Fig. 42.25** An intraoperative view showing completion of microvascular anastomose for both artery and vein in a superficial location.

identified and separated from the latissimus dorsi muscle. The dissection was continued toward the pedicle and its pedicle was identified once the muscle had been elevated. The dissection was continued toward the axilla. The muscle was detached from the humerus. The thoracodorsal nerve was divided and then several side branches of the thoracodorsal vessel were also divided. Once the dissection was close to the axillary vessels, the pedicle was divided and at this point the surgical dissection of the free latissimus dorsi muscle flap was completed. The pedicle of the muscle flap was prepared under loupe magnification. The artery and vein were identified and dissected free. The artery was flushed with heparinized saline solution. One artery and two veins were prepared for microvascular anastomoses (Fig. 42.24).

The muscle flap was temporarily inset into the popliteal wound. Under an operating microscope, an end-to-end arterial microanastomosis was performed with an interrupted 8-0 nylon suture. The venous microanastomosis was performed with a 2.5-mm coupler device in an end-to-end fashion (Fig. 42.25). After all clamps had been removed, the flap appeared to be well-perfused with a good Doppler signal.

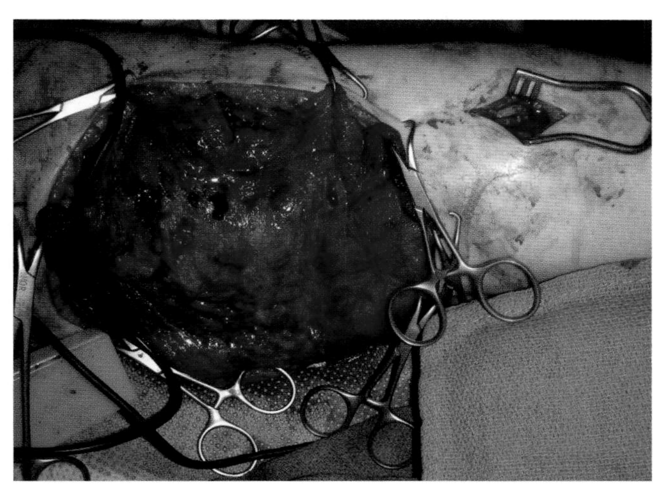

• **Fig. 42.26** An intraoperative view showing completion of the initial muscle flap inset.

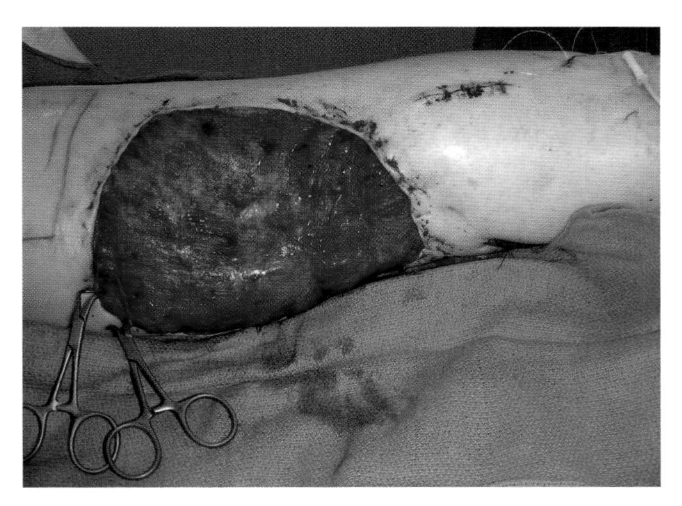

• **Fig. 42.27** An intraoperative view showing completion of a skin-grafted free latissimus dorsi muscle flap reconstruction for the popliteal wound.

The final inset of the muscle flap was performed once both microanastomoses were confirmed to be satisfactory (Fig. 42.26). A 10-mm flat JP was inserted into the wound under the flap. The muscle flap was sutured to the adjacent skin edge of the wound with interrupted 3-0 Monocryl sutures in a half-buried horizontal mattress fashion (Fig. 42.27). A split-thickness skin graft was harvested from the right posterior thigh. The skin graft was meshed to 1:1.5 ratio, placed over the muscle flap, and secured to the adjacent skin with skin staples. Several quilting sutures were placed with 5-0 chromic suture to immobilize the skin graft. The anterolateral leg incision for exposure of the anterior tibial vessel was closed in two layers (Fig. 42.28).

The right back latissimus flap donor site was closed in three layers after placing two 10-mm flat JP drains. The deep tissue layer was approximated with several interrupted 2-0 PDS sutures. The deep dermal layer was approximated with several interrupted 3-0 Monocryl sutures. The skin was closed with a 3-0 V-Loc suture in a running subcuticular fashion.

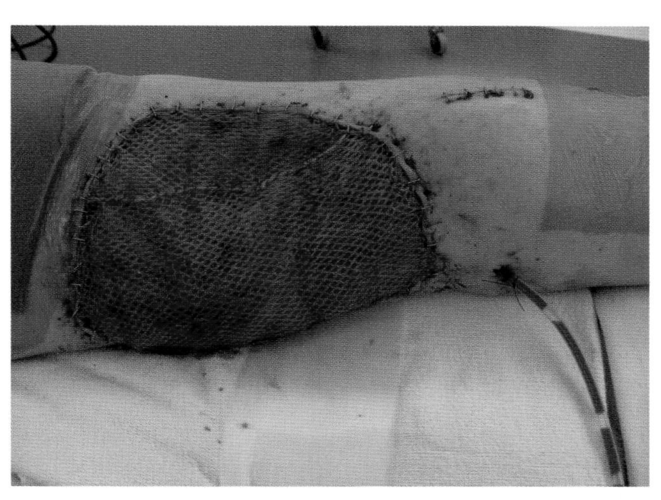

• **Fig. 42.28** An intraoperative view showing completion of the flap inset and the rest of the wound closure including a skin graft.

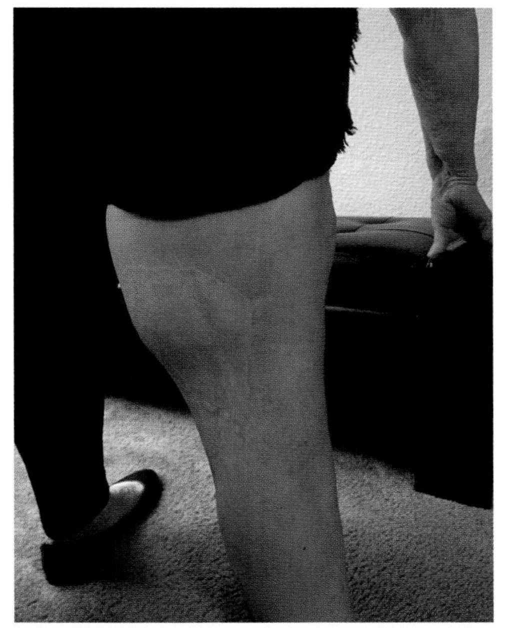

• **Fig. 42.29** The result at 4.5-year follow-up showing well-healed and stable right popliteal wound with good contour and minimal scarring.

Follow-Up Results

The patient did well postoperatively without any complications related to the free latissimus dorsi muscle flap reconstruction for her popliteal wound. She was discharged from hospital on postoperative day 14. All drains were removed during subsequent follow-up office visits. The right free latissimus dorsi muscle flap reconstruction site and the skin graft over the muscle flap healed well.

Final Outcome

The free flap reconstruction site for the popliteal wound coverage healed well with an excellent contour and minimal scarring

(Fig. 42.29). The patient has resumed her normal activities and been routinely followed by the surgical oncology service.

Pearls for Success

For a large complex knee wound when there is no good local reconstructive option available, a free flap, such as a free latissimus dorsi muscle flap, can be selected as a valid reconstructive option. However, selection of reliable recipient vessels is essential for successful microvascular free tissue transfer around the knee because of its unique vascular anatomy. In addition, selection of recipient vessels can be further complicated when patients have vascular trauma, a large zone of injury, or previous irradiation. As demonstrated in this case, an innovative creation of proper recipient vessels is possible for microvascular free tissue transfer around the knee with turnover of the anterior tibial vessels. In this way, a reliable recipient vessel is created and relatively straightforward microvascular anastomoses can be performed to ensure success. The anterior tibial vessels can be dissected for an adequate length and turned over to a superficial location near the popliteal wound for relatively easy microvascular anastomoses. The long vascular pedicle allows easy microvascular anastomosis and tension-free inset into the posterior knee wound. In addition, its pedicle vessel has good and there is no mismatch for microvascular anastomoses. In the event of microvascular thrombosis, risk to the distal extremity ischemia is mitigated by avoiding the popliteal and posterior tibial vessels. However, the anterior tibial vessel turnover for microvascular anastomosis cannot be used in cases of trauma or peripheral arterial disease where the anterior tibial vessels are not patent. A skin-grafted free latissimus dorsi muscle flap reconstruction for a popliteal wound can be significantly shrunk for an excellent long-term outcome.

Recommended Readings

Athey AG, Wyles CC, Carlsen BT, Perry KI, Houdek MT, Moran SL. Free flap coverage for complex primary and revision total knee arthroplasty. *Plast Reconstr Surg.* 2021;148:804e–810e.

Fang T, Zhang EW, Lineaweaver WC, Zhang F. Recipient vessels in the free flap reconstruction around the knee. *Ann Plast Surg.* 2013;71:429–433.

Louer CR, Garcia RM, Earle SA, Hollenbeck ST, Erdmann D, Levin LS. Free flap reconstruction of the knee: an outcome study of 34 cases. *Ann Plast Surg.* 2015;74:57–63.

Liau JE, Pu LL. Reconstruction of a large upper tibial wound extending to the knee with a free latissimus dorsi flap: optimizing the outcomes. *Microsurgery.* 2007;27:548–552.

Pu LL. Learning from our international colleagues: a US plastic surgeon's perspective. *Ann Plast Surg.* 2013;70:470–475.

Zeiderman MR, Bailey CM, Arora A, Pu LLQ. Anterior tibial vessel turnover as recipient vessel for complex free tissue transfer around the knee. *J Plast Reconstr Aesthet Surg.* 2020;73:1897–1916.

Zeiderman MR, Pu LLQ. Free-style free perforator flaps in lower extremity reconstruction. *Clin Plast Surg.* 2021;48:215–223.

43

Leg Reconstruction: Proximal Third

CASE 1

Clinical Presentation

An 11-year-old White male sustained a significant crush and avulsion injury to his right upper leg as a result of a motor vehicle accident. He had extensive full-thickness skin loss over the proximal third of his leg with the exposed underlying tibia measuring 7 × 2 cm. The soft tissue wound was debrided by the trauma service and his surgical care was then transferred to the plastic surgery service for definitive soft tissue reconstruction (Fig. 43.1). Soft tissue coverage was planned after definitive debridement.

Operative Plan and Special Considerations for Reconstruction

For this relatively large soft tissue wound with the exposed tibia in the proximal third of the leg, a classic local muscle flap, such as a medial gastrocnemius muscle flap, can be selected to cover the exposed tibia. The medial gastrocnemius muscle is a type I muscle flap and receives a blood supply primarily from the medial sural artery off the popliteal artery. The rest of the wound can be closed by an adjacent skin rearrangement and a split-thickness skin graft as a one-stage reconstruction. Because of significant crushing injury to the adjacent skin, any perforator-based skin flaps would not be an option. In addition, a distant flap, such as a reversed anterolateral thigh perforator flap, would not reach the proximal tibial location.

Operative Procedures

Under general anesthesia with the patient in the supine position, the right proximal tibial wound was debrided and unhealthy looking and traumatized skin was excised. All colonized tissues were sharply removed. The open wound appeared to be fresh and clean after a definitive debridement performed by the plastic surgery service (Fig. 43.2).

The proposed incision for exposure of the distal medial gastrocnemius muscle was marked and the flap dissection was performed under tourniquet control (Fig. 43.3). The skin incision was made through the skin, subcutaneous tissues, and fascia to expose the medial gastrocnemius muscle. In the proximal third of the leg, the medial surface of the medial gastrocnemius muscle was easily separated from the soleus muscle. The plantaris tendon was visualized between the gastrocnemius muscle and the underlying soleus muscle. The dissection went distally along the medial boarder of the medial gastrocnemius until its tendon joined the Achilles tendon. The tendon of the muscle was divided several centimeters distal to the muscle belly and the medial half of the gastrocnemius muscle was dissected from distal to proximal direction along the raphe between the medial and lateral gastrocnemius muscle bellies. During the flap dissection, the lessor saphenous vein and sural nerve were visualized and protected. Once the medial gastrocnemius muscle was elevated adequately, it was rotated medially to cover the exposed upper tibia. The flap was temporarily inset into the wound and the entire exposed upper tibial was completely covered. One drain was placed under the flap and another in the donor site.

The flap was approximated with the adjacent subcutaneous tissue with several interrupted half-buried 3-0 Monocryl sutures. Additional local skin rearrangements were done for some portions of wound closure and the rest of the wound including the muscle flap was covered with split-thickness skin grafts. Split-thickness skin grafts were harvested with a dermatome from the right lateral thigh and meshed to 1:1.5 ratio. The incision for the flap exposure was closed in two layers and all skin grafts were secured with skin staples (Fig. 43.4).

Follow-Up Results

The patient did well postoperatively without any issues related to the flap reconstruction and wound closure. He was discharged from hospital on postoperative day 5. The right upper leg wound healed uneventfully. He was followed by the plastic surgery service for routine postoperative care.

Final Outcome

During further follow-up, the right upper tibial wound flap reconstruction site has healed well with good contour and minimal scarring. There were no wound breakdown, recurrent infection, or contour issues related to the soft tissue reconstruction (Fig. 43.5). The patient has resumed his regular activities and has returned to school as a normal student.

Pearls for Success

This is a classic example where a medial gastrocnemius muscle flap is used to cover a complex proximal tibial wound. With a combination of the local muscle flap, local skin rearrangement, and skin graft, such a complex upper tibial wound can be reconstructed successfully. A medial gastrocnemius muscle flap is a

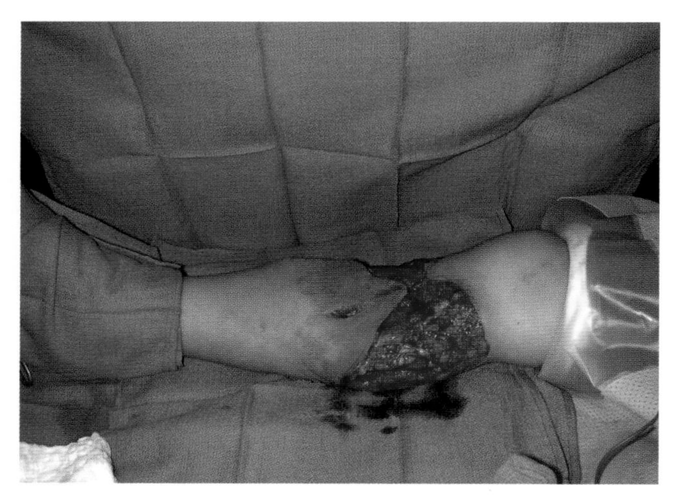

• **Fig. 43.1** A preoperative view showing a large and complex upper tibial crush and avulsion injury wound with exposed upper tibia.

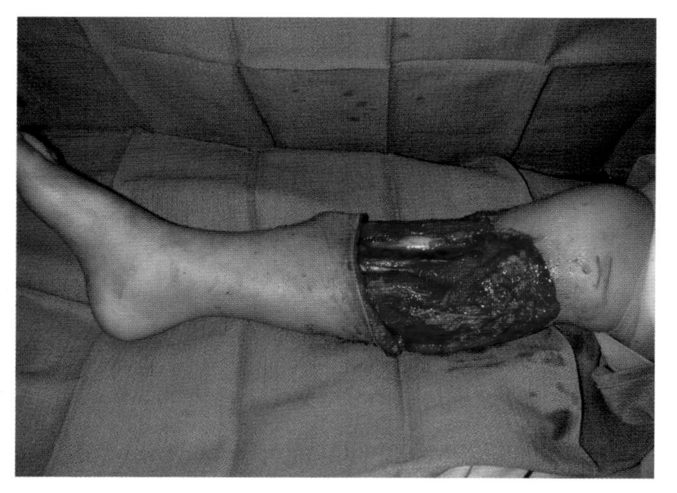

• **Fig. 43.2** An intraoperative view showing a fresh and clean proximal tibial wound after definitive debridement by the plastic surgery service.

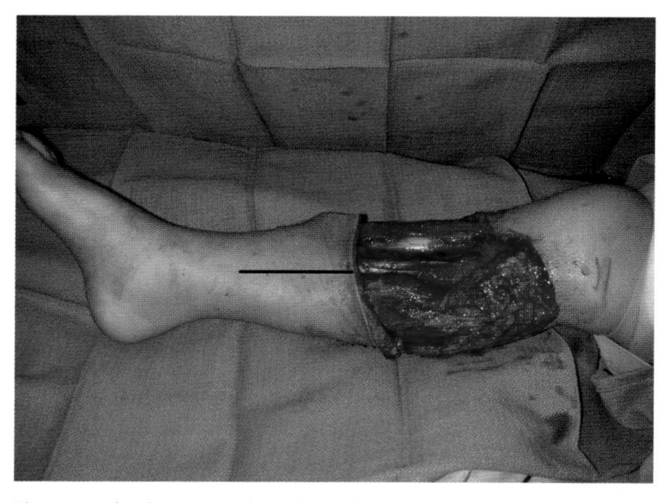

• **Fig. 43.3** An intraoperative view showing the planned incision for dissection of the medial gastrocnemius muscle flap.

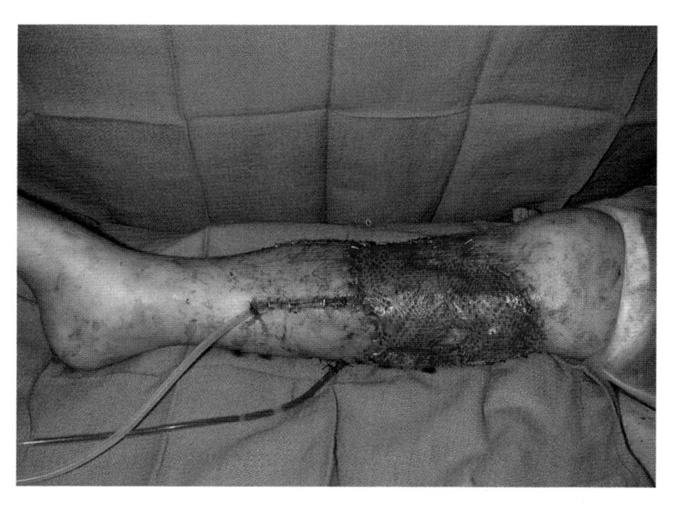

• **Fig. 43.4** An intraoperative view showing completion of the medial gastrocnemius muscle flap reconstruction. In this case, local skin rearrangement was performed and split-thickness skin grafts were added for the entire wound closure.

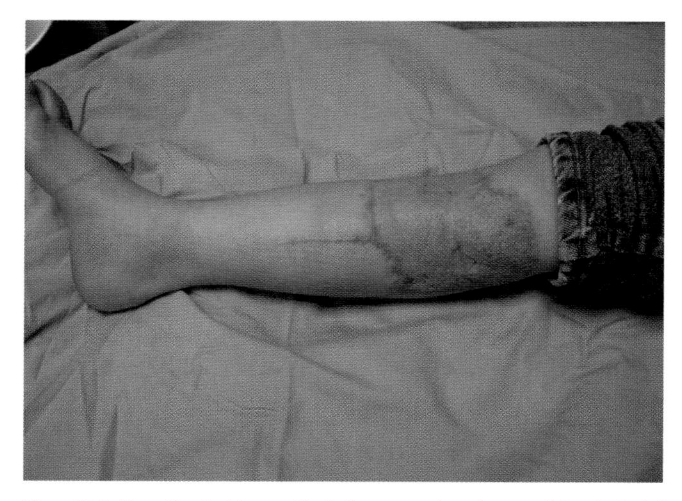

• **Fig. 43.5** Result at 11-month follow-up showing well-healed right proximal tibial wound after above flap reconstruction, local skin rearrangement, and skin grafts for the entire wound closure.

work horse to provide good soft tissue coverage for an upper tibial wound. If not traumatized, the muscle flap can be reliable and expanded several centimeters after fascial scoring on the surface of the muscle belly. If needed, the origin of the muscle flap can be divided from the medial condyle of the femur under direct vision once the medial sural artery has been identified. This maneuver can also add several centimeters to the flap advancement. Once the muscle origin has been divided, the flap's further advancement should be done very carefully to prevent avulsion injury to the pedicle because the pedicle length of the medial sural artery is quite short.

CASE 2

Clinical Presentation

A 58-year-old White female underwent orthopedic debridement of a previous left proximal tibial fracture site for nonunion. New

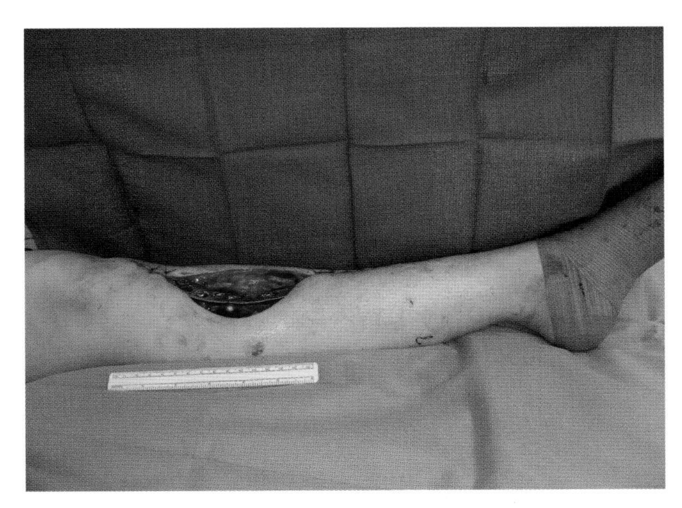

• **Fig. 43.6** A preoperative view showing the proximal third of the leg wound extended to the middle third, measuring 11 × 5.5 cm, with exposed fracture site and reconstruction plate.

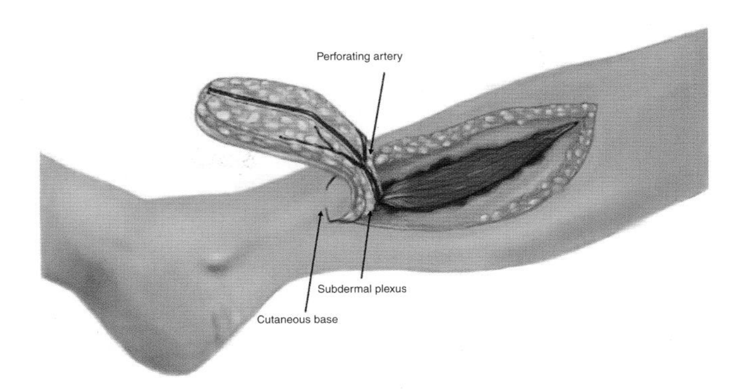

• **Fig. 43.7** A schematic diagram demonstrating the perforator-plus flap anatomy and design. Note the attached cutaneous base that allows a dual blood supply from the perforating vessel and the subdermal plexus.

open reduction and internal fixation with a large reconstruction plate were performed. Unfortunately, this left an 11 × 5.5 cm soft tissue wound mostly in the proximal third of the left leg with exposed fracture site and reconstruction plate. The plastic surgery service was asked by the orthopedic trauma service to provide soft tissue coverage for the fracture site and exposed reconstruction plate to facilitate wound closure (Fig. 43.6). The patient had several comorbidities including chronic occlusive pulmonary disease for which she received steroid therapy. Her leg was also relatively small with significant muscle atrophy and the fracture union and soft tissue healing therefore remained a challenge.

Operative Plan and Special Considerations for Reconstruction

For such a large proximal-third of leg wound extending to the middle-third of leg with exposed fracture site and hardware, a classic medial gastrocnemius muscle flap would normally not be large enough to provide coverage. In addition, the medial gastrocnemius muscle was also found to have atrophy and could not be used in this patient. A free flap reconstruction can be an option, but her multiple comorbidities would preclude her as a good candidate. With increasing knowledge and skill on perforator flap surgery, a local perforator-base skin flap can be attempted instead of a free flap reconstruction as an alternative option. The perforator-plus flap is a modification of the classic perforator-based fasciocutaneous flap. Instead of the skin paddle being supplied solely on the isolated perforator, the perforator-plus flap allows augmentation of the vascular supply to the perforating pedicle by keeping the skin edge attached to a cutaneous base (Fig. 43.7). Therefore, both the arterial inflow and venous outflow become more reliable. In exchange for a smaller arc of the flap rotation, a relatively larger and more robust local skin flap can be designed. The author prefers the use of intraoperative duplex scan in addition to a hand-held Doppler probe to identify target perforators accurately. In general, at least one good perforator is needed for the design of such a flap.

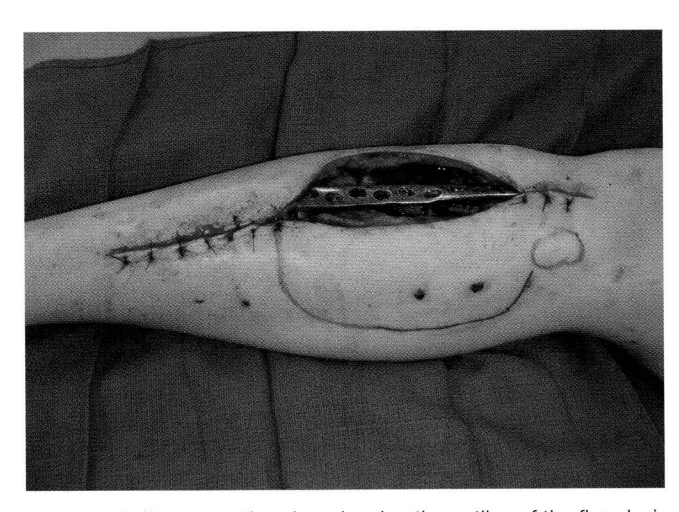

• **Fig. 43.8** An intraoperative view showing the outline of the flap design and two identified perforators within the flap territory and an intact skin portion as a bridge.

Operative Procedures

Under general anesthesia with the patient in the supine position, the left proximal leg wound was debrided. All unhealthy-looking skin edges and colonized tissues were removed. The open fracture wound appeared to be fresh and clean after more definitive soft tissue debridement performed by the plastic surgery service.

Two good perforators were identified by a duplex scan in the proximal aspect of the lateral leg adjacent to the soft tissue defect and used for the design of a free-style pedicled perforator-plus flap. An 11 × 5.5 cm skin flap was designed (Fig. 43.8). After the initial suprafascial dissection, the decision was made to follow the proposed incision for the flap design. The suprafascial dissection of the flap was completed with preservation of a small skin bridge so that it was not completely elevated as an island flap (Fig. 43.9). During the flap dissection, the two perforators were always visualized and well preserved (Fig. 43.10). The flap was elevated under direct vision, and as large as possible of the skin bridge was preserved, and the flap could easily be rotated into the defect without very much tension (Fig. 43.11).

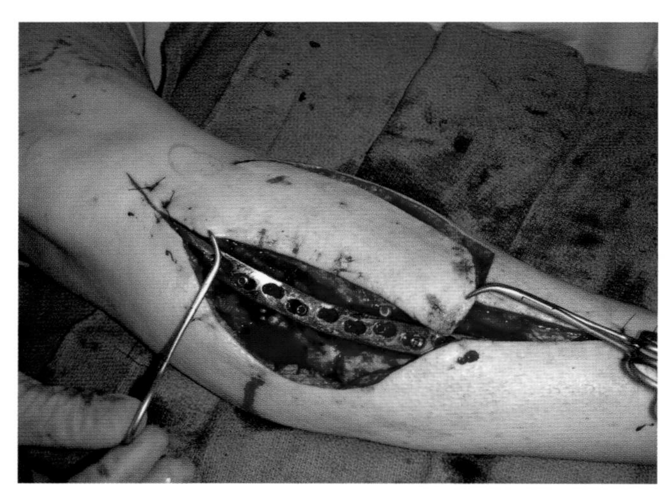

• **Fig. 43.9** An intraoperative view showing completion of the flap dissection with a sizable, connected skin bridge.

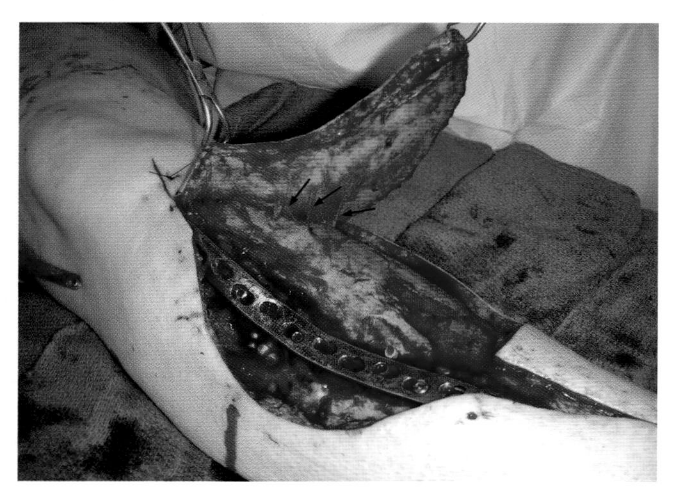

• **Fig. 43.10** An intraoperative view showing completion of the flap dissection and three well-preserved perforators *(arrows)* of the flap.

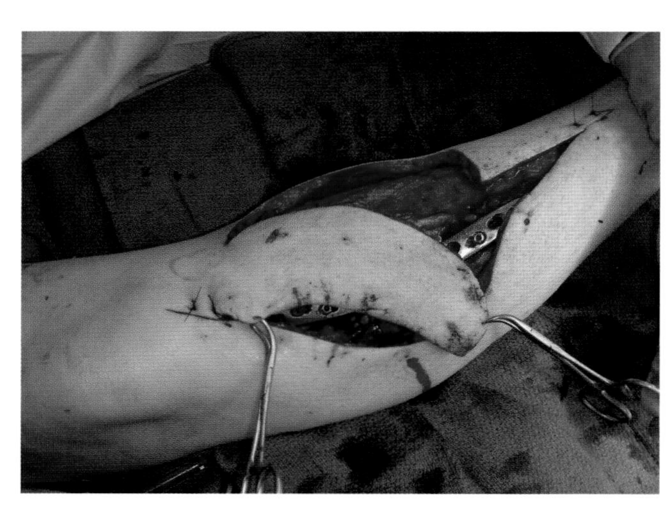

• **Fig. 43.11** An intraoperative view showing preliminary inset of the flap that could cover the wound in the left leg.

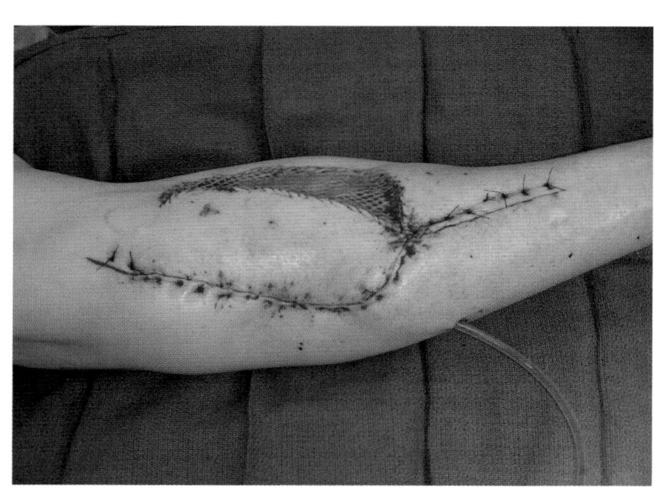

• **Fig. 43.12** An intraoperative view showing the completion of the flap inset and skin grafting to the flap donor site.

The medial aspect of the wound edge was also elevated in the suprafascial plane and significant undermining was performed to allow the flap to be approximated to the medial edge of the wound without too much tension. The flap was then easily inset into the soft tissue defect without any difficulty (Fig. 43.12).

After careful hemostasis, a 10-mm flat JP drain was inserted under the flap. The lateral leg skin flap donor site was sutured down to the deep fascia in order to reduce the size of the skin graft. Several tacking sutures were used to reduce the size of the skin flap donor site. The distal part of the wound was approximated directly with a two-layer closure. A split-thickness skin graft was harvested from the left lateral thigh. The skin graft was meshed to 1:1.5 ratio. The skin graft was placed on the flap donor site and sutured to adjacent skin edges with 5-0 chronic sutures.

Follow-Up Results

The patient did well postoperatively without any issues related to the flap reconstruction for the proximal leg wound closure. She was discharged from hospital on postoperative day 7. The left proximal leg wound after flap reconstruction healed uneventfully (Fig. 43.13). She was followed by the plastic surgery service for routine postoperative care and by the orthopedic trauma surgery for fracture healing.

Final Outcome

About 3 months after the flap reconstruction, the patient developed an infection of the fracture site under the flap even though the free-style perforator-plus flap survived completely. She was taken to the operating room by the orthopedic trauma service and the reconstruction plate was removed after flap elevation by the plastic surgery service. Because of the poor healing potential for the proximal tibial fracture and infection, the patient underwent a below-knee amputation and has been followed by the orthopedic trauma service.

Pearls for Success

When designing a free-style perforator skin flap, the identification of one or two more good perforators is important. The author

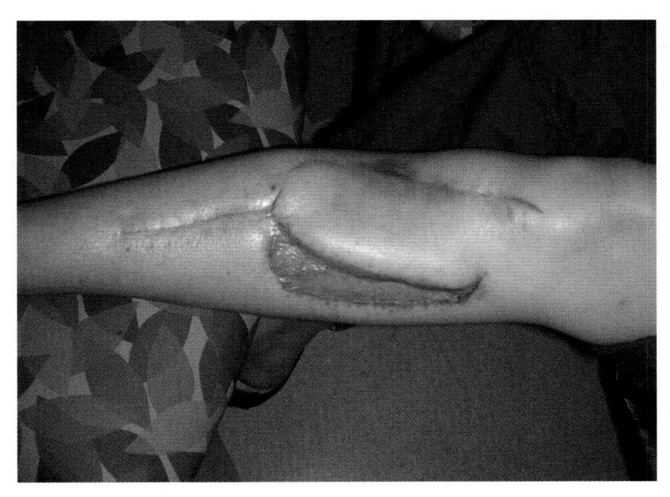

• **Fig. 43.13** Result at 2-month follow-up showing well-healed left proximal-third of leg wound extended to the middle-third after flap reconstruction.

prefers a preoperative duplex scan to map any adjacent perforators. In this way, an adjacent perforator flap can be reliably designed. The information on any given perforator such as the size, blood flow, and potential intramuscular dissection can be obtained. Each mapped perforator would also be confirmed intraoperatively by a handheld Doppler before elevation of the flap. In general, at least one good perforator is needed for the design of such a flap. The ad hoc nature of this step can be considered free-style, because it relies on the reconstructive surgeon's expertise to determine the planned approach. Preoperative CT angiogram may also act as adjunct to presurgical work-up. However, this cannot replace preoperative duplex scan or intraoperative Doppler to identify the exact locations of those cutaneous perforators. Because there may be several adjacent perforators, the flap design can be based on the most appropriate perforator. In addition, the arc of flap rotation while maintaining an adequate skin bridge and ensuring a tension-free closure can also be decided prior to the start of the flap dissection.

The perforator-plus flap can offer reliable soft tissue coverage for an appropriate wound if reliable perforators can be identified within the flap that is outside the zone of injury. The flap design should ensure readvancement is possible in case of distal flap separation or necrosis. Care should be taken with dissection close to the perforators but avoiding any direct trauma to those vessels. Postoperative care includes immobilization and bedrest if applicable to allow adequate reduction of leg swelling. Any signs of venous congestion can be managed with nonoperative methods (e.g., local nitroglycerin paste or leech therapy). In addition, incisional separation or flap tip necrosis can be successfully managed by readvancement of the flap after adequate debridement.

Recommended Readings

Buchner M, Zeifang F, Bernd L. Medial gastrocnemius muscle flap in limb-sparing surgery of malignant bone tumors of the proximal tibia: mid-term results in 25 patients. *Ann Plast Surg*. 2003;51: 266–272.

Gkiatas I, Korompilia M, Kostas-Agnantis I, Tsirigkakis SE, Stavraki M, Korompilias A. Gastrocnemius pedicled muscle flap for knee and upper tibia soft tissue reconstruction. A useful tool for the orthopaedic surgeon. *Injury*. 2021;52:3679–3684.

Pu LL. Soft-tissue coverage of an extensive mid-tibial wound with the combined medial gastrocnemius and medial hemisoleus muscle flaps: the role of local muscle flaps revisited. *J Plast Reconstr Aesthet Surg*. 2010;63:e605–e610.

Pu LL, Stevenson T. Principles of reconstruction for complex lower extremity wounds. *Techn Orthop*. 2009;24:78–87.

Song P, Pu LLQ. Perforator-Plus flaps in lower extremity reconstruction. *Clin Plast Surg*. 2021;48:183–192.

Thornton BP, Pu LLQ. Reconstruction of an extensive tibial soft-tissue defect with multiple local muscle flaps for limb salvage when free-tissue transfer was not an option. *Eur J Plast Surg*. 2004;27:217–221.

Zeiderman MR, Pu LLQ. Contemporary approach to soft-tissue reconstruction of the lower extremity after trauma. *Burns Trauma*. 2021;9:tkab024.

44

Leg Reconstruction: Middle Third

CASE 1

Clinical Presentation

A 40-year-old White male sustained chronic osteomyelitis secondary to an open middle tibial fracture 1 year ago from a motor vehicle accident. He had a longstanding smoking history. He had chronic drainage from the old fracture site about 2 months previously (Figs. 44.1 and 44.2). He had undergone debridement of the middle tibial wound, removal of hardware, and placement of an external fixator 2 weeks before. The plastic surgery service was consulted for soft tissue coverage of the middle tibial wound, measuring 11 × 7 cm, after the definitive bony fixation by the orthopedic trauma service (Fig. 44.3).

Operative Plan and Special Considerations for Reconstruction

For a typical middle-third wound of the leg with exposed fracture site or hardware, a classic local muscle flap, such as a soleus muscle flap, can be selected to cover the exposed fracture site and hardware. The soleus muscle is a type II muscle flap. However, only a medial hemisoleus muscle has been selected because it is not only able to provide adequate soft tissue coverage but also able to minimize functional loss of the foot plantar flexion. The bipenniform morphology of the soleus muscle and the independent neurovascular supply to either the medial or the lateral belly are important features that allow the surgeon to split the muscle longitudinally. Because the medial hemisoleus muscle is less bulky, the reconstructive outcome is usually much better than when a whole muscle is used as a flap. The medial half of the muscle receives blood supply throughout its length by minor pedicles (perforators) arising from the posterior tibial vessels. This constant feature makes the medial hemisoleus reliable as a proximally based flap.

Operative Procedures

Under general anesthesia with the patient in the supine position, the left middle tibial wound was debrided. All unhealthy-looking skin and colonized tissues were removed. The open tibial wound appeared to be fresh and clean after a definitive debridement performed by the plastic surgery service. The actual soft tissue wound was 11 × 7 cm (Fig. 44.4).

The proposed incision for exposure of the medial hemisoleus muscle flap was marked and the flap dissection was performed under tourniquet control. The existing open wound was extended proximally and distally through the skin, subcutaneous tissues, and fascia to expose the medial hemisoleus muscle. After the medial hemisoleus muscle had been identified and dissected free from the medial gastrocnemius muscle and the flexor digitorum longus, its insertion was divided distally at the level of the Achilles tendon based on the length of the flap rotation required. During dissection, the plantaris tendon was visualized between the gastrocnemius muscle and the underlying soleus muscle. The medial half of the soleus muscle was split along its anatomic midline. The medial hemisoleus muscle flap was elevated with emphasis on the preservation of as many minor pedicles from the posterior tibial vessels as possible to the flap in the middle third of the leg while allowing adequate arc rotation of the flap to cover the exposed tibia and hardware (Fig. 44.5). The flap was then transposed into the middle tibial wound and inset with interrupted 3-0 Monocryl horizontal mattress sutures. Scoring the fascia over the medial hemisoleus muscle belly was also performed to enhance the flap's arc of rotation for better soft tissue coverage of the tibial wound and hardware (Fig. 44.6).

One drain was placed under the flap and another drain was inserted into the flap donor site. The muscle flap was covered with split-thickness skin grafts. Split-thickness skin grafts were harvested with a dermatome from the left lateral thigh and meshed to 1:1.5 ratio. The incision for the flap exposure was closed in two layers and all skin grafts were secured with skin staples (Fig. 44.7).

Follow-Up Results

The patient did well postoperatively without any issues related to the flap reconstruction for the middle tibial wound closure. He was discharged from hospital on postoperative day 5. His left middle of leg wound healed uneventfully (Fig. 44.8). He was followed by the plastic surgery service for routine postoperative care and underwent an autologous bone graft procedure by the orthopedic trauma service 2 months after flap reconstruction.

Final Outcome

During further follow-up, the left middle tibial wound flap reconstruction site had healed well with good contour and minimal scarring. There was no wound breakdown, recurrent infection, or contour issues related to this soft tissue reconstruction (Fig. 44.10). The patient has resumed his weight-bearing status and has returned to work as a construction worker.

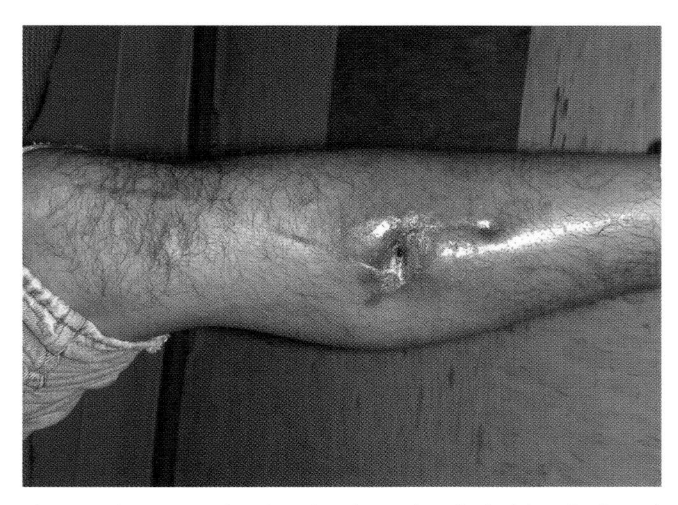

• **Fig. 44.1** A preoperative view showing a chronic draining site from the left tibial fracture wound.

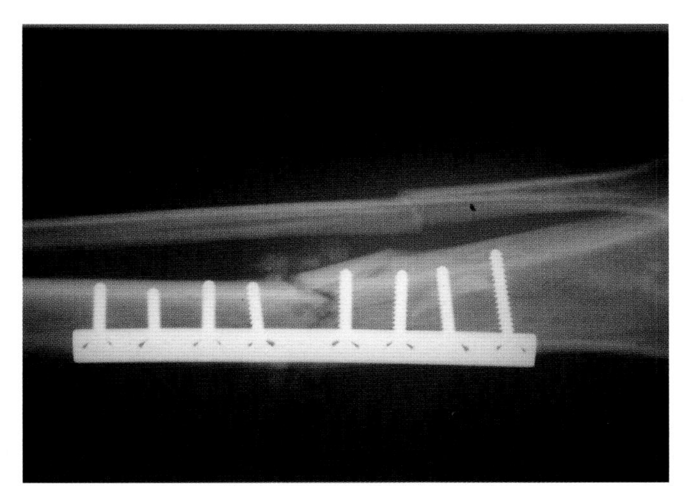

• **Fig. 44.2** A preoperative X-ray image showing nonunion of the left tibial fracture site even with an internal fixation.

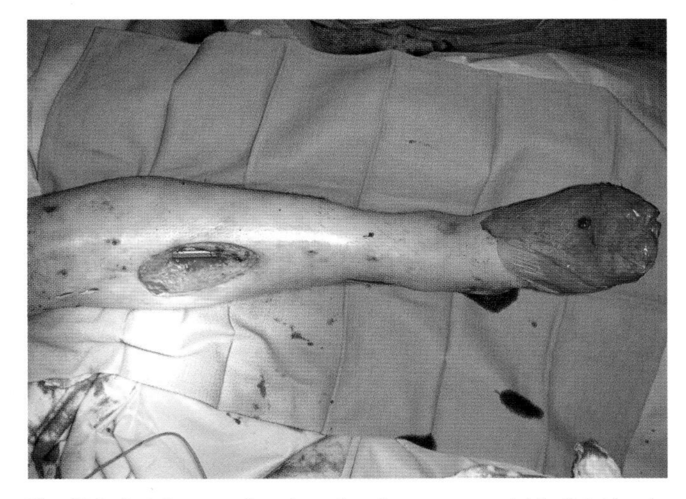

• **Fig. 44.3** An intraoperative view showing an open middle tibial fracture wound after an orthopedic debridement and internal fixation with a rod.

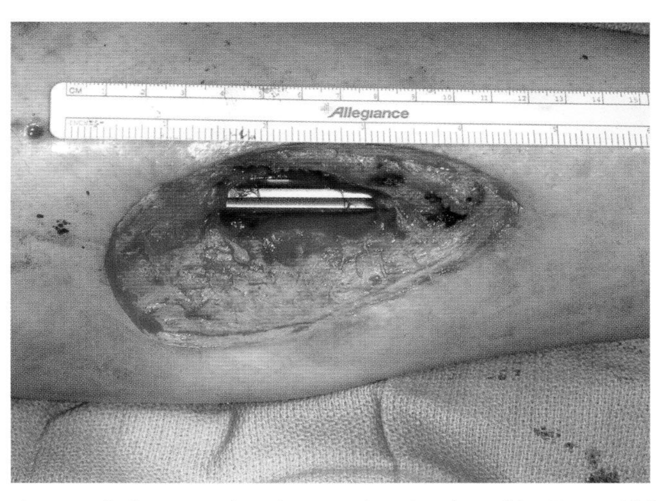

• **Fig. 44.4** An intraoperative close-up view showing a 11 × 7 cm middle tibial wound of the leg with the exposed tibia and hardware.

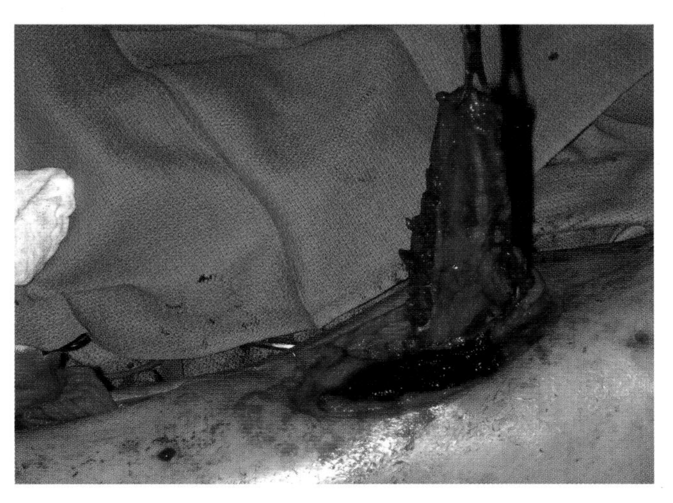

• **Fig. 44.5** An intraoperative view showing the elevated medial hemi-soleus muscle flap.

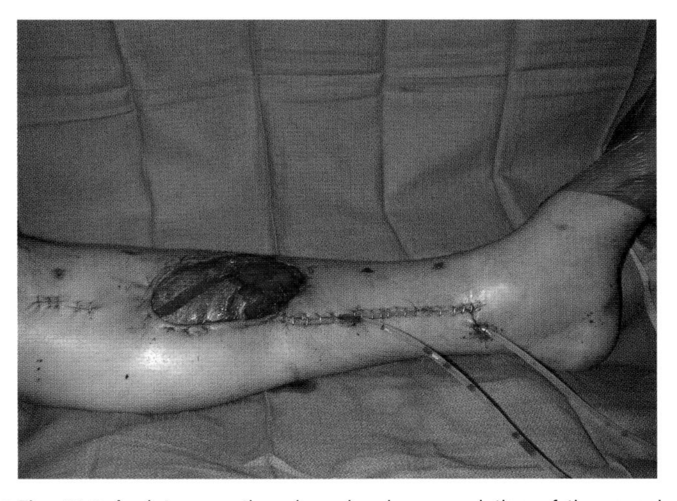

• **Fig. 44.6** An intraoperative view showing completion of the muscle flap inset before placement of a skin graft.

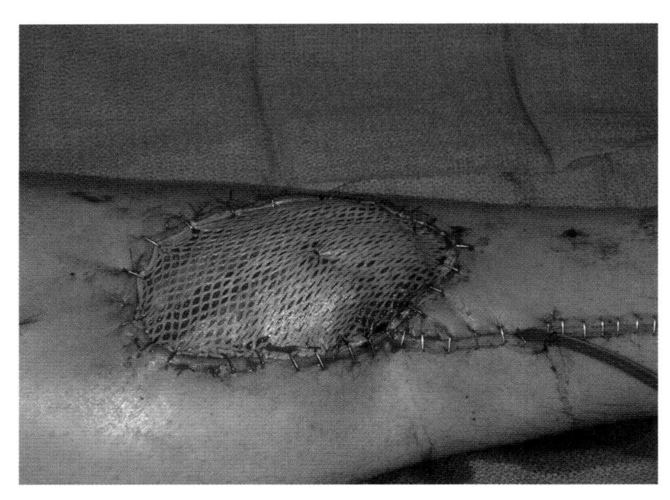

• **Fig. 44.7** An intraoperative close-up view showing completion of a skin graft placement over the muscle flap.

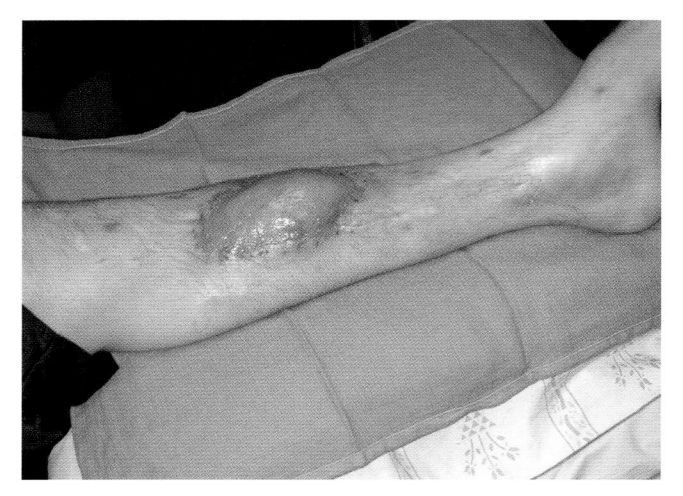

• **Fig. 44.8** Result at 5-week follow-up showing well-healed left middle-third tibial wound after the flap reconstruction.

Pearls for Success

A medial hemisoleus muscle flap, not a whole soleus muscle flap, can be used to cover a complex middle tibial wound with the exposed fracture site and hardware. The medial half of the muscle can be split longitudinally along its anatomic midline between the bellies of the soleus muscle. The medial hemisoleus muscle flap is elevated with emphasis on the preservation of as many minor pedicles (perforators) from the posterior tibial vessels as possible to the flap in the middle third of the leg while allowing adequate arc rotation of the flap to cover a wound in the middle third of the leg (Fig. 44.10). In this way, any adjacent perforators from the posterior tibial vessel to the flap can be preserved while allowing adequate arc of flap rotation. Only those perforators that are restricting the flap's arc of rotation for wound coverage can be divided during the flap dissection. In the author's practice, a medial hemisoleus muscle flap is a basis for soft tissue reconstruction of the middle-third leg wound. No total flap loss has been observed. Partial flap loss is also uncommon for a proximally based medial hemisoleus muscle flap and can be managed with additional flap advancement after proper debridement.

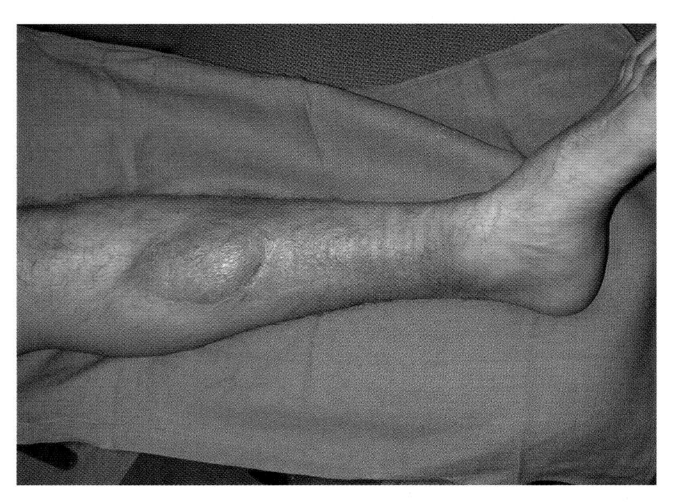

• **Fig. 44.9** Result at 6.5-month follow-up showing well-healed left middle third tibia wound after flap reconstruction with good contour and minimal scarring.

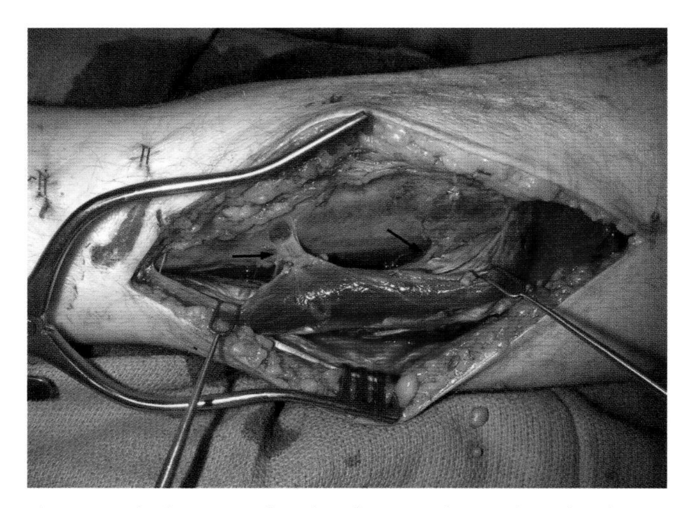

• **Fig. 44.10** An intraoperative view from another patient showing perforators *(arrows)* from the posterior tibial vessels to the medial half of the soleus muscle *(skin hooks)*. Preservation of as many of these perforators to the medial hemisoleus muscle flap as possible during the flap dissection is the key to ensuring adequate blood supply to the distal portion of the flap.

CASE 2

Clinical Presentation

A 31-year-old White female sustained an open tibial fracture wound of the right leg as a result of a motor vehicle accident. She sustained a 5 × 4 cm open fracture wound in the junction of the middle and distal thirds of the right leg with exposed tibial fracture site and hardware (Fig. 44.4). The orthopedic trauma service initially performed debridement of the open tibial fracture site and placement of an external fixator. The plastic surgery service was consulted for soft tissue coverage of the tibial wound after a

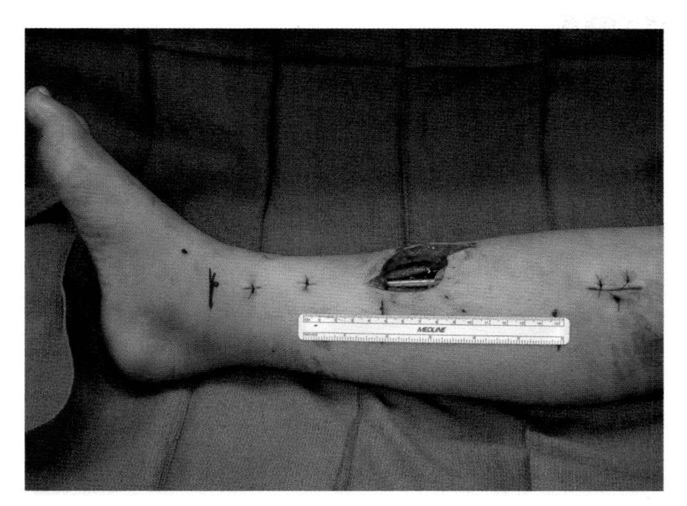

• **Fig. 44.11** A preoperative view showing a 5 × 4 cm open tibial wound at the junction of the middle and distal thirds of the right leg with exposed tibial fracture site and hardware.

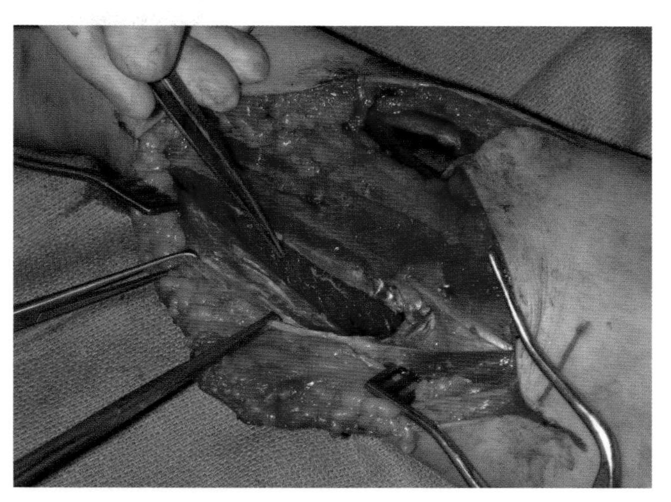

• **Fig. 44.12** An intraoperative view showing that only the muscular portion (indicated by *forceps*) of the medial hemisoleus muscle was dissected off the tendon of the medial gastrocnemius muscle (held by two *Allis clamps*) during the flap dissection.

definitive rigid fixation of the tibial fracture with an intramedullary rod placement (Fig. 44.11).

Operative Plan and Special Considerations for Reconstruction

For an open fracture wound in the junction of the middle and distal thirds of the leg with exposed fracture site and/or hardware, a proximally based medial hemisoleus muscle flap can be selected to cover the exposed fracture site and hardware. The soleus muscle is a type II muscle flap and only a medial hemisoleus muscle is elevated to provide adequate soft tissue coverage but also minimize functional loss of the foot plantar flexion. The bipenniform morphology of the soleus muscle and the independent neurovascular supply to either the medial or the lateral belly are important features so that the muscle can be split longitudinally. The medial half of the muscle receives blood supply throughout its length by perforators arising from the posterior tibial vessels. The medial hemisoleus muscle flap is elevated with emphasis on the preservation of as many minor pedicles (perforators) from the posterior tibial vessels as possible to the flap in the middle or distal third of the leg while allowing adequate arc rotation of the flap to cover the wound in the junction of the middle and distal thirds of the leg.

Operative Procedures

Under general anesthesia with the patient in the supine position, the open tibial fracture wound was debrided after a definitive orthopedic procedure for an internal fixation of the distal tibial fracture. All unhealthy-looking skin and colonized tissues were removed. The open tibial wound appeared to be fresh and clean after a definitive debridement performed by the plastic surgery service. The actual soft tissue wound measured 5 × 4 cm.

The flap dissection was performed under tourniquet control. An existing open wound was extended both proximally and distally as an incision. The distal skin incision was just above the Achilles tendon and the proximal incision was just distal to the junction of the proximal and middle thirds of the leg. After identifying the medial half of the proximal soleus muscle, it was dissected free from the medial gastrocnemius and flexor digitorum longus muscles. The medial half of the distal soleus muscle was sharply dissected with a knife from the tendon portion of the medial gastrocnemius muscle (Fig. 44.12). Only the muscular portion of the soleus was used as the flap and the tendon portion of the medial gastrocnemius muscle was left intact. The tendon was approximated to the remaining lateral half of the soleus muscle with 2-0 nonabsorbable sutures after the flap was elevated. The insertion of the medial half of the soleus muscle was divided distally close to the Achilles tendon, based on the required arc of the flap rotation. The medial half of the muscle was split longitudinally with a midline between the bellies of the soleus muscle.

The medial hemisoleus muscle flap was elevated only to just above the junction between the middle and distal thirds of the leg so that an adjacent perforator from the posterior tibial vessels to the flap was preserved while allowing adequate arc of flap rotation to cover the exposed tibia and hardware (Fig. 44.13). This

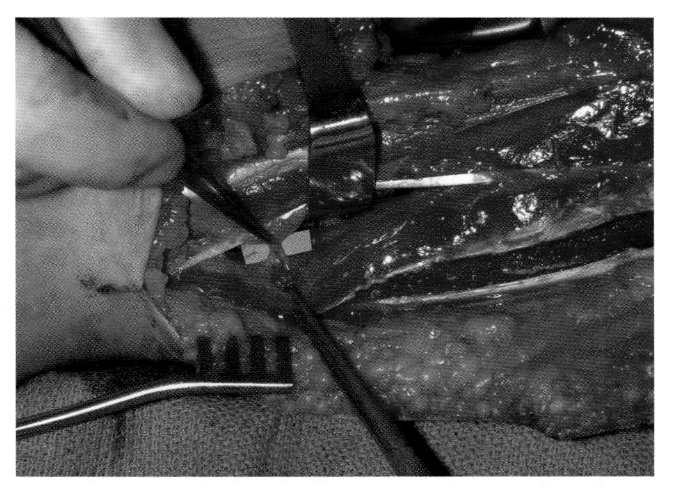

• **Fig. 44.13** An intraoperative view showing a distal perforator (indicated by *forceps*) from the posterior tibial vessels to the medial hemisoleus muscle flap. This perforator should be divided to allow adequate arc of the flap rotation to cover the distal tibial fracture wound.

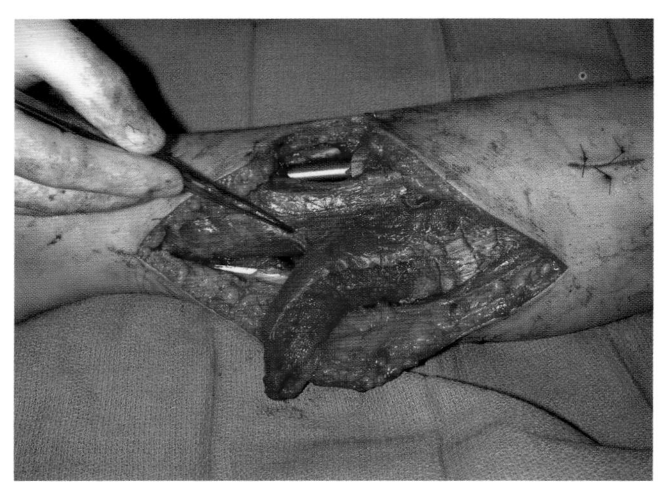

• **Fig. 44.14** An intraoperative view shows an adjacent perforator (indicated by *forceps*) from the posterior tibial vessels to the medial hemisoleus muscle flap. Preservation of this perforator may be critical to ensuring an adequate blood supply to the distal portion of the flap.

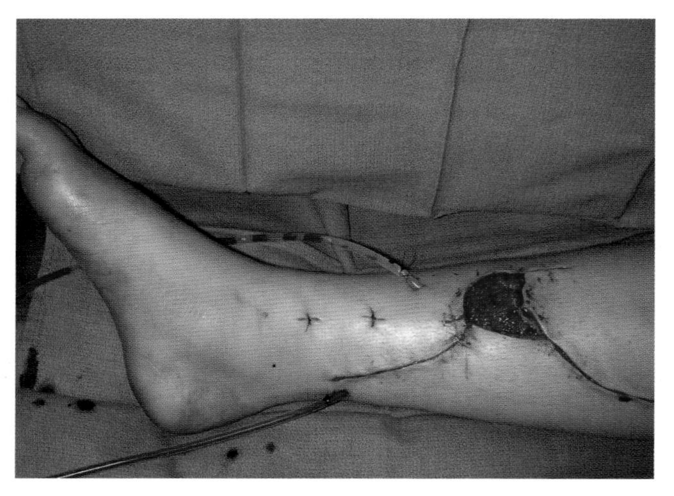

• **Fig. 44.15** An intraoperative view showing completion of the medial hemisoleus muscle flap inset before placement of a skin graft.

perforator could be a critical source of blood supply to the distal portion of the medial hemisoleus muscle flap and should be preserved whenever possible (Fig. 44.14). Scoring the fascia over the surface of the medial hemisoleus muscle belly was done to enhance a few centimeters more arc of flap rotation. The medial hemisoleus muscle flap was then transposed into the defect and inset with interrupted 3-0 Monocryl sutures in half-buried horizontal mattress fashion (Fig. 44.15).

One drain was placed under the flap and another was inserted into the flap donor site. The muscle flap was then covered with split-thickness skin grafts. A split-thickness skin graft was harvested with a dermatome from the right lateral thigh and meshed to 1:1.5 ratio. The incision for the flap exposure was closed in two layers and the skin graft was secured with staples (Fig. 44.16).

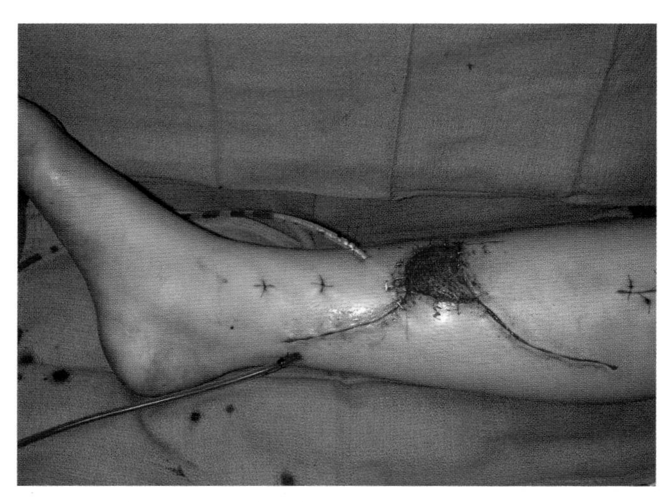

• **Fig. 44.16** An intraoperative view showing completion of a skin graft placement over the medial hemisoleus muscle flap.

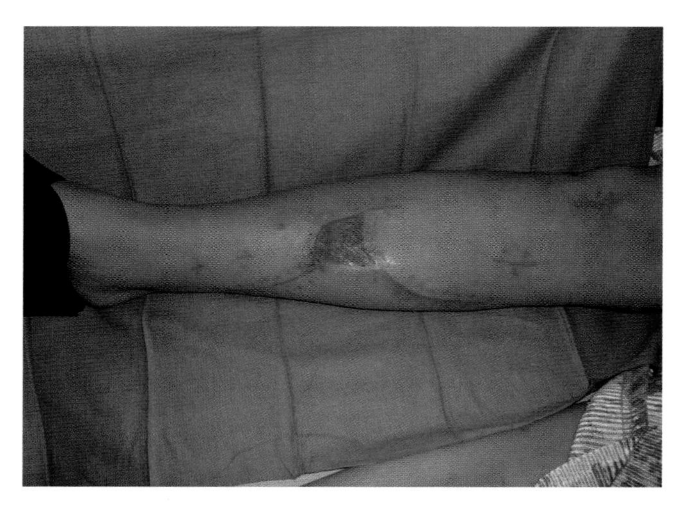

• **Fig. 44.17** Result at 5-week follow-up showing well-healed junction of the right middle and distal third tibial wound after flap reconstruction.

Follow-Up Results

The patient did well postoperatively without any issues related to the flap reconstruction for the junction of the middle and distal tibial wound closure. She was discharged from hospital on postoperative day 6. The right distal tibial wound healed uneventfully (Fig. 44.17). She was followed by the plastic surgery service for routine postoperative care and underwent an autologous bone graft procedure by the orthopedic trauma service 4 months after the flap reconstruction (Fig. 44.18).

Final Outcome

During further follow-up, the open tibial wound in the junction of the middle and distal thirds of the leg flap reconstruction site had healed well with good contour and minimal scarring. The patient also underwent a successful bone graft procedure by the orthopedic trauma service. There was no wound breakdown, recurrent infection, or contour issues related to the soft tissue

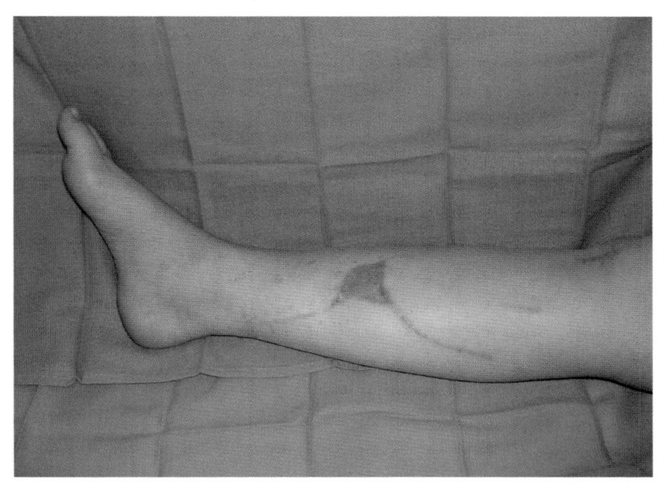

• **Fig. 44.18** Result at 4-month follow-up showing well-healed junction of the right middle and distal third tibial wound after flap reconstruction before autologous bone graft procedure.

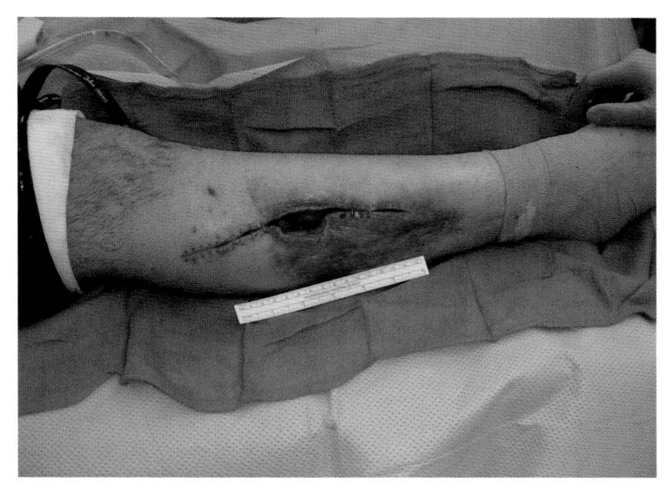

• **Fig. 44.20** A preoperative view showing a middle lateral leg soft tissue defect, measuring 5 × 3 cm, with the exposed underlying tibia.

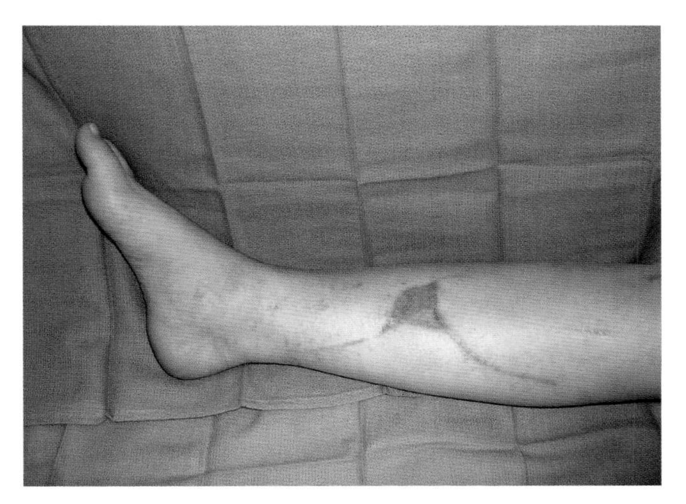

• **Fig. 44.19** Result at 7-month follow-up after the flap reconstruction showing well-healed junction of the right middle and distal third tibial wound and 3 months after autologous bone graft procedure with good contour and minimal scarring.

reconstruction (Fig. 44.19). She has resumed her weight-bearing status and has returned to her normal activities as instructed.

Pearls for Success

In the author's practice, all relatively limited soft-tissue defects (<50 cm^2) at the junction of the middle and distal thirds of the leg are covered with a medial hemisoleus muscle flap and thus free tissue transfer is not chosen. The medial half of the muscle can be split longitudinally along its anatomic midline between the bellies of the soleus muscle. The medial hemisoleus muscle flap is elevated with emphasis on the preservation of as many minor pedicles (perforators) from the posterior tibial vessels as possible to the flap in the middle and distal thirds of the leg while allowing adequate arc rotation of the flap to cover a wound in the junction of the middle and distal thirds of the leg. Once the medial half of the soleus muscle is identified and dissected free to just above the junction between the middle and distal thirds of the leg, any perforators from the posterior tibial vessels to the medial half of the soleus muscle adjacent to the junction of the middle and distal thirds of the leg should be preserved while allowing adequate arc of flap rotation to cover a distal tibial wound. The surgical technique in flap dissection refined by the author emphasizes the preservation of an adequate blood supply to the distal portion of the medial hemisoleus muscle flap. This technique may ensure viability of the medial hemisoleus muscle flap and expand its role in reconstruction of a relatively distal wound over the tibia. Only those perforators that are restricting the flap's arc of rotation for wound coverage need to be divided during the flap dissection. In addition, the approximation of the tendon of the medial gastrocnemius muscle to the remaining lateral half of the soleus muscle may minimize the functional loss of the leg after flap harvesting.

CASE 3

Clinical Presentation

A 29-year-old White male unfortunately developed heterotopic ossification of the right tibia and fibula following a previous soft tissue injury. This was resected with a resulting complication of hematoma and overlying skin breakdown along the incision. The evacuation of hematoma and debridement of necrotic tissue were performed by the orthopedic trauma service. This resulted in a 5 × 3 cm open area with the exposed tibia in the middle third of the lateral leg (Fig. 44.20). The plastic surgery service was consulted for soft tissue reconstruction in this unique location.

Operative Plan and Special Considerations for Reconstruction

For this middle-third wound of the lateral leg with the exposed tibia, because the surrounding skin was noted to be of poor quality, the use of a local bi-pedicled fasciocutaneous flap or any other local skin flaps for the wound closure was precluded. The anterior tibialis muscle is a type IV muscle located on the lateral

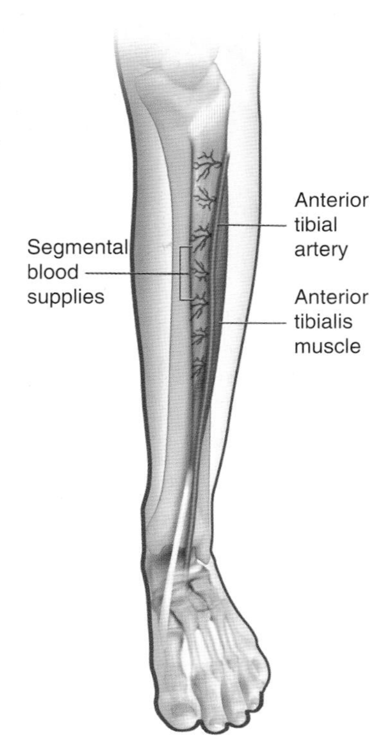

• **Fig. 44.21** A schematic diagram showing the segmental blood supplies to the anterior tibialis muscle from the anterior tibial vessels and the location of the muscle adjacent to the tibia in the leg.

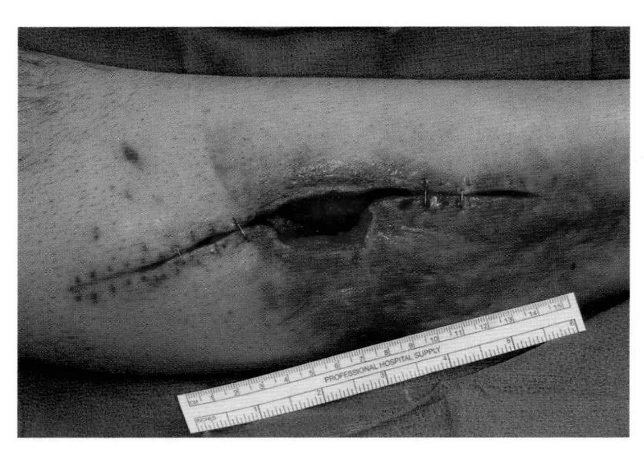

• **Fig. 44.22** An intraoperative close-up view showing the 5 × 3 cm middle tibial wound of the lateral leg with the exposed underlying tibia.

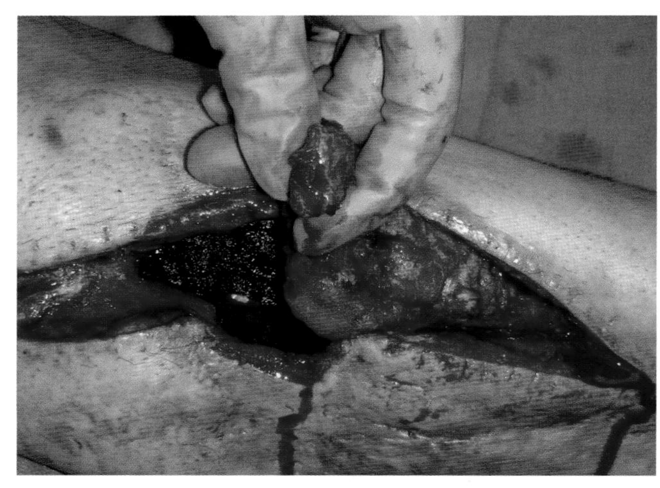

• **Fig. 44.23** An intraoperative view showing an elevated, distally based anterior tibialis muscle flap. Once the tourniquet was released, the tip of the flap appeared to be well perfused.

aspect of the tibia. It originates on the lateral tibial condyle as well as the upper lateral surface of the tibia and inserts onto the base of the first metatarsal. The muscle is innervated by deep branches of the peroneal nerve and functions to dorsiflex and invert the foot. The arterial supply is between 8 and 12 segmental pedicles from the anterior tibial artery that enters the muscle on its deep and lateral surface (Fig. 44.21). The flap may be used in coverage of small defects of the middle and lower third of the lateral leg. The muscle can be elevated conservatively based either proximally or distally. With limited elevation, the muscle can be used to cover a small lateral tibial wound with success.

Operative Procedures

Under general anesthesia with the patient in the supine position, the right lateral leg wound was debrided. The wound edge was then freshened with a blade and all colonized tissue was removed with a curette. The wound was then irrigated with Pulsavac and looked clean and fresh (Fig. 44.22).

The incision was extended both proximally and distally from the open wound. Under tourniquet control, the anterior tibialis muscle was identified and dissected free from the lateral tibia and the extensor hallucis longus muscle through extended incisions both proximally and distally. During exploration, the muscle was found to be transected proximally in the leg from previous orthopedic procedures. Therefore, the intraoperative decision was made to use the tibialis anterior muscle in the reverse fashion as a rotational muscle flap. At the higher level proximal to the wound, the anterior tibialis muscle was again divided and the attachment with the extensor hallucis longus muscle was dissected free. The further dissection was done to free the anterior tibialis muscle distally in order to have enough freedom of muscle flap rotation based distally. During the dissection, any potential segmental blood supplies from the anterior tibial vessels were preserved. The fascia on the anterior surface of the muscle was scored to expand the degree of the muscle flap's rotation without problems. The flap could be rotated to cover the wound and exposed tibia. At this point, the tourniquet was released. There was good bleeding to the tip of the muscle flap even in the reverse fashion (Fig. 44.23).

The flap was then inset into the defect and approximated to the adjacent soft tissue edges with several interrupted buried 2-0 PDS sutures. Two drains were inserted, one under the muscle flap and the other to the muscle flap donor site under the skin. All incisions were closed with several interrupted 3-0 Monocryl sutures for the deep dermal closure and with interrupted mattress 3-0 nylon sutures for the skin closure (Fig. 44.24).

A 5 × 3 cm area of the muscle flap was then skin grafted. The skin graft was harvested from the right anterior thigh with a dermatome. The split-thickness skin graft was meshed to 1:1.5

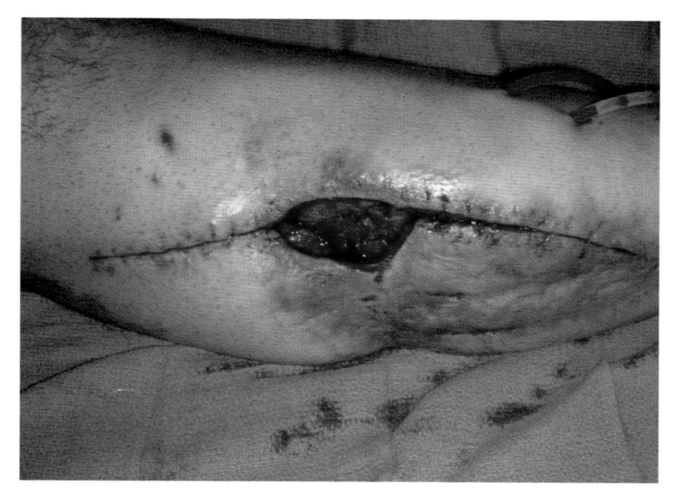

• **Fig. 44.24** An intraoperative view showing completion of the muscle flap inset before the placement of a skin graft.

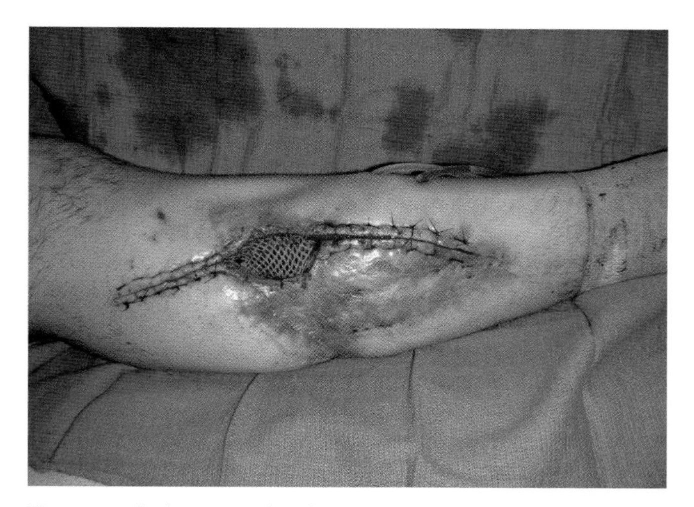

• **Fig. 44.25** An intraoperative view showing completion of a skin graft placement to the muscle flap and incisions closure.

ratio. It was placed on the muscle flap and secured with multiple 5-0-chromic sutures. The vacuum-assisted closure system was placed over the skin graft site for immobilization of the skin graft. The rest of the incision was then closed with several interrupted 3-0 nylon sutures (Fig. 44.25).

Follow-Up Results

The patient did well postoperatively without any issues related to the flap reconstruction for the middle lateral tibial wound closure. He was discharged from hospital on postoperative day 5. The right middle leg wound healed uneventfully. He was followed by the plastic surgery service for routine flap postoperative care and by the orthopedic trauma service for his orthopedic care.

Final Outcome

During further follow-up, the right lateral middle tibial wound flap reconstruction site had healed well with good contour and minimal scarring. There was no wound breakdown, recurrent infection, or contour issues related to this soft tissue reconstruction (Fig. 44.26). He has resumed his normal activities and has returned to work as a labor worker.

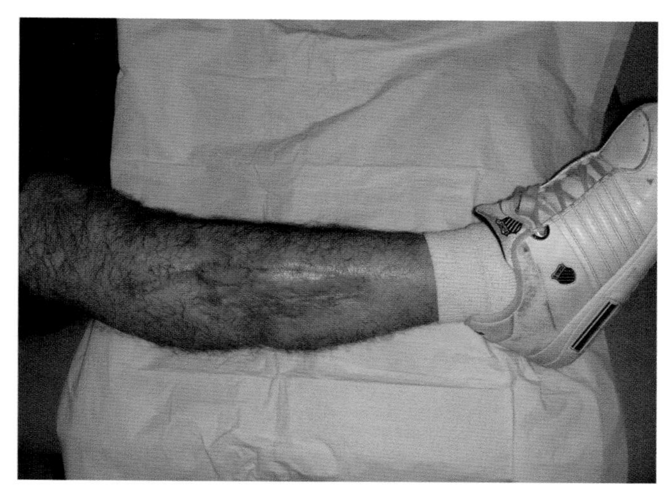

• **Fig. 44.26** Result at 3.5-month follow-up showing well-healed right middle third lateral leg wound after the flap reconstruction with good contour and minimal scarring.

Pearls for Success

The anterior tibialis muscle flap can be used for coverage of small defects of the middle and lower third of the lateral leg. Various usages of the muscle for coverage include standard proximally based flap, segmental flap, sagittal split flap, and longitudinal split muscle flap. Using the flap based on the distal segmental blood supply and in a turnover fashion as described in this case has illustrated the success of this reconstructive strategy. Therefore, familiarity with this muscle flap and its unique vascular anatomy and a possible arc of flap movement is key to success. The optimum amount of flap dissection and maintaining adequate segmental blood supply to the flap should be judged intraoperatively once the surgeon has gained clinical experience in flap dissection. In addition, the flap can only be used for a small soft tissue defect, that is, less than 20 cm^2 in the middle or distal third of the lateral leg. Such a limitation should be fully recognized by the surgeon. As with any distally based muscle flaps, partial muscle flap loss may occur even if the flap dissection is performed with all precautions. If tip necrosis of the flap occurs, the necrotic portion of flap can be debrided and readvancement of the flap may still be possible.

Recommended Readings

AlMugaren FM, Pak CJ, Suh HP, Hong JP. Best local flaps for lower extremity reconstruction. *Plast Reconstr Surg Glob Open*. 2020; 8:e2774.

Jitprapaikulsarn S, Patamamongkonchai C, Gromprasit A, Thremthakanpon W. Simultaneous internal fixation and soft tissue coverage by soleus muscle flap and variances: a reproducible strategy for managing open fractures of tibial shaft. *Eur J Orthop Surg Traumatol.* 2021;31:365–373.

Jaiswal R, Pu LL. The role of less commonly used local muscle flaps for soft tissue coverage of complex lower extremity wounds. *Ann Plast Surg*. 2015;74(Suppl 1):S22–S24.

Pu LL. Medial hemisoleus muscle flap: a reliable flap for soft tissue reconstruction of the middle-third tibial wound. *Int Surg*. 2006;91:194–200.

Pu LL. Soft-tissue coverage of an open tibial wound in the junction of the middle and distal thirds of the leg with the medial hemisoleus muscle flap. *Ann Plast Surg*. 2006;56:639–643.

Song P, Pu LLQ. The soleus muscle flap: an overview of its clinical applications for lower extremity reconstruction. *Ann Plast Surg*. 2018;81(6S suppl 1):S109–S116.

45

Leg Reconstruction: Distal Third (Local Flaps)

CASE 1

Clinical Presentation

A 57-year-old White female sustained an open tibial fracture of her left leg as a result of a motor vehicle accident. She had a 5 × 4 cm open fracture wound in the distal third of the leg with an exposed tibial fracture site. She initially had debridement of the open tibial fracture site and placement of an external fixator by the orthopedic trauma service. A rigid fixation of the distal tibial fracture with an intramedullary rod was planned by the primary service. The plastic surgery service was consulted to provide soft tissue coverage of the distal tibial wound following a definitive rigid fixation of the fracture (Fig. 45.1).

Operative Plan and Special Considerations for Reconstruction

For a relatively small open fracture wound in the distal third of the leg with the exposed fracture site and/or hardware, a proximally based medial hemisoleus muscle flap can be selected to cover the exposed fracture site and hardware. A medial hemisoleus muscle is selected to provide soft tissue coverage but also to minimize functional loss of the foot plantar flexion. The distal soleus muscle can be split longitudinally with some lateral extension so that the muscle flap would be large enough to cover adequately an open tibial fracture wound in the distal third of the leg (Fig. 45.2). Based on this author's clinical experience, the size of an open tibial wound in the distal third of the leg should be no more than 50 cm^2 when the wound is in the proximal part of the distal third leg. The distal medial half of the muscle receives blood supply primarily throughout its length by perforators arising from the posterior tibial vessels. Thus, the flap should be elevated with emphasis on the preservation of as many minor pedicles (perforators) from the posterior tibial vessels as possible to the flap while allowing adequate arc rotation of the flap to cover the wound in the distal third of the leg.

Operative Procedures

Under general anesthesia with the patient in the supine position, the open tibial fracture wound, measuring 5 × 4 cm, was debrided first after a definitive orthopedic procedure for an internal fixation of the distal tibial fracture by the orthopedic trauma service. All unhealthy-looking skin and colonized tissues were sharply debrided. The open tibial wound appeared to be fresh and clean after a definitive debridement performed by the plastic surgery service.

The flap dissection was performed under tourniquet control. An existing open wound was extended both proximally and distally. The proximal incision was extended to just above the junction of the distal and middle thirds of the leg and could be extended further proximally as needed. The distal skin incision was extended to just above the Achilles' tendon. After identifying the medial half of the soleus muscle, it was dissected free from the flexor digitorum longus muscle (Fig. 45.3). The entire distal soleus muscle near its insertion and the medial half of the soleus muscle were sharply dissected with a knife and freed from the tendon portion of the medial gastrocnemius muscle to the junction of the distal and middle thirds of the leg. Only the muscular portion of the soleus was used as the flap, while the tendon portion of both gastrocnemius muscles was left intact.

The insertion of the distal soleus muscle was divided close to the Achilles' tendon depending on the arc of the flap rotation required. The muscle flap was elevated only to the level just at or above the level of a tibial wound where a major perforator from the posterior tibial artery to the flap was identified (Fig. 45.4). This perforator served as a pivot point of the flap rotation and was carefully preserved. The flap dissection was completed with splitting the medial half (large portion) of the soleus muscle from the remaining lateral half (relatively small portion) of the muscle longitudinally to the level required by the exact location of the distal tibial wound (Fig. 45.5). Therefore, the flap was based proximally and received blood supply primarily from the distal perforators of the posterior tibial vessels in the area.

The intact tendon was approximated to the remaining lateral half of the soleus muscle with nonabsorbable sutures after the flap elevation. Scoring the fascia over the deep surface of the laterally extended medial hemisoleus muscle belly could often enhance a few centimeters more arc of flap rotation. The flap was transposed into the tibial wound and inset with 3-0 absorbable half-buried horizontal mattress sutures.

One drain was placed under the flap and another drain was inserted into the flap donor site. The muscle flap was covered with a split-thickness skin graft. A split-thickness skin graft was harvested with a dermatome from the left lateral thigh and meshed to 1:1.5 ratio. The incision for the flap exposure was closed in two layers and the skin graft was secured with skin staples (Fig. 45.6).

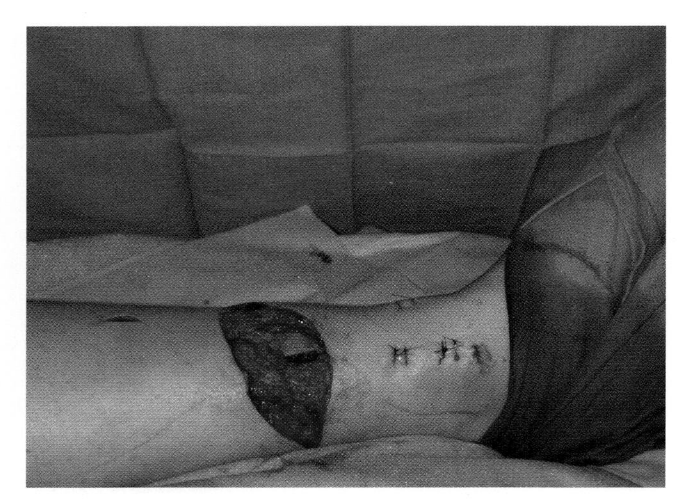

• **Fig. 45.1** A preoperative view showing a 5 × 4 cm open tibial wound in the distal third of the left leg with an exposed tibial fracture site.

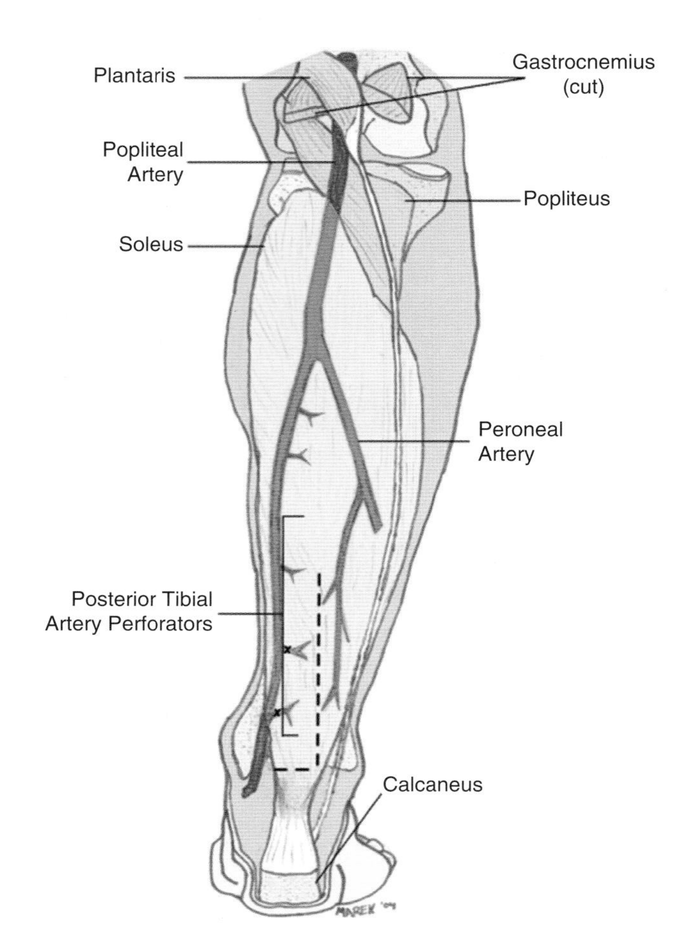

• **Fig. 45.3** A schematic diagram showing the blood supply to the medial and lateral halves of the soleus muscle as well as splitting of the muscle *(dotted line)* for the medial hemisoleus muscle flap dissection.

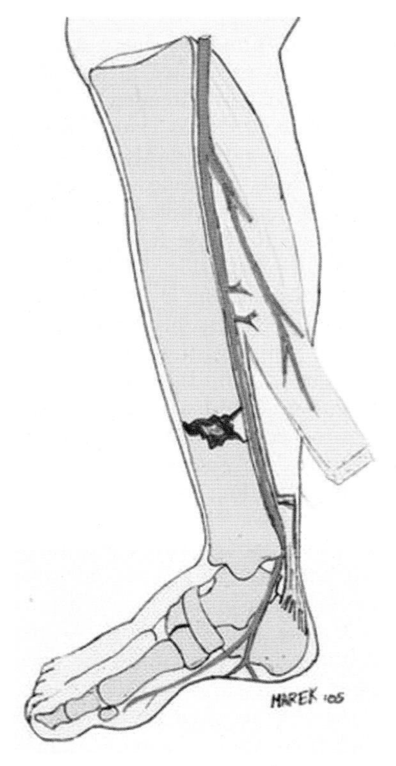

• **Fig. 45.2** A schematic diagram showing blood supplies to the laterally extended medial hemisoleus muscle flap. The flap is based proximally and receives blood supply primarily from the posterior tibial vessels. The flap also receives additional blood supply from one or two distal perforators of the posterior tibial vessels to its distal portion.

Follow-Up Results

The patient did well postoperatively without any issues related to the flap reconstruction for the distal third of the leg wound closure. She was discharged from hospital on postoperative day 5. The left distal open fracture wound healed uneventfully. She was followed by the plastic surgery service for routine postoperative care and underwent an autologous bone graft procedure by the orthopedic trauma service 4 months after the initial flap reconstruction.

Final Outcome

During further follow-up, the open tibial wound in the distal third of the leg after the flap reconstruction healed well with good contour and minimal scarring. The patient also underwent a successful bone graft procedure performed by the orthopedic trauma service. There was no wound breakdown, recurrent infection, or contour issues related to the soft tissue reconstruction (Fig. 45.7). She has resumed her weight-bearing status and returned to her normal activities as instructed.

Pearls for Success

In the author's experience, all relatively limited soft-tissue defects (<50 cm^2) in the distal third of the leg can be reconstructed with this laterally extended medial hemisoleus muscle flap as an alternative option to a free tissue transfer. The flap is elevated only to just at or above the level of a tibial wound where a major perforator from the posterior tibial artery to the flap is identified. This perforator often serves as a pivot point of the flap rotation and should be preserved whenever possible because it can be a critical

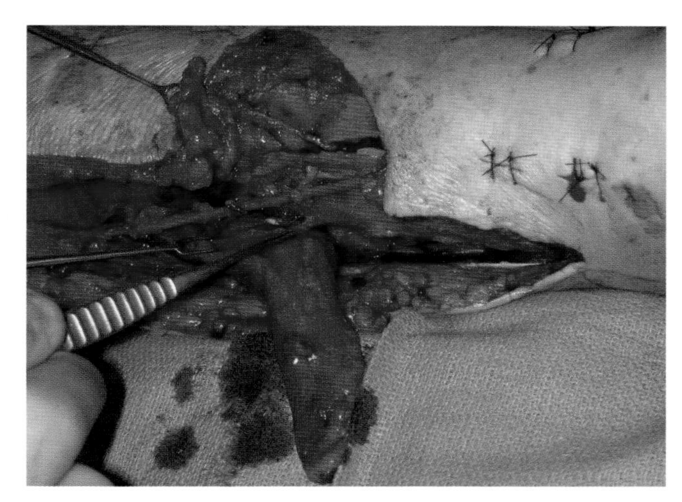

• **Fig. 45.4** An intraoperative view showing a perforator (indicated by *forceps*), adjacent to the distal tibial wound from the posterior tibial vessels to the medial hemisoleus, that should be preserved. This perforator may be critical to ensure an adequate blood supply to the distal portion of the flap.

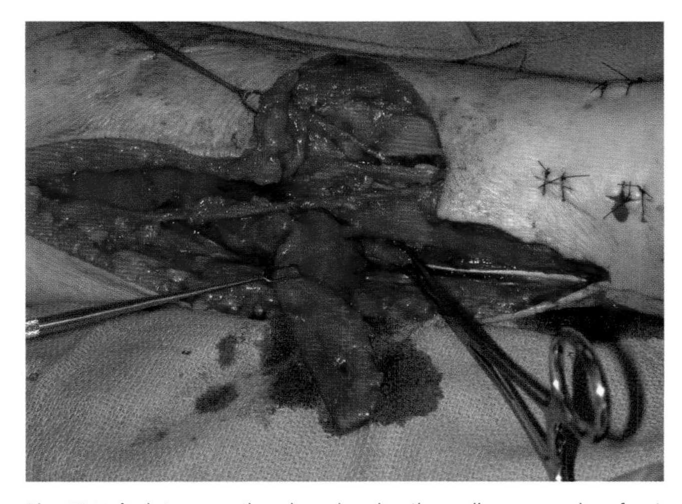

• **Fig. 45.5** An intraoperative view showing the well-preserved perforator from the posterior tibial vessels to the medial hemisoleus muscle flap. This perforator would not restrict the arc rotation of the flap.

source of blood supply to the distal portion of the flap. Preserving this important perforator, based on the author's experience, is often possible while allowing adequate arc of flap rotation to cover the exposed tibia fracture site and hardware.

The author prefers to free the entire distal soleus muscle during the flap dissection and then split the muscle longitudinally in a more laterally extended fashion than a standard medial hemisoleus muscle flap. In this way, the distal portion of the flap can be made bigger enough and used to cover adequately a relatively larger tibial wound in the distal third of the leg. Any perforators from the posterior tibial vessels to the distal medial half of the soleus muscle just at or above the tibial wound should be preserved while allowing adequate arc of flap rotation to cover the tibial wound in the distal third of the leg. In addition, the approximation of the tendon of the medial gastrocnemius muscle to the remaining soleus muscle may minimize the functional loss of the leg after

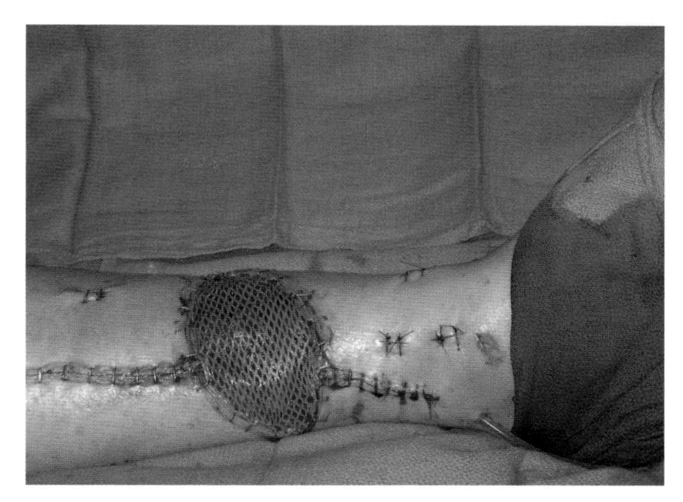

• **Fig. 45.6** An intraoperative view showing completion of flap inset and placement of a skin graft over the muscle flap as well as incision closure.

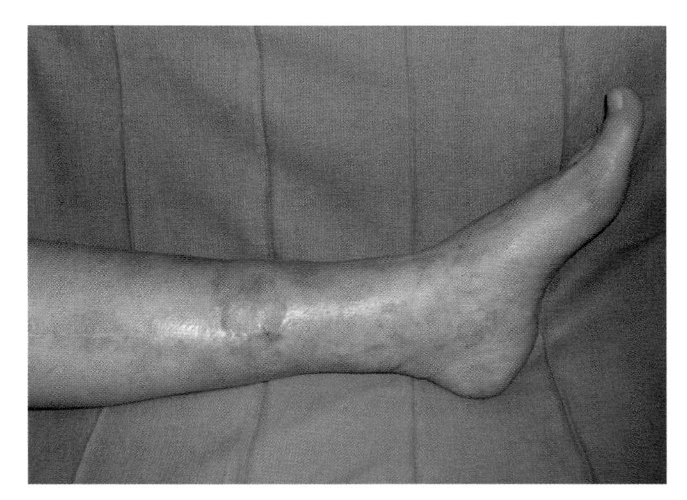

• **Fig. 45.7** Results at follow-up 2 years and 4 months after flap reconstruction showing well-healed distal-third tibial wound with excellent contour and minimal scarring.

harvesting the flap. The tip necrosis of the flap, if it occurs, can be managed successfully with subsequent debridement and flap readvancement. The laterally extended medial hemisoleus muscle flap may potentially offer an alternative approach to managing Gustilo IIIB open tibial fractures in the distal third of the leg.

CASE 2

Clinical Presentation

A 43-year-old White male developed a wound breakdown from a previous open reduction and internal fixation (ORIF) procedure of the left distal tibial after a fall. The left leg open wound was debrided by the orthopedic trauma service and left a 9×5 cm soft tissue defect in the distal third of the leg extending to the ankle with exposed hardware. The fracture fixation was satisfactory and there was no obvious infection. The plastic surgery service was consulted to provide soft tissue coverage for this open wound with

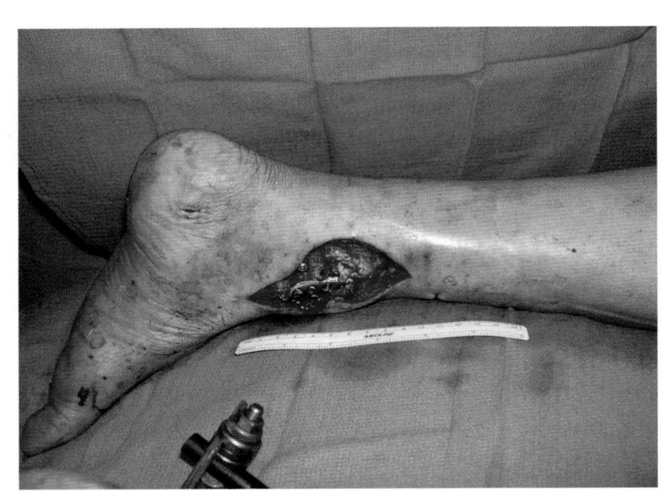

• **Fig. 45.8** A preoperative view showing a 9 × 5 cm open tibial wound in the distal third of the left leg extending to the ankle with exposed tibial fracture site and hardware.

the exposed hardware in the distal third of the leg extending to the proximal ankle (Fig. 45.8).

Operative Plan and Special Considerations for Reconstruction

The distally based sural artery flap, a distant skin island flap, has frequently been used to provide soft tissue coverage for a complex wound in the distal third of the leg, if the flap donor site is available, the pedicle of the flap in the lesser saphenous vein territory is not involved by previous trauma or surgery, and the peroneal artery is patent. The flap itself provides good skin coverage to a wound in both the medial and lateral aspects of the distal leg or ankle. The donor site of a distally based sural artery flap is centrally located in the posterior calf over the medial and lateral gastrocnemius muscles. The skin island can be harvested from the proximal two-thirds of the posterior leg. The safest size for the flap is about 12 × 8 cm, but the upper limit of the flap size remains unknown. The flap receives blood supply primarily from three to six septocutaneous perforators arising from the peroneal artery in a retrograde fashion. The most proximal end of those perforators is located 4 to 7 cm proximal to the lateral malleolus. It also receives a blood supply, again in a retrograde fashion, from the fasciocutaneous perforators from the posterior tibial artery, venocutaneous perforators from the lesser saphenous vein, and neurocutaneous perforators from the sural nerve (Fig. 45.9). Thus, the blood supplies to the flap are through the lesser saphenous vein and sural nerve systems that should all be included within the adipofascial pedicle when the flap is elevated. The venous outflow of the flap can either drain directly to the peroneal concomitant vein or drain back to the less saphenous vein.

Operative Procedures

Under general anesthesia with the patient in the prone position, the distal tibial wound, measuring 9 × 5 cm, was debrided. All unhealthy-looking skin edges and colonized tissues were sharply debrided. The wound appeared to be fresh

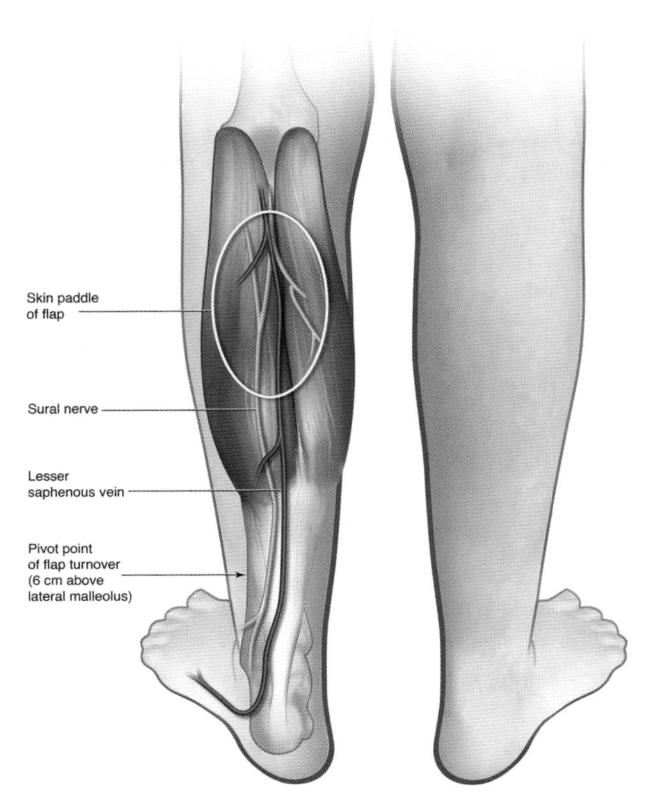

• **Fig. 45.9** A schematic diagram showing blood supplies to the distally based sural artery flap. The flap is based distally and receives blood supply primarily from vascular networks of both the lesser saphenous vein and the sural nerve.

and clean after a definitive debridement performed by the plastic surgery service.

The pivot point of the flap turnover was marked at 6 cm above the lateral malleolus. The entire course of the lesser saphenous vein was mapped with a handheld Doppler between the Achilles tendon and the lateral malleolus. The skin island flap was designed based on the size of soft tissue wound and the less saphenous vein should be included (Fig. 45.10). Under tourniquet control, the proximal incision of the flap was made first to explore the lesser saphenous vein and its accompanying vessels. The lesser saphenous vein and its accompanying vessels were divided. The sural nerve and its accompanying vessels were exposed next through the fascia and then divided. The skin island was elevated along the subfascial plane and the flap was elevated as a fasciocutaneous island flap. The adipofascial pedicle of the flap, about 2 cm wide, was dissected free after multiple zigzag incisions distal to the skin paddle. The flap was turned over and tunneled under the skin bridge to the medial aspect of the distal leg wound.

The flap was then inset into the soft tissue defect of the distal leg with interrupted 3-0 Monocryl sutures in a half-buried horizontal mattress fashion. One drain was placed under the flap (Fig. 45.11). The flap donor site in the middle leg was closed with a split-thickness skin graft. The split-thickness skin graft was harvested with a dermatome from the left lateral thigh and meshed to 1:1.5 ratio. The skin graft was approximated to the adjacent skin edges with skin staples. The remaining skin incisions for the flap dissection were closed in two layers with interrupted sutures.

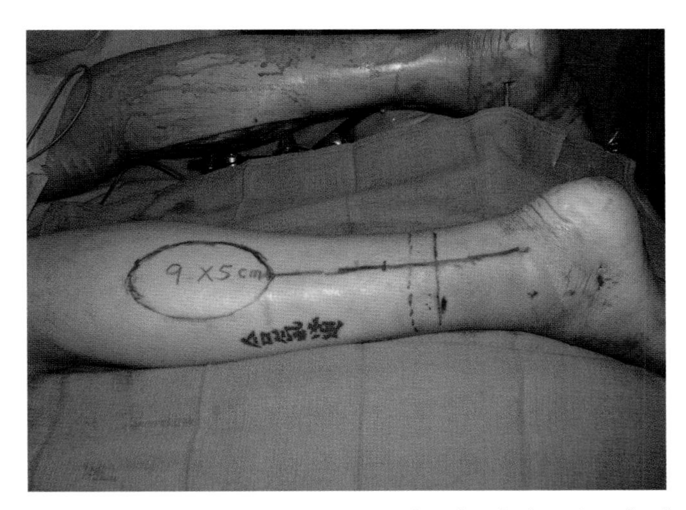

• **Fig. 45.10** An intraoperative view showing the design of a distally based sural artery flap as a turnover flap. The pivotal point of the flap turnover was 6 cm above the lateral malleolus.

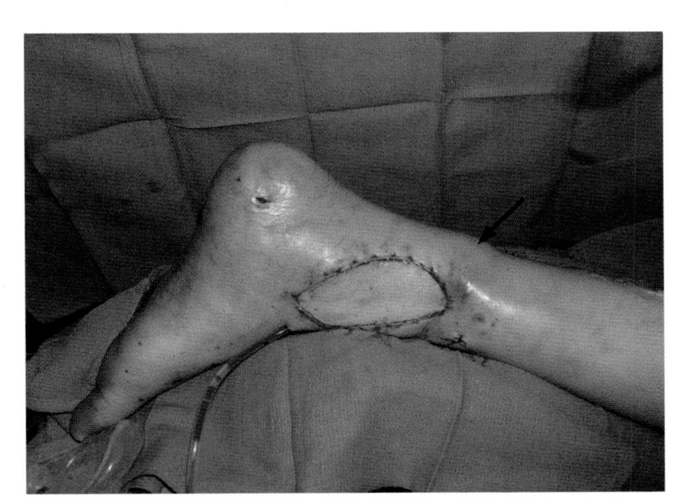

• **Fig. 45.11** An intraoperative view showing completion of the flap inset. In this case, the pedicle of the flap was tunneled through the skin bridge *(arrow)*.

Follow-Up Results

The patient did well postoperatively without any issues related to the distally based sural artery flap for the distal third of the leg wound closure (Fig. 45.12). He was discharged from hospital on postoperative day 5. The left distal tibial fracture also healed uneventfully. He was followed by the plastic surgery service for routine postoperative care and by the orthopedic trauma service for fracture healing after ORIF.

Final Outcome

During further follow-up, the open tibial wound in the distal third of the leg after the flap reconstruction had healed well with excellent contour and almost no scarring. There was no wound breakdown, recurrent infection, or contour issues related to the flap reconstruction (Fig. 45.13). The flap donor site after skin grafting also healed well (Fig. 45.14). He has resumed his weight-bearing status and returned to his normal activities as instructed.

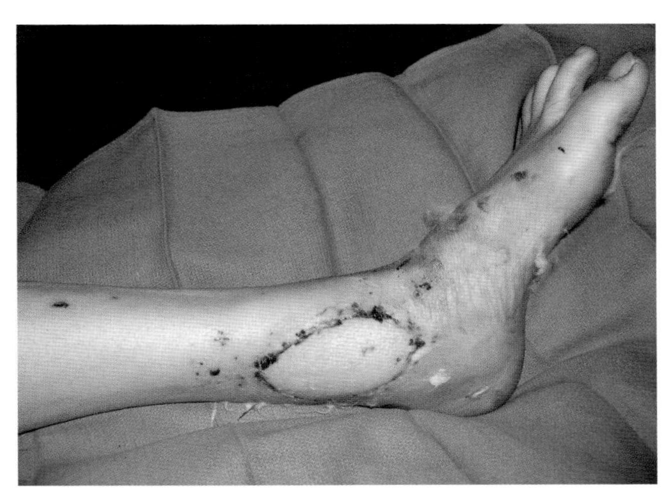

• **Fig. 45.12** Result at 4-week follow-up after flap reconstruction showing well-healed wound in the distal third of the leg with good contour and minimal swelling.

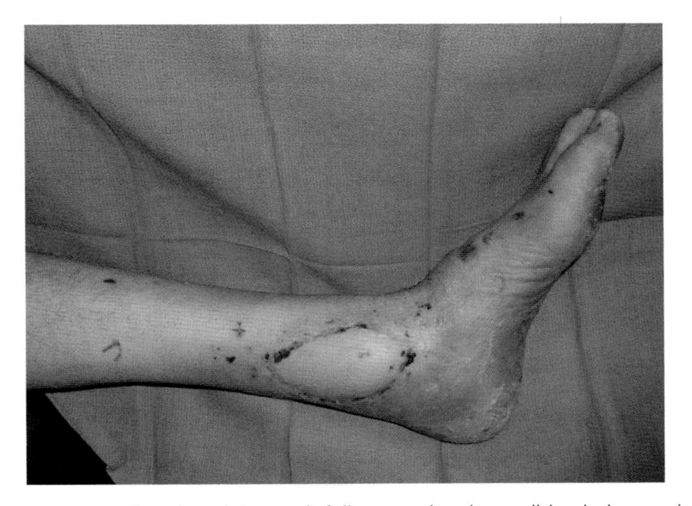

• **Fig. 45.13** Result at 2.5-month follow-up showing well-healed wound in the distal third of the leg with good contour and minimal scaring.

Pearls for Success

In the author's experience, a distal third of the leg wound can also be reconstructed with a distally based sural artery flap if only skin coverage is needed. The less optimal blood supply provided by a fasciocutaneous flap has been one of the main concerns for its routine use to replace a local muscle flap for soft tissue coverage of a complex wound in the distal third of the leg. The skin island is elevated under the fascia and the flap is elevated as a fasciocutaneous island flap. The adipofascial pedicle of the flap can be designed to about 2 cm wide as long as both the less saphenous vein and sural nerve systems are included and may be visualized (Fig. 45.15). The pedicle is dissected free and can be turned over and tunneled under the skin bridge or can be covered with the skin graft if such a tunnel is opened. The flap can be used to cover an exposed bone or hardware in the distal leg. The donor site can

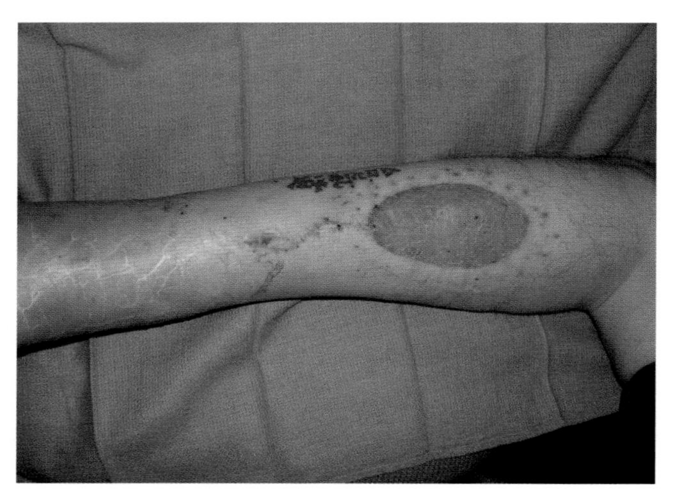

• **Fig. 45.14** Result at 2.5-month follow-up showing well-healed flap donor site with a skin graft closure and direct incision closure site.

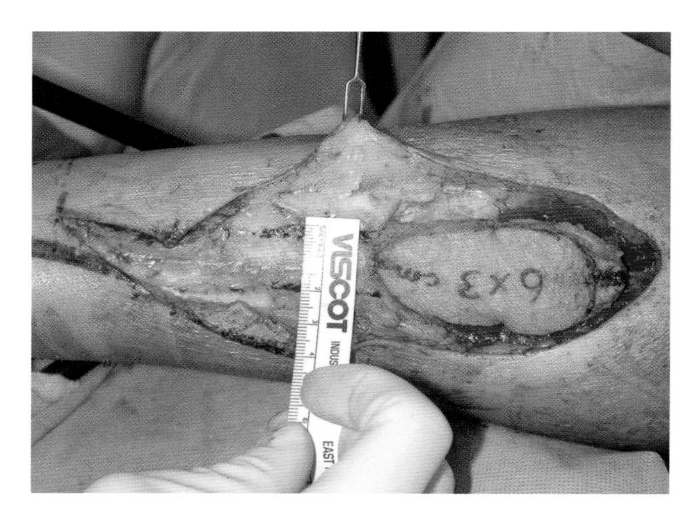

• **Fig. 45.15** An intraoperative view from a different patient showing the exposed pedicle of the flap after zigzag skin incisions. The pedicle can be as narrow as 2 cm and visible.

be closed primarily after undermining if it is less than 5 cm wide or closed with a skin graft.

Elevation of the affected leg in the postoperative period is critical because early venous congestion after a distally based sural artery flap is relatively common. In case of prolonged postoperative venous congestion, application of topical nitroglycerin paste or medicinal leech therapy can be used. Inspection of the flap pedicle is necessary to ensure there is no direct compression. If venous congestion persists or worsens, the flap can be placed back to the donor site or a supercharge to augment venous drainage between the proximal lesser saphenous vein and an adjacent vein in the ankle can be performed with microsurgical technique.

CASE 3

Clinical Presentation

A 32-year-old White male sustained infected nonunion in the left distal tibia. He underwent bony debridement by the orthopedic trauma service and multiple surgical debridements by the primary service, which resulted in a 6 × 3 cm open soft tissue wound in the distal third of the leg with an exposed old tibial fracture site (Fig. 45.16). An autologous bone graft procedure was planned by the primary service. The plastic surgery service was consulted to perform soft tissue reconstruction for the distal tibial wound coverage in preparation for a future bone graft procedure.

Operative Plan and Special Considerations for Reconstruction

For a relatively small open tibial wound in the distal third of the leg with exposed fracture site and/or hardware, a distally based medial hemisoleus muscle flap can be selected to cover such a wound. A medial hemisoleus muscle can be elevated, in reverse fashion, to provide adequate soft tissue coverage but also to minimize functional loss of the foot plantar flexion. The medial half of the soleus muscle can be partially divided at the junction between the proximal and middle thirds of the leg and can then be split longitudinally from proximal to distal and turned over to

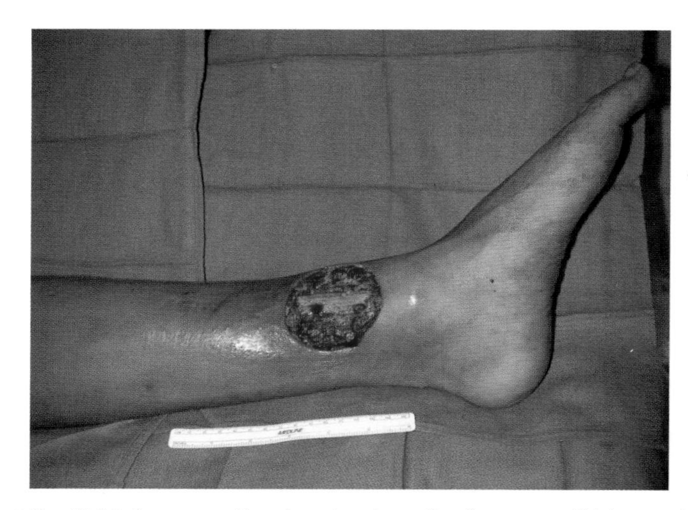

• **Fig. 45.16** A preoperative view showing a 6 × 3 cm open tibial wound in the distal third of the left leg with an exposed old tibial fracture site.

cover an open tibial wound in the distal third of the leg. The distally based medial soleus muscle flap receives blood supply primarily from two or three perforators from the posterior tibial vessels in the distal third of the leg. The distally based medial hemisoleus muscle flap is based primarily on the last two or three major perforators from the posterior tibial vessels. However, it also receives a blood supply from the proximal lateral half of the muscle in a reverse fashion. Therefore, the flap should not be considered a true distally based muscle flap. The flap can be elevated with preservation of as many minor pedicles (perforators) as possible from the posterior tibial vessels to the flap while allowing adequate arc of flap turnover to cover the wound in the distal third of the leg (Fig. 45.17). A preoperative angiogram may be necessary to determine the presence and location of those perforators from the posterior tibial vessels in the distal third of the leg. In general, based on this author's extensive clinical experience, the size of an open tibial wound in the distal third of the leg should not be more than 50 cm^2 if the wound is located in the distal third of the leg if the flap is selected for the wound coverage.

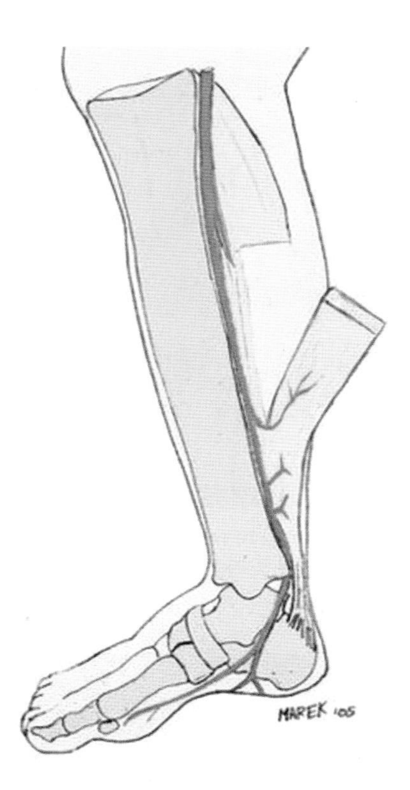

• **Fig. 45.17** A schematic diagram showing blood supplies to the distally based medial hemisoleus muscle flap. The flap is based distally and receives blood supply primarily from several distal perforators of the posterior tibial vessels. The flap also receives additional blood supply from the lateral half of the soleus muscle in a reverse fashion.

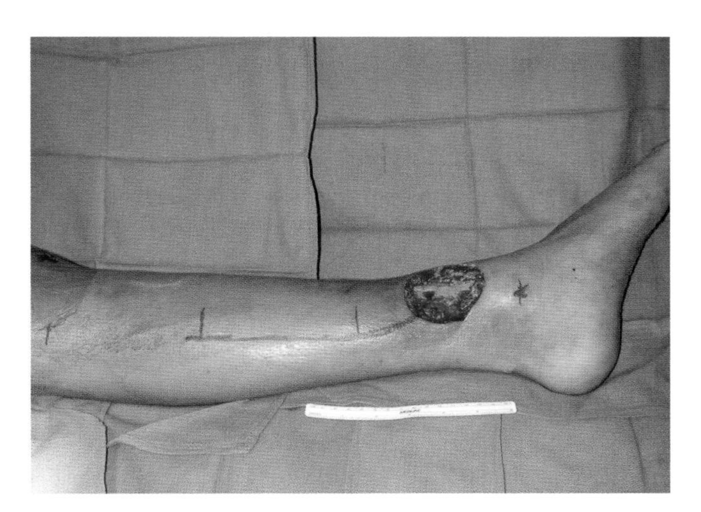

• **Fig. 45.18** An intraoperative view showing the planned surgical incision for dissection of the distally based medial hemisoleus muscle flap.

Operative Procedures

Under general anesthesia with the patient in the supine position, the open distal tibial wound, measuring 6 × 3 cm, was debrided. All unhealthy-looking skin and colonized tissues were sharply debrided. The wound was irrigated and appeared to be fresh and clean after a definitive debridement performed by the plastic surgery service.

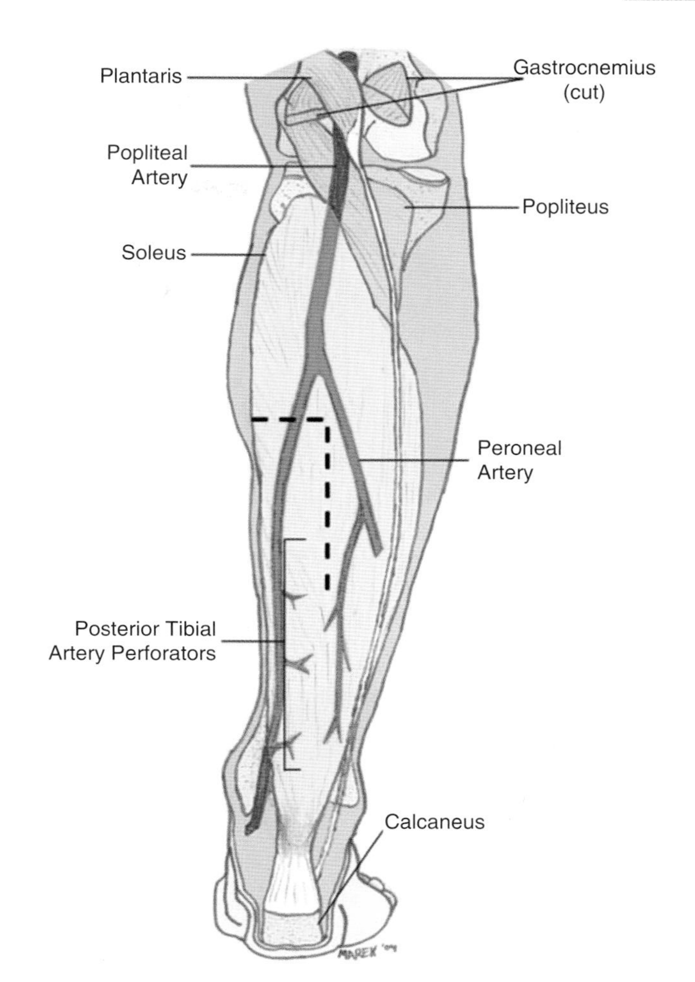

• **Fig. 45.19** A schematic diagram showing the blood supply to the distal part of the soleus muscle as well as splitting of the muscle *(dotted line)* for a distally based medial hemisoleus muscle flap dissection.

The flap dissection was performed under tourniquet control. From the existing open wound, a longitudinal skin incision was extended to about 2 cm medial to the medial border of the tibia and parallel to the tibia (Fig. 45.18). With this incision, the medial half of the soleus muscle in the middle third of the leg was dissected freely from the medial gastrocnemius and flexor digitorum longus muscles. At the junction of the proximal and middle thirds of the soleus muscle, the medial half of the muscle was partially divided and then split longitudinally with the midline of the soleus muscle to the junction of the middle and distal third of the leg (Fig. 45.19).

Care should be taken to preserve as many major perforators from the posterior tibial vessels to the flap as possible, even in the distal middle third of the tibia, while allowing an adequate arc of the flap turnover to cover the tibial wound in the distal third of the leg. The first large perforator from the posterior tibial vessels to the distal soleus muscle was identified and dissected relatively free. It would serve as a pivotal point in the flap turnover (Fig. 45.20).

Scoring the fascia over the deep surface of the reversed medial hemisoleus muscle belly could provide a few additional centimeters arc of flap turnover if needed. The flap was turned over into the defect and inset with several 3-0 absorbable half-buried horizontal mattress sutures. One drain was placed under the flap and another drain was inserted into the flap donor site.

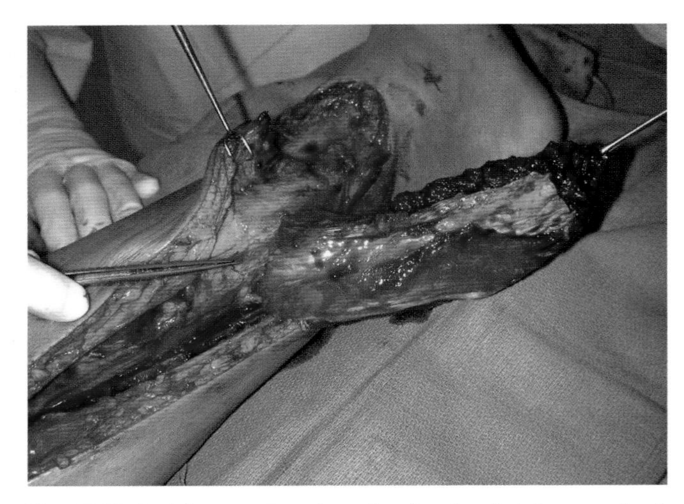

• **Fig. 45.20** An intraoperative view showing the first large perforator (indicated by *forceps*) from the posterior tibial vessels to the distally based medial hemisoleus muscle flap. This perforator served as a pivotal point of the flap turnover.

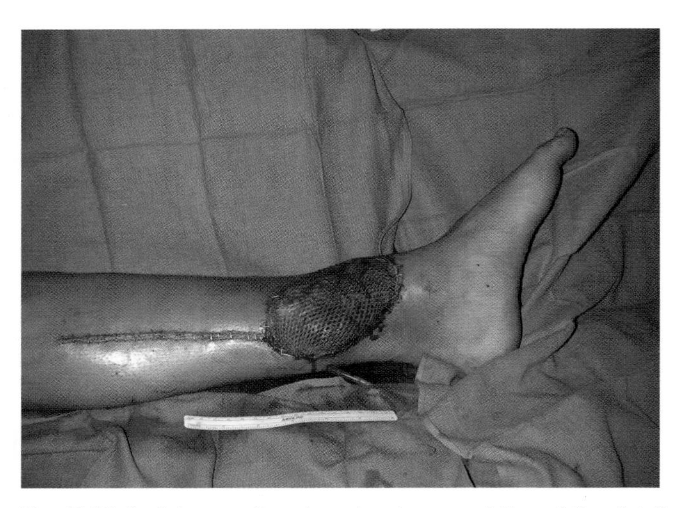

• **Fig. 45.21** An intraoperative view showing completion of the distally based medial hemisoleus muscle flap inset and placement of skin graft over the muscle flap at the end of the flap reconstruction.

The muscle flap was covered with a split-thickness skin graft. A split-thickness skin graft was harvested with a dermatome from the left lateral thigh and meshed to 1:1.5 ratio. The incision for the flap exposure was closed in two layers and the skin graft was secured with skin staples (Fig. 45.21).

Follow-Up Results

The patient did well postoperatively without any issues related to the flap reconstruction for the distal third of the leg wound closure. He was discharged from hospital on postoperative day 5. The left distal tibial wound healed uneventfully. He was followed by the plastic surgery service for routine postoperative care and underwent an autologous bone graft procedure by the orthopedic trauma service 4 months after the initial flap reconstruction (Fig. 45.22).

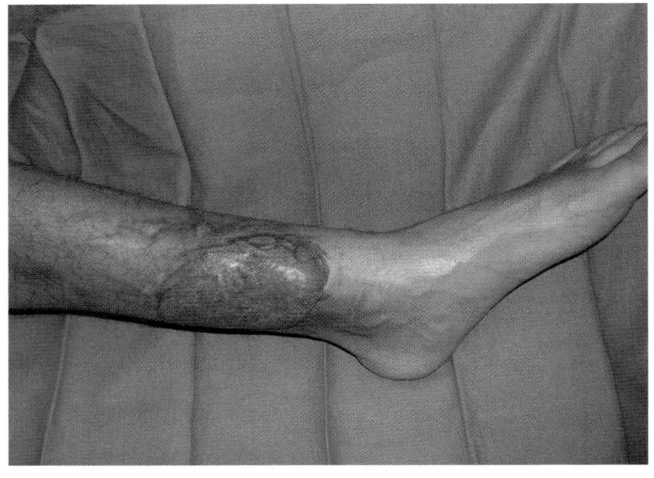

• **Fig. 45.22** Result at 4-month follow-up after the flap reconstruction showing well-healed distal-third tibial wound with reliable soft tissue coverage.

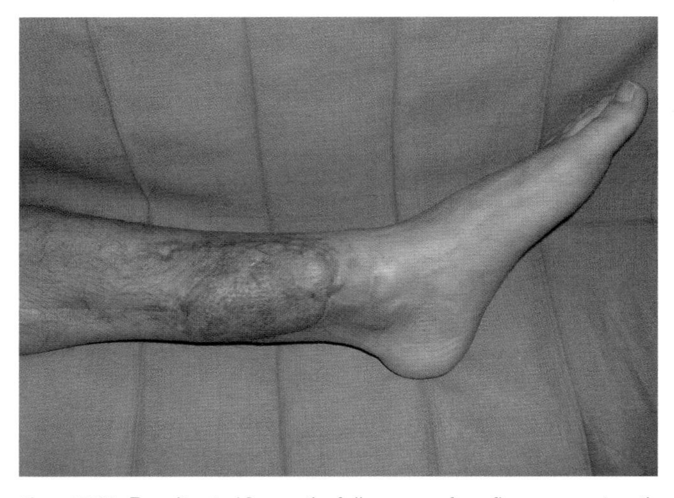

• **Fig. 45.23** Result at 10-month follow-up after flap reconstruction showing well-healed distal-third tibial wound with good contour and minimal scarring.

Final Outcome

During further follow-up, the open tibial wound in the distal third of the leg after the flap reconstruction healed well with good contour and minimal scarring. There has been union of the distal tibial fracture site and no wound breakdown, recurrent infection, or contour issues related to the soft tissue reconstruction (Fig. 45.23). The patient has resumed his weight-bearing status and has returned to his normal activities as instructed.

Pearls for Success

In the author's practice, all patients with a relatively limited soft tissue defect (<50 cm^2) in the distal third of the leg near the ankle can be reconstructed with this distally based medial hemisoleus muscle flap as an alternative option for a free tissue transfer. During flap dissection, all perforators to the distal soleus muscle are critical sources of blood supply to the distal portion of the medial hemisoleus muscle flap and should be preserved whenever possible. In addition, the first large perforator in the distal third of the leg is more critical because this perforator's location will determine how far the flap can reach to the distal leg wound.

The flap can be suitable for coverage of a sizable tibial wound in the distal third of the leg when it is turned approximately 180 degrees. Because the flap is still primarily based distally and normally turned approximately 180 degrees (reversed) to cover the tibial defect, it should not be recommended to smokers unless the flap has been previously delayed. Furthermore, the flap should not be considered if the portion of the soleus muscle has been severely traumatized. The flap may look bulky and present with some degree of venous congestion initially. However, venous congestion can be resolved in a couple of weeks. With time and prolonged leg elevation and ACE wrapping, the contour of the flap can be improved significantly and no debulking procedure is needed. Like any other pedicle flaps, distal flap necrosis may occur, but total flap loss should not happen if the procedure is performed properly. Fortunately, distal flap necrosis is usually insignificant and can be treated with debridement. The flap can then be readvanced to cover the tibial wound. Further advancement of the flap is possible by dividing the most proximal perforator that has served as a pivotal point because the flap has been "delayed" after initial flap elevation.

CASE 4

Clinical Presentation

A 42-year-old Hispanic male sustained a closed type C pilon fracture in the right distal leg as a result of a motor vehicle accident. He underwent multiple procedures, including an open reduction and internal fixation of the fibular and pilon fractures. Incisions used by the orthopedic trauma surgeon included a laterally based incision over the fibular shaft, a posterolateral incision in the Achilles tendon region, and an anteromedial incision over the ankle. He was followed in the orthopedics clinic and wound infections with purulent fluids were noted, requiring debridement in the operating room. He developed an exposed fracture site in addition to hardware and an area of 7 × 3 cm with exposed Achilles tendon as a result of orthopedic debridement. A free anterolateral thigh flap was performed for coverage of the exposed fracture and hardware wound in the distal third of the medial leg. The exposed Achilles tendon was treated using negative pressure wound therapy. However, this failed to improve the wound healing. The plastic surgery service was consulted again by the orthopedic trauma service 4 weeks later for soft tissue reconstruction in that location (Fig. 45.24).

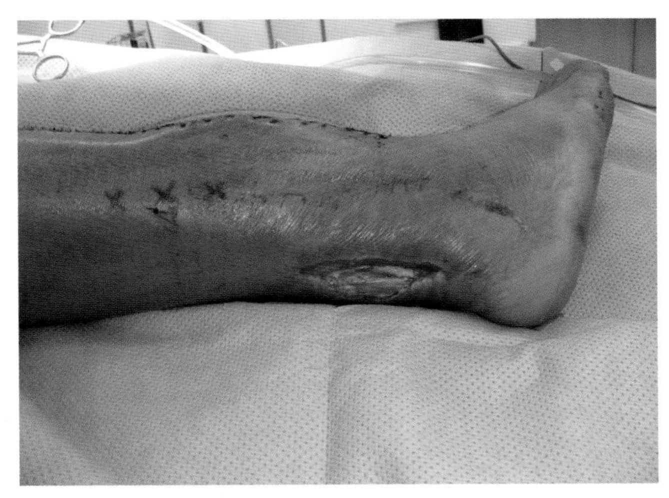

• **Fig. 45.24** A preoperative view showing a distal lateral leg soft tissue wound, measuring 7 × 3 cm, with exposed underlying tendon.

Operative Plan and Special Considerations for Reconstruction

Although a second free tissue transfer could be selected for soft tissue reconstruction of this open wound located in the distal third of the leg, a local reconstructive option would be better this time for the wound closure. The distally based peroneus brevis can be used to cover a complex wound in the distal third of the leg because the scar location in the lateral distal leg, the distally based sural artery flap cannot be performed safely. The peroneus brevis is a lateral compartmental muscle. It originates from the lower third of the lateral fibula and inserted to the fifth metatarsal. Its circulation pattern is type II. It receives blood supply primarily from muscular branches of the peroneal vessels. It also receives blood supply from anterior tibial vessels (Fig. 45.25). The muscle flap can also be elevated and based distally, and used as a turnover

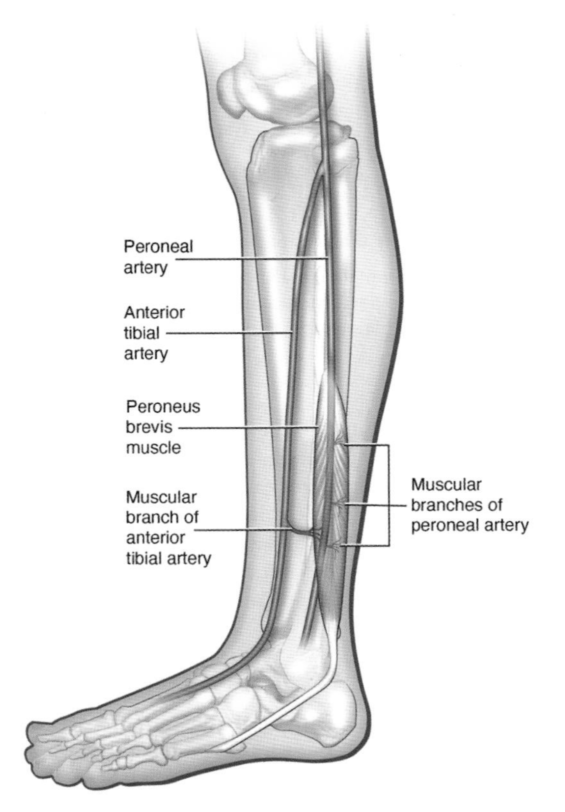

• **Fig. 45.25** A schematic diagram showing the segmental blood supplies to the peroneus brevis muscle primarily from the peroneal vessels. In addition, the muscle receives a blood supply from the anterior tibial vessels.

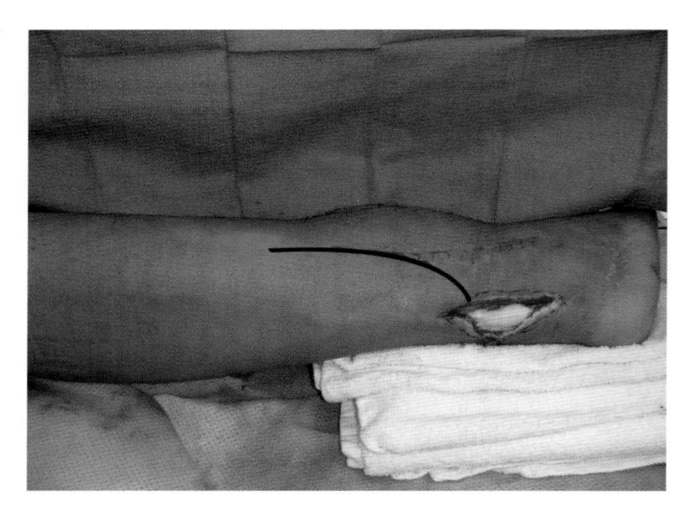

• **Fig. 45.26** An intraoperative view showing the design of the skin incision used to explore the distal peroneus brevis muscle after a definitive wound debridement.

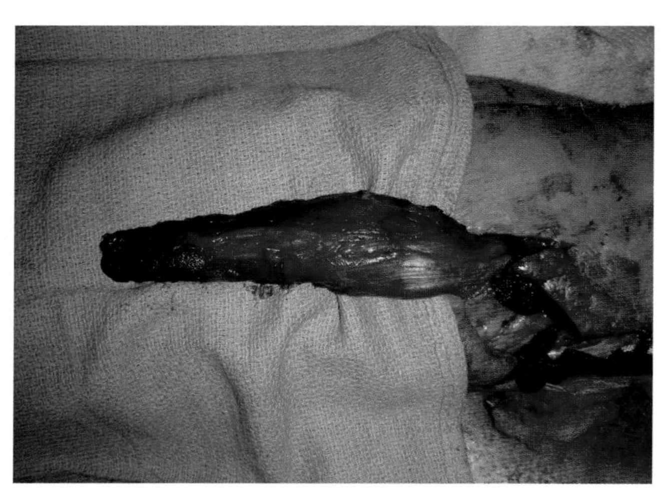

• **Fig. 45.27** An intraoperative view showing an elevated, distally based peroneus brevis muscle flap. The tip of the flap appeared to have good bleeding from venous congestion and was wrapped with Surgicel for hemostasis.

flap to cover a lateral wound in the distal third of the leg. The flap should be elevated with preservation of as many segmental pedicles (perforators) from the peroneal vessels as possible to the flap while allowing adequate arc of flap turnover to cover a lateral wound in the distal third of the leg. With limited dissection, the muscle can be turned over to cover a small lateral leg wound in the distal third of the leg with good success.

Operative Procedures

Under general anesthesia with the patient in the left decubitus position, the right lateral leg wound in the distal third of the leg was debrided. The wound edge was then freshened with a blade and all colonized tissue was removed with a curette. The wound was then irrigated with Pulsavac and looked clean and fresh.

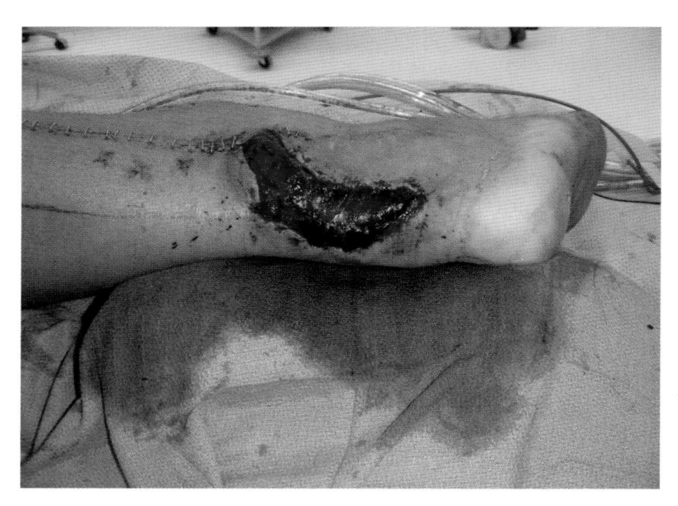

• **Fig. 45.28** An intraoperative view showing completion of the muscle flap inset before the placement of a skin graft. Venous congestion of the flap was still present.

The incision was extended proximally from the open wound and parallel to the fibula (Fig. 45.26). Once the skin incision had been made through the fascia, the peroneus brevis muscle was identified. The muscle's attachment to the fibula was dissected free distally and its proximal part was sharply dissected with a knife from the adjacent tissues. The proximal muscle was divided and the muscle flap was elevated in a reverse fashion. The muscle flap was further dissected distally enough to allow an adequate arc of the flap turnover. Unfortunately, this patient had undergone previous surgery around his lateral ankle; therefore, further dissection to have a longer arc rotation was not feasible because this might completely compromise circulation to the flap when it was based distally. The skin edge between the wound and the flap was incised. The muscle flap appeared to be somewhat congested (Fig. 45.27). The flap was wrapped with a warm saline lap. After about 1 hour, the flap appeared to be pinker, although the distal end was still somewhat congested. The muscle flap was turned over to cover the lateral wound in the distal third of the leg with an exposed Achilles tendon. The flap's inset was performed with several half-buried horizontal mattress 3-0 Monocryl sutures. Thus, the entire defect was covered with the flap in a reverse fashion (Fig. 45.28).

A JP drain was inserted into the flap's donor site. The incision for the flap dissection was closed in two layers. A split-thickness skin graft was harvested from the right lateral thigh. It was meshed to a 1:1.5 ratio. It was then placed over the muscle flap and secured to the adjacent tissue with multiple skin staples (Fig. 45.29). A 5-0 chromic suture was placed as multiple quilting sutures to immobilize the skin graft.

Follow-Up Results

The patient did well postoperatively without any issues related to the flap reconstruction for the wound closure. The initial venous congestion resolved several days postoperatively and he was discharged from hospital on postoperative day 7. The right distal lateral leg wound healed uneventfully (Fig. 45.30). He was followed by the plastic surgery service for routine flap postoperative care and by the orthopedic trauma service for orthopedic care.

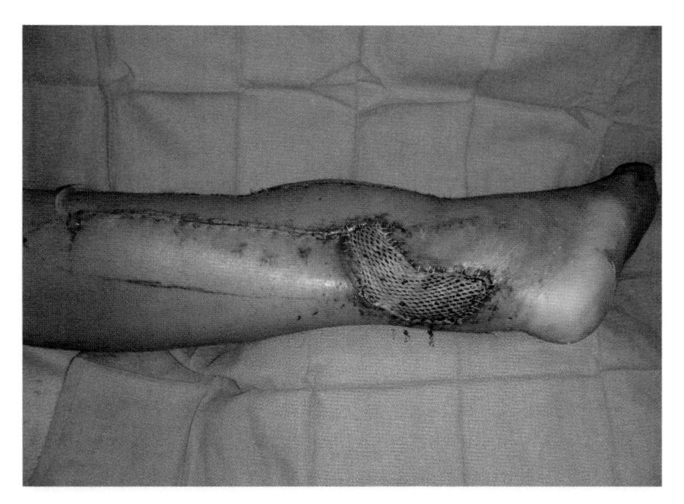

• **Fig. 45.29** An intraoperative view showing completion of a skin graft placement to the muscle flap and incisions closure.

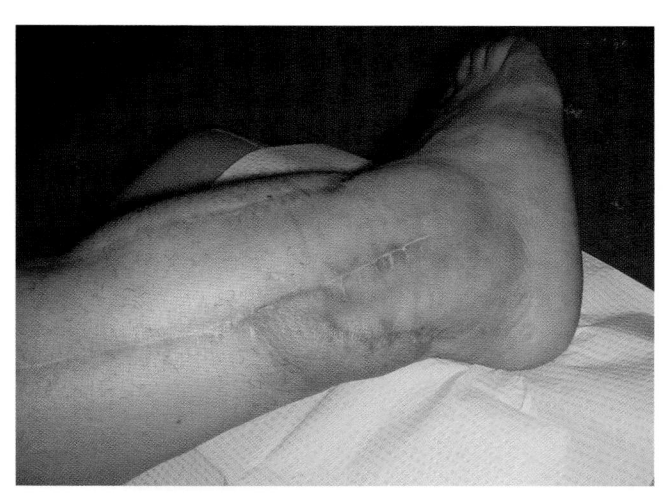

• **Fig. 45.31** Result at 10-month follow-up showing well-healed wound in the distal third of the lateral leg after flap reconstruction with good contour and minimal scarring.

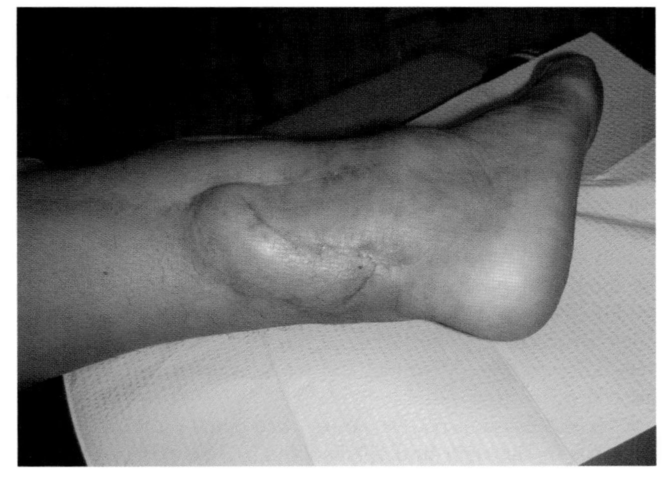

• **Fig. 45.30** Result at 6-month follow-up showing well-healed wound in the distal third of the lateral leg after flap reconstruction.

Final Outcome

During further follow-up, the right lateral leg wound after the flap reconstruction had healed well with acceptable contour and minimal scarring with no wound breakdown, recurrent infection, or contour issues related to the soft tissue reconstruction (Fig. 45.31). He has resumed his normal weight-bearing status and has returned to his normal activities.

Pearls for Success

The distally based peroneus brevis muscle flap can be used in coverage of a small defect in the distal third of the lateral leg. The dominant pedicle is the muscular branch of the peroneal artery that enters the deep surface of the proximal portion of the muscle. The muscular branch of the anterior tibial artery serves as a minor pedicle and enters the deep surface of the muscle in the distal portion. The distally based flap can be raised by separating the proximal origins of the muscle from the fibula as well as the neighboring peroneus longus and flexor digitorum longus muscles. During the flap dissection, the minor pedicle can be identified and protected so that the flap can be dissected freely allowing adequate turnover to cover a distal-third lateral leg wound. Because it is distally based, venous congestion of the flap is common, but it can be resolved in the next few days with proper management. Keeping the flap warm with more consistent and reliable leg elevation can be key for postoperative care. If tip necrosis of the flap occurs, the necrotic portion of flap can be debrided and readvancement of the flap may still be possible.

Recommended Readings

Buluç L, Tosun B, Sen C, Sarlak AY. A modified technique for transposition of the reverse sural artery flap. *Plast Reconstr Surg*. 2006; 117:2488–2492.

Pu LL. Successful soft-tissue coverage of a tibial wound in the distal third of the leg with a medial hemisoleus muscle flap. *Plast Reconstr Surg*. 2005;115:245–251.

Pu LLQ. Locoregional flaps in lower extremity reconstruction. *Clin Plast Surg*. 2021;48:157–171.

Pu LLQ. Further experience with the medial hemisoleus muscle flap for soft-tissue coverage of a tibial wound in the distal third of the leg. *Plast Reconstr Surg*. 2008;121:2024–2028.

Pu LL. Soft-tissue reconstruction of an open tibial wound in the distal third of the leg: a new treatment algorithm. *Ann Plast Surg*. 2007;58:78–83.

Pu LL. The reversed medial hemisoleus muscle flap and its role in reconstruction of an open tibial wound in the lower third of the leg. *Ann Plast Surg*. 2006;56:59–63.

Schmidt K, Jakubietz M, Djalek S, Harenberg PS, Zeplin PH, Jakubietz R. The distally based adipofascial sural artery flap: faster, safer, and easier? A long-term comparison of the fasciocutaneous and adipofascial method in a multimorbid patient population. *Plast Reconstr Surg*. 2012;130:360–368.

Song P, Pu LLQ. The soleus muscle flap: an overview of its clinical applications for lower extremity reconstruction. *Ann Plast Surg*. 2018;(6S suppl 1):S109–S116.

Troisi L, Wright T, Khan U, Emam AT, Chapman TWL. The distally based peroneus brevis flap: the 5-Step technique. *Ann Plast Surg*. 2018;80:272–276.

46

Leg Reconstruction: Distal Third (Free Flaps)

CASE 1

Clinical Presentation

A 54-year-old White male unfortunately developed a wound dehiscence in the left distal third of his leg after an open reduction and internal fixation for a distal tibial fracture. The distal tibial wound measured 12 × 6 cm with the exposed fracture site, reconstruction plate, and antibiotic beads. The wound was located quite distally and extended to the ankle (Fig. 46.1). Clearly, there was no reliable local option for soft tissue reconstruction of the wound. The plastic surgery service was consulted for a free tissue transfer as a first option for soft tissue reconstruction. The preoperative angiogram showed some atherosclerotic disease of the arteries in the left leg.

Operative Plan and Special Considerations

For this relatively large soft tissue wound in the distal third of the leg extending to the ankle, the primary soft tissue reconstructive option would be a free tissue transfer because there was no reliable local option available to meet the reconstructive need in this case. As most reconstructive plastic surgeons know more and feel comfortable with the anterolateral thigh (ALT) perforator flap, it could be selected to provide a good and reliable soft tissue coverage for this distal tibial open fracture wound. The flap has a long pedicle and can provide a relatively large amount of fasciocutaneous tissue for reliable soft tissue coverage of the wound. As far as selection of recipient vessels for microvascular anastomoses, it has been this author's preference to select the anterior tibial vessels, if possible, for an end-to-end microvascular anastomosis. In this way, it would be relatively easy to perform microvascular anastomosis with potentially improved patency rate so that a free tissue transfer to the lower extremity might be less complicated. In addition, a preoperative duplex scan is routinely performed to determine which side of the thigh should be selected as a donor site based on the size and blood flow of the perforator identified as well as the amount of intramuscular perforator dissection required.

Operative Procedures

Under general anesthesia with the patient in the supine position, the duplex scan was performed first to identify which side would be better for the ALT perforator free flap donor site. Based on duplex scan findings, there was no obvious perforator on the left side. However, on the right side, there was a single good perforator that measured 1.5 mm in diameter and was about 1.5 cm deep. Anticipated intramuscular dissection was less extensive. Therefore, the intraoperative decision was made to harvest the right ALT perforator flap (Fig. 46.2).

The procedure started by debriding the left distal tibial wound. All colonized tissues were removed. The skin edge was freshened with a blade and the wound was irrigated with Pulsavac. The anterior tibial vessels were exposed as the recipient vessels. The skin incision was extended more laterally and parallel to the lateral tibia. The anterior tibial vessels were identified between the peroneus and anterior tibialis muscles. The anterior tibial artery appeared to be somewhat calcified. After retracting the deep peroneal nerve, both artery and vein were identified and were dissected free. Each vessel was wrapped with a vessel loop.

A 15 × 7 cm skin paddle was marked based on location of the perforator in the right anterolateral thigh. The skin incision was made around the skin paddle through the deep fascia down to the muscle. The subfascial dissection was performed to explore the perforator. During dissection, one major perforator and two small perforators were identified (Fig. 46.3). The space between the rectus femoris and vastus lateralis muscles was opened. The large perforator was followed and gradually dissected free. It traveled through the vastus lateralis muscle and jointed to the descending branch of the lateral circumflex femoral vessels. The vessels were divided distal to the perforator/descending branch junction. The dissection followed the descending branch in a retrograde fashion until it reached the profunda. The pedicle was then divided off the profunda vessel (Fig. 46.4).

The flap was prepared under loupe magnification. Both artery and vein were dissected free from each other. The arterial pedicle was flushed with heparinized saline solution. After that, the pedicle of the flap was ready for microvascular anastomoses. The flap was first inset into the defect and secured with towel clips. The anterior tibial vein was divided distally with hemoclips. The proximal part of it was prepared under the microscope. The anterior tibial artery was also divided distally with hemoclips and further dissection was done to remove all the adventitious tissues under the microscope. The pedicle to the anterior tibial artery was anastomosed with interrupted end-to-end 8-0 nylon sutures. The pedicle to the anterior tibial vein was anastomosed with a 2-mm coupler device in an end-to-end fashion. After all clamps had

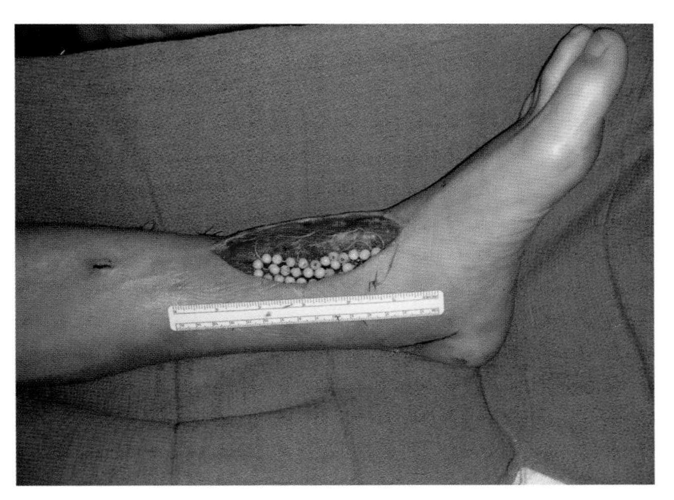

• **Fig. 46.1** An intraoperative view showing a 12 × 6-cm complex soft tissue wound in the distal tibial of the left leg extending to the ankle with the exposed fracture site, reconstruction plate, and antibiotic beads.

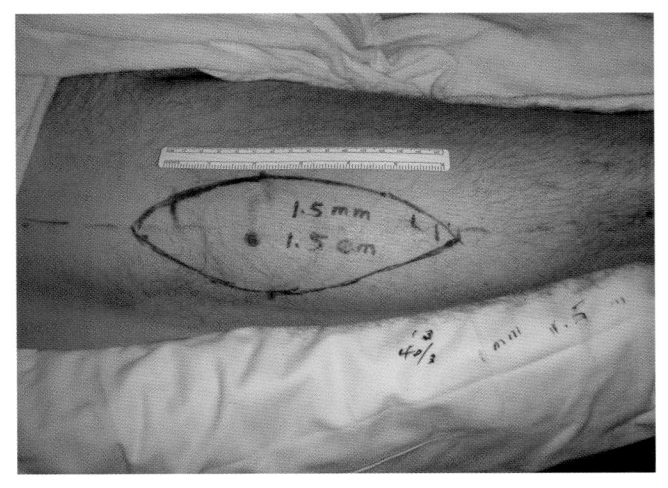

• **Fig. 46.2** An intraoperative view showing the design of the right anterolateral thigh perforator flap. The skin paddle of the flap was 16 × 7 cm. The single large perforator was identified by preoperative duplex scan.

been removed, the flap appeared to have good arterial inflow and venous outflow.

The flap was inset into the distal leg wound and approximated with adjacent skin with interrupted 3-0 Monocryl sutures in a half-buried horizontal mattress fashion. Prior to the flap inset, a drain was placed under the flap but was kept away from the pedicle vessels. The proximal leg incision was approximated with skin staples (Fig. 46.5).

The flap donor site of the right thigh was closed last. A small portion of divided muscle was approximated with 3-0 Vicryl suture in a figure-of-eight fashion. The deep dermal closure was done with interrupted 2-0 PDS sutures. The skin was closed with 3-0 Monocryl sutures in a running subcuticular fashion.

Follow-Up Results

The patient did well postoperatively without any complications related to the free ALT flap transfer. He was discharged from

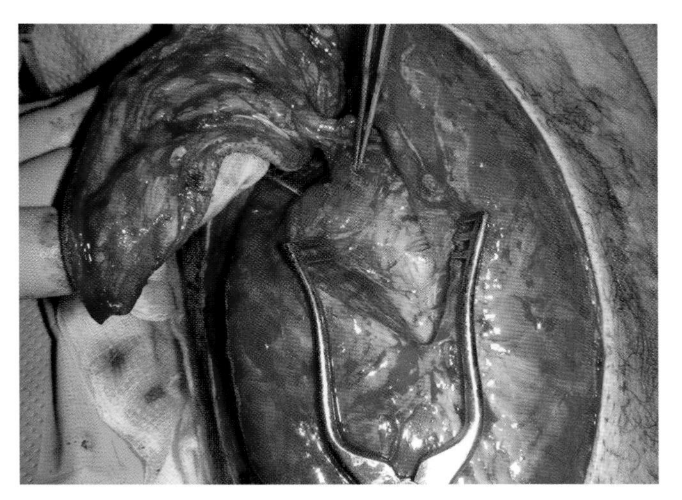

• **Fig. 46.3** An intraoperative view showing the large perforator of the flap that was dissected free. It traveled through the vastus lateralis muscle and joined to the descending branch of the lateral circumflex femoral artery.

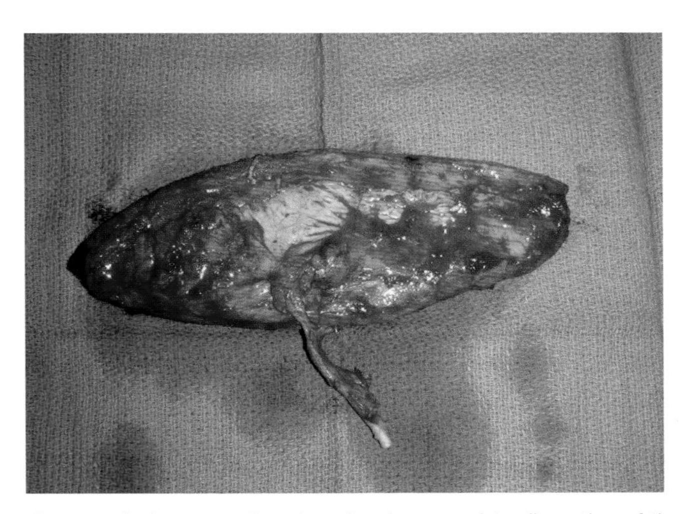

• **Fig. 46.4** An intraoperative view showing complete dissection of the anterolateral thigh flap. The flap was based on a single large perforator.

hospital on postoperative day 10 once he tolerated flap dangling. The drain was removed during subsequent follow-up visits. The reconstruction site over the left distal third of the leg healed well (Fig. 46.6).

Final Outcome

The left distal third of the leg wound after free ALT flap reconstruction healed well with good contour and minimal scarring. The distal tibial fracture site also healed well. No flap debulking procedure was needed. The patient has resumed his normal activities and is being routinely followed by the orthopedic trauma service.

Pearls for Success

A free ALT perforator flap can be a valid reconstructive option as long as the surgeon feels comfortable to perform a perforator flap

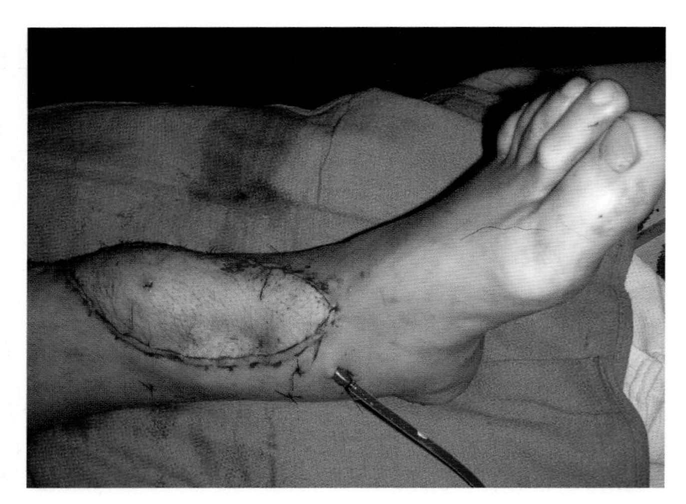

• **Fig. 46.5** An intraoperative view showing completion of the flap inset at the end of the procedure.

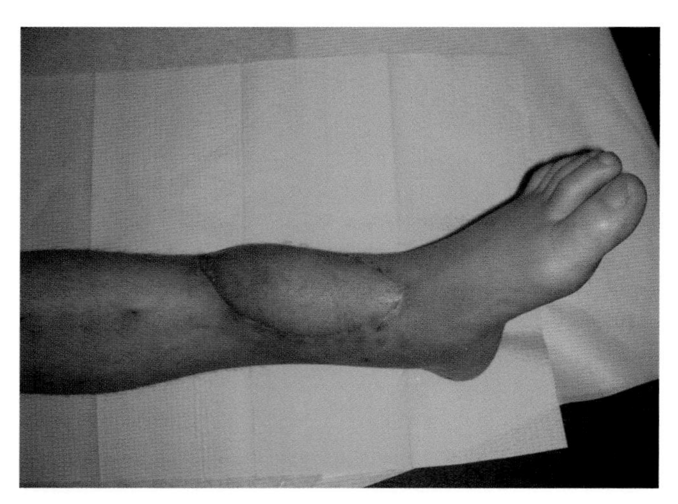

• **Fig. 46.6** Results at 3-week follow-up showing well-healed and stable left distal third of the leg wound after the flap reconstruction with some flap bulking and minimal scarring.

surgery. The flap is large enough and can be harvested as a fasciocutaneous or cutaneous flap to provide reliable soft tissue coverage in the distal third of the leg. However, the ALT flap dissection can be challenging if the patient is obese and the flap may remain bulky after it heals in the recipient site. Thus, compared with a free muscle flap, a subsequent debulking procedure may be necessary to improve the contour in the distal leg. It has been the author's preference to perform a preoperative duplex scan routinely to determine the best and easiest site as an ALT flap donor site. Such information is critical because the size, blood flow, and location of a perforator as well as the potential amount of intramuscular dissection for the perforator can be determined. This has made the ALT perforator dissection more predictable and less time-consuming. In addition, because an end-to-end microvascular anastomosis would be easier than an end-to-side anastomosis, the author routinely selects the anterior tibial vessels, if possible, as the recipient vessels for a less complicated microvascular free tissue transfer in the distal leg. After 1 year, flap debulking procedure may be necessary in certain patients to improve leg contour. It can be performed via liposuction followed by a direct excision of excess flap tissue.

CASE 2

Clinical Presentation

A 37-year-old Indian female sustained a closed distal tibia fracture during a fall while vacationing out of state. The patient was initially treated at an outside facility with Steinmann pin fixation of the tibial fracture and casting. Six weeks after the initial injury, she was transferred to our hospital for definitive orthopedic care. At that time, she had a large area of necrotic soft tissue over the fracture site with purulent drainage. She was taken to the operating room emergently by the orthopedic trauma service for debridement and removal of hardware. The patient returned to the operating room later for debridement and definitive fixation of the tibia fracture with an intramedullary nail. The soft tissue wound was 8 × 6 cm after debridement with the exposed fracture site in the distal third of the left leg (Fig. 46.7). The plastic surgery service was consulted for soft tissue coverage of the wound.

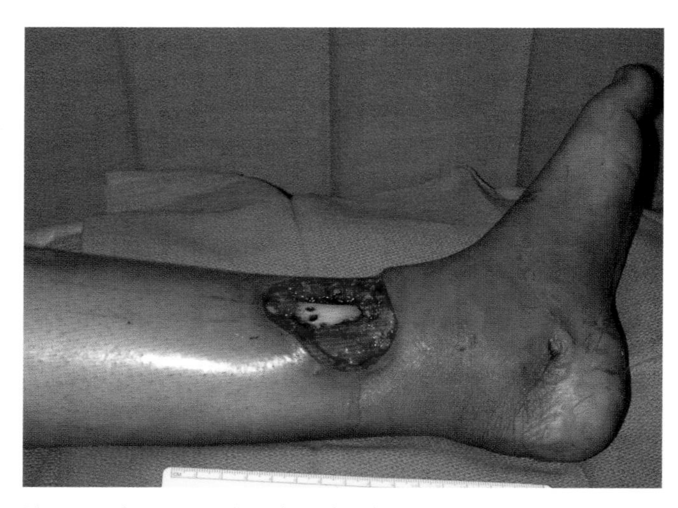

• **Fig. 46.7** A preoperative view showing an 8 × 6-cm complex soft tissue wound in the distal third of the left leg.

Operative Plan and Special Considerations

For a complex wound in the distal third of the leg, a classic approach to soft tissue reconstruction would be a free tissue transfer. This patient had a relatively small wound in the distal third of the leg and thus, a small muscle flap, such as a free gracilis muscle flap, could be selected to provide a reliable soft tissue reconstruction to the distal tibial wound. The gracilis muscle is a type II muscle flap. It is a narrow straplike muscle (24 × 5 × 1.5 cm) with a pedicle length averaging 6 cm. The gracilis muscle can be an excellent choice for small- to medium-sized defects. It has become the author's first choice to cover a small to medium defect of the distal third tibial wound. With many advances in surgical technique for muscle harvesting, the gracilis muscle can be used for various reconstructive needs as a free muscle flap. Its flap dissection can be relatively straightforward and a pedicle length and size can be improved by dividing the branches of the medial circumflex femoral vessels to the adductor longus and brevis muscles.

Operative Procedures

Under general anesthesia with the patient in the supine position, the left distal tibial wound was debrided. All colonized tissues were removed and the skin edge was freshened with a blade. The wound was then irrigated with Pulsavac and looked clean and fresh after more definitive wound debridement by the plastic surgery service (Fig. 46.8).

The posterior tibial vessels were exposed as the recipient vessels for this case. The skin incision was extended more proximally and parallel to the anterior edge of the tibia. The posterior tibial vessels were identified between the soleus and flexor digitorum longus muscles. After retracting the tibial nerve, both artery and vein were identified and dissected free under loupe magnification. Each vessel was then wrapped with a vessel loop.

A 15-cm longitudinal incision was made in the left medial thigh along a line between the pubic tubercle and the medial femoral condyle. The skin and subcutaneous tissue were incised and the fascia was opened. Once the anterior border of the gracilis muscle had been identified and dissected free, the adductor longus muscle was retracted laterally to expose the main pedicle vessels. After identifying the main pedicle of the gracilis muscle, all minor pedicles in the distal portion of the muscle were divided. The distal muscle was also divided near the origin. Proximally, the muscle insertion to the pubic tubercle was also divided. With careful retraction, the pedicle dissection was performed under loupe magnification and during its dissection, all small branches on the pedicle vessels were divided with microclips. The branches of the medial circumflex femoral vessels to the adductor longus and brevis were divided, which would obtain an additional 2 to 3 cm in pedicle length with a possible vessel diameter greater than 2.0 mm for the artery. The pedicle vessels were divided with hemoclips from the profunda and ready for free tissue transfer.

The pedicle of the muscle flap was prepared under loupe magnification. The artery and vein were dissected free. The artery was flushed with heparinized saline solution. One artery and two veins were prepared for microvascular anastomoses (Fig. 46.9). After further preparation of the pedicle vessels under a microscope, the muscle flap was temporarily inset into the distal tibial wound. Again, under a microscope, an end-to-side arterial microanastomosis was performed between the pedicle and the posterior tibial artery with an interrupted 8-0 nylon suture. The venous microanastomosis was performed with a 2.0-mm coupler device in an end-to-end fashion. Once all clamps had been released, the muscle flap appeared to be well perfused with a good Doppler signal.

The final inset of the muscle flap was performed. A drain was inserted into the wound under the flap. The muscle flap was sutured to the adjacent skin edge of the wound with interrupted 3-0 Monocryl sutures in a half-buried horizontal mattress fashion (Fig. 46.10). A split-thickness skin graft was harvested from the left lateral thigh. The skin graft was meshed to 1:1.5 ratio, placed over the muscle flap, and secured to the adjacent skin with skin staples. The anteromedial leg incision for exposure of the posterior tibial vessel was closed in two layers. The deep dermal layer was approximated with several interrupted 3-0 Monocryl sutures. The skin was closed with skin staples (Fig. 46.11).

The left thigh gracilis muscle flap donor site was closed in two layers after placing a JP drain. The deep dermal layer was approximated with interrupted 3-0 Monocryl sutures. The skin was closed with skin staples.

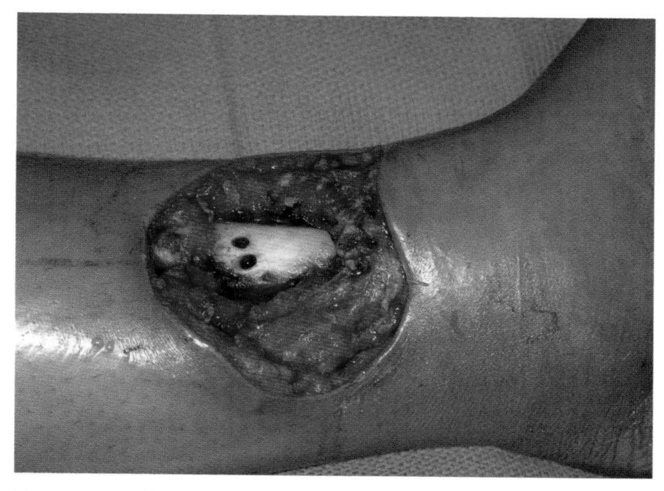

• **Fig. 46.8** An intraoperative close-up view showing this complex soft tissue wound in the distal third of the left leg with the exposed tibial fracture site.

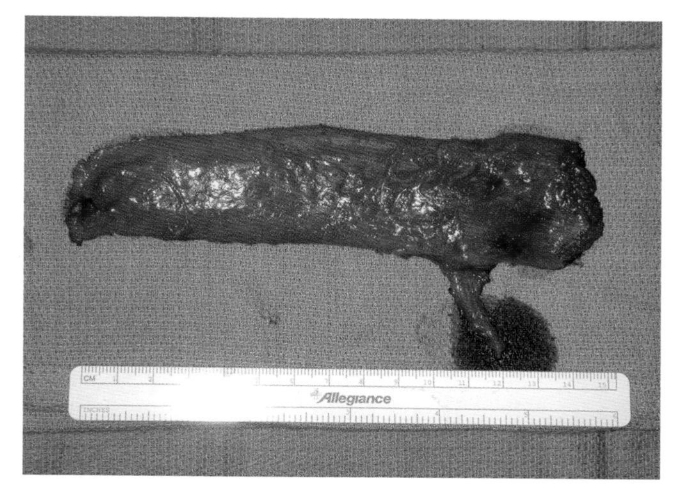

• **Fig. 46.9** An intraoperative view showing completion of the flap dissection for the left free gracilis muscle flap and its pedicle.

Follow-Up Results

The patient did well postoperatively without any complications related to the free gracilis muscle flap reconstruction for the distal tibial wound closure. She was discharged from hospital on postoperative day 7 after tolerating the flap dangling. All drains were removed during subsequent follow-up visits. The left free gracilis muscle flap reconstruction site and the skin graft over the muscle flap healed well.

Final Outcome

The free gracilis muscle flap reconstruction for coverage of the distal tibial wound healed well with an excellent contour but minimal scarring (Fig. 46.12). With a good soft tissue coverage, the distal tibial fracture also healed well. No bone graft was needed. The patient has resumed her normal activities and been routinely followed by the orthopedic trauma service.

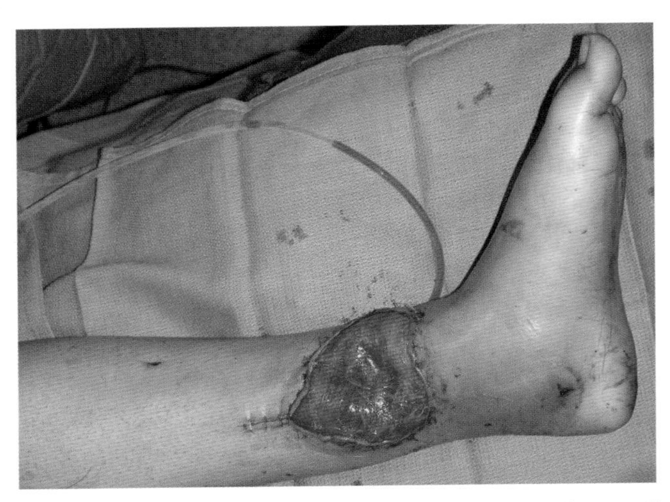

• **Fig. 46.10** An intraoperative view showing completion of free gracilis muscle flap inset and incision closure.

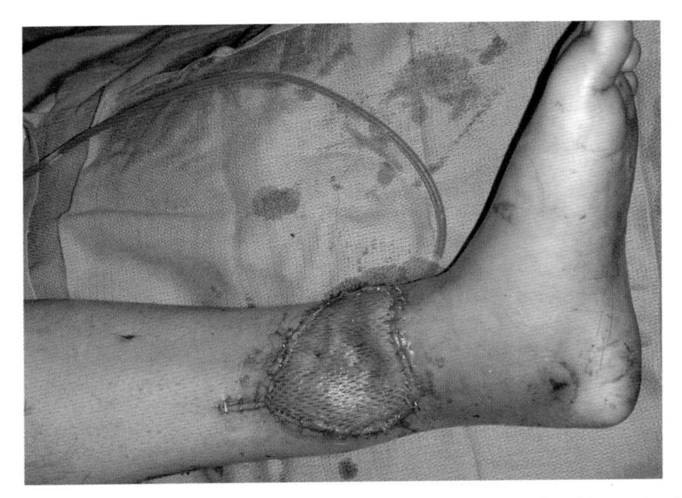

• **Fig. 46.11** An intraoperative view showing completion of a skin-grafted free gracilis muscle flap reconstruction for the distal tibial wound.

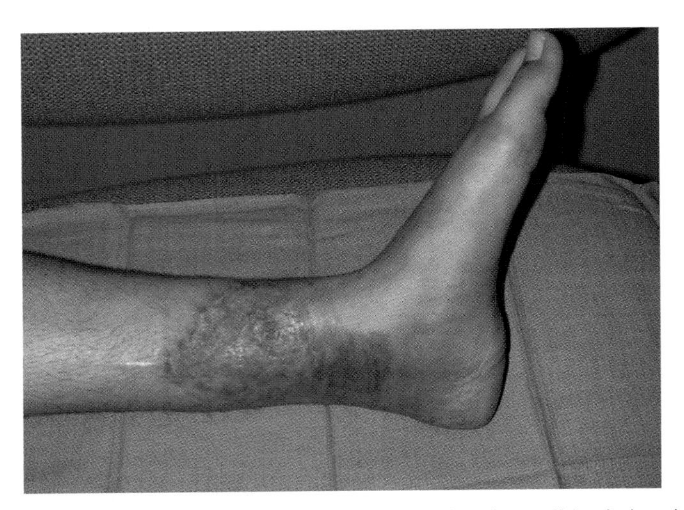

• **Fig. 46.12** The result at 7-month follow-up showing well-healed and stable distal third of the left leg wound with excellent contour and minimal scarring.

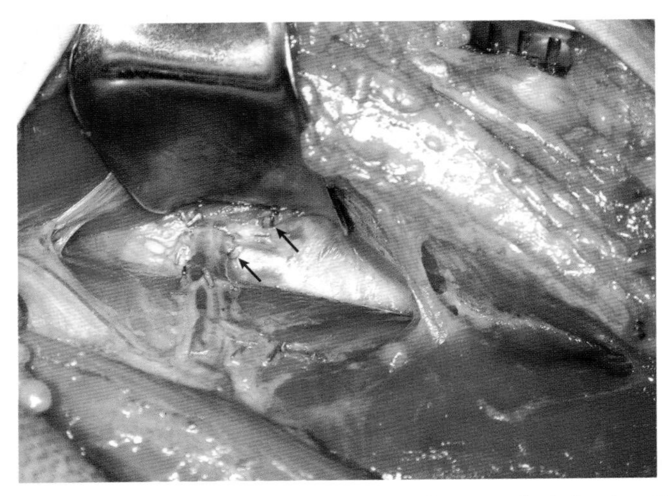

• **Fig. 46.13** An intraoperative view from a different patient showing division of the branches of the medial circumflex femoral vessels to the adductor longus and brevis muscles *(arrows)*. In this way, the pedicle length could be increased by 2 cm and the size of the pedicle could be at least 2 mm in diameter.

Pearls for Success

A free gracilis muscle flap can be an excellent choice for a small or medium soft tissue defect in the distal third of the leg. It is a small muscle, averaging 24 cm in length, 5 cm in width, and 1.5 cm in thickness. The proximal two-thirds of the muscle is reliable based on the dominant pedicle vessels. The muscle can be harvested relatively quickly and has few donor site problems. Its pedicle dissection can be difficult because it is small. Once again, the pedicle length and size can be improved by dividing the branches of the medial circumflex femoral vessels to the adductor longus and brevis muscles. In this way, the pedicle length can be extended by an additional 2 cm and the diameter of the vessel can be greater than 2 mm (Fig. 46.13). This would make free gracilis muscle transfer less difficult and challenging and could potentially expand the flap's clinical applications. It is the author's preference to inset the muscle flap into the soft tissue defect with multiple absorbable horizontal mattress sutures. This technique would allow a more uniformed contour between muscle and normal skin edge of the defect prior to skin grafting. Two advantages of free gracilis muscle transfer are worth mentioning: there are almost no donor site morbidities in the thigh except a surgical scar; the muscle flap can be shrunk over 6 months and the contour after such a free muscle flap reconstruction in the lower extremity can be excellent.

CASE 3

Clinical Presentation

A 62-year-old White female developed chronic osteomyelitis from a nonunion tibial fracture of the right distal leg after previous open reduction and internal fixation of a tibial fracture (Fig. 46.14). The wound was debrided by the orthopedic trauma service, which resulted in a 10-cm bony defect in the distal tibia and an 18 × 8 cm soft tissue wound. An external fixator for

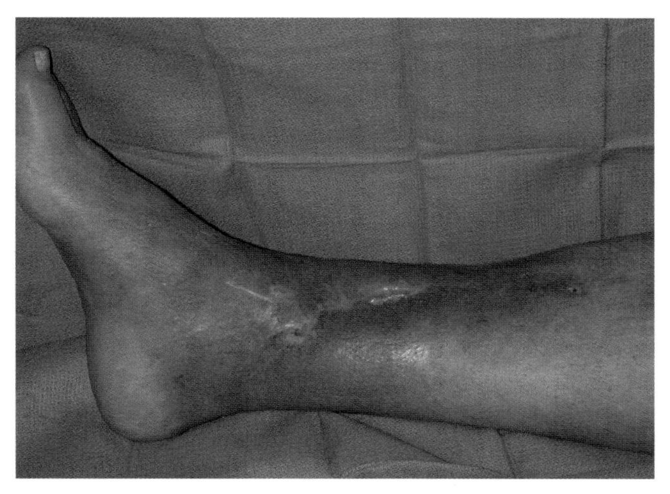

• **Fig. 46.14** A preoperative view showing a chronic draining site from the right distal tibia with associated skin changes.

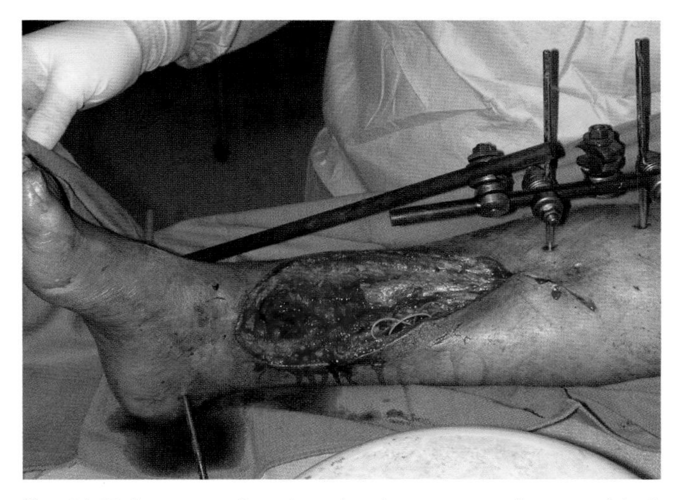

• **Fig. 46.15** A preoperative view showing a composite wound in the right distal third of the leg with a 10-cm large bony gap and an 18 × 8 cm soft tissue wound.

temporary stabilization of the distal leg (Fig. 46.15) was placed. The plastic surgery service was consulted for reconstruction of this composite defect because limb salvage for this patient was still highly desirable by both the patient and the orthopedic surgeon.

Operative Plan and Special Considerations

For a composite defect of the distal leg with a large bony gap (>10 cm) and soft tissue wound (18 × 8 cm), a free fibula osteocutaneous flap from the contralateral leg would provide a one-stage reconstruction for this large composite defect. The flap could provide a vascularized fibular bone, after internal fixation with a reconstructive plate, for the best chance of bony union in the distal tibia and a large skin paddle for wound coverage in the distal third of the leg. Because a preoperative angiogram had confirmed a normal vascular anatomy of both lower extremities, a free fibula osteocutaneous flap could be harvested safely from her left leg and transferred to her right leg after microvascular anastomoses.

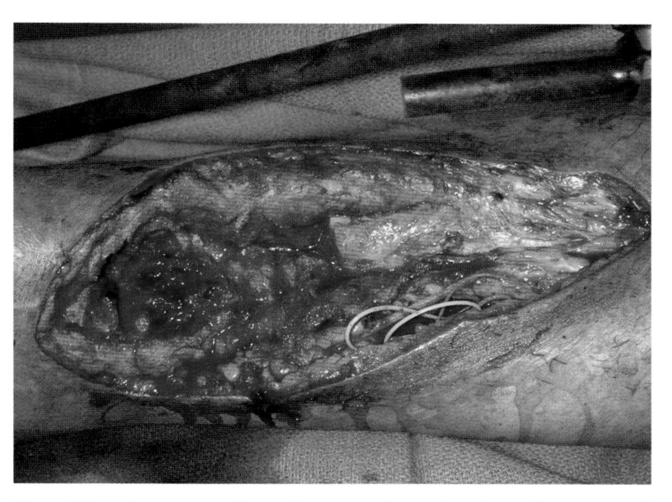

• **Fig. 46.16** A preoperative close-up view showing the composite wound in the right distal third of the leg. In this case, the posterior tibial vessels were exposed through an extended incision and dissected free *(red and blue vessel loops)*.

Operative Procedures

Under general anesthesia with the patient in the supine position, the right distal tibial wound was debrided by the plastic surgery service. All colonized tissues and skin edges were sharply debrided and the wound was then irrigated with Pulsavac. The wound appeared to be clean and fresh after a definitive debridement (Fig. 46.16).

An incision was extended from the right distal leg wound to explore the posterior tibial vessels as recipient vessels for microvascular anastomoses. The skin incision was extended proximally and parallel to the anterior edge of the tibia. The posterior tibial vessels were identified between the soleus and flexor digitorum longus muscles. After retracting the tibial nerve, both artery and vein were identified, dissected free, and wrapped with vessel loops under loupe magnification.

The left free fibula osteocutaneous flap was harvested. An 18 × 8 cm of the skin paddle was designed and two septocutaneous perforators were mapped by a handheld Doppler (Fig. 46.17). Under tourniquet control, the skin paddle was incised down to the fascia. The subfascial dissection was performed toward the posterior intermuscular septum. At least one septocutaneous perforator was identified within the septum (Fig. 46.18). Care was taken to avoid direct or indirect injury to the perforator. The dissection was performed to release the muscle attachment to the fibula from the soleus muscle. After identifying the peroneal vessels close to the fibula, the distal osteotomy was performed at least 6 cm proximal to the lateral malleolus. By further dissection of the hallucis longus muscle's attachment, the peroneal vessels along with the fibula were dissected free. The proximal osteotomy was then performed and a 10.5-cm segment of the fibula was obtained. A longitudinal skin incision was extended proximally toward the fibular head. Following more dissection around the pedicle, the peroneal vessels were dissected free toward its bifurcation. Once the bifurcation was visualized, the pedicle was divided and the flap's dissection was completed (Fig. 46.19).

The free fibular osteocutaneous flap was inset into the distal tibial bony gap and soft tissue defect. The fibular bone was placed into the bony gap and fixed to the proximal and distal native tibia with a reconstruction plate and multiple screws. After completing

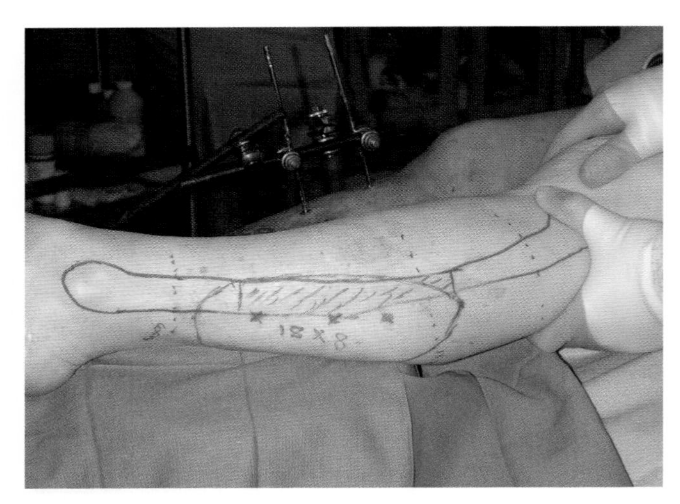

• **Fig. 46.17** Intraoperative view showing the design of a left free fibular osteocutaneous flap. In this case, two septocutaneous perforators were mapped by an intraoperative handheld Doppler.

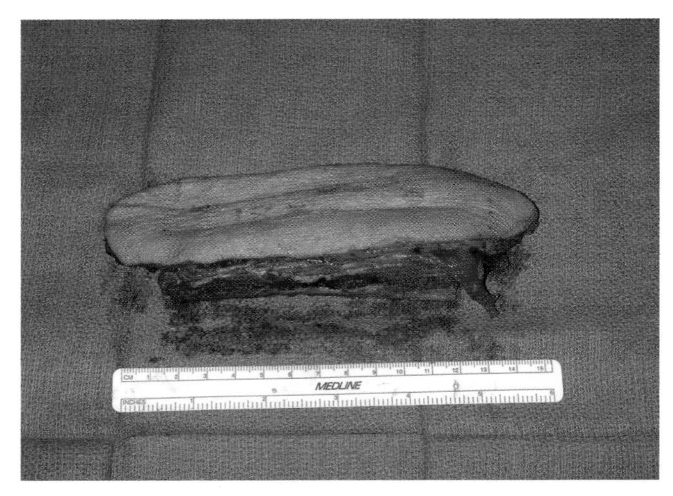

• **Fig. 46.19** Intraoperative view showing completion of the left free osteocutaneous flap dissection.

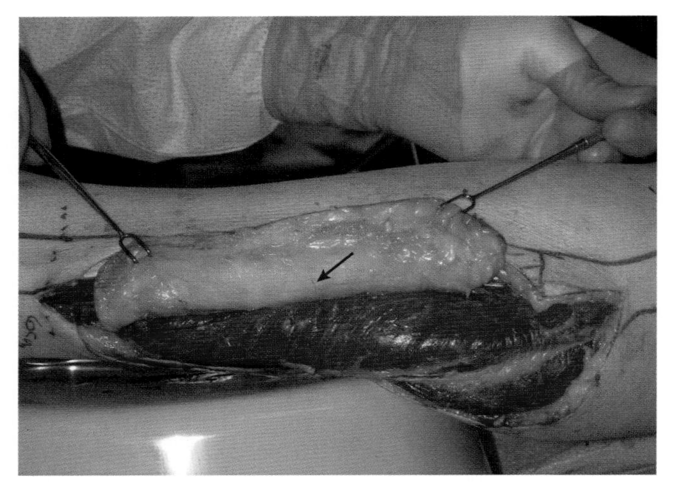

• **Fig. 46.18** Intraoperative view showing at least one septocutaneous perforator *(arrow)* within the posterior septum of the free fibular osteocutaneous flap.

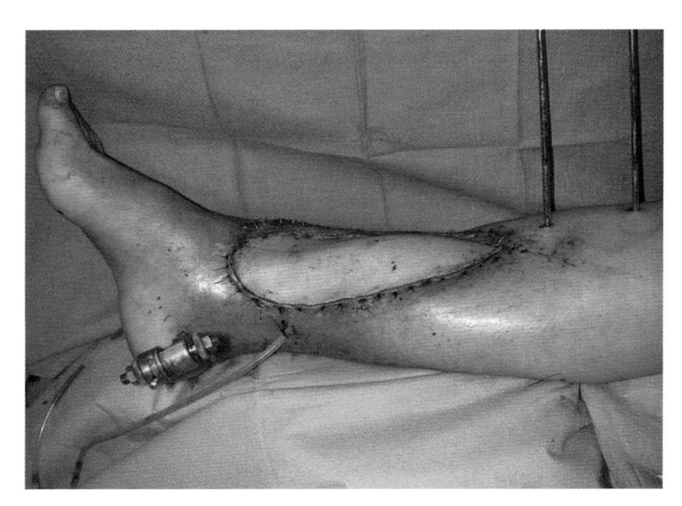

• **Figs. 46.20** Intraoperative view showing completion of the skin paddle inset of the free fibular osteocutaneous flap, placement of a skin graft, and closure of the incision for exposure of the posterior tibial vessels.

the rigid fixation, both microvascular anastomoses were performed. With loupe magnification, both pedicle and recipient vessels were prepared. Under an operating microscope, the arterial microvascular anastomosis was performed between the pedicle artery and the posterior tibial artery in an end-to-side fashion with interrupted 8-0 nylon sutures. The venous microvascular anastomosis between the pedicle vein and the posterior tibial vein was performed with 2.5-mm coupler device in an end-to-end fashion. After all clamps had been released, the flap appeared to be well perfused with good arterial and venous Doppler signals.

The skin paddle of the flap was then inset into the right distal leg soft tissue wound to cover the entire vascularized fibular bone graft and the large distal tibial wound. It was approximated with adjacent skin edges with interrupted half-buried horizontal sutures. A drain was inserted under the skin paddle of the flap. A long, narrow piece of a split-thickness skin graft was harvested from the lateral thigh of the same leg and placed on the lateral part of the wound and secured with skin staples. The rest of the incision was closed in two layers (Fig. 46.20).

The left leg fibular flap donor site was closed primarily with a skin graft after all muscles were approximated with several interrupted 2-0 Vicryl sutures. Once again, a split-thickness skin graft was harvested from the left lateral thigh and meshed to 1:1.5 ratio. The skin graft was placed over the underlying muscle bed and secured with multiple skin staples. A bolster dressing was used to immobilize the skin graft.

Follow-Up Results

The patient did well after the initial free fibular osteocutaneous flap reconstruction as a one-stage procedure for the composite defect in the distal third of the right leg after radical debridement for osteomyelitis. There was no recurrent infection or wound dehiscence in the right distal leg. The skin paddle of the flap and skin graft site healed well (Fig. 46.21). No further operation was required and no complications related to the free fibular osteocutaneous flap reconstruction were observed. Early postoperative X-ray examination showed good alignment and early bony healing

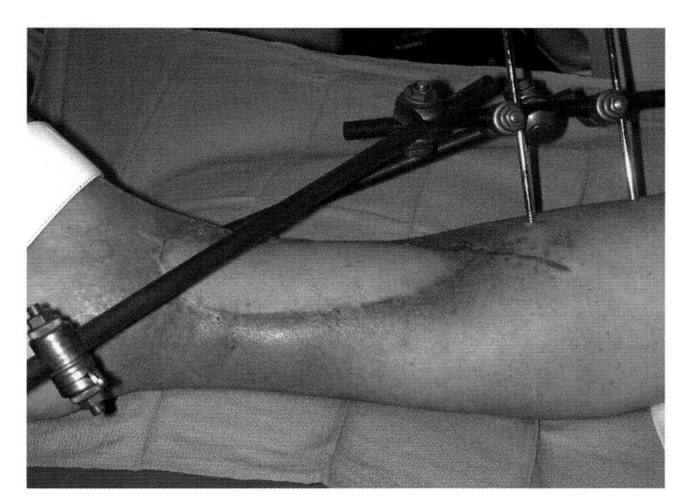

• **Fig. 46.21** Results at 2-month follow-up showing good contour of the right distal leg and the well-healed skin paddle of the free fibular osteocutaneous flap, skin graft, and incision.

of the fibular vascularized bone graft. The left leg fibular flap donor site also healed well after skin grafting.

Final Outcome

The right distal leg wound healed after a successful one-stage free fibular osteocutaneous flap reconstruction including both vascularized bony reconstruction and soft tissue coverage. No further bone grafts were needed. The patient has returned to her weight-bearing and normal activities and has been routinely followed by the orthopedic trauma service.

Pearls for Success

A large composite defect in the distal third of the leg can be reconstructed with a free fibular osteocutaneous flap from the contralateral leg as a one-stage reconstruction. It is very important to map the septocutaneous perforators prior to the flap elevation because the viability of the skin paddle is based on these perforators. During the flap dissection, the surgeon should visualize the perforators and avoid any traction injury to them. The fibular osteocutaneous flap can provide a large amount of vascularized bone graft that can be used to bridge a sizable tibial bony gap after fixation with a reconstructive plate. The blood supply to the fibular bone flap is usually quite good because no additional osteotomy is needed for long bone reconstruction. Bony fixation should be performed before microvascular anastomoses so that they can be done under the most controlled condition with a good set-up for the pedicle vessels. If the skin paddle is less than 5 cm in width, the flap donor site can be closed primarily for better cosmetic outcome. However, a skin graft should be used initially for the leg donor site closure if attempted primary closure is under more than moderate amount of tension. A preoperative angiogram should be performed to evaluate vascular anatomy in both donor and recipient legs.

Recommended Readings

Marek CA, Pu LL. Refinements of free tissue transfer for optimal outcome in lower extremity reconstruction. *Ann Plast Surg*. 2004;52:270–275.

Nazerali RS, Pu LL. Free tissue transfer to the lower extremity: a paradigm shift in flap selection for soft tissue reconstruction. *Ann Plast Surg*. 2013;70:419–422.

Pu LL, Medalie DA, Lawrence SJ, Vasconez HC. Reconstruction of through-and-through gunshot wounds to the feet with free gracilis muscle flaps. *Ann Plast Surg*. 2003;50:286–291.

Pu LL, Stevenson TR. Principles of reconstruction for complex lower extremity wounds. *Tech Orthop*. 2009;24:78–87.

Pu LL. A comprehensive approach to lower extremity free-tissue transfer. *Plast Reconstr Surg Glob Open*. 2017; 9:5, e1228.

Pu LL. Free flaps in lower extremity reconstruction. *Clin Plast Surg*. 2021;48:201–214.

Wallace CG, Chang YM, Tsai CY, Wei FC. Harnessing the potential of the free fibula osteoseptocutaneous flap in mandible reconstruction. *Plast Reconstr Surg*. 2010;125:305–314.

47

Complex Leg Reconstruction

CASE 1

Clinical Presentation

A 21-year-old White male had an extensive middle tibia wound of his right leg associated with an open fracture as a result of a motor vehicle accident. He had a 13 × 6 cm middle tibia wound of the right leg with exposed tibial fracture site. A rigid fixation of the tibia fracture was performed with an intramedullary rod by the orthopedic trauma service after the initial wound debridement (Fig. 47.1). The plastic surgery service was consulted for soft tissue reconstruction of this large middle tibia wound within 1 week after the definitive bony reconstruction performed by the primary service.

Operative Plan and Special Considerations for Reconstruction

For this large middle tibia wound with exposed fracture site and hardware, a single adjacent local muscle flap, such as a medial gastrocnemius or medial hemisoleus muscle flap, is not large enough to provide adequate soft tissue coverage for the exposed fracture site and hardware. However, because both local muscle flaps are commonly used for lower extremity soft tissue reconstruction, the combination of both local muscle flaps has been used by the author as an alternative approach to a free tissue transfer for a large middle tibia wound. The medial gastrocnemius muscle could be used to cover a relatively proximal middle tibia wound and the medial hemisoleus muscle could be used to cover a relatively distal middle tibia wound. The combined medial gastrocnemius and medial hemisoleus muscles flaps can be a valid and less extensive reconstructive option for a large middle tibia wound and can be performed in 2 to 3 hours by most surgeons without microsurgical expertise.

Operative Procedures

Under general anesthesia with the patient in the supine position, the right middle tibia wound was debrided. All unhealthy-looking skin and colonized tissues were removed. The open tibia wound appeared to be fresh and clean after a definitive debridement performed by the plastic surgery service (Fig. 47.2).

Both flap dissections were performed under tourniquet control. The existing open wound was extended into the incision both proximally and distally. The proximal incision was made toward the knee. The distal skin incision was made just above the Achilles' tendon. After opening the fascia of the posterior compartment, both the medial gastrocnemius and the medial half of the soleus muscles were identified. The gastrocnemius muscle was easily separated from the underlying soleus muscle. The proximally based medial gastrocnemius muscle was dissected free and then split from the lateral gastrocnemius muscle along its raphe. The tendon portion of the gastrocnemius muscle was divided from the conjoined tendon. The fascial layer over the medial gastrocnemius muscle belly was scored. With the aid of this maneuver, the medial gastrocnemius muscle could reach the proximal portion of the middle tibia wound.

The medial half of the soleus muscle was dissected free from the flexor digitorum longus muscle. The medial half of the distal soleus muscle was sharply dissected with a knife and freed from the conjoint tendon distally. Only the muscular portion of the soleus was used as the flap and the remaining conjoint tendon was left intact. The insertion of the distal soleus muscle was divided close to the Achilles' tendon depending on the arc of the flap rotation required to cover a more distal part of the middle tibia wound. The flap was based proximally and its dissection was completed with additional splitting of the medial half of the soleus muscle from the remaining lateral half of the muscle longitudinally depending on the need for coverage of the distal part of the middle tibia wound. The flap was only elevated to just at or above the level of the distal middle tibia wound where two major perforators from the posterior tibial vessels to the flap were identified (Fig. 47.3). One of the adjacent perforators acted as a pivot point of the flap rotation and was preserved while allowing adequate arc of flap rotation to cover the middle tibia wound (Fig. 47.4). The fascia was scored over the surface of the medial hemisoleus muscle belly to facilitate flap rotation. The left intact conjoint tendon from the distal medial half of the soleus muscle was then approximated to the remaining lateral half of the soleus muscle with nonabsorbable sutures (Fig. 47.5).

Both muscle flaps were transposed into the middle tibia wound sequentially. The medial gastrocnemius muscle flap was placed proximally to cover the most proximal portion of the middle tibia wound and the medial hemisoleus muscle flap was placed distally to cover the most distal portion. Both flaps were inset into the medial tibia wound using absorbable half-buried horizontal mattress sutures (Fig. 47.6).

A drain was placed under both muscle flaps. All muscle flaps were covered with split-thickness skin grafts. Split-thickness skin grafts were harvested with a dermatome from the right lateral thigh and meshed to 1:1.5 ratio. They were placed over the muscle flaps and secured with skin staples. All incisions for each flap dissection were closed in two layers (Fig. 47.7).

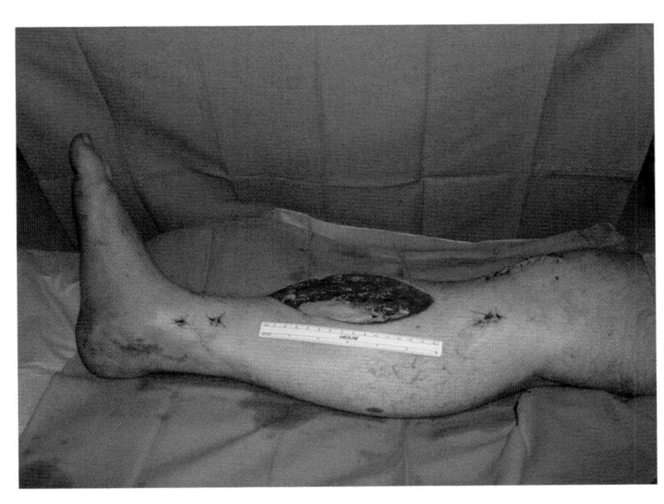

• **Fig. 47.1** A preoperative view showing an extensive middle tibia wound, measuring 13 × 6 cm, on the right leg with an exposed tibial fracture site and hardware.

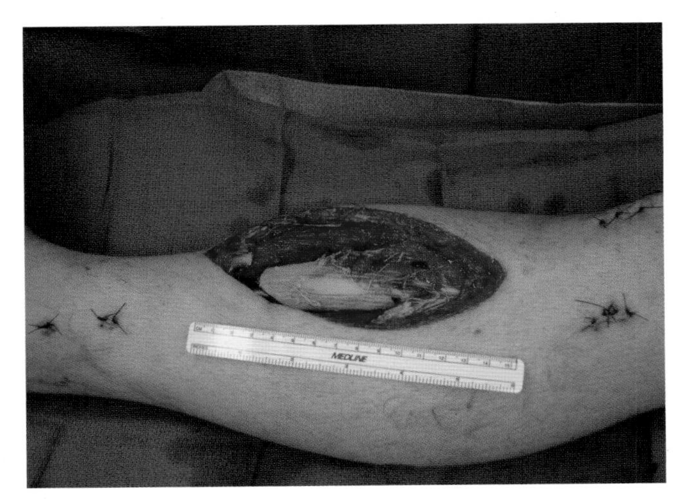

• **Fig. 47.2** An intraoperative close-up view showing the exposed tibial fracture site and hardware after definitive debridement.

Follow-Up Results

The patient did well postoperatively without any issues related to the two-muscle flap reconstruction for the extensive middle tibia wound closure. He was discharged from hospital on postoperative day 5. The right middle tibia wound healed well and the skin grafts took uneventfully. He was followed by the plastic surgery service for routine postoperative care and by the orthopedic trauma service for fracture healing.

Final Outcome

During further follow-up, the right middle tibia wound after the two-muscle flap reconstruction healed well with good contour and minimal scarring. There were no wound breakdown, recurrent infection, or contour issues (Fig. 47.8). The patient has resumed his weight-bearing status and has returned to work as instructed.

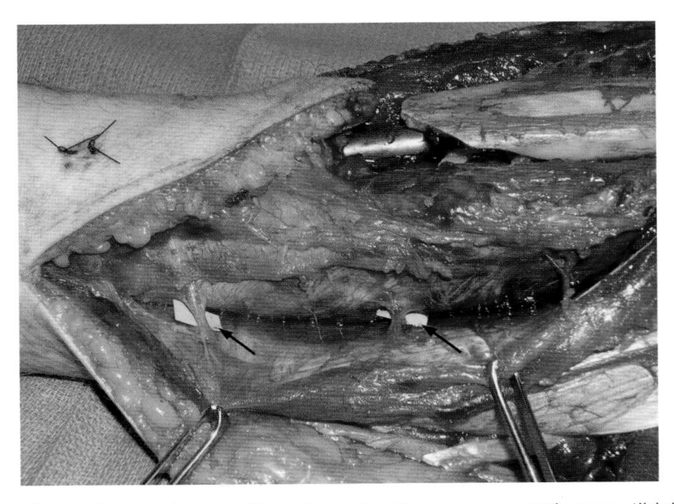

• **Fig. 47.3** An intraoperative view showing an exposed open tibial fracture site of the middle leg in relation to two major perforators from the posterior tibial vessels to the medial half of the distal soleus muscle (*arrows*). Only the distal perforator might be divided to allow adequate arc of flap rotation to cover the exposed hardware and open tibial fracture site.

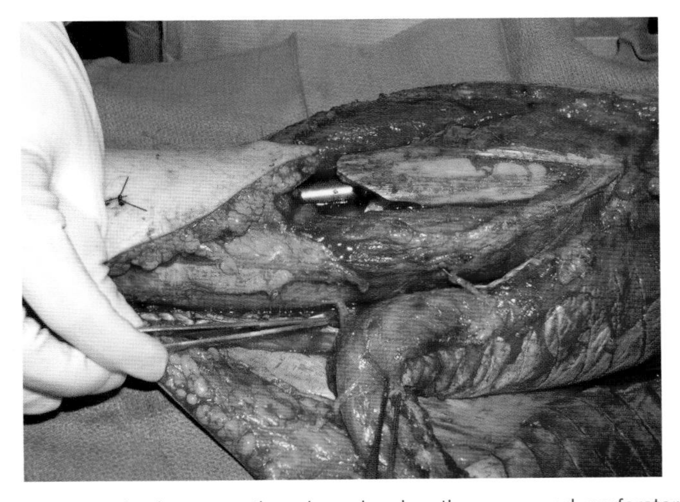

• **Fig. 47.4** An intraoperative view showing the preserved perforator from the posterior tibial vessels to the medial hemisoleus muscle flap (indicated by *forceps*) after the flap was completely elevated. This perforator would be critical to ensure adequate blood supply to the distal medial hemisoleus muscle flap.

Pearls for Success

The combined medial gastrocnemius and medial hemisoleus muscle flaps may provide the same quality of soft-tissue coverage for an extensive middle tibia wound as a free tissue transfer. Its cosmetic outcome after such local muscle flap reconstructions can also be quite pleasing. In general, a medial gastrocnemius muscle flap can be used to cover the proximal part of the wound and a medial hemisoleus muscle flap can be used to cover the more distal portion of the wound even to the junction of the middle and distal thirds of the leg. Obviously, in certain orthopedic trauma patients, these muscles may frequently be within the zone of injury, especially the soleus muscle. It has been the author's preference to explore this muscle for its feasibility as a local muscle

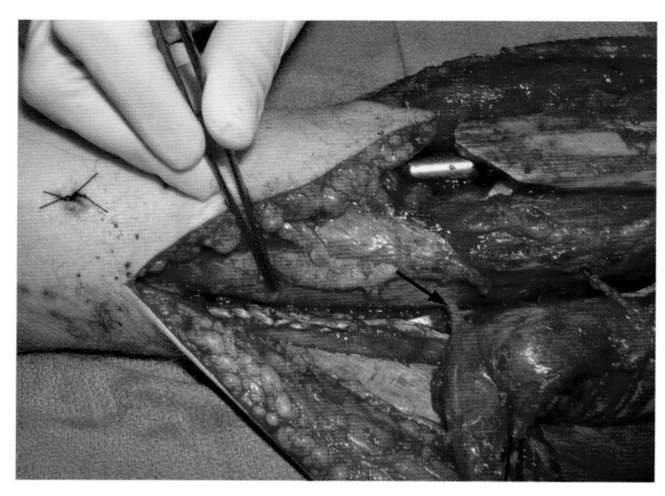

• **Fig. 47.5** An intraoperative view showing the preserved perforator from the posterior tibial vessels to the medial hemisoleus muscle flap (*arrow*). The left intact conjoint tendon from the distal medial half of the soleus muscle is approximated to the remaining lateral half of the soleus muscle with nonabsorbable sutures (indicated by *forceps*) after the flap dissection has been completed.

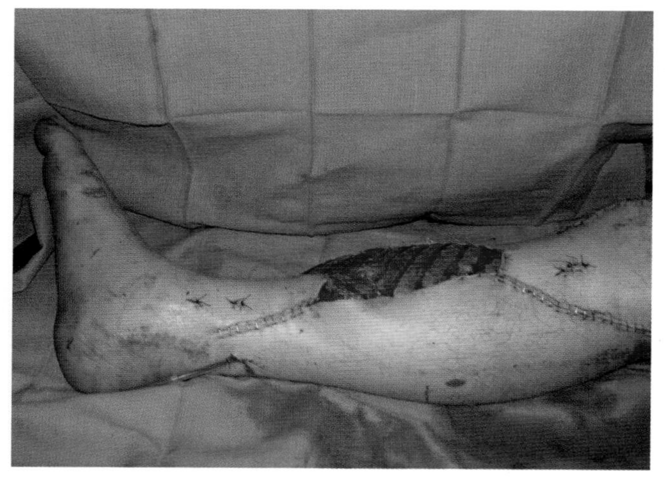

• **Fig. 47.6** An intraoperative view showing completion of both muscle flap insets before placement of a skin graft.

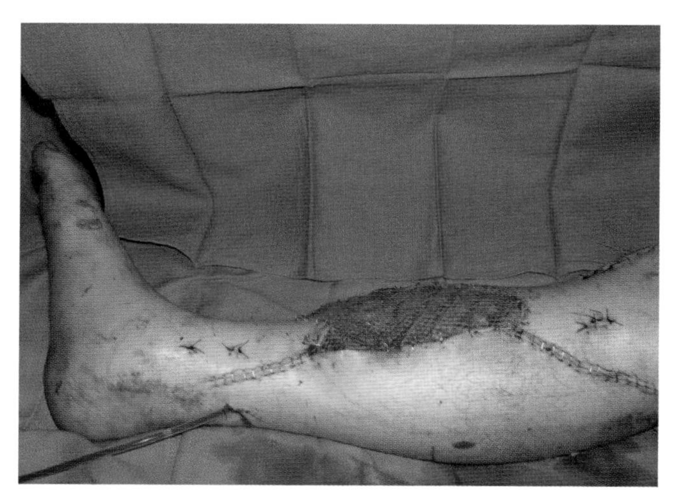

• **Fig. 47.7** An intraoperative view showing completion of a skin graft placement over both muscle flaps.

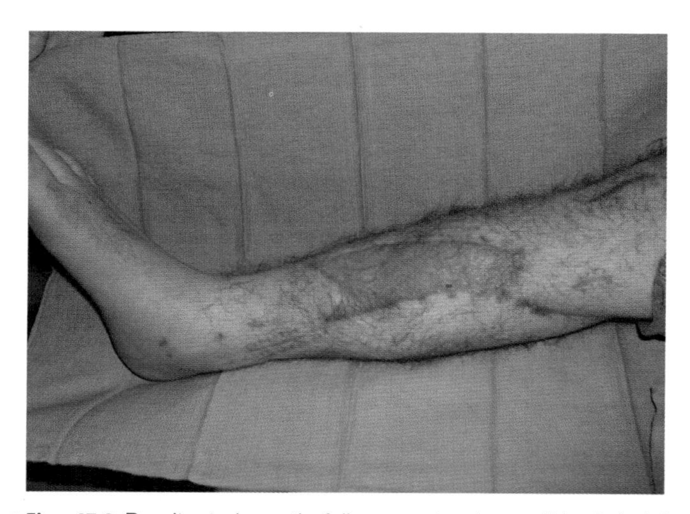

• **Fig. 47.8** Result at 4-month follow-up showing well-healed right middle tibia wound after combined muscle flap reconstructions with good contour and minimal scarring.

flap. If the medial gastrocnemius or the medial soleus muscle appears to be hemorrhagic and swollen, neither muscle can be used as a local flap. A preoperative magnetic resonance imaging scan of the muscles may be helpful to provide such information.

Scarifying both medial gastrocnemius and medial hemisoleus muscles as local flaps for soft-tissue coverage of an extensive tibia wound may lead to functional donor-site morbidity of the leg. Because only half of the gastrocnemius muscle and half of the soleus muscle are sacrificed and the remaining lateral halves of the gastrocnemius muscle and the soleus muscle are still intact, such a function loss may not be significant and can be well tolerated by most patients. In addition, the left intact conjoint tendon from the distal medial half of the soleus muscle is approximated to the remaining lateral half of the soleus muscle with nonabsorbable sutures. With this repair, potential functional impairment of the leg may be reduced.

CASE 2

Clinical Presentation

A 55-year-old White male, with severe cirrhosis of liver, sustained a traumatic injury to his right leg from a motor vehicle accident. He was initially managed by the orthopedic trauma service for bony and soft tissue debridement. He had a composite tissue loss in the middle third of the leg with a large soft tissue wound, measuring 15 × 6 cm and a segmental middle tibial fracture with a potential bony gap measuring 10 cm (Fig. 47.9). He had also sustained a distal fibular fracture (Fig. 47.10). An external fixator was placed for temporary bony stabilization and the patient was admitted to hospital for possible limb salvage procedure. The plastic surgery service was consulted for soft tissue reconstruction of the middle tibia wound immediately after the definitive bony fixation by the primary service. Because of his underlying medical conditions, more extensive limb salvage procedures, such as free

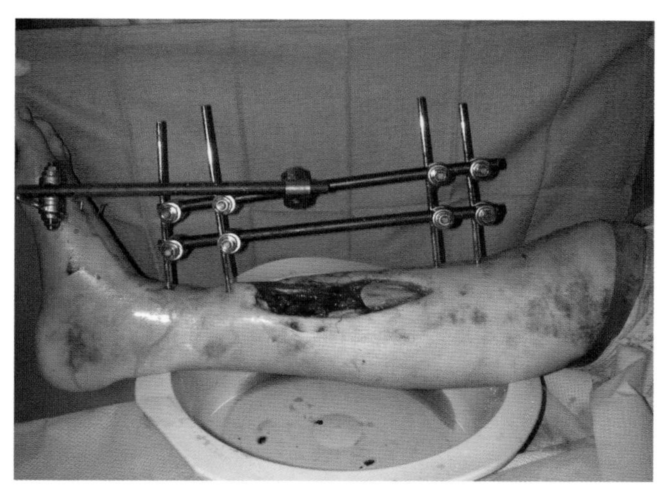

• **Fig. 47.9** A preoperative view showing a large composite soft tissue defect and potential bony gap in the middle third of the right leg.

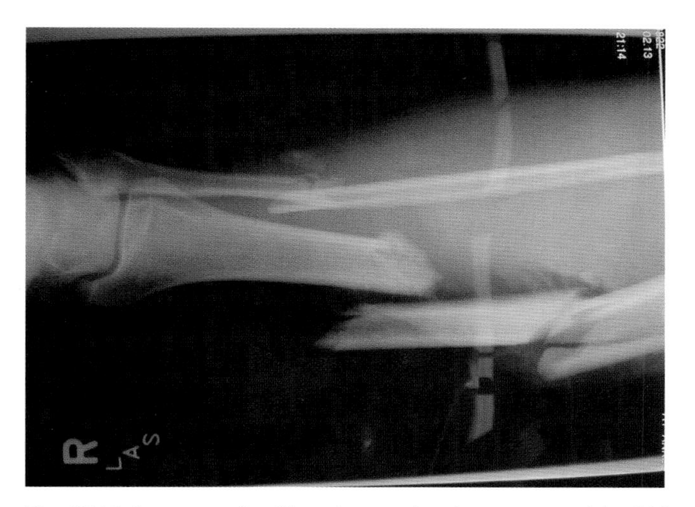

• **Fig. 47.10** A preoperative X-ray image showing a segmental middle tibial fracture and a distal fibular fracture.

tissue transfer, might not be indicated and the possibility of a below knee amputation (BKA) could be high.

Operative Plan and Special Considerations for Reconstruction

For a composite defect of the middle third tibia wound with a large soft tissue defect and tibial gap, a free fibular osteocutaneous flap from the contralateral leg would be the classic option as a one-stage procedure for a composite reconstruction. However, this would be a lengthy operation involving microvascular free tissue transfer. In addition, the donor leg may be weakened after a free fibular osteocutaneous flap harvest. It might present a significant problem if this patient eventually has to undergo a BKA as a result of infected nonunion or an unsuccessful free flap reconstruction. After several extensive discussions with the orthopedic trauma surgeon, we all agreed that a less lengthy and extensive procedure would be more appropriate for the limb salvage procedure and a classic option, such as a free fibular osteocutaneous flap from the contralateral leg, would not be a good option for this patient. One

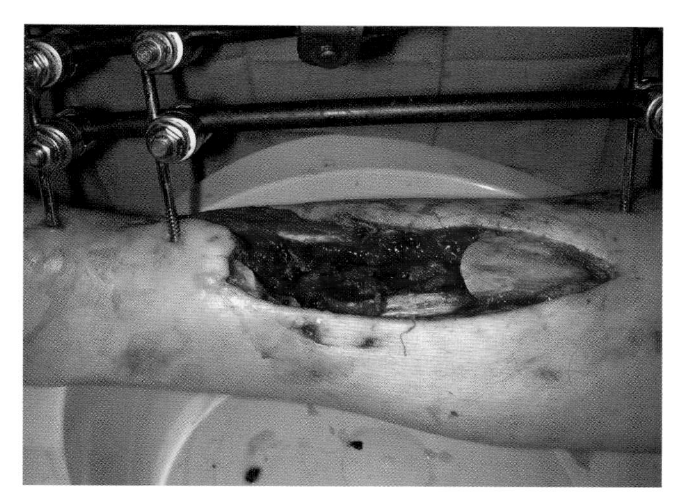

• **Fig. 47.11** An intraoperative close-up view showing an open middle tibial fracture wound with significant soft tissue loss and bony loss.

of the interesting findings for this patient was that he also had a distal fibular fracture. Could the fibula be harvested as a pedicled vascularized bone flap to reconstruct the middle tibial bony defect? If this were feasible, the soft tissue defect in the middle third of the leg could also be reconstructed with a pedicled medial hemisoleus muscle flap. Thus, this composite tissue defect could be reconstructed as a one-stage orthoplastic approach from the same leg. No free tissue transfer would be needed and no donor site morbidity would result in the contralateral leg. The pedicled fibular flap could provide a vascularized bone for the best chance of bony union in the middle tibia after internal fixation with a reconstructive plate. The medial hemisoleus muscle flap would also provide an adequate soft tissue reconstruction for the middle tibia wound. A preoperative angiogram should be performed to evaluate patency of the peroneal artery as well as of the posterior and anterior tibial arteries.

Operative Procedures

Under general anesthesia with the patient in the supine position, the open tibia fracture wound was debrided by the plastic surgery service. All colonized tissues and skin edges were sharply debrided and the wound was then irrigated with Pulsavac (Fig. 47.11). This was a combined orthoplastic procedure with close interaction between the plastic surgery and orthopedic surgery services in the operating room.

The ipsilateral pedicled fibula bone flap was designed and a 12-cm fibular segment in the middle leg was marked (Fig. 47.12). Under tourniquet control, the skin incision was made over the lateral leg down to the fascia. After opening the fascia , the surgical dissection was performed to free the muscle attachment to the fibula from the soleus muscle. The distal fibular fracture site was dissected free. Once the peroneal vessels close to the fibular fracture site had been identified, further surgical dissection was performed to release the hallucis longus muscle's attachment to the fibula. The peroneal vessels and the fibula were dissected free and protected. The proximal osteotomy was performed 10 cm distal to the fibular head. A 12-cm segment of the pedicled fibular bone flap was obtained (Fig. 47.13). At this point, the fractured segmental tibia was removed by the orthopedic trauma service. Once the proximal peroneal vessels had already been dissected free, this pedicled fibular

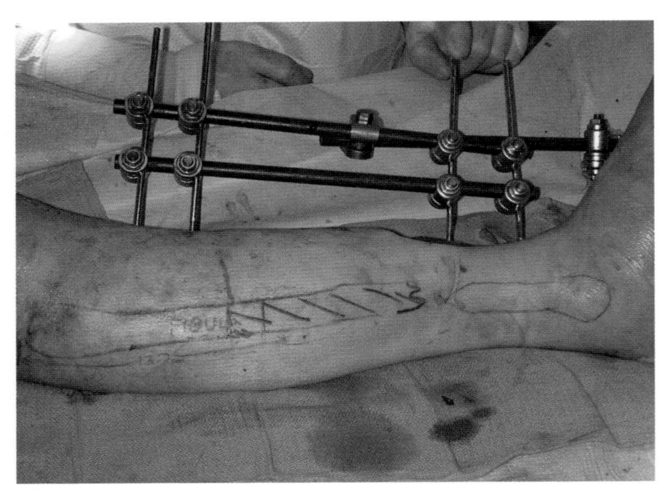

• **Fig. 47.12** An intraoperative view showing the design of the fibular bone flap. The proximal osteotomy should be performed about 10 cm distal to the medial femoral condyle.

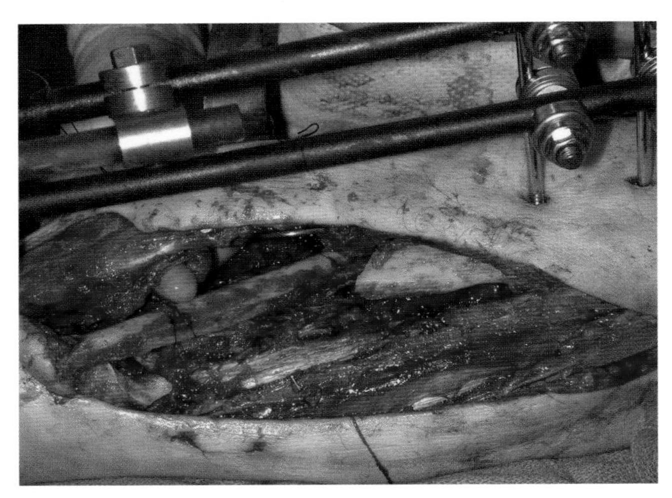

• **Fig. 47.14** An intraoperative view showing the pedicle fibular bone flap that could easily be transferred into the tibial bony defect of the right leg.

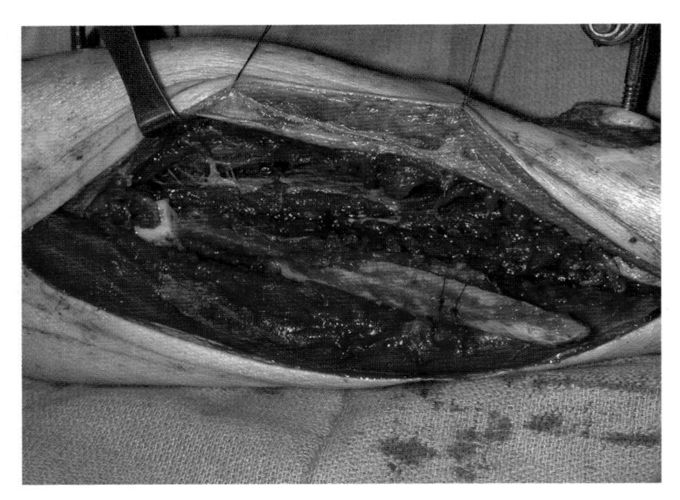

• **Fig. 47.13** An intraoperative view showing completion of the pedicled fibular bone flap dissection.

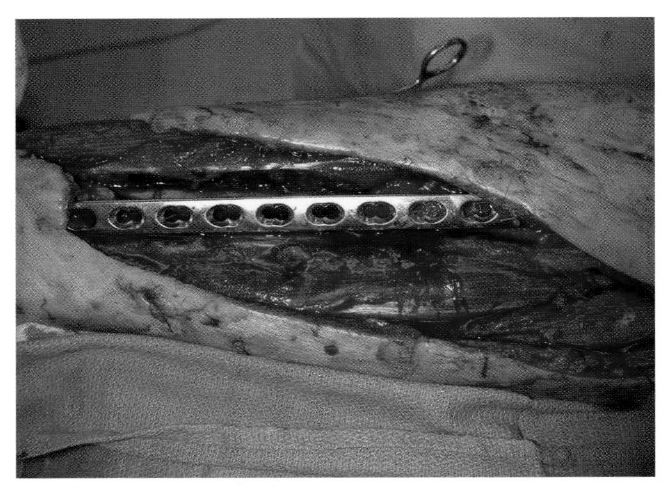

• **Fig. 47.15** An intraoperative view showing completion of the internal fixation for the fibular bone flap with a large reconstructive plate.

bone flap could easily be moved parallel to the tibial bony defect without difficulty (Fig. 47.14).

The fibular bone flap was placed into the tibial bony gap after trimming each end and was then fixated to proximal and distal native tibia with a reconstruction plate and multiple screws by the orthopedic trauma service (Fig. 47.15). Such a rigid fixation of the fibular bone flap appeared to be satisfactory.

The exposed fibular bone flap and reconstruction plate were then covered with the proximally based medial hemisoleus muscle flap. Under tourniquet control, the skin incision for the flap elevation was extended from the existing open wound in the middle tibia proximally and distally and through the skin, subcutaneous tissues, and fascia to expose the medial hemisoleus muscle. Once the medial hemisoleus muscle had been identified and dissected free from the medial gastrocnemius muscle and the flexor digitorum longus, its insertion was divided distally at the Achilles tendon. During dissection, the plantaris tendon was visualized between the gastrocnemius muscle and the underlying soleus muscle. The medial half of the soleus muscle was split along its anatomic midline. The medial hemisoleus muscle flap was elevated with emphasis on the preservation of as many minor pedicles from the posterior tibial vessels as possible to the flap in the middle tibia wound while allowing adequate arc rotation of the flap to cover the exposed fibular bone flap and reconstruction plate. Scoring the fascia over the medial hemisoleus muscle belly was also performed to enhance the flap's arc of rotation. The flap was inset into the soft tissue defect with interrupted 3-0 Monocryl horizontal mattress sutures (Fig. 47.16).

One drain was inserted into the flap donor site. The muscle flap was then covered with split-thickness skin grafts. Split-thickness skin grafts were harvested with a dermatome from the right lateral thigh and meshed to 1:1.5 ratio. The incision for the flap dissection was closed in two layers and all skin grafts were secured with skin staples (Fig. 47.17). The entire orthoplastic procedure by two services took only 6 hours.

Management of Complications

The patient tolerated the procedure well and remained medically stable. Unfortunately, he developed a distal tip necrosis of the

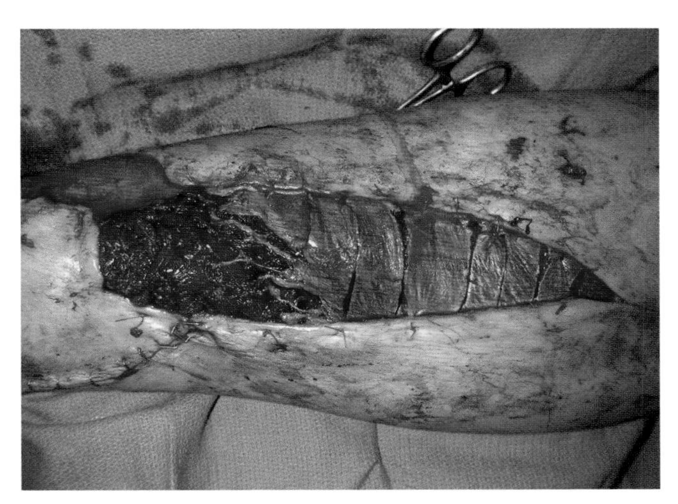

• **Fig. 47.16** An intraoperative view showing completion of the medial hemisoleus muscle flap inset in the same operation to cover the exposed fibular bone flap, reconstructive plate, and large middle tibia wound.

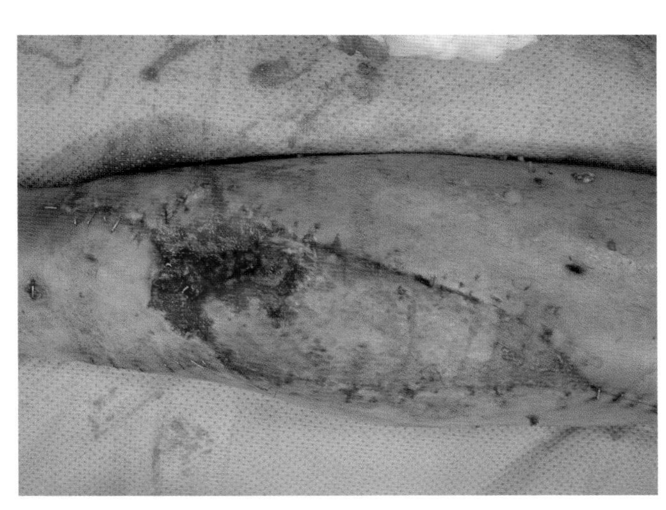

• **Fig. 47.18** Results at 3 weeks postoperative showing distal tip necrosis of the medial hemisoleus muscle flap.

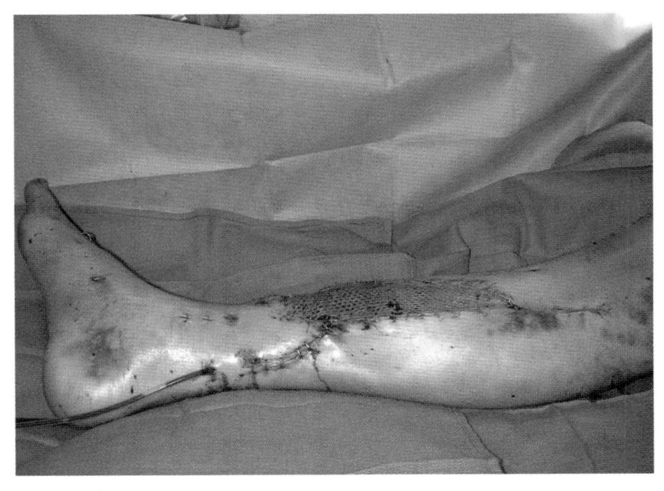

• **Fig. 47.17** An intraoperative view showing placement of the split-thickness skin graft to the medial hemisoleus muscle flap and completion of the rest of incision closure.

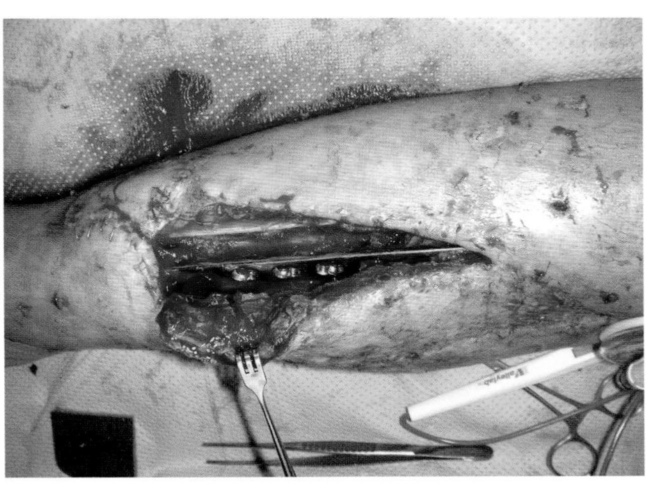

• **Fig. 47.19** An intraoperative view showing the elevated medial hemisoleus muscle flap after debridement and the viable pedicled fibular bone flap.

medial hemisoleus muscle flap over the next 3 weeks presumably as a result of trauma to the distal muscle (Fig. 47.18). He was taken back to the operating room by the two services 3 weeks later. The necrotic portion of the flap was debrided and the flap was largely elevated again (Fig. 47.19). The fibular bone flap appeared to be viable and the medial hemisoleus muscle flap after debridement was inset into the soft tissue defect and approximated with interrupted sutures in the same fashion and a small area over the muscle flap was covered with a split-thickness skin graft (Fig. 47.20).

Follow-Up Results

The patient did well postoperatively after the second operation without any issues related to the medial hemisoleus muscle flap reconstruction for the middle tibia wound closure. He was finally discharged from hospital. The right middle tibia wound healed well after the flap debridement, elevation, and advancement, and skin grafting (Fig. 47.21). The patient was followed by the plastic

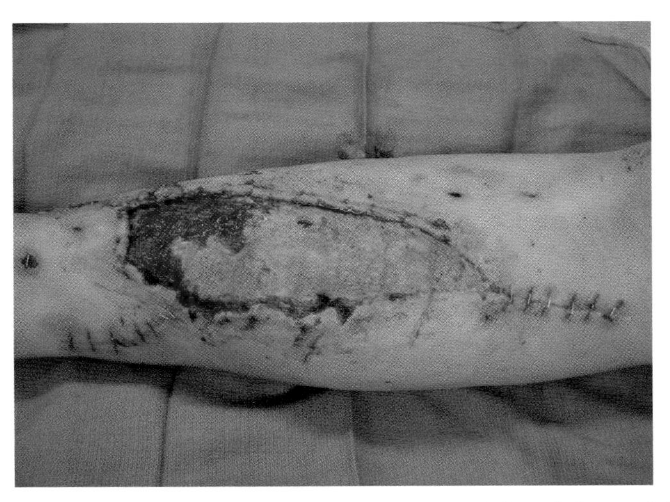

• **Fig. 47.20** An intraoperative view showing completion of the medial hemisoleus muscle flap inset before placement of additional skin graft.

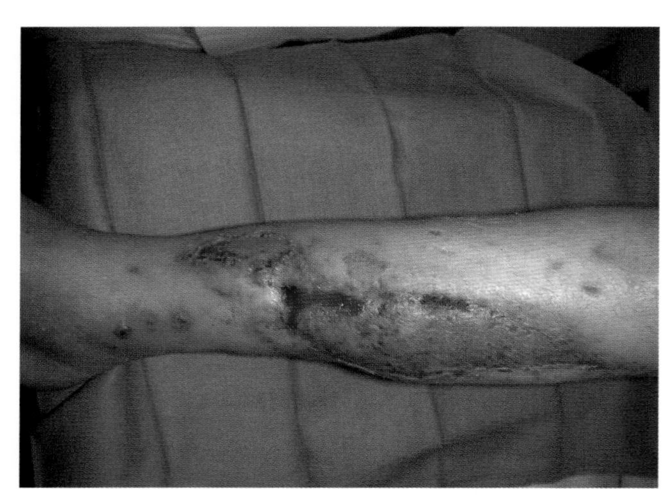

• **Fig. 47.21** Results at 6 weeks after reoperation showing well-healed flap site of the medial hemisoleus muscle flap.

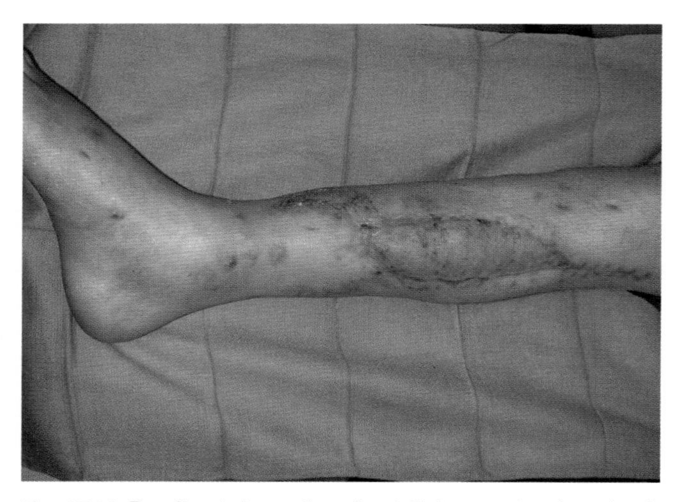

• **Fig. 47.22** Results at 4 months after initial reconstruction showing well-healed middle tibia wound after medial hemisoleus muscle flap reconstruction.

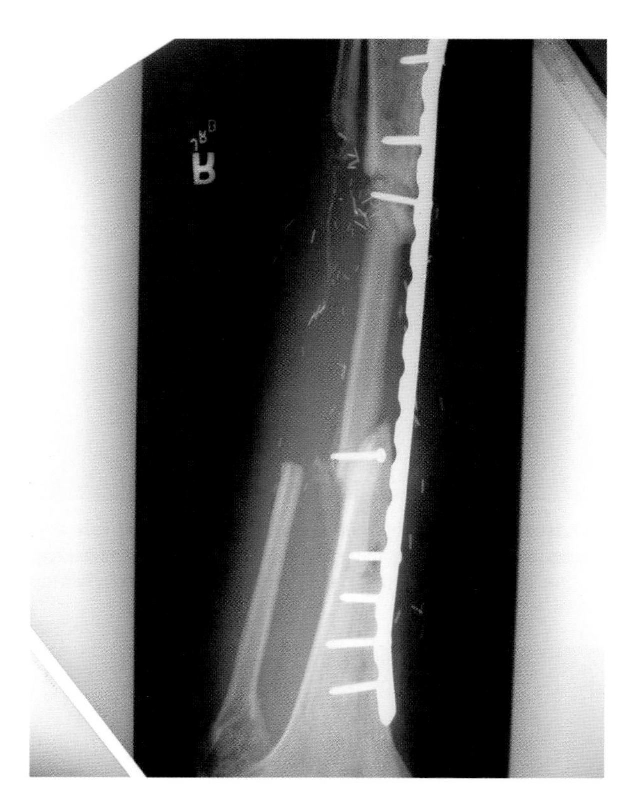

• **Fig. 47.23** An X-ray image 4 months after initial reconstruction showing good healing of the pedicled fibular bone flap.

surgery service for routine postoperative care and by the orthopedic trauma service for fibular bone graft healing.

Final Outcome

During further follow-up, the left middle tibial flap reconstruction site had healed well with good contour, minimal scarring, and no wound breakdown, recurrent infection, or contour issues (Fig. 47.22). The fibular bone flap had also healed well (Fig. 47.23). The patient eventually underwent removal of the reconstruction plate because it was no longer needed. He resumed his weight-bearing status. The follow-up X-ray examination at 17 months postoperatively showed complete bony union of the fibular bone flap with compensated hypertrophy (Fig. 47.24).

Pearls for Success

A large composite defect in the leg, deconstructed in this case, can be reconstructed with the combination of a pedicled fibular bone flap and a medial hemisoleus muscle flap as a one-stage local orthoplastic approach. During the pedicled fibular bone flap dissection, the proximal peroneal vessels should be dissected free so that the pedicle is not under tension or stretching once the flap has been transferred and placed into the meddle tibial bony gap. A preoperative angiogram can be performed to determine whether the peroneal artery would be patent. The medial hemisoleus muscle flap is elevated with emphasis on the preservation of as many minor pedicles (perforators) from the posterior tibial vessels as possible to the flap while allowing adequate arc rotation of the flap to cover such a wound in the middle third of the leg. In this way, any adjacent perforators from the posterior tibial vessel to the flap can be preserved while allowing adequate arc of flap rotation. Only those perforators that are restricting the flap's arc of rotation for wound coverage can be divided during the flap dissection. Partial flap loss is not common for a proximally based medial hemisoleus muscle flap and can be managed with additional flap advancement with or without a skin graft after proper debridement.

CASE 3

Clinical Presentation

A 54-year-old African-American female with severe schizophrenia was hit by a car while walking on the street at night. She underwent open reduction and internal fixation with a large reconstruction plate for multiple segmental tibial fractures by the orthopedic trauma service. However, her initial hospital course was complicated by diabetes, anemia, poorly controlled blood

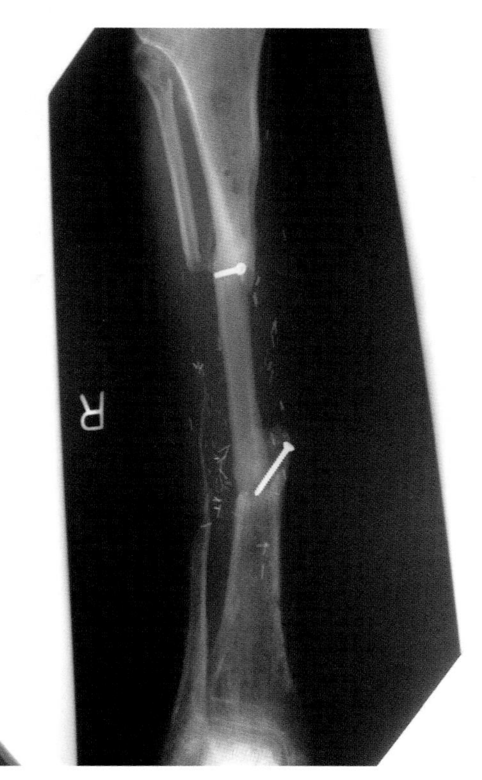

• **Fig. 47.24** An X-ray image 17 months after initial reconstruction showing well-healed fracture sites after the pedicled fibular bone flap reconstruction. There was significant hypertrophy of the fibular bone flap.

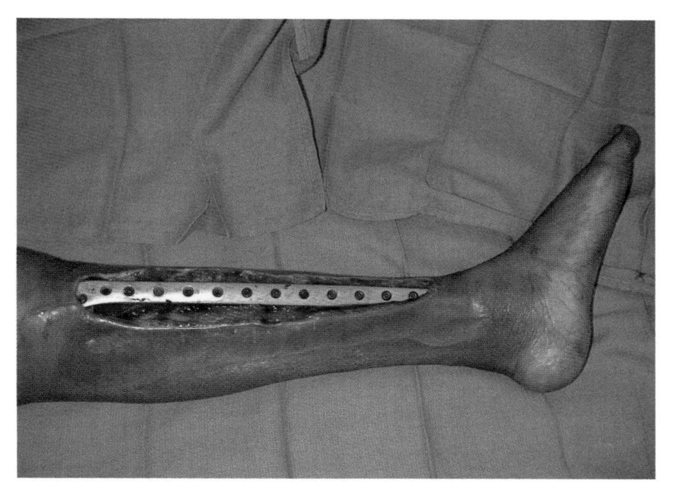

• **Fig. 47.25** A preoperative view showing the entire tibia wound, measuring 25 × 6 cm, of the left leg with the exposed tibial fracture sites and large reconstruction plate.

pressure, and lack of family support. She was eventually discharged to a rehabilitation hospital but missed several follow-up appointments. At her first follow-up, approximately 4 months after her orthopedic surgery, she was noted to have exposed the entire tibia and hardware of the left leg, measured 25 × 6 cm (Fig. 47.25). She underwent multiple wound debridement by the primary service prior to the plastic surgery consultation for soft-tissue reconstruction. Because of her significant psychiatric problems and predicted noncompliance for the postoperative follow-ups, the soft tissue reconstruction for this extensive large tibia wound with the exposed fracture sites and reconstructive plate remained challenging.

Operative Plan and Special Considerations for Reconstruction

For this extensively large open fracture wound of the leg with the exposed entire tibia, fracture sites, and reconstructive plate, a single free flap may not be large enough to cover such a complex wound of the entire leg. In the author's experience, the combination of a free rectus abdominis muscle flap and a pedicled medial gastrocnemius muscle flap would normally be selected as the best option for such an extensive soft tissue reconstruction. However, because of her significant psychiatric problems and predicted noncompliance in postoperative follow-up if a free tissue transfer were to be performed, she was offered a palliative soft tissue reconstruction with multiple local muscle flaps for limb salvage. Therefore, for reconstruction of the entire tibial soft tissue wound, three pedicled local muscle flaps (medial gastrocnemius, medial hemisoleus, and flexor digitorum longus [FDL]) could be used to cover the entire tibia wound of the left leg. The combination of the medial gastrocnemius and medial hemisoleus muscles flaps has previously been used successfully by the author to reconstruct a large middle tibia wound. The FDL may also be used for soft tissue coverage of a small distal tibia wound. It is a type IV muscle flap and receives the blood supply primarily from the branches of the posterior tibial vessels. No more than four branches could be sacrificed during the flap's dissection in order to ensure the reliability of the muscle flap. The FDL muscle flap can be used in combination with the medial gastrocnemius and hemisoleus muscle flaps as three sequential local muscle flaps to cover an entire tibial soft tissue defect of the leg.

Operative Procedures

Under general anesthesia with the patient in the supine position, the entire left tibia wound was debrided. All unhealthy-looking skin and colonized tissues were then sharply debrided. The open tibia wound appeared to be fresh and clean after the definitive debridement performed by the plastic surgery service.

A tourniquet was placed in the distal thigh and inflated to allow a bloodless field during dissection. The existing open wound was extended into the incision both proximally and distally. The proximal incision was made obliquely toward the medial femoral condyle. The distal skin incision was also made obliquely toward to the medial malleolus. After opening the posterior compartment of the leg, both medial gastrocnemius and medial half of the soleus muscles were identified. The medial gastrocnemius muscle was dissected free from the soleus muscle and then split longitudinally from the lateral gastrocnemius along its raphe. The origin of the medial gastrocnemius muscle was divided under direct vision with protection of the medial sural vessels. The fascial layer over the muscle was also scored. With the aid of these maneuvers, the medial gastrocnemius muscle was able to cover the proximal third and the proximal portion of the middle third of the tibia wounds (Fig. 47.26).

The medial half of the soleus muscle was dissected free from the flexor digitorum longus muscle. The medial half of the distal

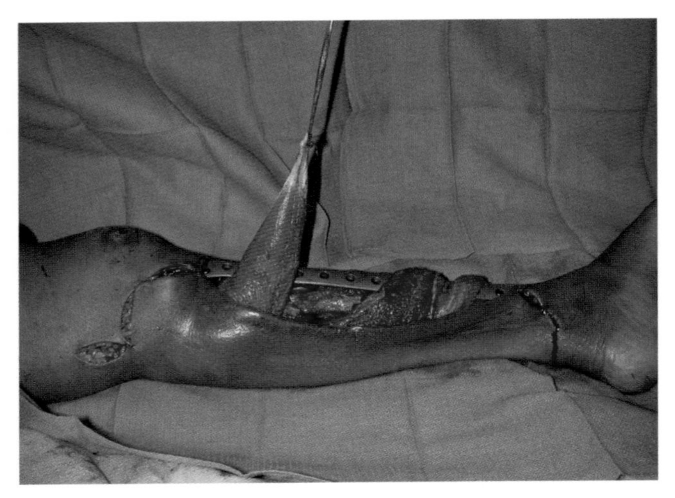

• **Fig. 47.26** An intraoperative view showing an elevated medial gastrocnemius muscle flap after the division of its proximal insertion to the medial femoral condyle and scoring of the fascia over the muscle belly.

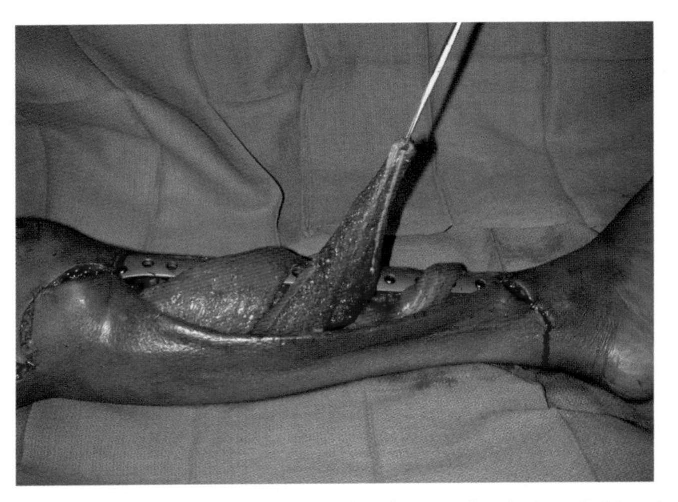

• **Fig. 47.27** An intraoperative view showing an elevated medial hemisoleus muscle flap after scoring of the fascia over the muscle belly.

soleus muscle was sharply dissected with a knife and freed from the conjoint tendon distally. Only the muscular portion of the soleus was used as the flap and the remaining conjoint tendon was left intact. The insertion of the distal soleus muscle was divided close to the Achilles tendon with care taken to preserve the Achilles tendon. The medial hemisoleus muscle was split near its midline longitudinally and any major perforators from the posterior tibial vessels were preserved while allowing an adequate arc of the flap rotation during dissection. Scoring the fascia over the surface of the medial hemisoleus muscle belly was done to facilitate the flap rotation. A large portion of the middle third and a portion of the distal third of the tibia wound could be covered by the medial hemisoleus muscle flap (Fig. 47.27). The left intact conjoint tendon from the distal medial half of the soleus muscle was then approximated to the remaining lateral half of the soleus muscle with nonabsorbable sutures.

The FDL tendon was identified and its distal insertion was divided. The muscle flap was dissected from distal to proximal. During dissection, only two branches from the posterior tibial

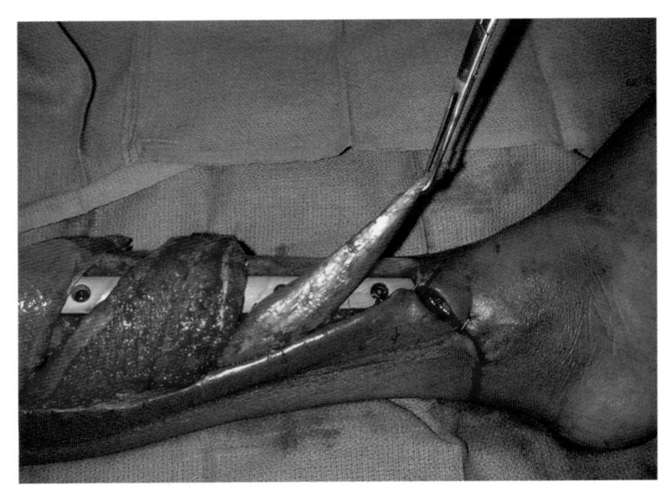

• **Fig. 47.28** An intraoperative view showing an elevated flexor digitorum longus muscle flap after dividing only two branches from the distal posterior tibial vessels.

vessels to the distal portion of the FDL were divided while allowing adequate flap rotation. In this way, the flap was able to cover the rest of the distal third of the leg wound without problems (Fig. 47.28).

All three muscle flaps were transposed into the entire tibia wound of the left leg sequentially. The medial gastrocnemius muscle flap was placed proximally to cover the primary third and the proximal portion of the middle third tibia wound. The medial hemisoleus muscle flap was placed after that to cover the rest of the middle third and the proximal portion of the distal third tibia wound. The FDL was then placed to cover the distal portion of the distal third tibia wound. All muscle flaps were attached with absorbable half-buried horizontal mattress sutures (Fig. 47.29).

Two drains were placed under the three muscle flaps. All muscle flaps were covered with split-thickness skin grafts. Split-thickness skin grafts were harvested with a dermatome from the left lateral thigh and meshed to 1:1.5 ratio. They were placed on all muscle flaps and secured with skin staples. The proximal and distal leg incisions were closed in two layers (Fig. 47.30).

Follow-Up Results

The patient did well postoperatively without any surgical issues related to the three local muscle flap reconstructions for this extensive open wound involving the entire tibia with the exposed fracture sites and reconstructive plate. She was admitted to a medical floor under psychiatric nursing care in addition to regular surgical nursing care. She was discharged from hospital on postoperative day 10 to a nursing home. The entire left tibia wound healed uneventfully. The postoperative follow-up has been difficult because of her psychiatric problems. She missed her regular follow-up by the orthopedic trauma service for nearly 3 months.

Final Outcome

During further orthopedic follow-up visits, the tibial fractures of the left leg had healed. She has resumed her weight-bearing status and normal activities. There was no wound breakdown, recurrent infection, or contour issues related to this combined multiple local

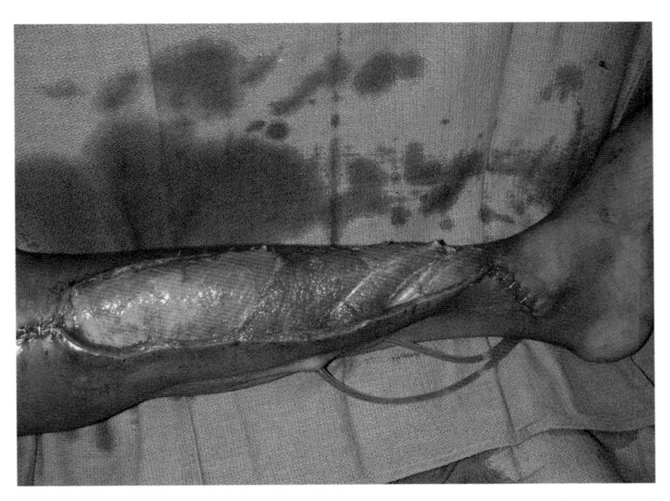

• **Fig. 47.29** An intraoperative view showing the sequential use of the medial gastrocnemius, medial hemisoleus, flexor digitorum longus muscle flaps for soft tissue reconstruction of an entire tibia wound of the left leg and completion of all three muscle flap insets before placement of skin grafts.

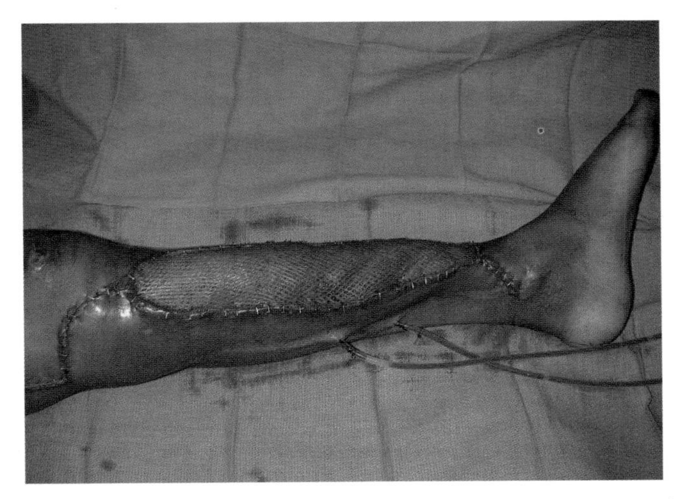

• **Fig. 47.30** An intraoperative view showing completion of skin graft placement over three muscle flaps.

muscle flap reconstructions (Fig. 47.31). The large reconstructive plate for fixation of the multiple tibial fractures was no longer needed. The orthopedic trauma service removed the plate 3.5 months later. All three muscle flaps were elevated under tourniquet control and sutured back to the leg once the plate was removed. The entire left leg wound healed well with good contour and minimal scarring.

Pearls for Success

The use of multiple local muscles for coverage of the lower-extremity wound has been overshadowed in recent years by the excitement of microvascular free tissue transfers. There are several advantages of multiple local muscle flaps over microvascular free tissue transfer for soft tissue coverage of an entire tibia wound. They are: (1) shorter operative time, (2) relatively straightforward surgical technique, (3) less intensive requirements for flap monitoring, (4) shortened hospital stay, (5) avoidance of perioperative anticoagulation, (6) less vigorous postoperative care, and (7) often no need for additional soft tissue debulking procedure.

The medial gastrocnemius muscle is reliable for soft tissue coverage of the proximal third of a tibial defect. By division of its insertion and scoring of the underlying fascia, the muscle may be expanded to cover a portion of the middle third of the tibial defect. The medial hemisoleus muscle has an increased arc of rotation of 8 to 10 cm in the middle leg and 3 to 5 cm in the distal leg. In the acute setting, the uninjured medial gastrocnemius and hemisoleus muscles are malleable enough and together they can provide adequate soft tissue coverage for at least the proximal two-thirds of a tibia wound. However, for chronic tibia wounds, both muscles may be indurated or edematous and may not be suitable to provide adequate soft-tissue coverage for the similar tibia wound. The FDL may be used for soft tissue coverage of a small distal tibia wound. No more than four branches can be sacrificed in order to ensure the reliability of the muscle flap. The FDL muscle flap can be used in combination with medial gastrocnemius and hemisoleus muscle flaps to cover an entire tibial soft tissue defect of the lower extremity, as demonstrated in this case. The combination of three medially located muscle flaps represents an alternative approach to free tissue transfer to reconstruct an entire tibia wound of the lower extremity. The sequential use of the medial gastrocnemius, hemisoleus, and FDL muscles for coverage of an entire tibial soft tissue defect may weaken some functions of the leg and foot, such as plantar flexion of the foot and flexion of the toes. Because the conjoint tendon of the leg is still intact, adequate ankle stabilization during ambulation may be maintained.

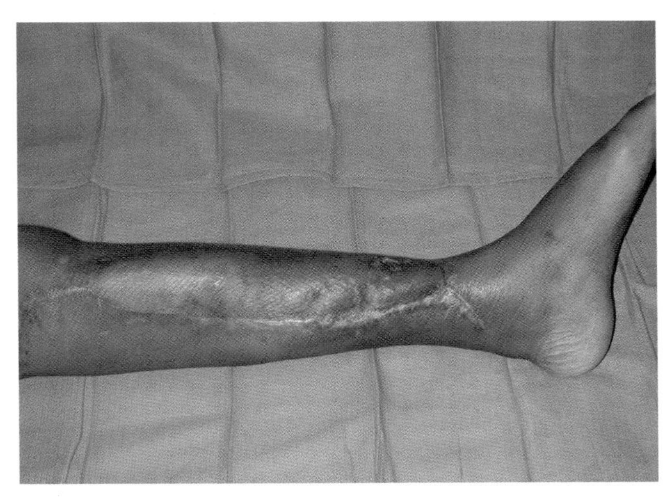

• **Fig. 47.31** Results at 3.5-month follow-up before elevation of all three muscle flaps for removal of the reconstruction plate showing well-healed entire tibia wound after the three sequential muscle flap reconstructions with good contour and minimal scarring.

CASE 4

Clinical Presentation

A 34-year-old White male unfortunately developed a complex left knee wound complicated from previous knee surgery. The open wound measured 7 × 4 cm with the exposed patella tendon,

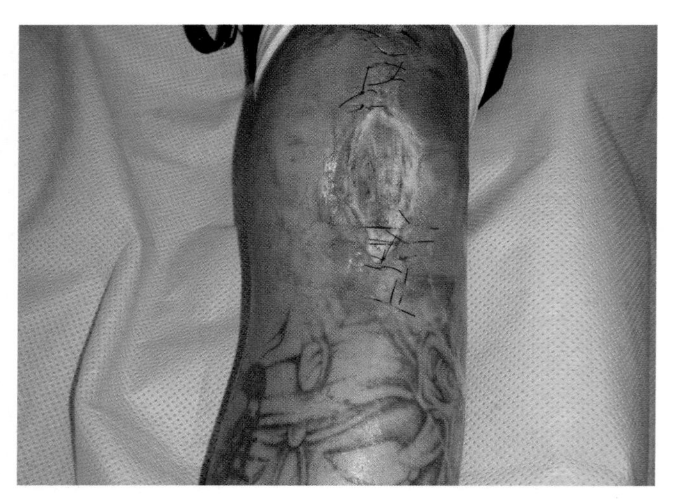

• **Fig. 47.32** A preoperative view showing an anterior knee wound of the left leg, measuring 7 × 4 cm, with the exposed patella tendon.

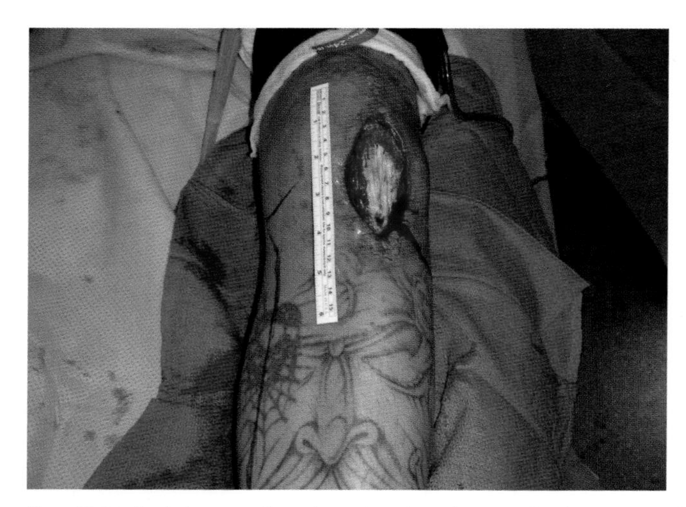

• **Fig. 47.33** An intraoperative view showing the anterior knee wound after surgical debridement of necrotic patella tendon and wound by the plastic surgery service.

which became necrotic (Fig. 47.32). He was referred by an outside orthopedic surgeon for knee soft tissue coverage. In addition, the patient was very motivated to have the left knee wound closed. Soft tissue coverage was planned after further definitive debridement.

Operative Plan and Special Considerations for Reconstruction

For this relatively large complex soft tissue wound in the knee, a classic local muscle flap, such as a medial gastrocnemius muscle flap, could be selected. The medial gastrocnemius muscle is a type I muscle flap and receives a blood supply primarily from the medial sural artery off the popliteal artery. The flap, in general, can be quite reliable and with scoring of the fascia over the muscle's belly, it can be used to cover this anterior knee wound without difficulty. A split-thickness skin graft would also be needed as a one-stage reconstruction for the anterior knee wound.

Operative Procedures

Under general anesthesia with the patient in the supine position, the anterior knee wound was debrided. The necrotic portion of the patellar tendon was sharply excised and the entire wound was curetted and the skin edge freshened with a knife. After debridement, the wound measured 7 × 4 cm and was irrigated with Pulsavac (Fig. 47.33).

The medial gastrocnemius muscle flap dissection was done under tourniquet control. The incision was made through the skin and subcutaneous tissue down to the fascia. Once the fascia was incised, the medial gastrocnemius muscle was identified. By finger dissection, the medial half of the muscle was dissected free from the medial half of the soleus muscle after identifying the plantaris tendon between two muscles. The incision was extended more distally to the area where the gastrocnemius muscle ended with its tendon. The muscle was divided with a 2-cm portion of its tendon and was longitudinally split with its raphe between the medial and lateral halves of the gastrocnemius muscle. Some dissection was also done to release the medial gastrocnemius muscle more proximally. The muscle belly was also scored with a knife 1 cm apart to improve the length of the flap's advancement.

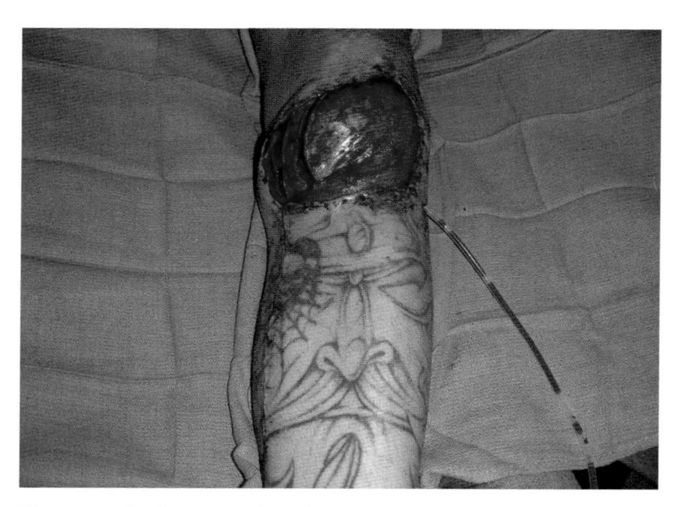

• **Fig. 47.34** An intraoperative view showing completion of the medial gastrocnemius muscle flap inset before skin graft placement over the muscle flap.

After releasing the tourniquet, the entire muscle flap appeared to be viable with good bleeding from the tip. One drain was inserted under the flap. The excess skin from the medial aspect of the left leg between the wound and the flap was excised to facilitate the flap inset. The flap was inset into the defect and secured with several 3-0 Monocryl sutures in a half-buried horizontal mattress fashion. A drain was inserted into the flap donor site. All incisions were closed in two layers. The deep dermal layer was approximated with several interrupted 3-0 Monocryl sutures. The skin was closed with 3-0 Monocryl sutures in a running subcuticular fashion (Fig. 47.34).

A split-thickness skin graft was harvested from the left lateral thigh with a dermatome and then meshed to 1:1.5 ratio. It was precisely placed over the muscle flap and secured with multiple skin staples to the skin edges. Several quilting sutures to the muscle were also placed (Fig. 47.35).

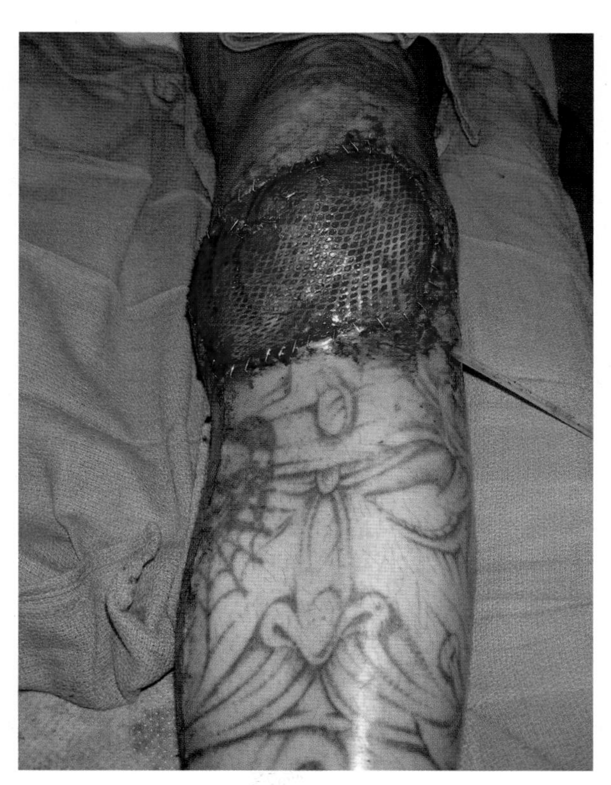

• **Fig. 47.35** An intraoperative view showing completion of the medial gastrocnemius muscle flap reconstruction. In this case, split-thickness skin grafts were used for the entire wound closure.

Management of Complications

Unfortunately, on postoperative day 4 the patient was found to have developed cellulitis around the flap site. There was some purulent drainage from under the flap. He was brought to the operating room for elevation of the flap and appropriate debridement. All sutures were removed and the flap was again elevated. The entire medial gastrocnemius muscle flap appeared to be healthy and viable. There were some purulent material under the flap along with the patellar tendon. Additional debridement was performed to remove all potential necrotic patella tendon. All the infected purulent material under the flap was removed manually. After vigorous irrigation, the flap was placed back on the wound and was approximated to the adjacent skin with sutures. Additional debridement of unhealthy-looking proximal knee skin was also performed, leaving a 3 × 2 cm open area that was covered with an allogenic skin graft as a temporary dressing.

The patient was taken back to the operating room 1 week later for definitive soft tissue coverage for the resulting knee wound (Fig. 47.36). A reverse anterolateral thigh (ALT) perforator flap was designed after a large perforator had been identified. It had only a superficial intramuscular course based on intraoperative duplex study (Fig. 47.37). A 15 × 7 cm skin paddle was designed and elevated. The descending branch of the lateral circumflex femoral vessels was identified. After intramuscular dissection, the perforator was found to join the descending branch. Prior to the division of the descending branch, its proximal end was clamped with an atraumatic vascular clamp. The flap appeared to have

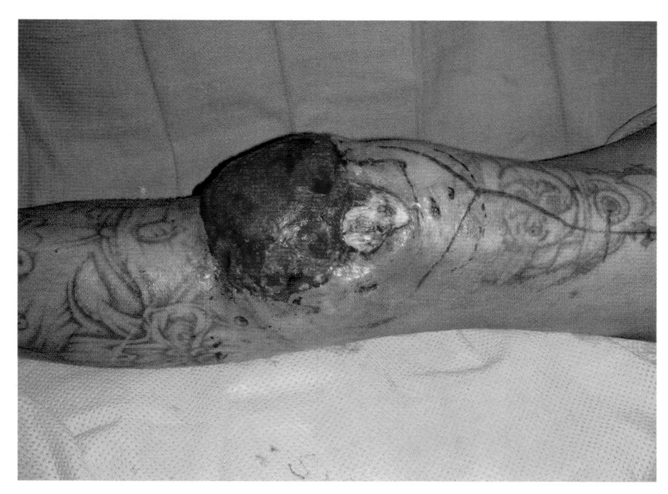

• **Fig. 47.36** A preoperative view showing a newly developed knee wound of the left leg, measuring 3 × 2 cm, with the exposed joint capsule of the knee.

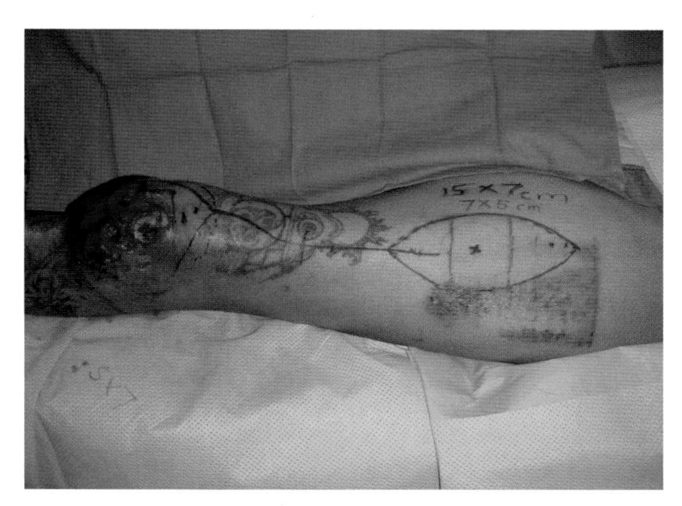

• **Fig. 47.37** An intraoperative view showing the design of a reverse anterolateral thigh perforator flap.

adequate perfusion with a reverse blood flow. The pedicle dissection was performed to follow the descending branch to about 10 cm above the lateral border of the patella. The flap was turned over in a reverse fashion to be inset into the soft tissue wound with sutures (Fig. 47.38). The left thigh flap donor site was closed primarily in two layers (Fig. 47.39). Additional skin grafts were placed over the rest of the medial gastrocnemius muscle flap and secured with skin staples (Fig. 47.40).

Follow-Up Results

The patient did well this time and there were no issues related to the final flap reconstruction. The left knee wound healed well (Fig. 47.41). He was eventually discharged from hospital and was followed by the plastic surgery service for routine postoperative care and an outside orthopedic surgeon for follow-up of the left knee reconstruction.

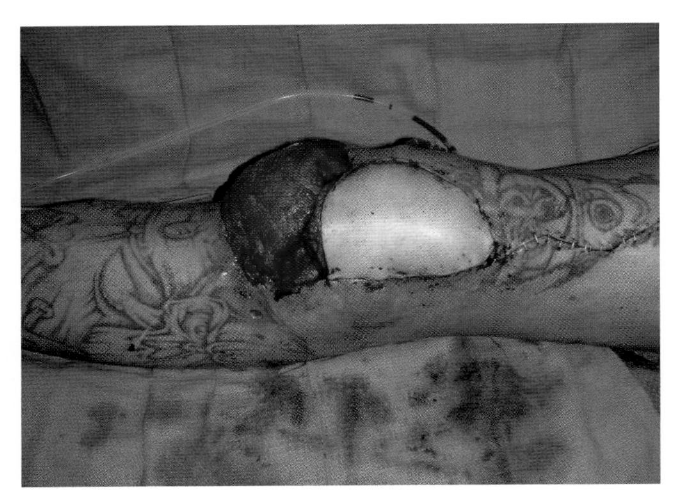

• **Fig. 47.38** An intraoperative view showing completion of the reverse anterolateral thigh perforator flap inset.

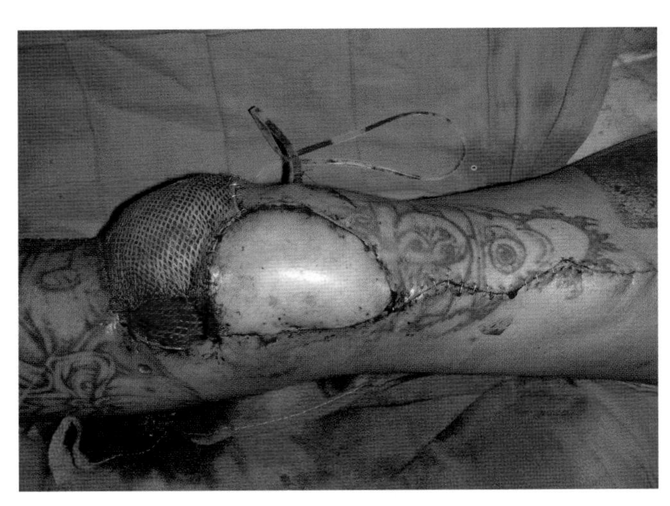

• **Fig. 47.40** An intraoperative view showing placement of new skin grafts to the medial gastrocnemius muscle flap after completion of the reverse anterolateral thigh perforator flap inset.

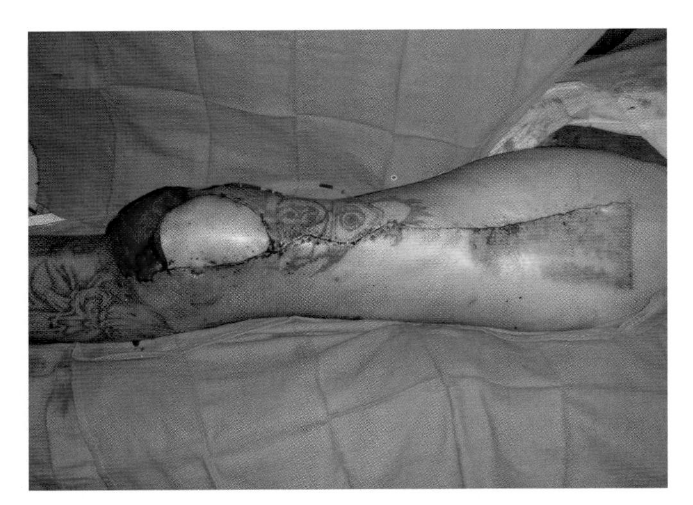

• **Fig. 47.39** An intraoperative view showing the primary closure of the anterolateral thigh flap donor site.

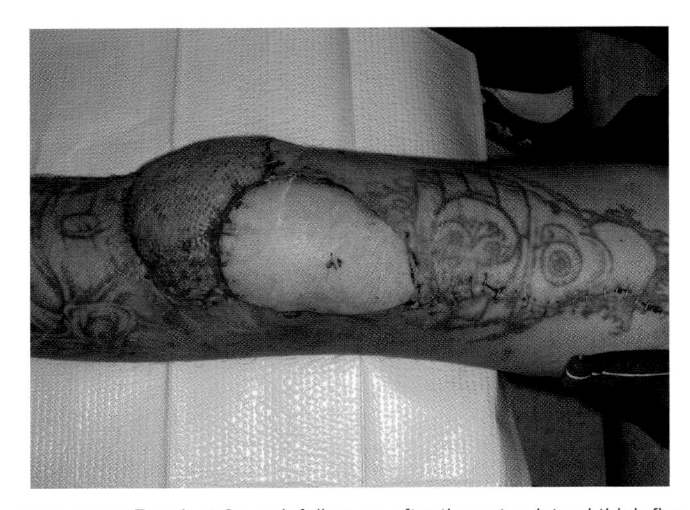

• **Fig. 47.41** Result at 2-week follow-up after the anterolateral thigh flap reconstruction showing well-healed left knee wound with good contour and the intact left thigh flap's donor site closure.

Final Outcome

During additional follow-up, after the combination of a medial gastrocnemius muscle flap and a reversed ALT perforator flap reconstruction, the left knee wound healed well (Fig. 47.42). The left thigh ALT flap donor site also healed well (Fig. 47.43) with no wound breakdown, recurrent infection, or contour issues related to the soft tissue reconstruction. The patient has resumed his regular activities and has been followed by his orthopedic surgeon for future left knee surgery.

Pearls for Success

Although a medial gastrocnemius muscle flap can be used to cover a complex knee wound, a larger knee wound may need more than one flap for adequate soft tissue coverage. A reverse ALT perforator flap can replace a lateral gastrocnemius muscle flap for such wound coverage. As with a free ALT perforator flap, a preoperative duplex study should be performed to provide reliable information on the perforator including its size, blood flow, and intramuscular course. With this information, an ALT perforator flap can be dissected quickly with less intraoperative difficulty. Before the pedicle is divided proximally, it should be temporary occluded to ensure that the flap receives adequate blood supply based on the reverse pedicle. The pivot point of the flap turnover is about 10 cm above the lateral border of the patella. If the flap appears to have venous congestion, a supercharge can be performed between the proximal pedicle vein and an adjacent native vein in the area.

CASE 5

Clinical Presentation

A 43-year-old White male presented to our hospital with a mangled left lower extremity after a motorcycle collision. He had a near circumferential left Gustilo IIIC middle and distal thirds

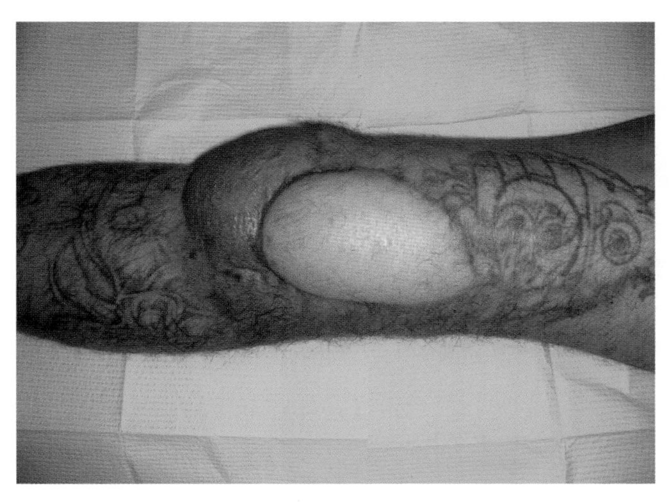

• **Fig. 47.42** Results at 3-month follow-up showing well-healed left knee wound after two flap reconstructions with good contour.

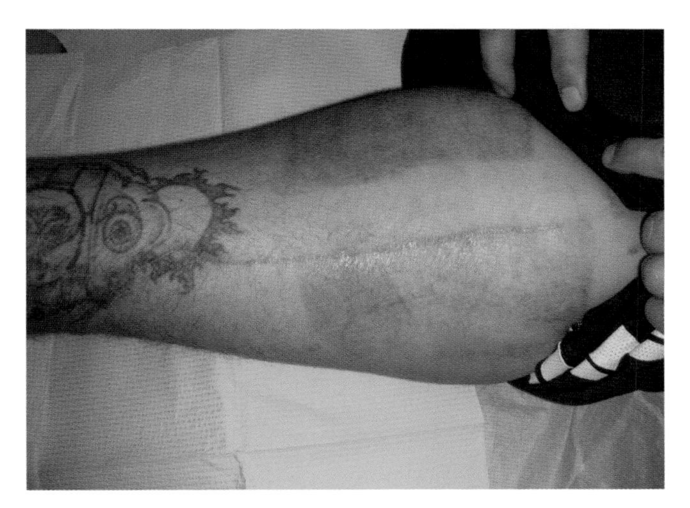

• **Fig. 47.43** Results at 3-month follow-up showing well-healed left thigh anterolateral thigh flap donor site.

open fracture wound, measuring 30 × 15 cm, with transection of the posterior tibial artery and vein in the middle leg (Figs. 47.44 and 47.45A). The peroneal artery was also not patent on the initial preoperative CT angiogram (Fig. 47.45B). His significant medical history included myocardial infarct within the previous 6 months. The patient was hemodynamically unstable and underwent exploratory laparotomy with splenectomy for splenic laceration on admission. Afterward, the patient's multiple orthopedic injuries were stabilized by the orthopedic trauma service. After the initial postsplenectomy, the patient developed acute segmental pulmonary emboli of the right lung. The plastic surgery service was consulted for soft tissue reconstruction of this near circumferential open fracture wound in the middle and distal thirds of the left leg.

Operative Plan and Special Considerations

This was a challenging lower extremity reconstructive case for limb salvage. The large size of the soft tissue defect in the left leg

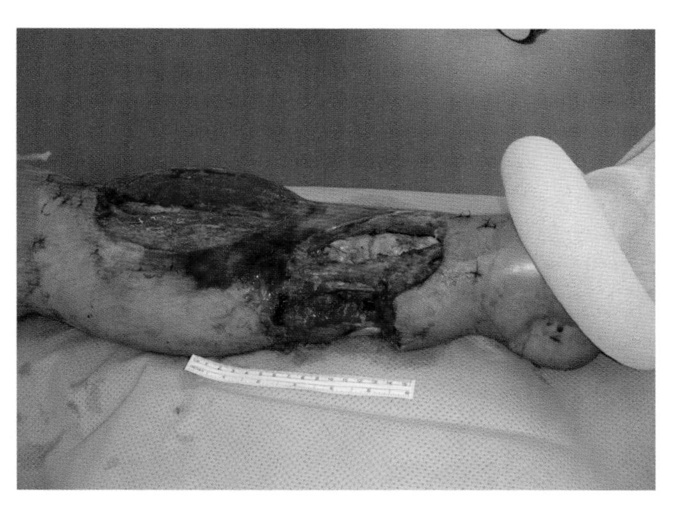

• **Fig. 47.44** A preoperative view showing an extensive soft tissue defect, measuring 30 × 15 cm, in the left leg at the time of initial consultation.

would need a large free muscle flap, such as a free latissimus dorsi muscle flap for lower part of the open tibial fracture wound coverage with a combination of a medial gastrocnemius muscle flap for the upper tibia wound coverage. In terms of selection of the recipient vessels for the free latissimus dorsi muscle flap, the proximal posterior tibial vessels above the transacted level were outside the zone of the injury and could be selected for both end-to-end arterial and venous anastomoses. In this way, the only patent artery, the anterior tibial artery, could remain undisturbed to ensure adequate blood supply to the foot. The definitive reconstructive procedure could be performed in two stages. The first procedure would be performed to explore the stump of the posterior tibial vessels and to evaluate whether those vessels could still be used as good recipient vessels. The medial gastrocnemius muscle flap could be performed at the same time. The second procedure would be performed for the free latissimus dorsi muscle transfer within a few days. Determining the status of the potential recipient vessels could potentially shorten the length of the free tissue transfer for coverage of the complex distal leg wound. Clearance from the trauma service would be needed to ensure the patient's stability and more optimal conditions to proceed following complex reconstructive procedures.

Operative Procedures

Under general anesthesia, the patient's entire left lower extremity wound was debrided and irrigated with Pulsavac during the first-stage procedure. The posterior tibial artery and vein were then explored as potential recipient vessels for future microvascular free flap transfer. Ligation site of the posterior tibial vessels was identified between the medial soleus muscle and the flexor digitorum longus muscles. By further dissection along the vessels proximally, both artery and vein apparently looked normal and outside the zone of injury. Both the artery and the vein were wrapped with a vessel loop separately for future use (Fig. 47.46).

The medial gastrocnemius muscle flap was then elevated. Once the fascia had been opened, the muscle was identified. It was dissected free from the medial soleus muscle. The dissection was done sharply to free the tendon portion of the medial

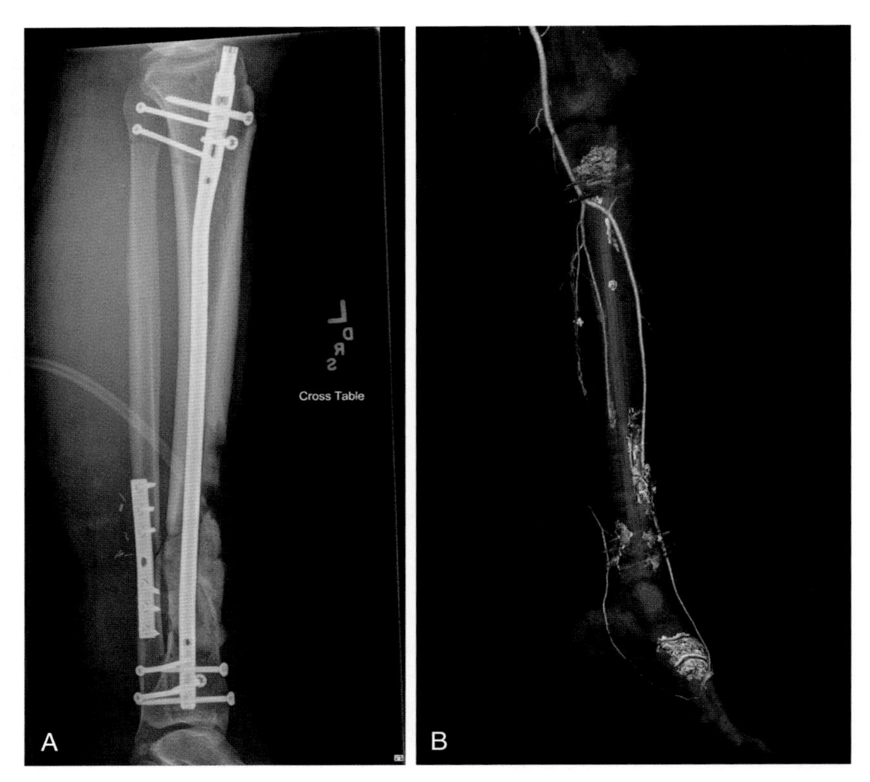

• **Fig. 47.45** (A) An X-ray image showing a large distal tibial gap that has been filled with an antibiotic bead. (B) Preoperative CT angiogram showing the transected posterior tibial artery. In addition, the peroneal artery has also been transected.

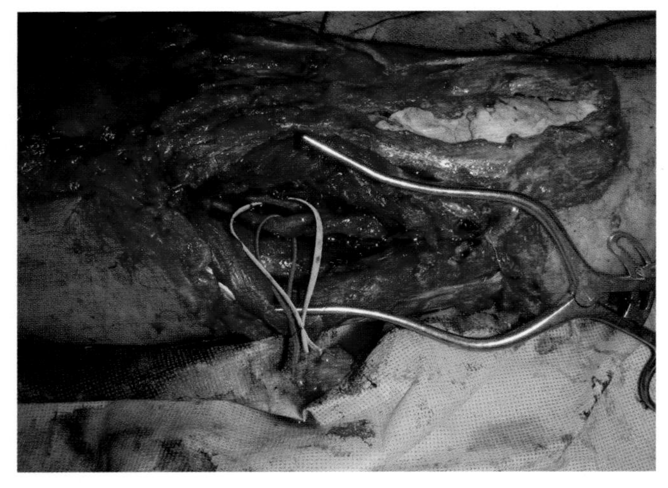

• **Fig. 47.46** An intraoperative view showing completion of surgical dissection for the posterior tibial vessel above the vessel transection. Both vessels were wrapped with vessel loops.

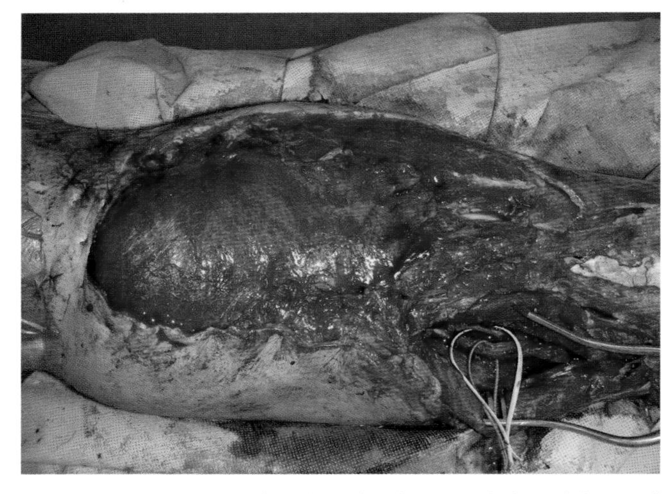

• **Fig. 47.47** An intraoperative view showing completion of the medial gastrocnemius muscle inset for soft tissue coverage of the proximal tibia wound.

gastrocnemius muscle from the conjoint tendon. The muscle was divided distally with a 2-cm cuff of the tendon and split longitudinally along with its raphe. The fascia of the muscle belly was scored with a knife to provide additional flap advancement for coverage of the exposed proximal tibia. The flap was completely secured with interrupted 3-0 Monocryl sutures (Fig. 47.47). The split-thickness skin graft was harvested with a dermatome from the left lateral thigh. The skin graft was meshed to 1:1.5 ratio, placed on the muscle flap, and secured with multiple skin staples. A vacuum-assisted closure (VAC) dressing was placed over the skin graft and connected with a VAC machine.

Two days later the patient was taken back to the operating room for the second-stage procedure again under general anesthesia. He was placed in the left lateral decubitus position. The right latissimus dorsi muscle flap was harvested first. An oblique incision was made down to the muscle. The latissimus dorsi

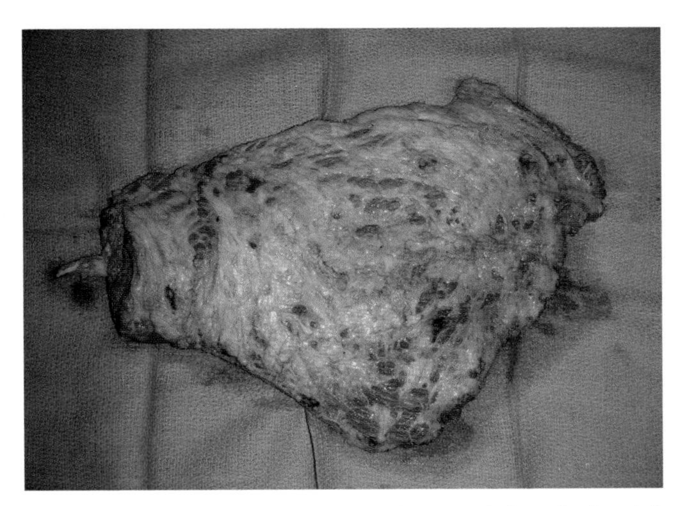

• **Fig. 47.48** An intraoperative view showing completion of a free latissimus dorsi muscle flap dissection.

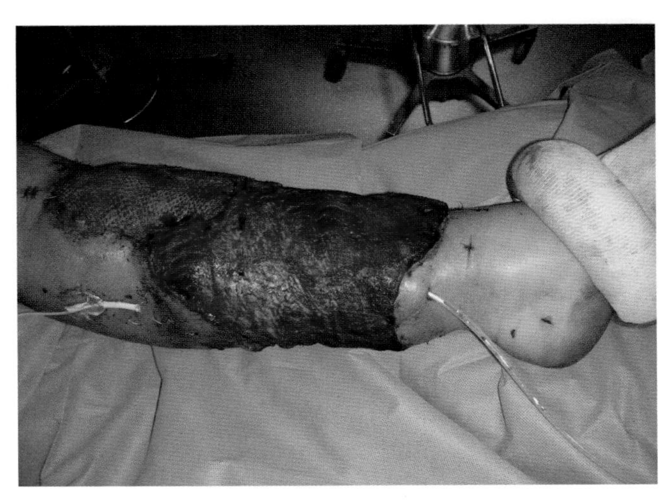

• **Fig. 47.49** An intraoperative view showing completion of a free latissimus dorsi muscle flap transfer to the left lower extremity before placement of a skin graft.

muscle was identified and skin flaps were raised superiorly and inferiorly and then medially and laterally. The superior medial border of the latissimus dorsi muscle was identified and it was then elevated off the chest wall and the medial attachment was divided under direct vision followed by the division of the inferior attachment a centimeter above the posterior iliac spine. Once the lateral border of the latissimus dorsi muscle was identified and detached, the muscle was elevated off the chest wall toward the axilla, but the serratus muscle was left on the chest wall. The thoracodorsal vessels were identified by a handheld Doppler and then marked. With further traction and dissection of the flap toward the axilla, the thoracodorsal pedicle was dissected free and a space between the pedicle and the muscle insertion was created. The muscle insertion was divided with finger protection of the pedicle. The pedicle dissection was then performed under loupe magnification. The thoracodorsal nerve was identified and divided. The dissection was performed for the artery and vein toward the axillary vessels. The pedicle artery and vein were dissected free and then divided individually with large hemoclips.

The pedicle vessel was prepared under loupe magnification. There were one artery and two venae comitantes and they all appeared to be relatively small. They were flushed with heparinized saline solution. The flap was then wrapped with cold saline lap to prevent further ischemic damage (Fig. 47.48).

The right back donor site was closed after hemostasis. Two drains were inserted and the incision was closed with 2-0 PDS sutures for the deep tissue layer followed by 3-0 Monocryl suture for the deep dermal closure. The skin was closed with skin staples.

The patient was then turned to the supine position. The procedure started by opening the area between the soleus muscle and the flexor digitorum longus muscle. The previous vessel loops were identified and both the posterior tibial artery and vein stumps were identified. There was good inflow from the posterior tibial artery. The flap was temporarily inset into the defect. Under a microscope, both pedicle and recipient vessels were prepared. The arterial microanastomosis was performed with interrupted end-to-end 8-0 nylon sutures. Although the recipient vein appeared to be quite large, the pedicle vein appeared to be small. A 2-mm coupler device was selected for the venous microanastomosis in an end-to-end fashion.

Once all atraumatic microvascular clamps had been removed, the flap appeared to be well perfused.

The flap was inset into the defect to cover the rest of the wound in the left leg. Before the final inset, the Cook Doppler probe was wrapped around the pedicle artery distal to the anastomosis. A drain was placed under the flap. The rest of the flap was secured to the adjacent skin edges with half-buried horizontal mattress 3-0 Vicryl sutures (Fig. 47.49). The split-thickness skin graft was harvested with a dermatome from the left thigh and meshed to 1:1.5 ratio. The skin graft was placed over the muscle flap and wound bed and secured with multiple skin staples.

Management of Complications

The free latissimus dorsi flap surgery was uneventful and the patient was monitored in the surgical intensive care unit on oral aspirin and intravenous dextran. On postoperative day 4, he developed an infected hematoma of the left knee with systemic signs of fever and hypotension. Clinical exam indicated anastomotic thrombosis of the flap and the patient was taken back to the operating room for exploration (Fig. 47.50). Intraoperatively, it was noted that both arterial and venous anastomoses thrombosed (Fig. 47.51). Thromboembolectomy was performed with a 2-mm Fogarty catheter after all platelet blood clots within the vessels had been manually removed with micro instruments under a microscope. After repeating the arterial and venous microvascular anastomoses, both pedicle artery and vein were patent (Fig. 47.52). However, while the patient was still in the recovery room less than 1 hour after reoperation, both microanastomoses thrombosed again even on a systemic heparin drip. At this point, the flap became unsalvageable and was removed after clamping both the posterior tibial artery and vein with hemoclips (Fig. 47.53). A temporary VAC device was placed after removal of the necrotic flap.

In light of the failure of the first free tissue transfer, the patient's platelet count was found to have a coincidental peak that exceeded more than 1,000,000/mL at the time of the initial free tissue transfer. After appropriate consultation, the apheresis service was involved to aid the perioperative management of thrombocytosis. Thus, the decision was made to treat the thrombocytosis

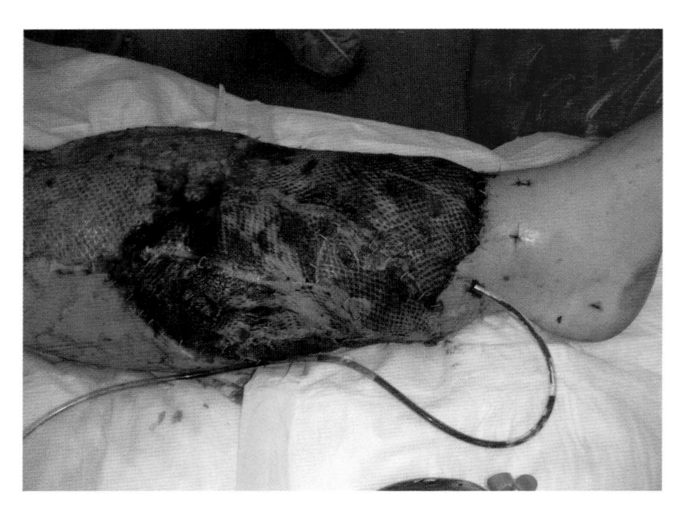

• **Fig. 47.50** A preoperative view showing obvious ischemia of a free latissimus dorsi muscle flap caused by thrombosis of microvascular anastomoses.

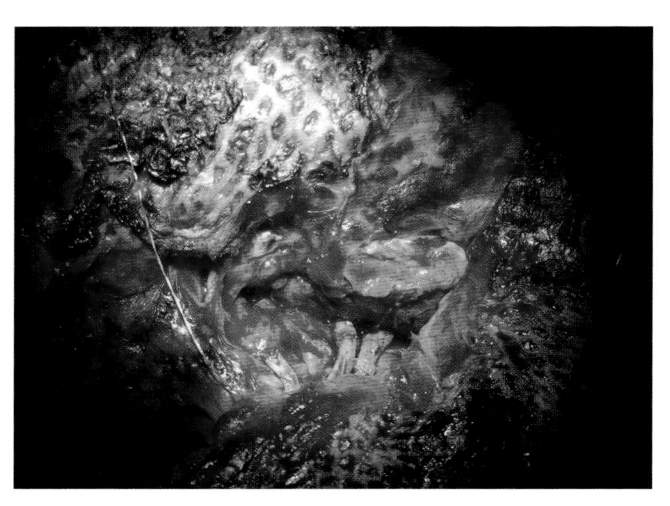

• **Fig. 47.52** An intraoperative view showing both patent arterial and venous microanastomoses under a microscope after repeating both arterial and venous microanastomoses under a microscope.

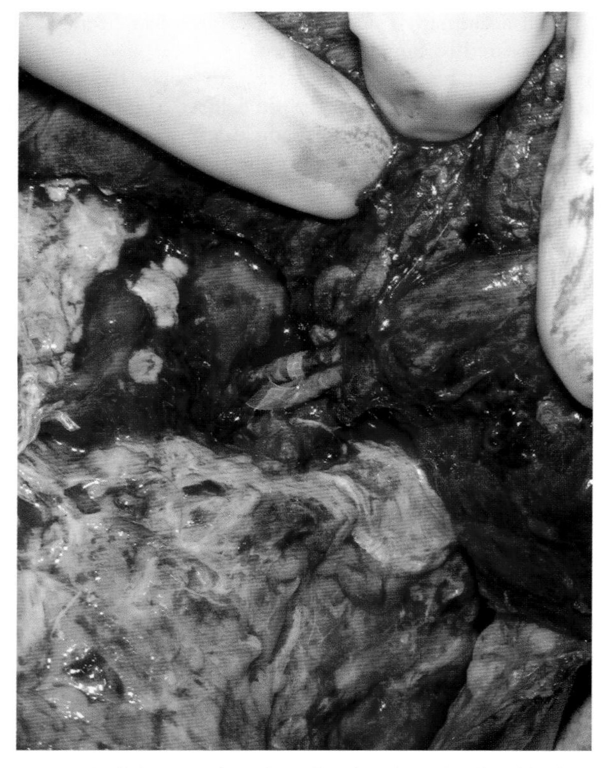

• **Fig. 47.51** An intraoperative view showing thrombosis of both arterial and venous microanastomoses.

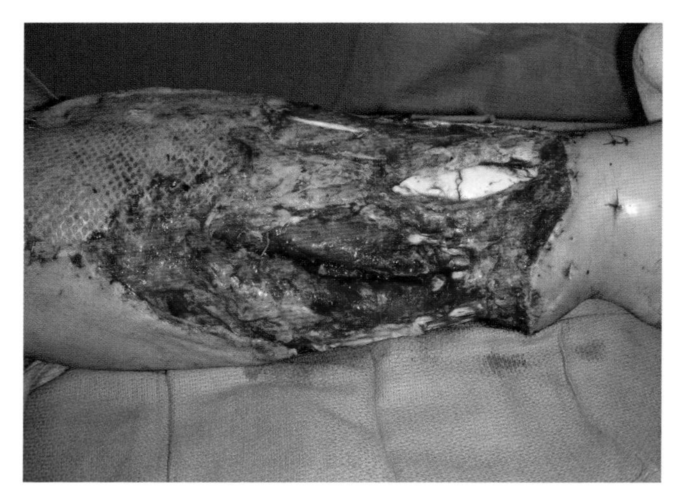

• **Fig. 47.53** An intraoperative view showing the appearance of the left lower extremity wound after removal of the free latissimus dorsi muscle flap.

with platelet apheresis before performing a second free flap. While waiting for the second free tissue transfer, the patient was taken back to the operating room twice a week for wound debridement and placement of a new VAC.

After the first apheresis session, platelet counts reached a nadir of 197,000/mL, it was felt that this would be a good opportunity for the second free tissue transfer (Fig. 47.54). Again under general anesthesia, the left leg wound was debrided, followed by Pulsavac irrigation (Fig. 47.55).

Exploration of the posterior tibial artery and vein stumps was carried out because they were still patient proximally based on the CT angiogram findings. The dissection was performed to open the space between proximal medial hemisoleus and flexor digitorum longus muscles. The previous well-healed gastrocnemius muscle flap was elevated distally in order to have a better exposure of the posterior artery and vein. Once the posterior artery and vein were identified proximal to the scarred areas, they were dissected free about 4 cm proximal to both vessel stumps. There was a good inflow of the posterior tibial artery and vein appeared to be healthy with an adequate size. After further preparation under loupe magnification, both artery and vein were ready as recipient vessels for microvascular anastomoses (Fig. 47.56).

A right paramedian incision was made to harvest the right free rectus abdominis muscle flap. The skin, subcutaneous tissue, and anterior rectus sheath were incised. By further dissection of the anterior rectus sheath more medially and laterally, the outline of the rectus abdominis muscle was identified and the anterior

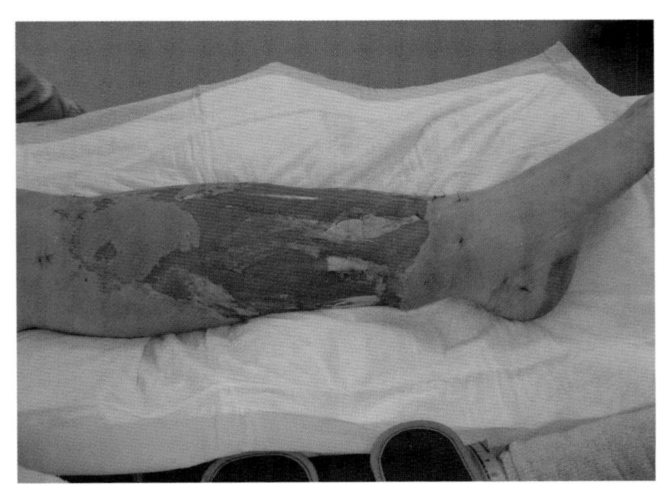

• **Fig. 47.54** A preoperative view showing the appearance of the left lower extremity wound after repeated wound debridement and vacuum-assisted closure treatment.

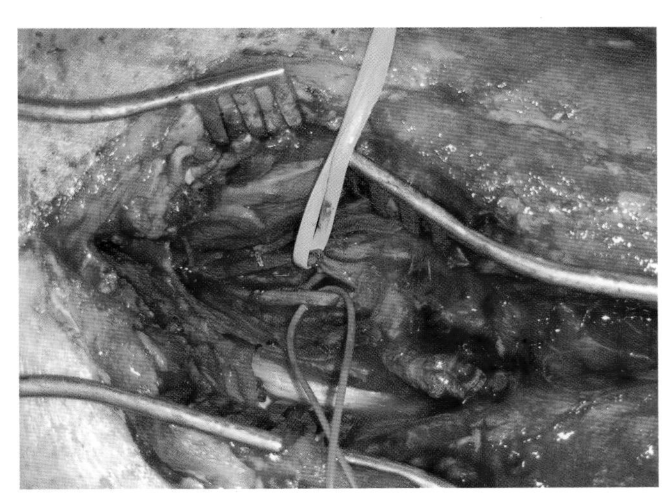

• **Fig. 47.56** An intraoperative view showing completion of surgical dissection for the posterior tibial vessel above the previous surgery site. Each vessel was wrapped with a vessel loop.

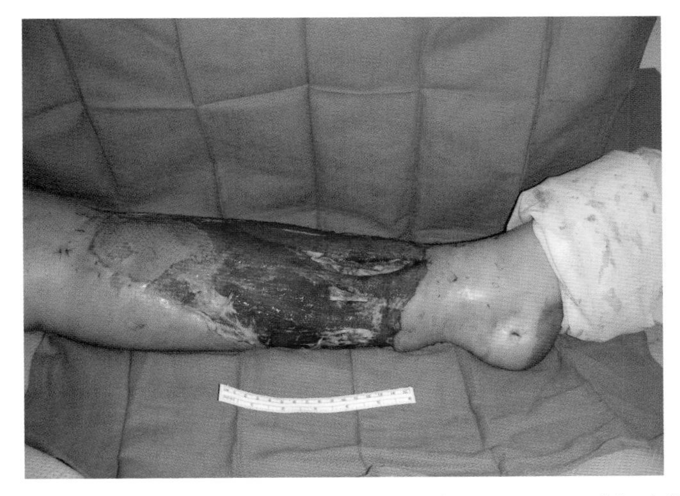

• **Fig. 47.55** An intraoperative view showing the appearance of the left lower extremity wound right after serial debridement before the second free tissue transfer.

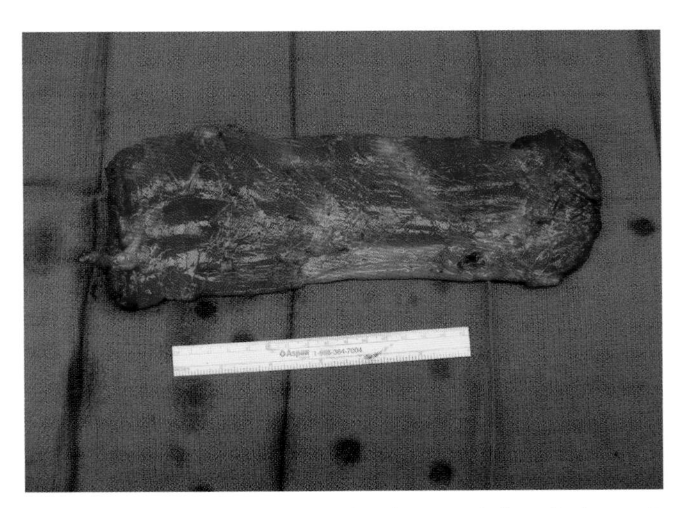

• **Fig. 47.57** An intraoperative view showing completion of a free rectus abdominis muscle flap dissection.

dissection of the muscle was done all the way up to about 2 cm below the costal margin. The insertion of the muscle was divided and the muscle was easily elevated off the posterior rectus sheath. The origin of the muscle was divided under direct vision. Dissection around the pedicle vessels was performed toward the external iliac vessels. Both pedicle artery and vein were divided with medium size hemoclips near the external iliac vessels (Fig. 47.57).

With the aid of loupe magnification, both pedicle artery and vein were prepared with micro instruments. Both pedicle vessels were flushed with heparinized saline solution. The muscle flap was inset into the defect of the left leg wound. The arterial microanastomosis was performed between the pedicle artery and the posterior tibial artery stump. It was done in an end-to-end fashion with interrupted 8-0 nylon sutures. The venous microanastomosis was performed with a 2.5-mm coupler device in end-to-end fashion. The additional vein in the pedicle was clipped. A Cook Doppler probe was wrapped around the pedicle artery (Fig. 47.58). A drain was inserted under the flap but away from the pedicle vessels. The entire flap was approximated to the adjacent wound edges with 3-0 Monocryl sutures in half-buried horizontal mattress fashion (Fig. 47.59). The split-thickness skin graft was harvested from both thighs with a dermatome and meshed to 1:1.5 ratio. The skin grafts were placed on the muscle flap and the rest of the wound and secured with multiple skin staples (Fig. 47.60).

The right abdominal muscle donor site was closed in three layers. The anterior rectus sheath was repaired with several interrupted figure-of-eight 3-0 PDS sutures. A drain was inserted under the abdominal skin. The dermal deep closure was

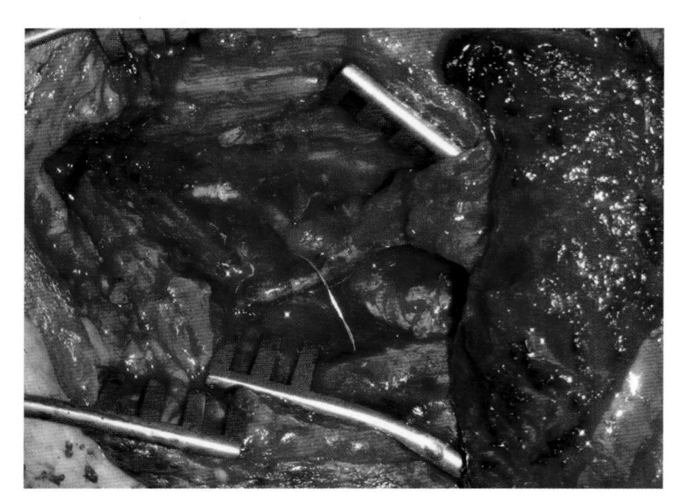

• **Fig. 47.58** An intraoperative view showing both successful arterial and venous microanastomoses under a microscope. Both microanastomoses were performed at least 5 cm proximal to the previous anastomotic sites.

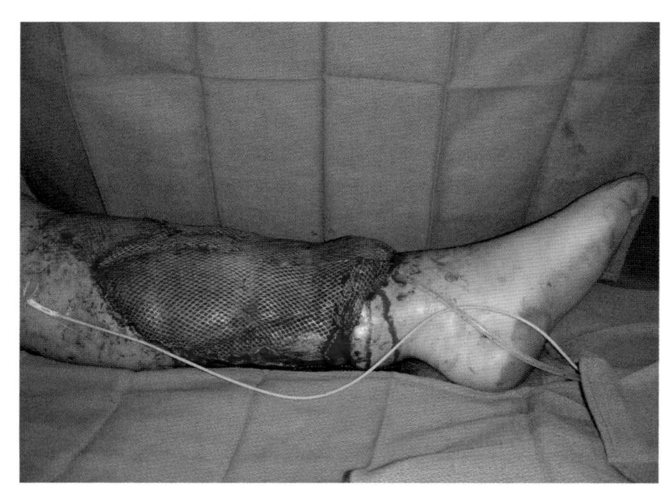

• **Fig. 47.60** An intraoperative view showing completion of a free rectus abdominis muscle flap transfer to the left lower extremity and the skin graft placement.

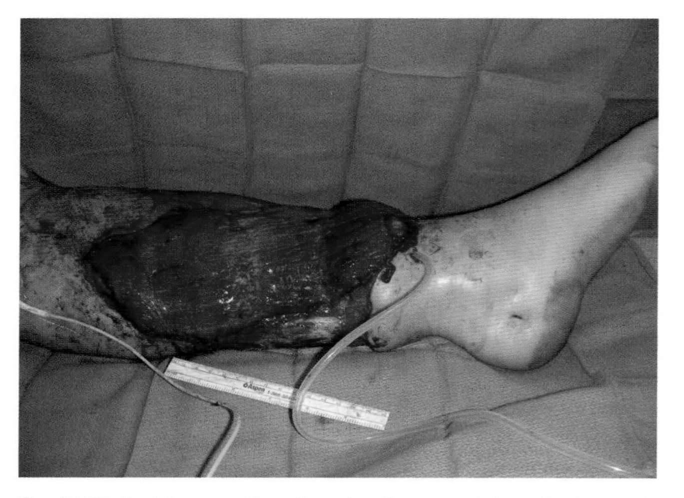

• **Fig. 47.59** An intraoperative view showing completion of a free rectus abdominis muscle flap transfer to the left lower extremity before skin graft placement.

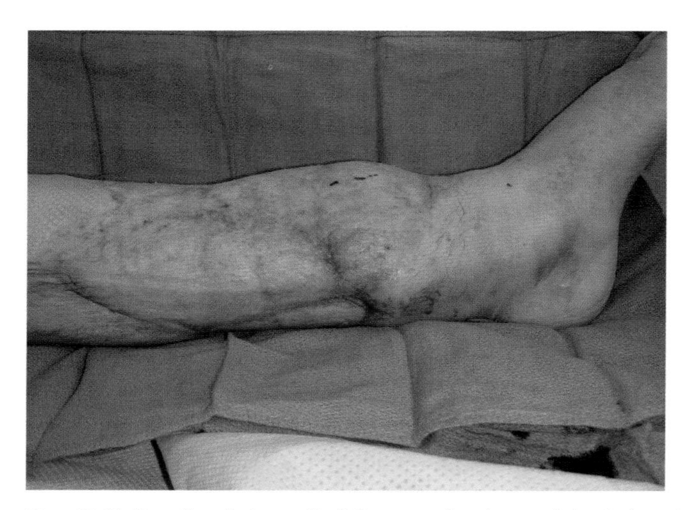

• **Fig. 47.61** Results at 4-month follow-up showing well-healed and stable left distal leg wound with minimal scarring.

performed with several interrupted 3-0 Monocryl sutures and the skin was closed with skin staples.

Follow-Up Results

The patient did well this time postoperatively without any complications related to the free rectus abdominis muscle flap transfer to the large distal tibia wound. He underwent two more sessions of platelet apheresis within 2 weeks postoperatively and the platelet level was maintained at less than 600,000/mL during that period. Although his platelet level gradually increased to 600,000/mL or higher, the second free tissue transfer remained successful and there were no microvascular complications during the perioperative period. He was discharged home 4 weeks after the second free tissue transfer and all drains were removed during subsequent follow-up visits. The free rectus abdominis muscle flap reconstruction site healed well and the skin graft over the muscle flap also took well (Fig. 47.61).

Final Outcome

About 10 months after the second free tissue transfer, an autologous bone graft procedure was performed (Fig. 47.62). The free rectus abdominis muscle flap was elevated by the plastic surgery service and the autologous bone graft procedure was performed by the orthopedic trauma service (Fig. 47.63). The patient did well after the bone graft procedure and again the free rectus abdominis muscle flap healed well (Fig. 47.64). Subsequently, the left distal tibial fracture site also healed well about 7 months later (Fig. 47.65). He has resumed his normal activities and been routinely followed by the orthopedic trauma service.

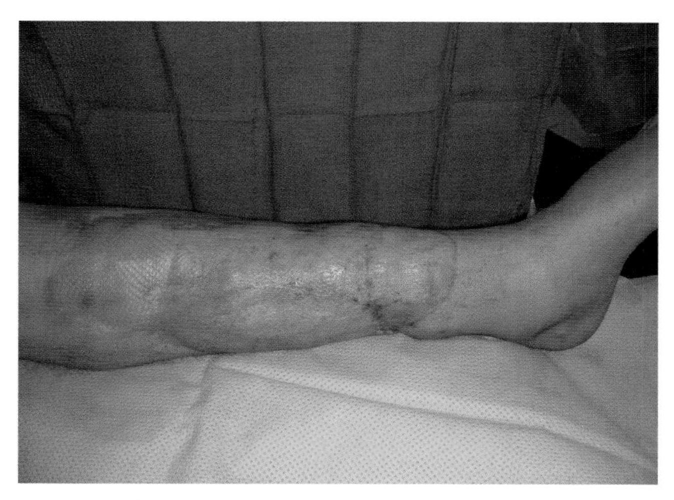

• **Fig. 47.62** Results at 10 months before a bone graft procedure showing well-healed and stable left distal leg wound with good contour and minimal scarring.

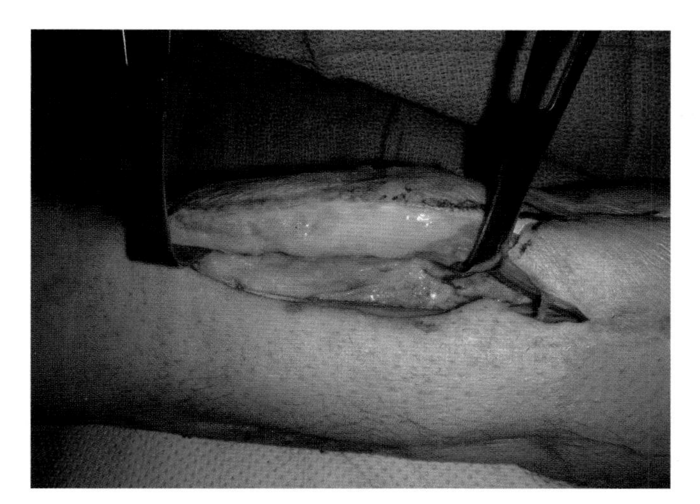

• **Fig. 47.63** An intraoperative view showing a healthy soft tissue coverage after the second free tissue transfer before a bone grafting procedure.

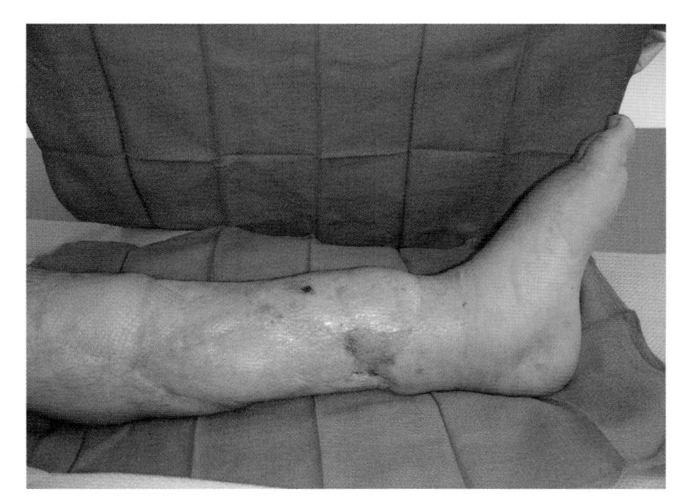

• **Fig. 47.64** Results at 13 months (3 months after a bone grafting procedure) showing the well-healed and stable distal leg wound with good contour and minimal scarring.

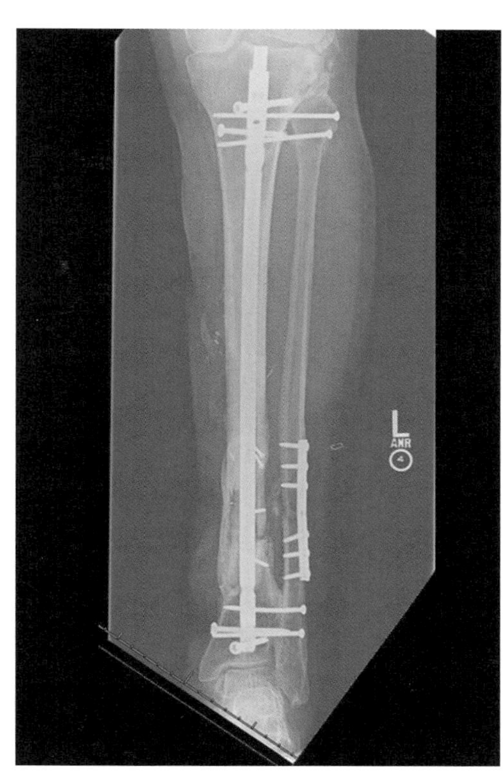

• **Fig. 47.65** A follow-up X-ray image showing appropriate healing of the tibial fracture site 2 years after bone grafting.

Pearls for Success

Either a free latissimus dorsi or a free rectus abdominis muscle flap can be an excellent choice for a large soft tissue reconstruction in the distal leg. In this case, even though the posterior tibial vessels were ligated after orthopedic trauma, their stumps could still be used as recipient vessels as long as they are outside the zone of injury. This would be much safer than to explore the anterior tibial vessels as receipt vessels and the arterial anastomosis would have been performed in an end-to-side fashion.

The treatment strategy to counter thrombocytosis-induced flap failure in lower extremity microsurgical reconstruction is demonstrated here (Fig. 47.66). This patient initially developed thrombocytosis-associated flap failure in the setting of routine free flap protocol. In addition, the patient developed preoperative pulmonary emboli, which should alert the surgeon that the patient would be at high risk of thrombocytosis. One preoperative platelet apheresis session and two additional postoperative sessions were needed to maintain platelet counts within relatively normal physiologic range until 2 weeks postoperatively. Any patients with thrombocytosis, who demonstrate one or more signs of spontaneous thrombotic events before microsurgical reconstruction, should be considered at high risk and should undergo the appropriate platelet apheresis therapy for thrombocytosis. Platelet apheresis can be an effective option and should be considered by the surgeon when a microsurgical patient presents with thrombocytosis especially after splenectomy. Platelet apheresis should be included in a microsurgeon's armamentarium when managing perioperative thrombocytosis.

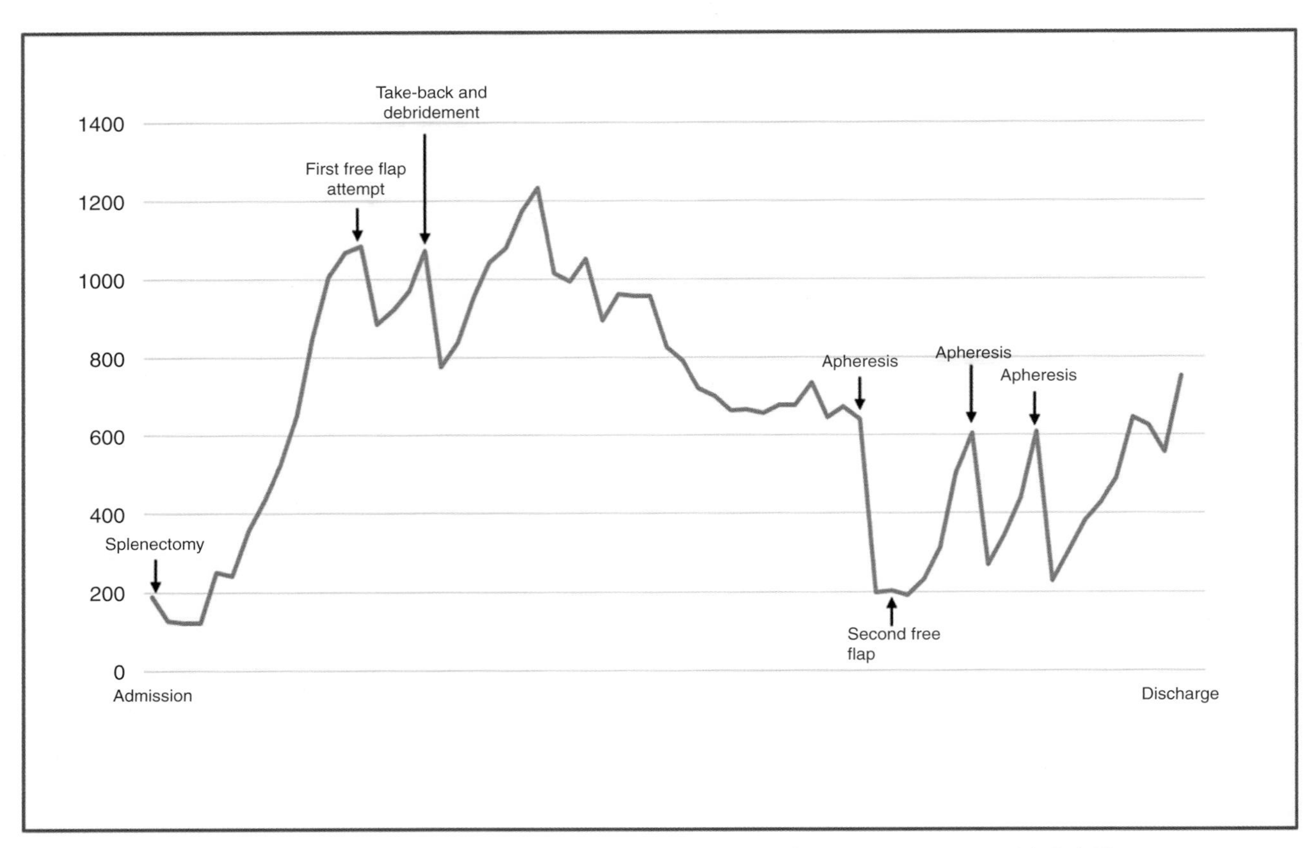

• **Fig. 47.66** Platelet counts throughout the hospital admission. Significant events were labeled. Note the reactive thrombocytosis and the peak in platelet count during initial reconstruction.

Recommended Readings

Bigdeli AK, Thomas B, Falkner F, Radu CA, Gazyakan E, Kneser U. Microsurgical reconstruction of extensive lower extremity defects with the conjoined parascapular and latissimus dorsi free flap. *Microsurgery*. 2020;40:639–648.

Demirseren ME, Efendioglu K, Demiralp CO, Kilicarslan K, Akkaya H. Clinical experience with a reverse-flow anterolateral thigh perforator flap for the reconstruction of soft-tissue defects of the knee and proximal lower leg. *J Plast Reconstr Aesthet Surg*. 2011;64:1613–1620.

Heller L, Phillips K, Levin LS. Pedicled osteocutaneous fibula flap for reconstruction in the lower extremity. *Plast Reconstr Surg*. 2000; 109:2037–2042.

Pu LL. Soft-tissue coverage of an extensive mid-tibia wound with the combined medial gastrocnemius and medial hemisoleus muscle flaps: the role of local muscle flaps revisited. *J Plast Reconstr Aesthet Surg*. 2010;63:e605–e610.

Song P, Patel N, Pu LLQ. Reoperation of lower extremity microsurgical reconstruction when facing postsplenectomy thrombocytosis. *Plast Reconstr Surg Glob Open*. 2019;7:e2492.

Song P, Pu LLQ. The soleus muscle flap: an overview of its clinical applications for lower extremity reconstruction. *Ann Plast Surg*. 2018;81(6S suppl 1):S109–S116.

Thornton BP, Pu LL. Reconstruction of an extensive tibial soft-tissue defect with multiple local muscle flaps for limb salvage when free-tissue transfer was not an option. *Euro J Plast Surg*. 2004;27:217–221.

48 Ankle Reconstruction

CASE 1

Clinical Presentation

A 68-year-old Asian male sustained left ankle open fracture and dislocation as a result of a motorcycle collision. He had a complex open wound over the medial malleolus with an exposed flexor digitorum longus tendon. He was managed initially by the orthopedic trauma service for wound debridement and placement of an external fixator. The critical part of the wound measured 7 × 4 cm and the rest of the wound measured 5 × 6 cm (Fig. 48.1). The plastic surgery service was consulted to provide soft tissue coverage for this complex ankle wound. No further orthopedic procedures were needed after soft tissue reconstruction.

Operative Plan and Special Considerations for Reconstruction

The distally based sural artery flap can also be used to cover a complex wound in the ankle if the flap donor site is available and the pedicle of the flap in the territory of the lesser saphenous vein is not involved with previous trauma or surgery. The flap can provide good skin coverage to a wound in both the medial and lateral aspects of the ankle. The donor site of a distally based sural artery flap is centrally located in the posterior calf over the medial and lateral gastrocnemius muscles. The skin island can be harvested from the proximal two-thirds of the posterior leg with a skin paddle up to 12 × 8 cm. The flap receives blood supply primarily from three to six septocutaneous perforators arising from the peroneal artery in a retrograde fashion. The most proximal end of those perforators is located about 6 cm proximal to the lateral malleolus. Therefore, preoperative evaluation to determine the patency of the peroneal artery is critical. The flap also receives a blood supply, again in a retrograde fashion, from the fasciocutaneous perforators from the posterior tibial artery, venocutaneous perforators from the lesser saphenous vein, and neurocutaneous perforators from the sural nerve. Thus, the blood supplies to the flap through both the lesser saphenous vein and sural nerve systems should all be included within the adipofascial pedicle to ensure adequate blood supply when the flap is used to cover an ankle wound (see Chapter 45, Case 2; Fig. 45.9). In addition, a venous supercharge should also be prepared if the flap becomes congested after its inset.

Operative Procedures

Under general anesthesia with the patient in the prone position, the medial ankle wound, measuring 7 × 4 cm with the exposed underlying tendon and joint capsule, was debrided. All unhealthy-looking skin edges and colonized tissues were sharply debrided and the wound was then irrigated with Pulsavac. The wound appeared to be fresh and clean after a definitive debridement performed by the plastic surgery service.

The whole course of the lesser saphenous vein was mapped with a handheld Doppler between the Achilles tendon and the lateral malleolus. Although the scar presented in the lateral aspect of the distal leg, the pedicle of the less saphenous vein appeared to be intact and could be used for the flap. The pivot point of the flap turnover was marked about 6 cm above the lateral malleolus. A 7 × 4 cm of the flap's skin island was designed based on the size of soft tissue wound and two triangular extensions were also included because they acted as a dog ear for each end and would normally be excised during the closure of the flap's donor site (Fig. 48.2).

Under tourniquet control, the proximal incision of the flap was made to explore the lesser saphenous vein and its accompanying vessels distal to the flap. The lesser saphenous vein and its accompanying vessels were then divided with hemoclips. The sural nerve and its accompanying vessels were exposed and then divided again with hemoclips after incising the fascia. The skin island was elevated along the subfascial plane and it was then completely elevated as a fasciocutaneous island flap. The adipofascial pedicle of the flap, about 2 cm wide, was dissected free after multiple zigzag skin incisions proximal to the skin paddle. After releasing the tourniquet, the flap was turned over and tunneled under the skin bridge to place over the medial aspect of the ankle wound. The flap was then inset into the medial ankle wound to cover the exposed tendon with interrupted 3-0 Monocryl sutures in a half-buried horizontal mattress fashion. One drain was placed under the flap (Fig. 48.3).

The flap donor site in the middle of the leg was closed primarily with a split-thickness skin graft after undermining the adjacent skin edge to reduce the size of the needed skin graft. The split-thickness skin graft was harvested with a dermatome from the left lateral thigh and meshed to 1:1.5 ratio. The skin graft was approximated to the adjacent skin edges with interrupted chromic sutures. The less critical part of the wound was also covered by a skin graft. The rest of the skin incision for the flap dissection was closed in two layers with interrupted sutures (Fig. 48.4).

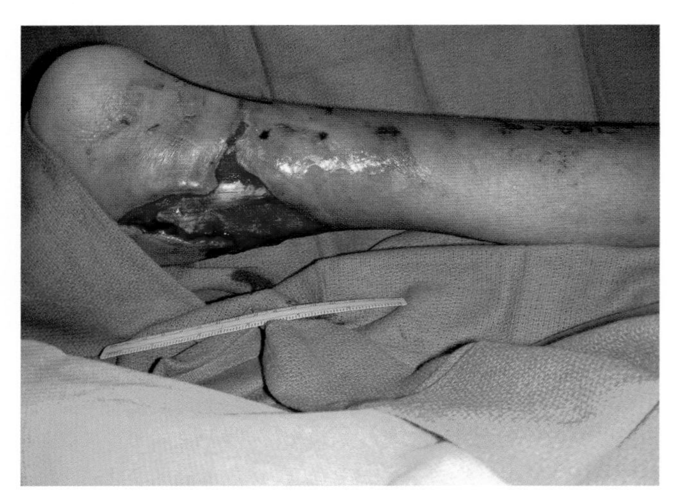

• **Fig. 48.1** A preoperative view showing a 7 × 4 cm complex wound over the left medial ankle with the exposed flexor digitorum longus tendon and joint capsule. The rest of the wound with just the skin defect measured 5 × 6 cm.

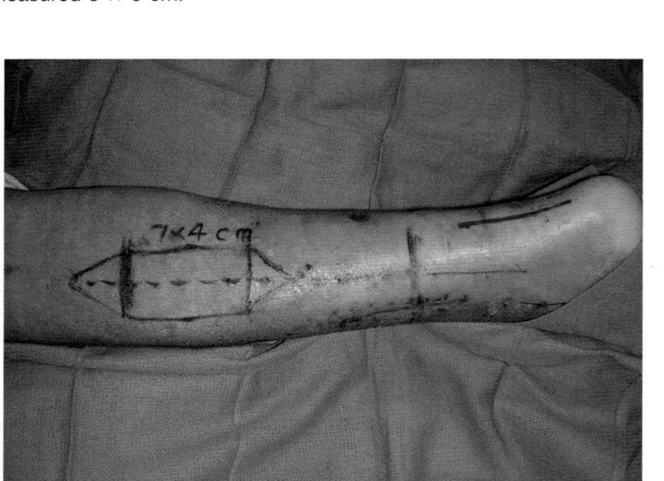

• **Fig. 48.2** An intraoperative view showing the design of the distally based sural artery flap as a turnover flap. The pivotal point of the flap turnover was 6 cm above the lateral malleolus. The lesser saphenous vein and its accompanying vessels were found to be intact based on the Doppler study even though there was a surgical scar in the lateral leg.

Follow-Up Results

The patient did well postoperatively without any issues related to the distally based sural artery flap for soft tissue coverage of the medial ankle wound. He was discharged from the hospital on postoperative day 5. His left medial ankle wound healed uneventfully. He was followed by the plastic surgery service for routine postoperative care and by the orthopedic trauma service for left ankle fracture and dislocation.

Final Outcome

During further follow-up, the complex left anterior ankle wound after the distally based reverse sural artery flap reconstruction had healed well with excellent contour and minimal scarring. The rest

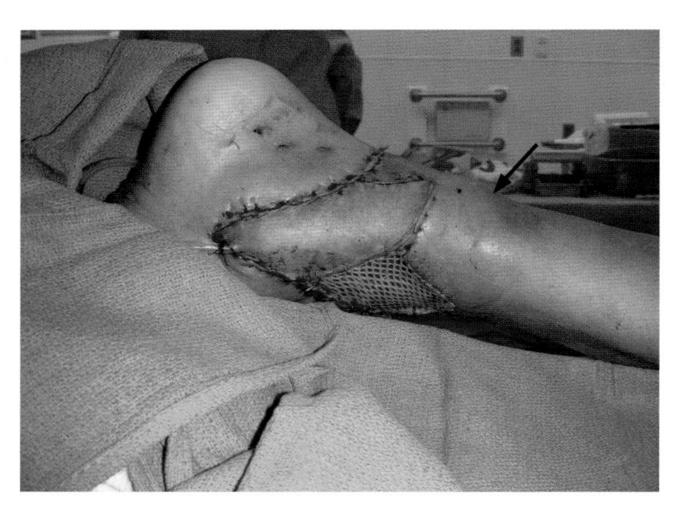

• **Fig. 48.3** An intraoperative view showing completion of the flap inset. In this case, the pedicle of the flap was also tunneled through the skin bridge (*arrow*).

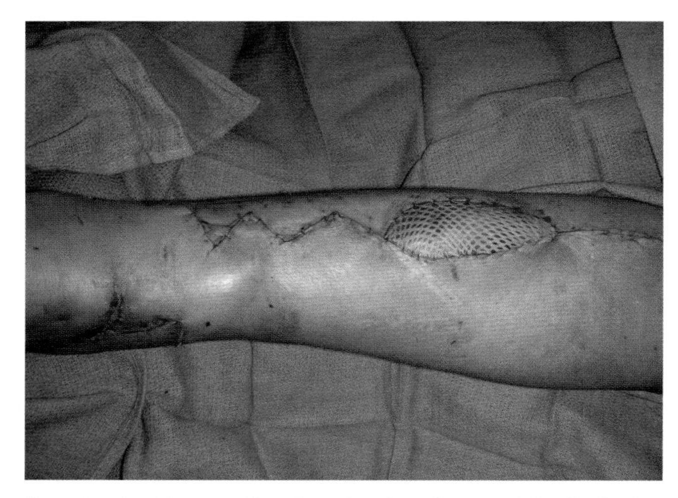

• **Fig. 48.4** An intraoperative view showing closure of the flap's donor site with a skin graft after undermining. The rest of the incisions were closed with interrupted sutures in two layers.

of the wound after skin grafting also healed well with no wound breakdown, recurrent infection, or contour issues related to the soft tissue flap reconstruction (Fig. 48.5). The flap donor site after skin grafting and primary closure also healed well (Fig. 48.6). The patient has resumed his weight-bearing status and returned to his normal activities as instructed.

Pearls for Success

An ankle complex soft tissue wound can also be reconstructed with a distally based sural artery flap if only skin coverage is needed. The skin island is elevated as a fasciocutaneous island flap with dual blood supplies: one is based on the lesser saphenous vein system and the other is based on the sural artery system. The adipofascial pedicle of the flap can be designed as narrow as 2 cm wide as long as both the lesser saphenous vein and the sural nerve systems are included and can be visualized. The pedicle is dissected free and can be tunneled under the skin bridge if there is

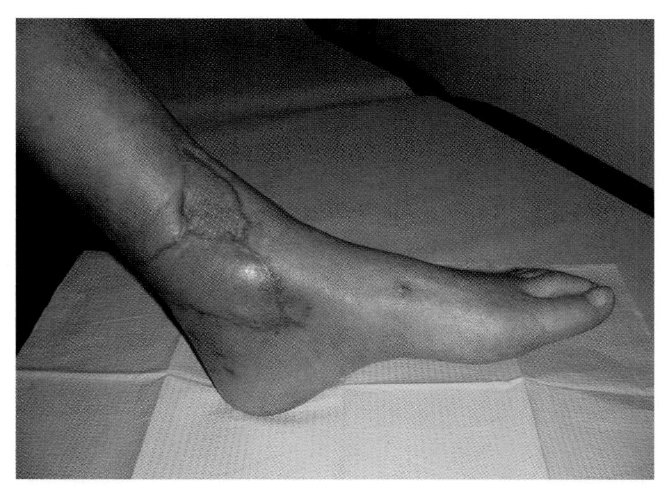

• **Fig. 48.5** Results at 5-month follow-up showing the well-healed left medial ankle wound with good contour and minimal scarring.

no significant compression to the pedicle of the flap. The donor site can be closed primarily after undermining if it is less than 5 cm wide or closed with a skin graft. Early venous congestion after a distally based sural artery flap is relatively common because the flap has been turned over. In case of prolonged postoperative venous congestion, application of topical nitroglycerin paste or medicinal leech therapy may be used. Inspection of the flap pedicle is required to ensure there is no direct compression. If venous congestion persists or worsens, the flap can be placed back to the donor site or a supercharge can be performed with microsurgical technique to augment venous drainage between the proximal lesser saphenous vein and an adjacent vein in the foot.

CASE 2

Clinical Presentation

A 29-year-old White male had a ruptured left Achilles tendon and underwent repair of the tendon by the orthopedic foot and ankle service. He unfortunately developed an open wound over the repaired tendon site with the exposed tendon (Fig. 48.7). The plastic surgery service was consulted to provide a soft tissue reconstruction for this posterior ankle wound as a first-stage reconstruction so that there would be a better soft tissue coverage over the future tendon repair site for a better chance of success after subsequent tendon reconstruction.

Operative Plan and Special Considerations

The primary requirement for soft tissue coverage in the posterior ankle over the Achilles tendon is a well-vascularized skin flap that should be thin, malleable, reliable, and resistant to direct trauma and sheer force. A free radial forearm skin flap can be selected for the purpose. It is versatile, and could provide reliable soft tissue coverage in the area with good contour after an easy flap inset and long-term healing. The flap has a long pedicle and both microvascular anastomoses to the posterior tibial vessels can be performed easily and comfortably. A preoperative angiogram was performed to determine a normal vascular anatomy with three vessels to the left foot.

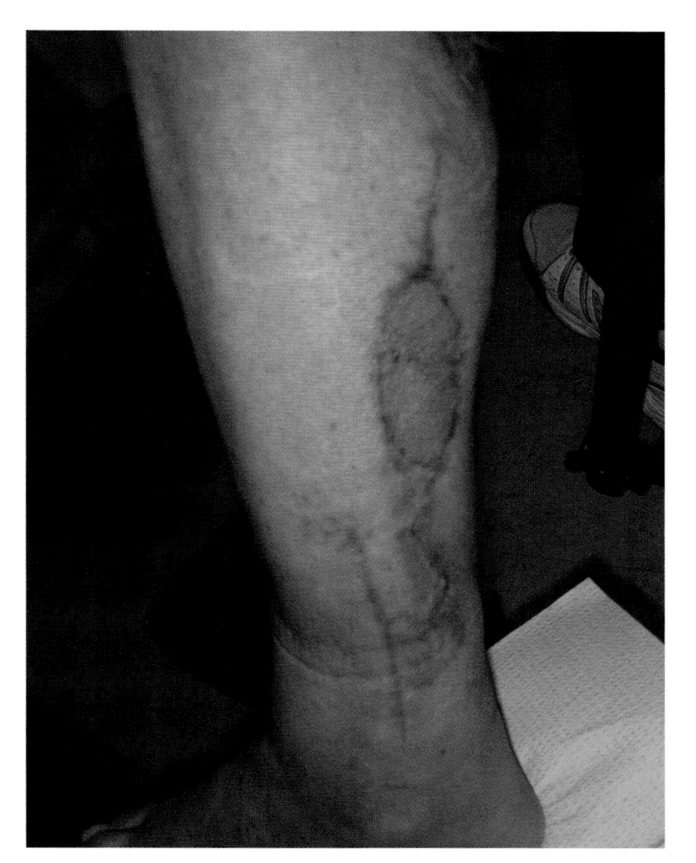

• **Fig. 48.6** Results at 5-month follow-up showing well-healed flap donor site with a skin graft and direct closure for the pedicle dissection site.

Operative Procedures

Under general anesthesia with the patient in the oblique position, the Achilles wound was debrided and all unhealthy-looking skin and the underlying necrotic tendon were excised. This left a posterior ankle wound, measuring 5 × 4 cm (Fig. 48.8). A free radial forearm skin flap was designed on the nondominant side of the left forearm after a negative Allen's test. A 7 × 6 cm skin paddle of the flap, oriented longitudinally, was marked (Fig. 48.9). The flap dissection was performed under tourniquet control. Once the skin incision had been made through the fascia, subfascial dissection was performed to elevate the skin paddle including the pedicle vessels that contained the cephalic vein. With a zigzag incision, the dissection of the pedicle in the forearm between the flexor carpi radialis muscle and brachioradialis muscle was performed toward the antecubital fossa. The radial artery and its venae comitantes as well as the cephalic vein were dissected free and ready to be divided before microvascular anastomoses.

The left posterior tibial vessels were explored in the left distal leg via an incision from the ankle wound extended proximally and longitudinally parallel to the medial board of the tibia. The posterior tibial artery and vein were easily identified between the medial soleus and flexor digitorum long muscles, were found to be in good condition, and were dissected out for an adequate length. Under a microscope, the arterial microanastomosis was performed between the pedicle artery and the posterior tibial artery in an end-to-side fashion with interrupted 8-0 nylon sutures. The venous microanastomosis was performed between the cephalic

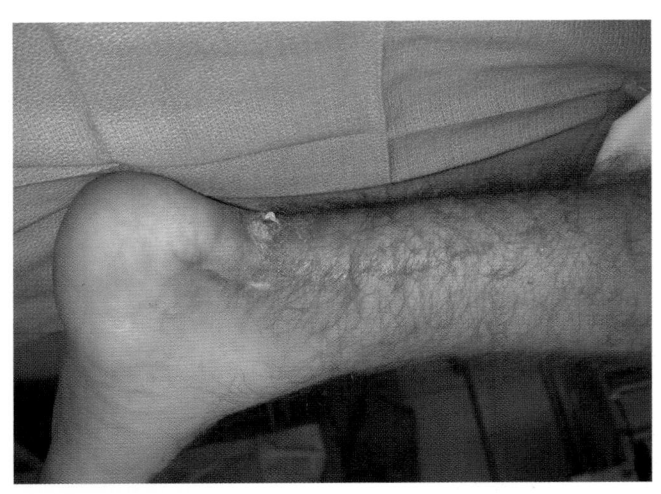

• **Fig. 48.7** A preoperative view showing a wound breakdown over the reconstructed Achilles tendon site with unhealthy-looking skin in the area.

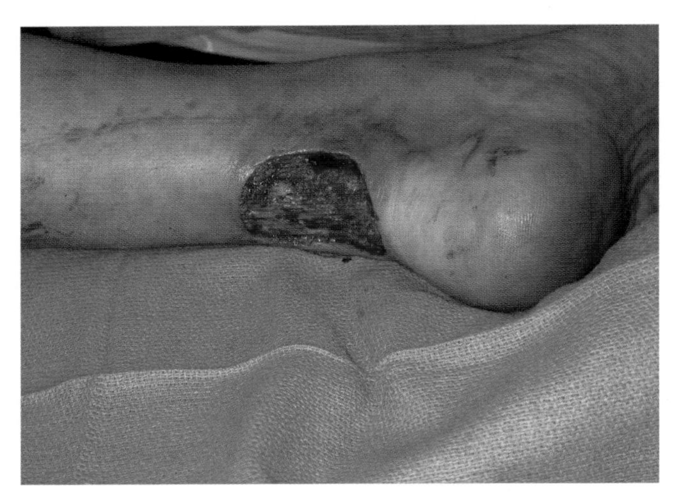

• **Fig. 48.8** Intraoperative view showing the completion of the wound debridement that had left a 5 × 4 cm skin defect in the posterior ankle.

vein and the posterior tibial vein in an end-to-end fashion with interrupted 8-0 nylon sutures (Fig. 48.10).

The flap inset was performed next. The flap was approximated to the adjacent wound edges with a 3-0 Vicryl suture in an interrupted half-buried horizontal mattress fashion. One drain was placed under the flap. A portion of the flap's pedicle, measuring 3 × 2 cm, was covered with a skin graft (Fig. 48.11).

The forearm skin incision for the pedicle dissection was closed in two layers. A unmeshed split-thickness skin graft, harvested from the left lateral thigh, was placed on the flap donor site and secured with a tie-over dressing.

Follow-Up Results

The patient did well postoperatively without any complications related to the free radial forearm flap reconstruction. He was discharged from the hospital on postoperative day 7 after successful dangling. The drain was removed during the first-week follow-up. The posterior ankle wound flap site and the left forearm flap donor site healed well. The patient underwent a delayed

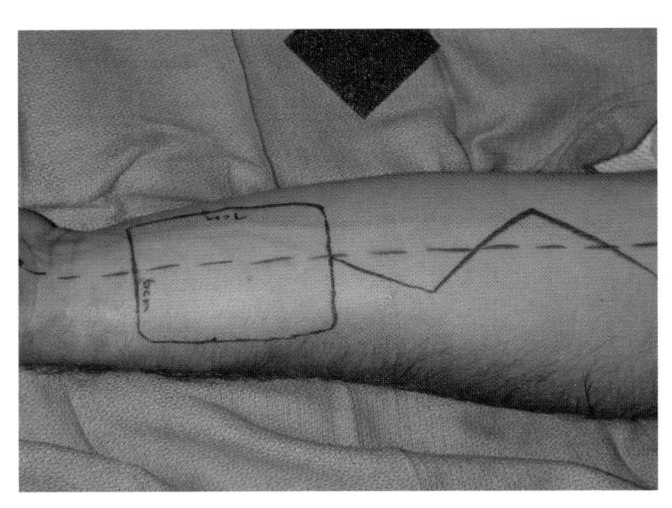

• **Fig. 48.9** Intraoperative view showing the design of the left radial forearm free flap and the incision for the pedicle dissection.

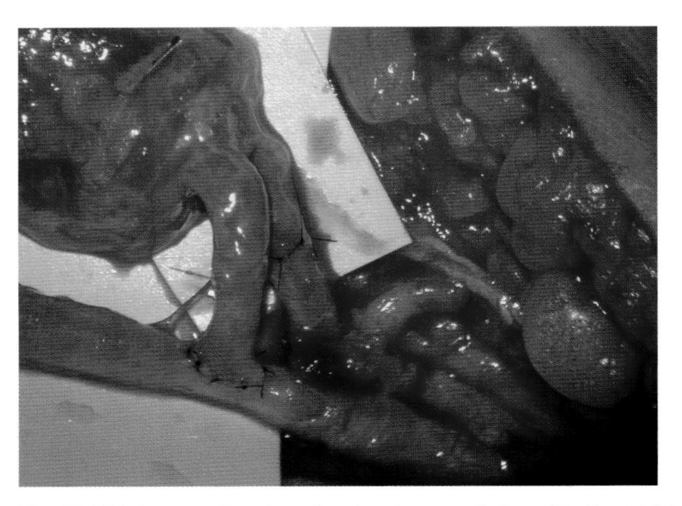

• **Fig. 48.10** Intraoperative view showing the completion of both arterial (end-to-side) and venous (end-to-end) microvascular anastomoses under a microscope.

Achilles tendon reconstruction by the orthopedic foot and ankle service 6 weeks after the initial soft tissue reconstruction. The flap was elevated again by the plastic surgery service for the tendon reconstruction by the orthopedic foot and ankle service.

Final Outcome

The left posterior ankle wound healed well with good contour and minimal scarring (Fig. 48.12). The left forearm flap donor site also healed well with minimal scarring (Fig. 48.13). His left ankle looked almost normal after the two-stage reconstruction including soft tissue coverage and tendon reconstruction. He has returned to his normal activities and has been routinely followed by the orthopedic foot and ankle service.

Pearls for Success

A free radial forearm skin flap can be an excellent choice for soft tissue coverage of a complex ankle wound. The flap can be

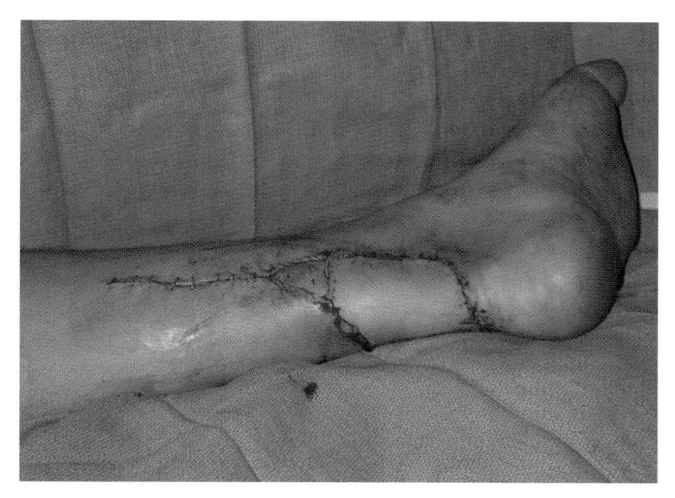

• **Fig. 48.11** Intraoperative view showing the completion of the flap reconstruction for the left posterior ankle wound, skin graft to the portion of the pedicle, and closure of the incision.

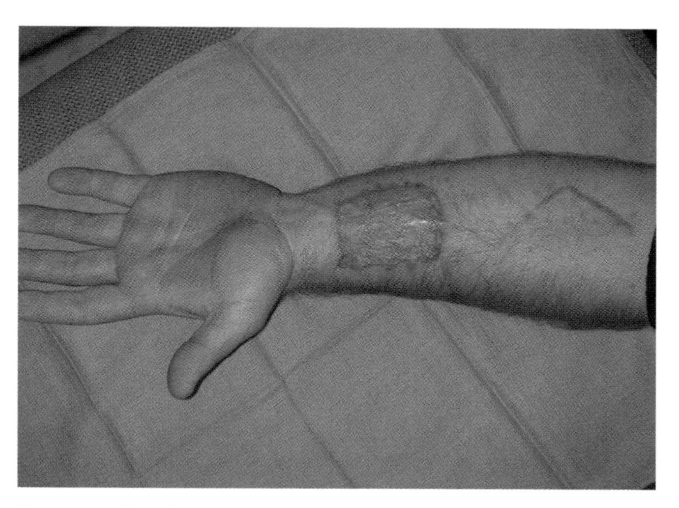

• **Fig. 48.13** Results at 4-month follow-up showing a well-healed radial forearm flap donor site with good contour and minimal scaring.

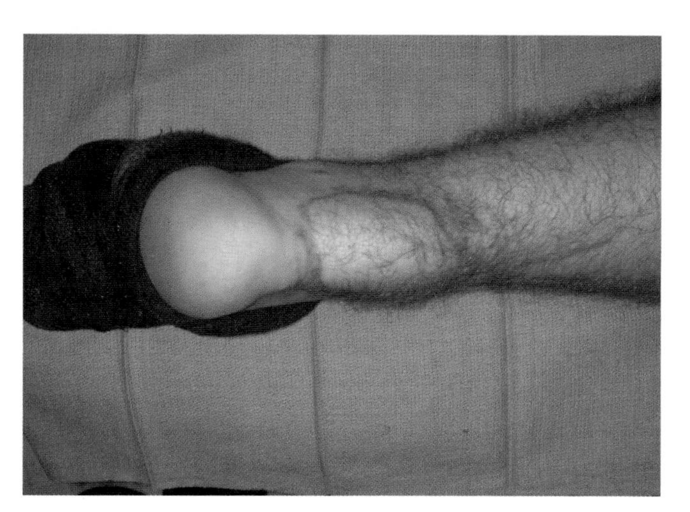

• **Fig. 48.12** Results at 4-month follow-up showing a stable soft tissue reconstruction over the posterior ankle with good contour and minimal scarring.

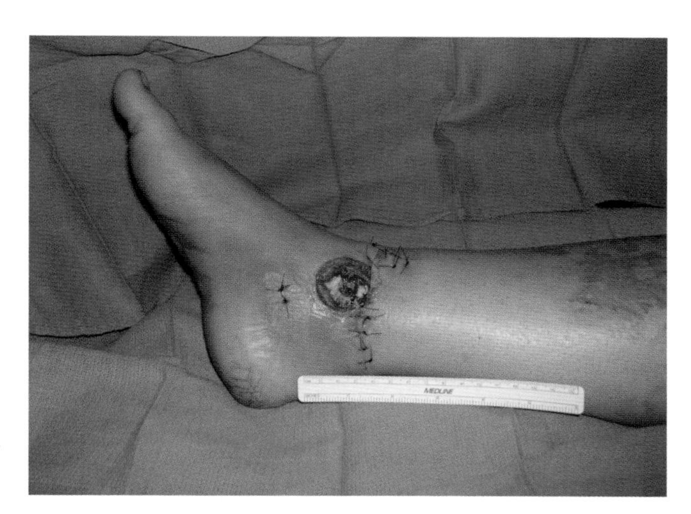

• **Fig. 48.14** A preoperative view showing a 3 × 3 cm complex soft tissue wound over the right medial malleolus with exposed underlying tibia.

harvested quickly and provide a thin and malleable soft tissue coverage for the area. The fascia can be included via a subfascial dissection. It may provide a gliding service for future tendon reconstruction. The cephalic vein is generally considered a dominant vein of the radial forearm flap and should be used for venous drainage. The contour of the flap several months after reconstruction can be quite good, with no further flap debulking needed. The flap to adjacent wound edges can be closed in a single layer. A small portion of the pedicle can be skin-grafted if needed. Delayed wound healing may develop in the flap donor site if subfascial dissection is used for the entire flap harvest. The flap donor site after a subfascial dissection can be closed temporarily with Integra and vacuum-assisted closure (VAC) and then subsequent skin grafting. Such a composite tissue defect in the posterior ankle can also be reconstructed with a free anterolateral thigh perforator flap with fascial component as a one-stage procedure.

CASE 3

Clinical Presentation

A 52-year-old White female was involved in a motor vehicle accident and sustained a right ankle fracture associated with soft tissue loss, in addition to a closed head injury and left acetabular fracture. She had a 3 × 3 cm open wound over the right medial malleolus with an exposed underlying tibia (Fig. 48.14). She had several major medical conditions that would limit a lengthy reconstructive option for soft tissue coverage. A lateral leg incision between the lateral malleolus and the midline of the posterior leg had been made by the orthopedic foot and ankle service for open reduction and internal fixation of the ankle fracture. The plastic surgery service was consulted to provide soft tissue coverage over the medial malleolus as a definitive reconstruction.

Operative Plan and Special Considerations for Reconstruction

Although a free tissue transfer could be an option for this type of wound, the patient's multiple major medical conditions would prevent her from such an extensive and lengthy reconstructive operation for soft tissue coverage of this small medial malleolar wound. One of the good options, such as a distally based sural artery flap, would not be reliable because there was a surgical scar along the course of the lesser saphenous vein in the lateral leg. Both VAC and artificial dermis (Integra, Integra LifeSciences, NJ) have been used by reconstructive surgeons in the management of a complex wound in the lower extremity with some success. Therefore, artificial dermis and VAC, and subsequent skin graft can serve as an alternative approach for soft-tissue reconstruction of a complex wound in the foot and ankle with the exposed bone. These combined procedures could be an innovative approach to this complex wound coverage and would be much simpler and less extensive for the patient.

Operative Procedures

Under general anesthesia, with the patient in the supine position, the medial malleolus wound of the right leg was debrided. The wound edge was freshened with a blade and all colonized tissue was removed with a curette. The exposed tibia was also debrided with a powered burr. The wound was then irrigated with Pulsavac (Fig. 48.15).

A proper size of artificial dermis was prepared and placed over the medial malleolus wound according to the instructions provided by the manufacturer. The silicone sheet was facing out and the Integra was approximated to the adjacent skin edge of the wound with skin staples. Several small openings through the silicone sheet were made with a knife for possible drainage (Fig. 48.16). A VAC sponge (KCI, TX) was placed directly over the silicone sheet of the Integra and the wound was maintained at continuous subatmospheric pressure (125 mmHg) provided by a VAC machine (KCI Inc., San Antonio, TX).

The patient was discharged immediately after the procedure for home VAC therapy. The VAC sponge was changed every 3 days by the patient supervised by home health nurses. The wound was examined every week by the surgeon in the clinic. It took 3 weeks until a well-vascularized tissue bed was noted under the silicone sheet.

After 3-week serial outpatient follow-ups, a simple skin-grafting procedure was planned subsequently at an outpatient surgery. The patient was taken back to the operating room. Again, under general anesthesia, with the patient in the supine position, the VAC sponge was removed. After removing the silicone sheet, the previously exposed bone was covered with the neodermis and such a well-vascularized wound bed would clearly take a skin graft (Fig. 48.17). A proper size of a split-thickness skin graft was harvested from the right lateral thigh with a dermatome. The skin graft was meshed to 1:1.5 ratio and placed on the wound bed and approximated to the wound skin edges with multiple skin staples (Fig. 48.18). An occlusive dressing was placed on the skin graft and no further VAC therapy was needed.

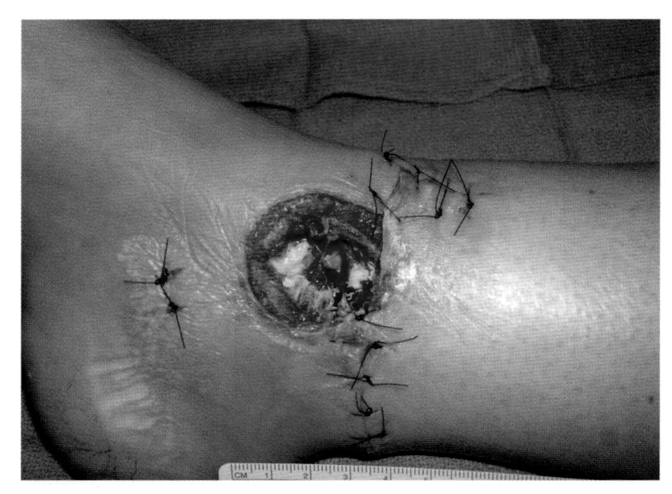

• **Fig. 48.15** An intraoperative close-up view showing completion of definitive wound debridement including the underlying tibia.

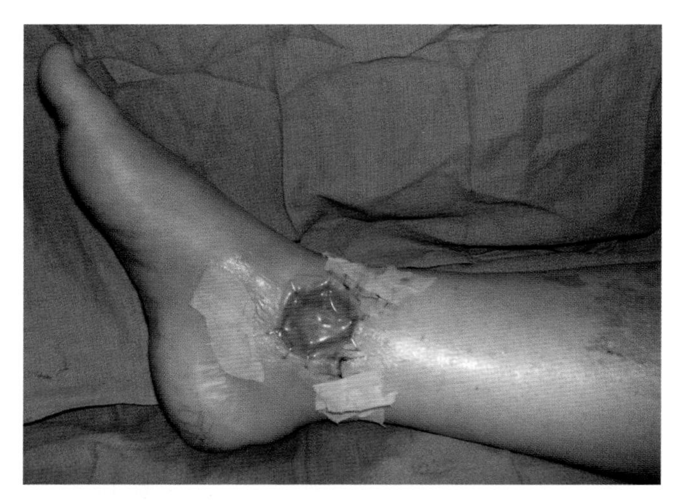

• **Fig. 48.16** An intraoperative view showing that an Integra was securely placed over the medial malleolar wound after adequate wound debridement.

Follow-Up Results

The patient did well postoperatively without any issues related to the skin graft site. She was discharged from hospital after the outpatient procedure. The medial malleolus wound of the right leg healed uneventfully (Fig. 48.19). She was followed by the plastic surgery service for routine postoperative skin graft care and by the orthopedic trauma service for orthopedic care.

Final Outcome

During further follow-up, the right medial malleolus wound after the combination of Integra placement and continuous VAC treatment, and subsequent skin graft had healed well with good contour and minimal scarring. There was no wound breakdown, recurrent infection, or contour issues related to the soft tissue reconstruction with this innovative technique (Fig. 48.20). She has resumed her normal weight-bearing status and returned to her normal activities.

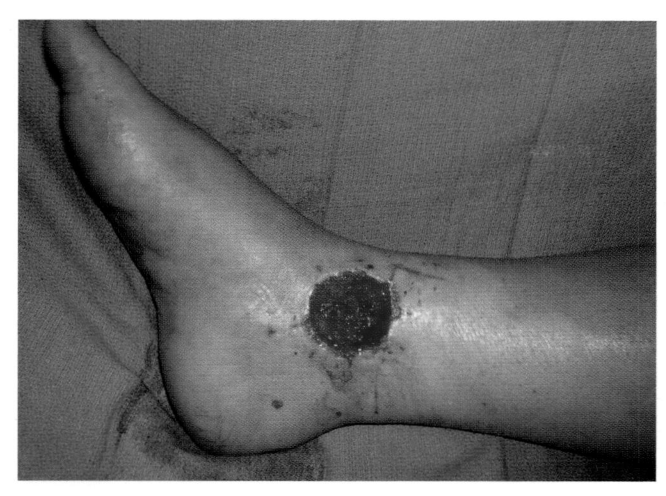

• **Fig. 48.17** An intraoperative view showing that a well-vascularized wound bed had developed after removal of the silicone sheet 3 weeks after the VAC therapy over the Integra.

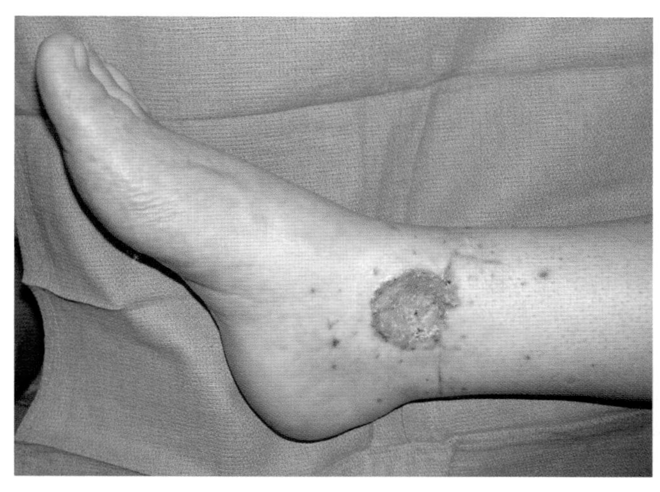

• **Fig. 48.19** Results at 4-week follow-up showing a well-healed wound in the right medial ankle.

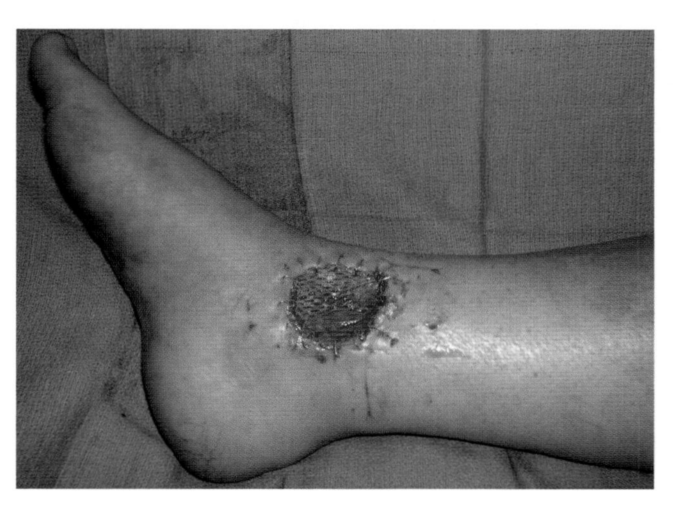

• **Fig. 48.18** An intraoperative view showing completion of a split-thickness skin graft placement over the wound bed.

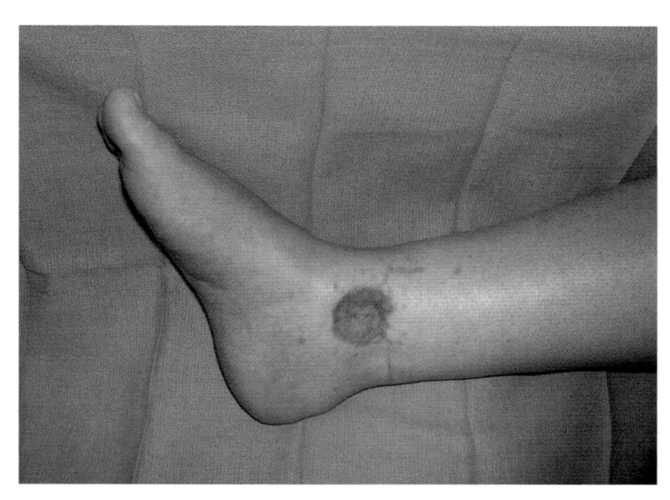

• **Fig. 48.20** Results at 3.5-month follow-up showing a well-healed and stable wound coverage over the medial malleolus with excellent contour.

Pearls for Success

The VAC therapy over artificial dermis and subsequent skin graft can be an alternative approach to a free-tissue transfer for soft tissue coverage of a limited foot and ankle wound associated with an exposed bone, especially when free-tissue transfer is not an option due to the patient's medical conditions. It may offer a simplified approach to managing such a unique but complex clinical problem. VAC therapy has been demonstrated to improve vascularity, to decrease edema and infection rates, to speed up wound closure, and to optimize skin-graft take by enhancing its contact with the wound bed. The application of the VAC to the tissue-engineered skin substitute, such as Integra, might result in fast healing of a wound where Integra is placed for a temporary wound closure. A well-vascularized wound bed can be developed usually within 3 weeks after Integra placement for a cutaneous wound. However, it may take longer in certain areas of the body if a wound bed has less potential to become fully vascularized. Based on the author's clinical experience, the application of the VAC to a wound with the underlying bone exposed where Integra is placed for temporary coverage, a true vascularization of the wound bed requires more time than a cutaneous wound for the development of an optimal recipient bed for the skin graft to take.

Recommended Readings

Gazzini L, Dallari V, Fazio E. How I do it: harvesting of radial forearm free flap. *Eur Ann Otorhinolaryngol Head Neck Dis.* 2021;138(suppl 2):47–48.

Korompilias A, Gkiatas I, Korompilia M, Kosmas D, Kostas-Agnantis I. Reverse sural artery flap: a reliable alternative for foot and ankle soft tissue reconstruction. *Eur J Orthop Surg Traumatol.* 2019;29:367–372.

Pu LLQ. Locoregional flaps in lower extremity reconstruction. *Clin Plast Surg*. 2021;48:157–171.

Pu LL. An alternative approach for soft-tissue coverage of a complex wound in the foot and ankle with vacuum-assisted closure over artificial dermis and subsequent skin graft. *J Plast Reconstr Aesthet Surg*. 2009;62:e682–e684.

Weinzweig N, Davies BW. Foot and ankle reconstruction using the radial forearm flap: a review of 25 cases. *Plast Reconstr Surg*. 1998;102: 1999–2005.

49

Complex Ankle Reconstruction

CASE 1

Clinical Presentation

A 28-year-old White male had a complex left foot open fracture wound as a result of a motor vehicle accident. He suffered an avulsion injury of the left medial ankle with underlying comminuted fractures. There was significate bone loss and lack of continuity of bony structures with an open wound measuring 15 × 8 cm (Fig. 49.1). The plastic surgery service was consulted for soft tissue coverage because the limb salvage would depend on it. He was brought to the operating room by the orthopedic foot and ankle service for ankle orthopedic reconstruction with primary bony fusion followed by a free tissue transfer to this large medial ankle wound by the plastic surgery service.

Operative Plan and Special Considerations

For such a large and complex soft tissue wound in the medial ankle, the primary soft tissue reconstructive option would be a free tissue transfer because there was no local option available to provide the reliable soft tissue coverage critical for limb salvage. As a contemporary reconstructive option, an anterolateral thigh (ALT) perforator flap can be selected to provide a good and reliable soft tissue coverage for this large open fracture ankle wound. The flap has a long pedicle and can provide a relatively large amount of the fasciocutaneous tissue for reliable soft tissue coverage of such a wound. Because a preoperative CT angiogram showed that the patient had a normal three vessels' leg, the distal posterior tibial artery could be selected as a recipient vessel for an end-to-side arterial microanastomosis near the ankle soft tissue defect. A preoperative duplex scan could be performed to determine which side of the thigh should be selected as a donor site for an ALT perforator flap based on the size and blood flow of the perforator identified and the amount of intramuscular perforator dissection required.

Operative Procedures

Under general anesthesia, with the patient in the supine position, the soft tissue reconstructive procedure started by debriding the wound located in the medial ankle. All unhealthy-looking skin edges were freshly debrided and the wound was then irrigated with Pulsavac.

The posterior tibial artery and vein were explored first. The skin incision was extended proximally from the medial ankle wound and both vessel dissections were performed between the medial soleus and flexor digitorum longus muscles. Both the posterior tibial artery and vena comitans were carefully prepared under loupe magnification and were ready for microvascular anastomoses.

Based on a preoperative duplex scan finding, the left ALT perforator flap was designed. A 20 × 8 cm skin paddle was marked (Fig. 49.2). Two perforators were confirmed by an intraoperative Doppler scan. The incision was made around the skin paddle down to the fascia. Suprafascial dissection was performed toward the perforators. Around those two medially located perforators, the intramuscular dissection was performed through the rectus femoris muscle. After at least 7 cm of intramuscular dissection with proper traction of the pedicle and by splitting the muscles between the rectus femoris and vastus lateralis muscles, the perforator was found to join the descending branch of the lateral circumflex femoral vessels (Fig. 49.3). The distal descending branch of the circumflex femoral vessels was divided and dissection was continued further along the pedicle toward the profunda vessels. A 12-cm pedicle of the flap was obtained and divided with medium-sized clips off the profunda (Fig. 49.4). During dissection, motor nerves to the vastus lateralis muscle were completely spared. The pedicle of the flap was then prepared under loupe magnification and the artery was flushed with heparinized saline.

The flap was temporarily inset into the wound. The pedicle and recipient vessels were prepared for microvascular anastomoses under an operating microscope. The arterial microanastomosis was performed between the pedicle artery and the posterior tibial artery in an end-to-side fashion with interrupted 8-0 nylon sutures after the correct size of arteriotomy on the posterior tibial artery was well prepared. The venous microanastomosis was performed between the pedicle vein and the posterior tibial vein with a 2.5-mm coupler device in an end-to-end fashion (Fig. 49.5). After releasing all clamps, the flap appeared well perfused with a strong Doppler signal.

A drain was placed under the flap and the entire flap was inset into the left medial ankle wound and sutured to the adjacent skin edges with several interrupted 3-0 Monocryl sutures in half-buried mattress fashion as a single-layer closure. The skin incision in the distal leg over both microvascular anastomoses was approximated with several interrupted 3-0 Monocryl sutures (Fig. 49.6).

The left thigh flap donor site was closed primarily. The transected portion of the rectus femoris muscle was approximated with several interrupted 2-0 Vicryl sutures. A fascial layer opening was approximated with several interrupted 3-0 PDS sutures and

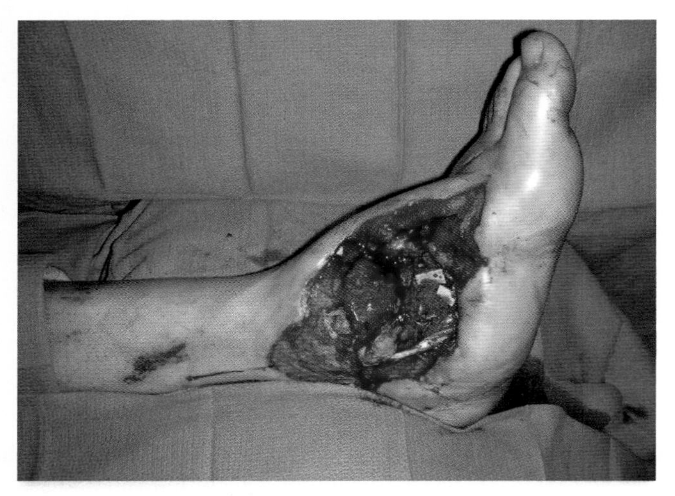

• **Fig. 49.1** A preoperative view showing a 15 × 8 cm complex soft tissue wound in the left medial ankle associated with underlying comminuted fractures.

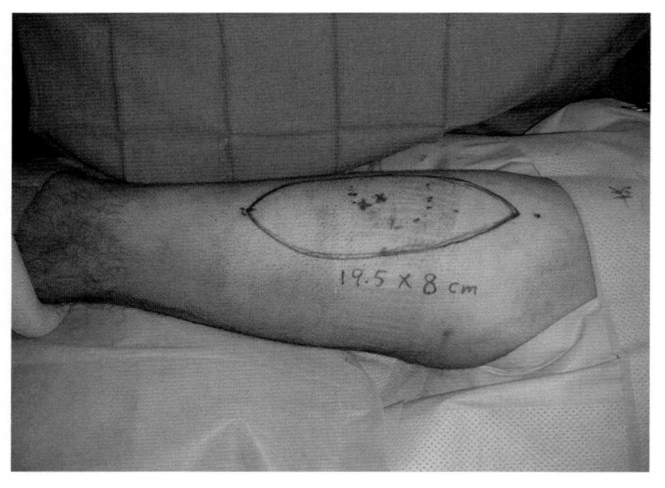

• **Fig. 49.2** An intraoperative view showing the design of the left anterolateral thigh perforator flap. The skin paddle of the flap was 20 × 8 cm. Two large perforators were identified by the preoperative duplex scan.

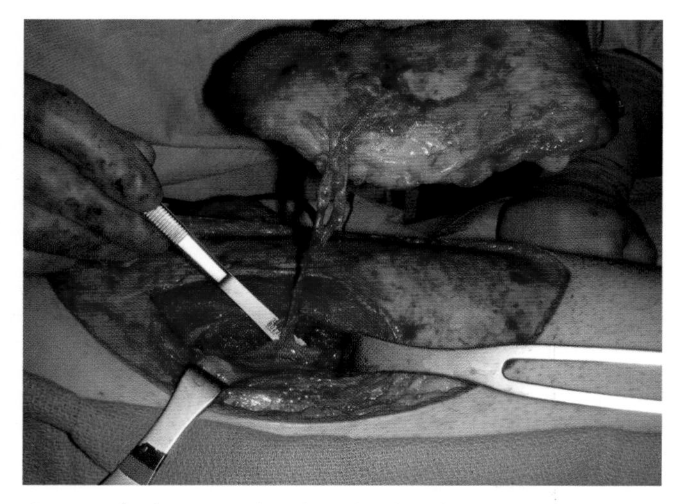

• **Fig. 49.3** An intraoperative view showing the successful perforator dissection. Both perforators formed a single perforator that joined the descending branch of the lateral circumflex femoral artery.

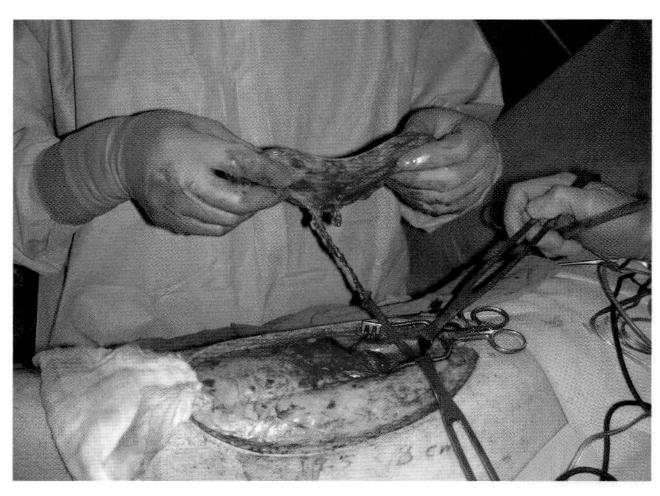

• **Fig. 49.4** An intraoperative view showing near completion for the anterolateral thigh flap dissection. The pedicle length of the flap was 12 cm.

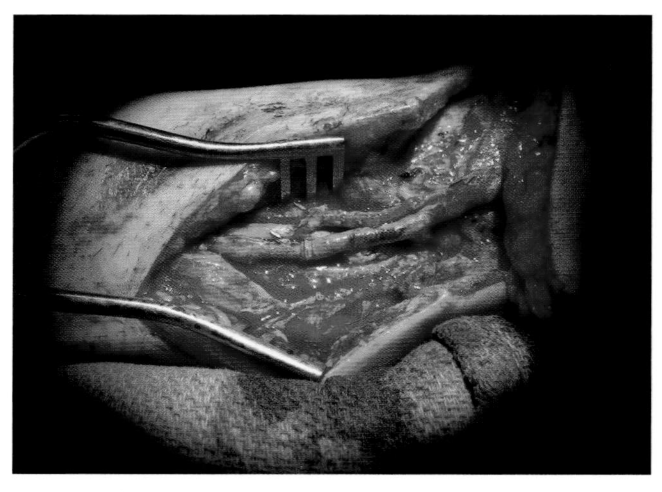

• **Fig. 49.5** An intraoperative view showing completion of successful microvascular anastomoses. The arterial microanastomosis was end-to-side with 8-0 nylon sutures and the venous microanastomosis was end-to-end with a coupler device.

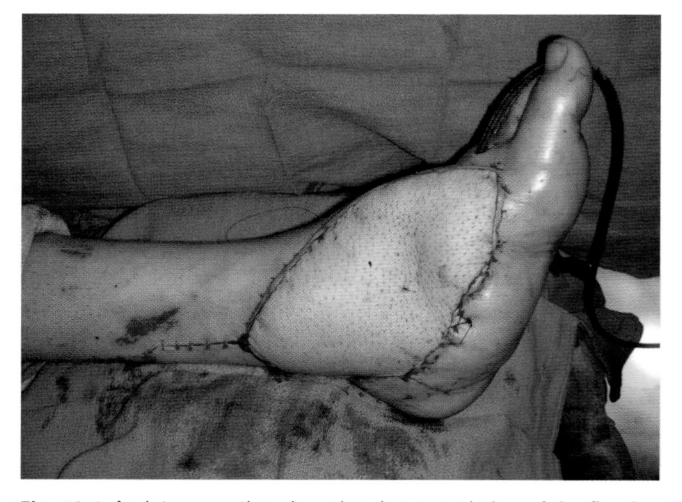

• **Fig. 49.6** An intraoperative view showing completion of the flap inset and incision closure at the end of the procedure.

the subcutaneous closure was performed with interrupted 3-0 Monocryl sutures. The skin closure was performed with 3-0 Monocryl in a running subcuticular fashion (Fig. 49.7).

Follow-Up Results

The patient did well postoperatively without any complications related to the free ALT flap transfer. He was discharged from hospital on postoperative day 12 after tolerating dangling protocol. The drain was removed during a subsequent follow-up office visit. The flap reconstruction site over the left medial ankle healed well (Fig. 49.8).

Final Outcome

The left medial ankle wound after a free ALT flap reconstruction healed well with good contour and minimal scarring (Fig. 49.9). The patient underwent further autologous bone grafting for the ankle bony reconstruction. Eventually, the ankle fracture site also healed. No flap debulking procedure was needed (Fig. 49.10). The left thigh ALT flap donor site also healed well with minimal scarring (Fig. 49.11). He has resumed his normal activities and has routinely been followed by the orthopedic foot and ankle service.

Pearls for Success

A free ALT perforator flap can be an excellent option for soft tissue reconstruction of a complex ankle wound. The flap is large enough and can be harvested as a cutaneous flap to provide reliable soft tissue coverage of a large and complex ankle wound. The ALT perforator flap can been replace a free muscle as the first line reconstructive option as long as the surgeon feels comfortable to perform the flap dissection. A preoperative duplex scan can be performed to determine the best and easiest site that can be selected as an ALT flap donor site for free tissue transfer because the size, blood flow, and location of a perforator as well as potential course of intramuscular perforator dissection can be determined and selected. This has made the ALT perforator dissection more predictable and less time-consuming. An end-to-side arterial microanastomosis could also be performed without difficulty because the posterior tibial artery is located adjacent to the ankle. In a relatively slim young adult patient, a future flap debulking procedure may not be necessary and the contour of the ankle after such a flap reconstruction can be quite good in the long term.

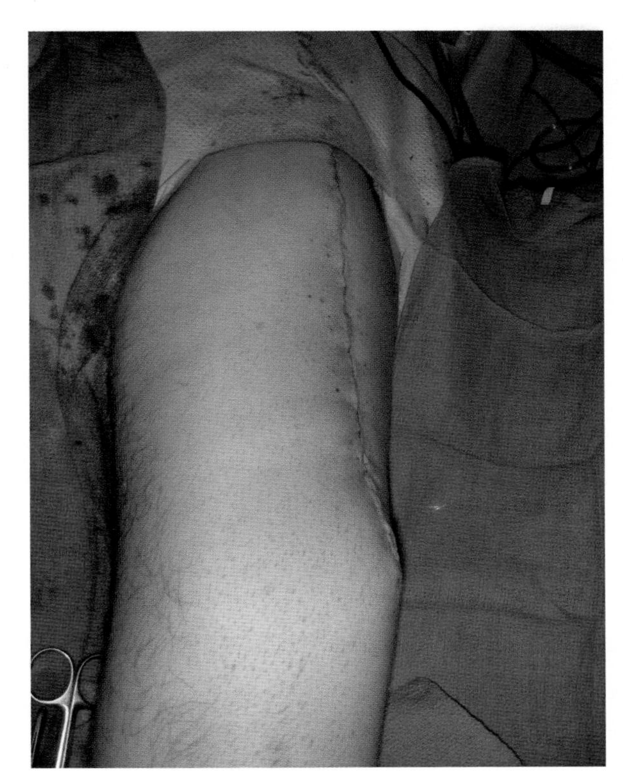

• **Fig. 49.7** An intraoperative view showing completion of the left thigh flap donor site closure.

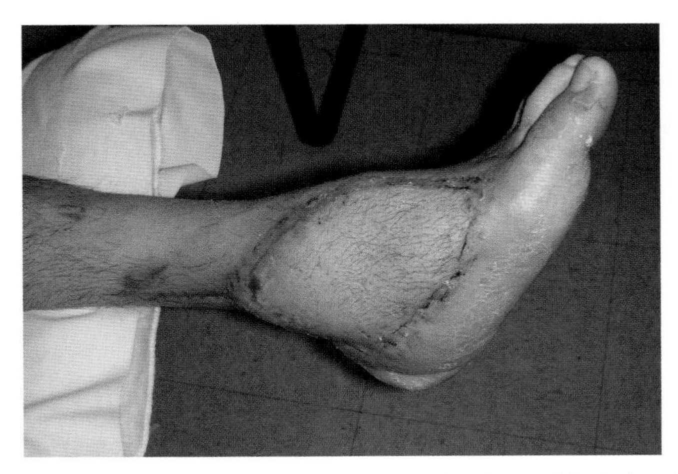

• **Fig. 49.8** The result at 7-week follow-up showing well-healed and stable left medial ankle wound after a successful free anterolateral thigh flap transfer.

CASE 2

Clinical Presentation

A 17-year-old African-American male had type I neurofibromatosis with multiple subcutaneous neurofibromas throughout his body. He presented to the plastic surgery service complaining of pain and deformity of his left foot and ankle, where a large, recurrent plexiform neurofibroma affected his left medial ankle and heel. The mass was interfering with walking and wearing shoes. A debulking procedure with a primary closure had been performed by another surgeon approximately 5 years previously for the same complaints, but local recurrence had developed gradually over the years. He now experienced increased symptoms and deformity of the affected area. On physical examination, there was a large, 24 × 22 cm plexiform neurofibroma involving most of the left medial ankle and heel (Fig. 49.12). A neurovascular examination of the left foot confirmed that the vessels were not compromised. The range of motion of the left ankle was within normal limits. Preoperative plain X-ray images showed a slightly flattened calcaneus without bony involvement (Fig. 49.13). A magnetic resonance image showed a large mass involving the medial and posterior aspects of the foot and ankle, which extended to the tibialis posterior, flexor hallucis longus, and flexor

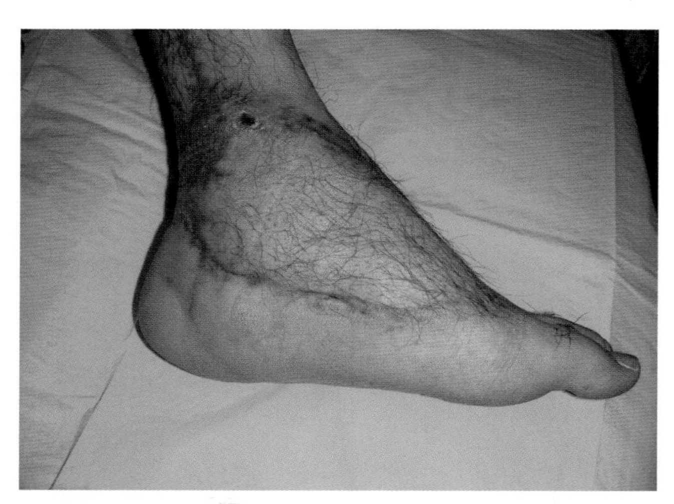

• **Fig. 49.9** The result at 4-month follow-up showing well-healed and stable left medial ankle wound after a free anterolateral thigh flap transfer with good contour and minimal scarring.

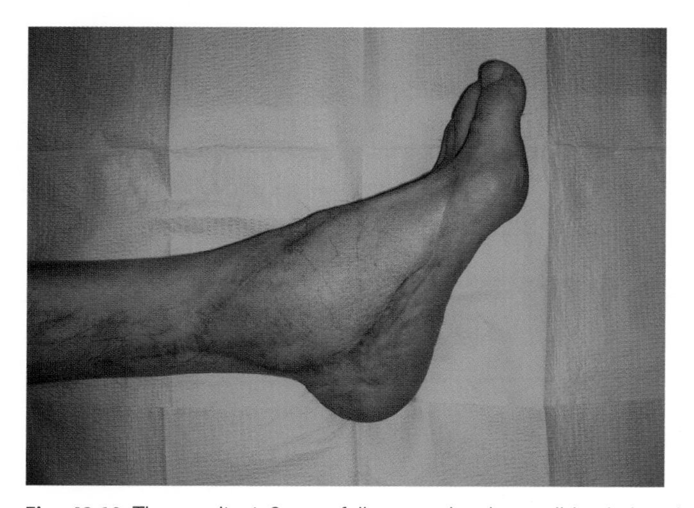

• **Fig. 49.10** The result at 8-year follow-up showing well-healed and stable left medial ankle wound after a free anterolateral thigh flap transfer with excellent contour.

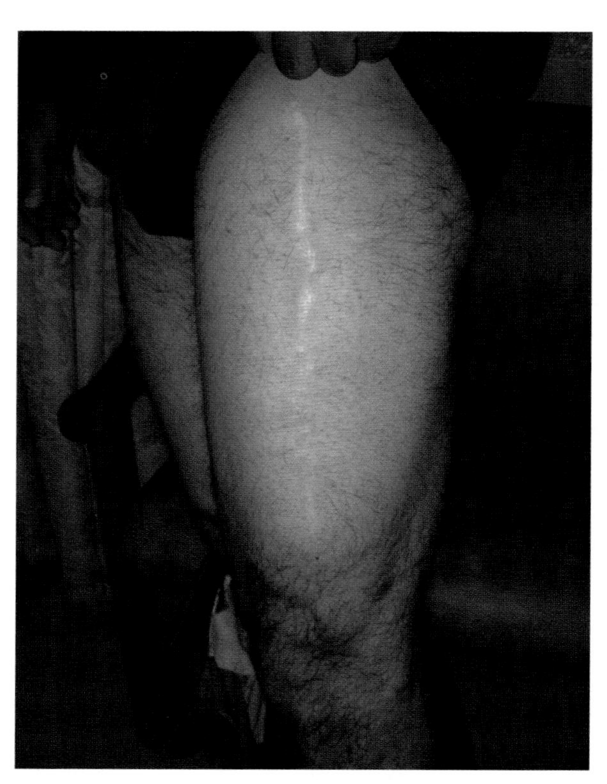

• **Fig. 49.11** The result at 8-year follow-up showing the appearance of the left thigh flap donor site with almost no scarring.

digitorum longus (Fig. 49.14). The left lower extremity angiogram showed a patent but hypertrophied and distorted distal posterior tibial artery (Fig. 49.15). The clinical diagnosis of the left foot and ankle mass was consistent with recurrent plexiform neurofibroma. A radical resection of the recurrent neurofibroma and subsequent soft tissue reconstruction were planned.

Operative Plan and Special Considerations

Because this patient had recurrent neurofibroma after the previous debulking procedure, a radical resection should be performed this time to prevent future recurrence as long as there would be no injury to the posterior tibial vessels and tibia nerve during resection. It would be an anticipated large soft tissue defect with the exposed ankle joint, underlying bones, and vital neurovascular structures. A free latissimus dorsi muscle flap could be selected to provide good and reliable soft tissue coverage for potentially exposed underlying structures. The flap should be large enough to cover the soft tissue defect after resection of the recurrent neurofibroma. Surgical dissection of the posterior tibial vessels would be involved during the surgical resection of the neurofibroma. These vessels could be dissected further proximally to the area outside the zone of the neurofibroma and be prepared as recipient vessels for microvascular anastomoses. Because of anticipated length of the operation for both resection and reconstruction, two-stage procedures were planned for this patient. Future flap debulking procedures may be necessary if the flap remains bulky for a long time.

Operative Procedures

The first-stage procedure focused on radical resection of neurofibroma in the foot and ankle. Under general anesthesia, with the patient in the supine position, the resection was performed under tourniquet control. The posterior tibial vessels and tibial nerve were first identified in the unaffected area proximal to the tumor. A lengthy dissection was carried out in order to free neurovascular structures from the tumor in an antegrade fashion. Last, a formal neurolysis of the tibia nerve was performed. In order to achieve complete resection of the tumor, the dissection actually went into the ankle joint capsule. Additional resection of the tumor was performed around the tibialis posterior, flexor hallucis longus, and flexor digitorum longus, and a formal tenolysis was performed for each of the tendons. The entire resection of the tumor took approximately 6 hours with inflation and deflation of the tourniquet three times. The surgical resection was quite difficult because the neurofibroma tissues were diffuse, hard, adherent to the tibial nerve or joint

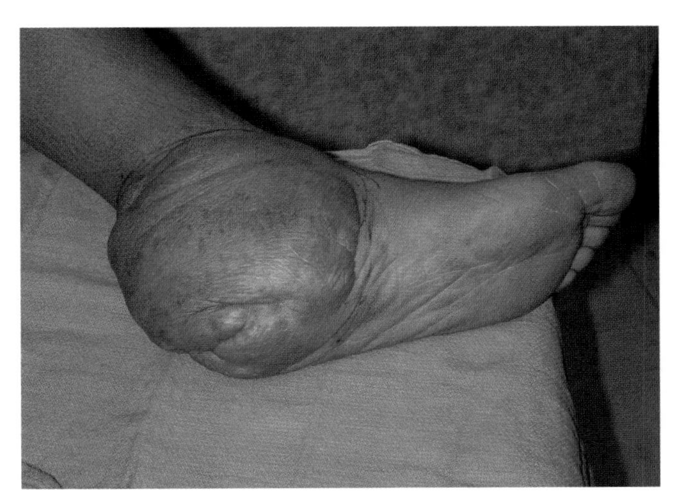

• **Fig. 49.12** Preoperative view of the left foot and ankle showing a large recurrent plexiform neurofibroma, measuring 24 × 22 cm, involving both medial and posterior aspects of left ankle and heel.

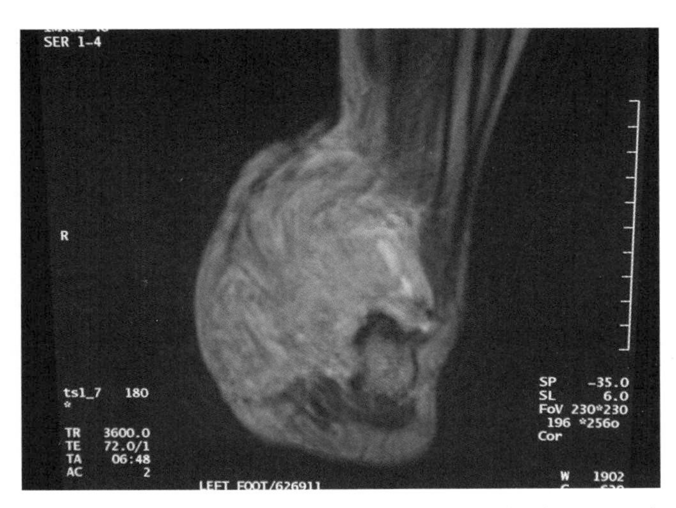

• **Fig. 49.14** Preoperative MRI of coronal view showing extensive involvement of plexiform neurofibroma in left foot and ankle.

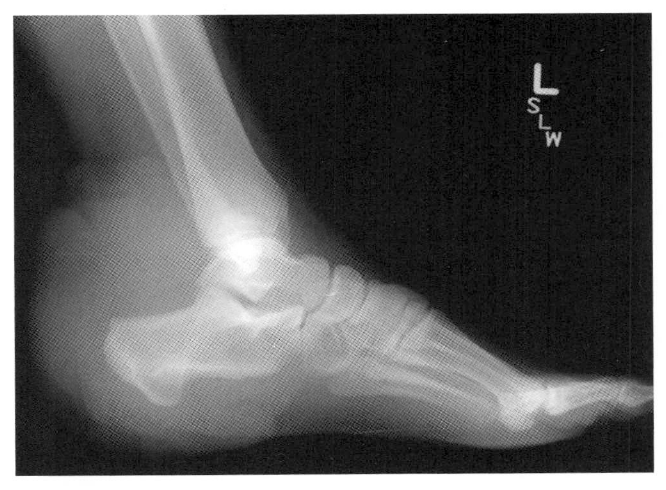

• **Fig. 49.13** Preoperative X-ray image showing a large soft tissue mass in left foot and ankle but with no bony involvement.

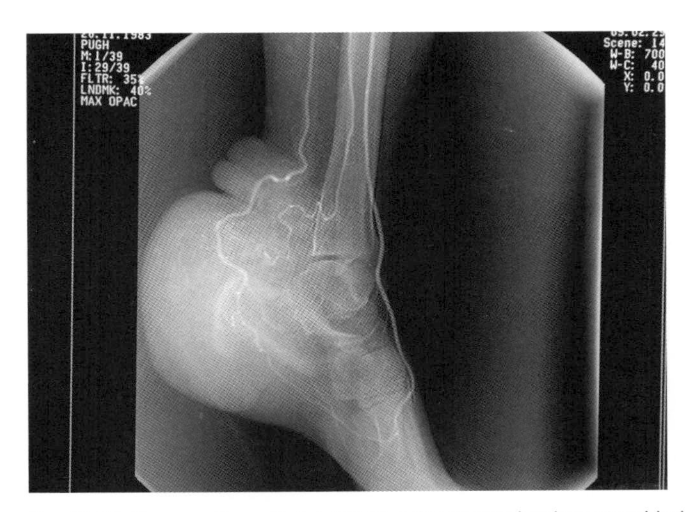

• **Fig. 49.15** Preoperative arteriogram showing patent but hypertrophied and distorted distal posterior tibial artery.

capsule, and bleeding extensively even under tourniquet control. There was significant blood loss during the neurofibroma resection.

A complete resection of this recurrent neurofibroma was accomplished. The posterior tibial vessels in the distal leg were dissected free and could serve as recipient vessels for the subsequent free tissue transfer. The proximal skin incision was closed with skin staples (Figs. 49.16A and B). At the end of the resection, a skin allograft was used to cover the patient's ankle and heel soft-tissue defect temporarily. Only clear gross margins were accomplished during the resection and negative microscopic margins were not attempted. The final pathology report confirmed the clinical diagnosis of plexiform neurofibroma.

Because there would be significantly prolonged surgery for resection of the tumor and subsequent soft tissue reconstruction of the foot and ankle defect in one operation, the soft tissue reconstruction was delayed. The patient was brought back to the operating room 2 days later, when a free left latissimus dorsi muscle flap from his nondominant side was harvested.

Under general anesthesia, with the patient in the right lateral decubitus position, an incision was made down to the latissimus dorsi muscle fascia. After identifying the medial and lateral borders of the latissimus muscle, the muscle was divided medially, inferiorly, and laterally. Under direct vision, the latissimus dorsi muscle was elevated from the chest wall and the serratus muscle was left in place. The serratus branch of the artery was divided with hemoclips and the muscle attachment to the humerus was divided with electrocautery. The pedicle dissection was performed under direct vision with proper retraction. The thoracodorsal nerve was divided first and both thoracodorsal artery and vein were divided off the axillary vessels after further pedicle dissection. The latissimus flap donor site was closed in three layers after placement of two drains.

The patient was then repositioned to the supine position. The pedicle vessels of the flap were prepared under loupe magnification. Both pedicle artery and vein were flushed with heparinized saline solution. The additional preparation of the pedicle artery and vein were performed under an operating microscope after the flap had been temporarily inset into the ankle wound. Using a standard microsurgical technique, an end-to-side anastomosis was

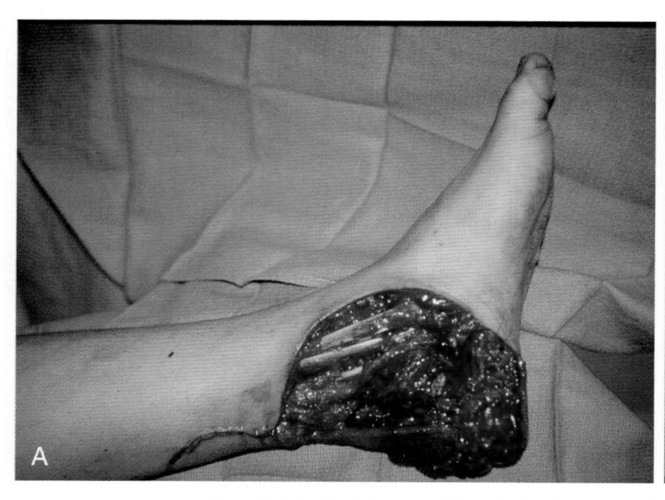

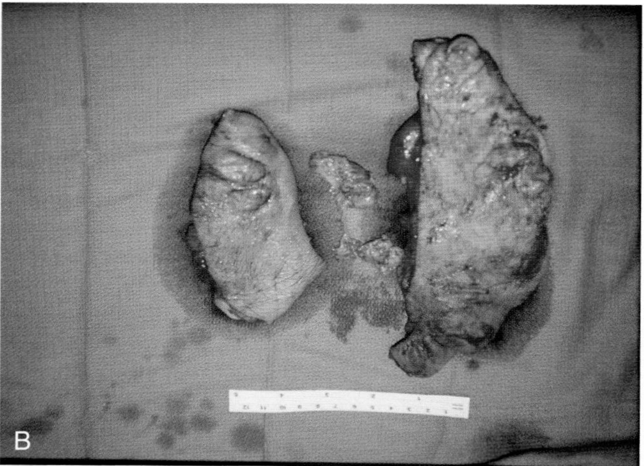

• **Fig. 49.16** (A) Intraoperative view showing a large soft tissue defect of left foot and ankle after complete resection of plexiform neurofibroma, with exposed tendons, posterior tibial vessels, tibial nerve, and ankle joint. (B) Intraoperative view showing specimens from complete resection of left foot and ankle plexiform neurofibroma.

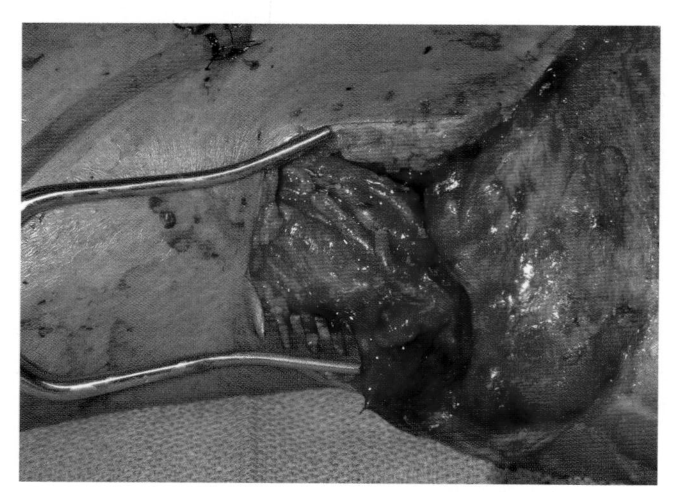

• **Fig. 49.17** Intraoperative view showing completion of microvascular anastomoses to the distal posterior tibial vessels.

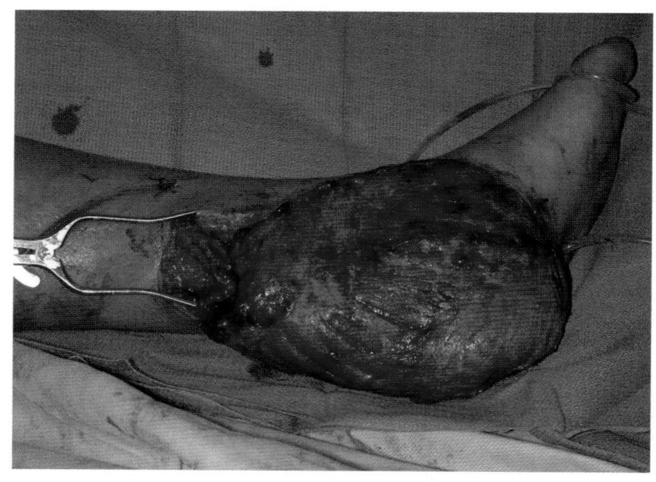

• **Fig. 49.18** Intraoperative view showing completion of a free latissimus dorsi muscle flap inset before skin graft placement.

performed with interrupted 8-0 nylon sutures between the pedicle artery and the posterior tibial artery and an end-to-end anastomosis between the pedicle vein and the posterior tibial vein was performed with interrupted 8-0 nylon sutures. Once all clamps had been released, the flap appeared to be well perfused with a strong Doppler signal (Fig. 49.17).

The flap was approximated to the adjacent ankle wound skin edges with several interrupted 3-0 Vicryl sutures in half-buried horizontal mattress fashion. Two drains were placed under the flap (Fig. 49.18). Split-thickness skin grafts were harvested from the left lateral thigh with a dermatome and meshed to 1:1.5 ratio. The skin graft was placed over the muscle flap and secured with multiple skin staples (Fig. 49.19).

Follow-Up Results

The patient did well postoperatively without any complications related to the free latissimus dorsi muscle flap transfer for the large

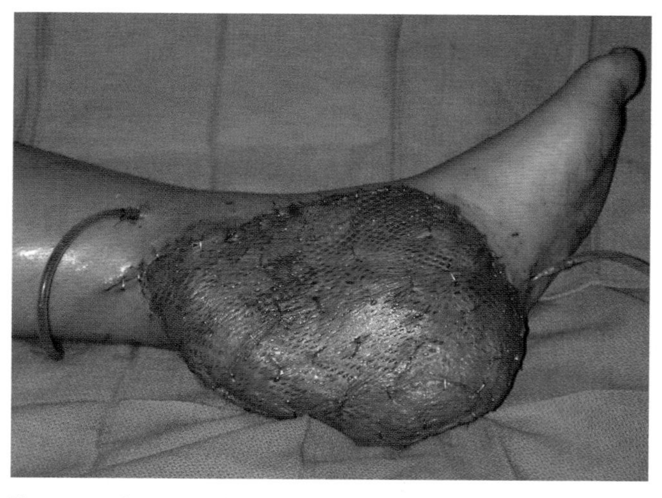

• **Fig. 49.19** Intraoperative view showing completion of skin graft placements over the free latissimus dorsi muscle flap.

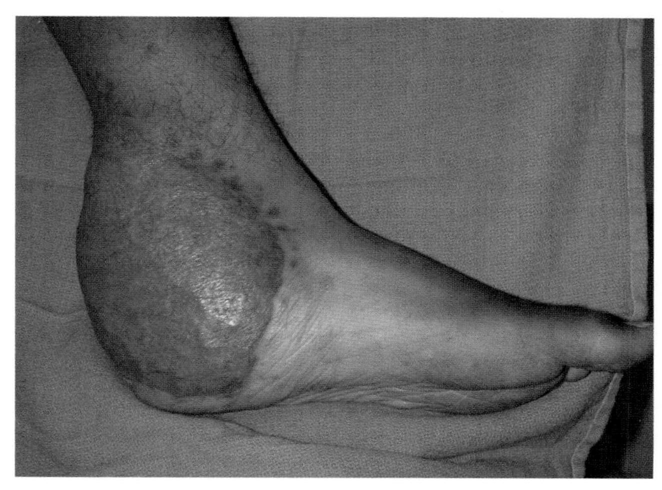

• **Fig. 49.20** The result at 3-month follow-up showing well-healed skin-grafted free latissimus dorsi muscle flap to the left foot and ankle.

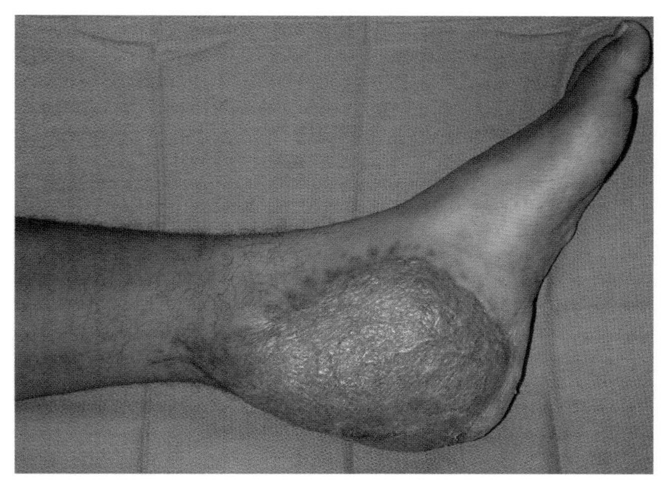

• **Fig. 49.21** Preoperative view showing well-healed skin-grafted free latissimus dorsi muscle flap to the left foot and ankle but with a persist contour deformity at 5 months after initial transfer.

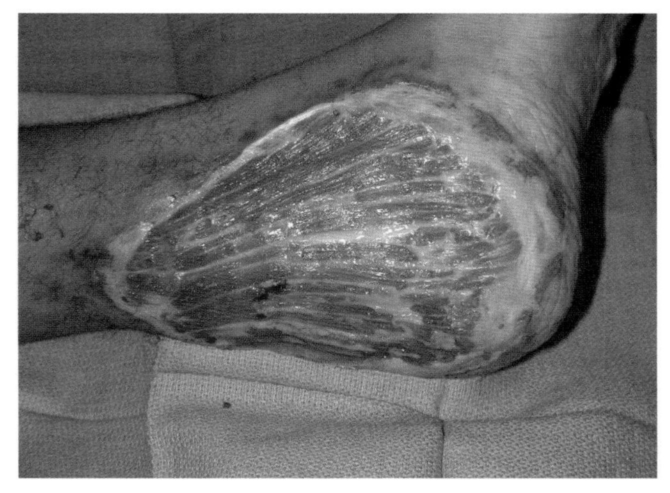

• **Fig. 49.22** Intraoperative view showing completion of debulking procedure by a tangential excision of the excess flap tissue under tourniquet control.

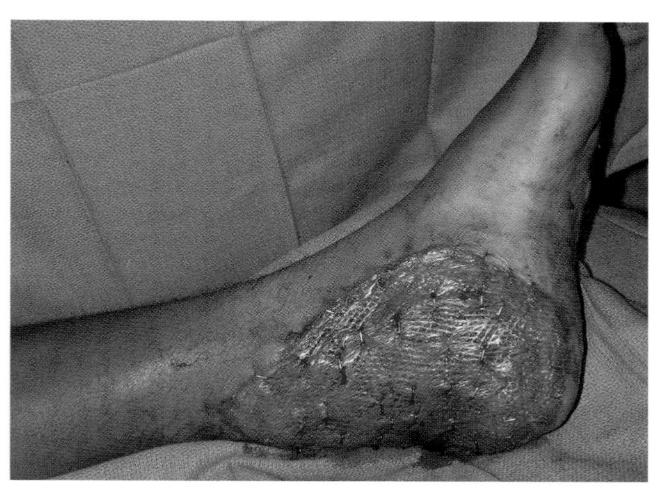

• **Fig. 49.23** Intraoperative view showing completion of placement of new skin grafts over the raw surface of the flap after a debulking procedure.

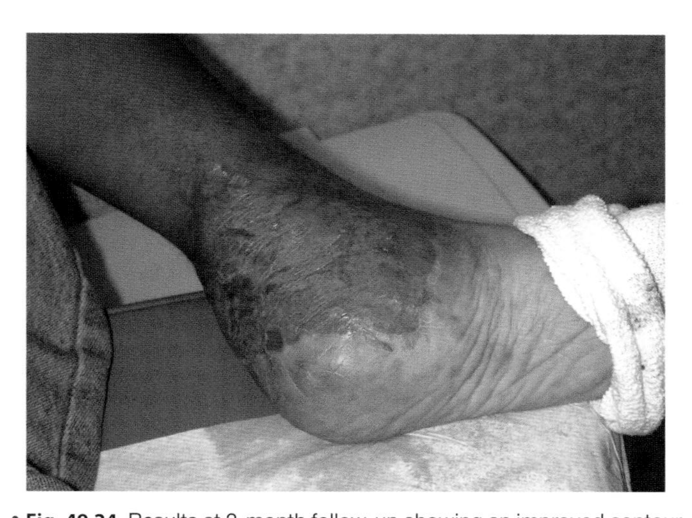

• **Fig. 49.24** Results at 2-month follow-up showing an improved contour of the left foot and ankle after the debulking procedure.

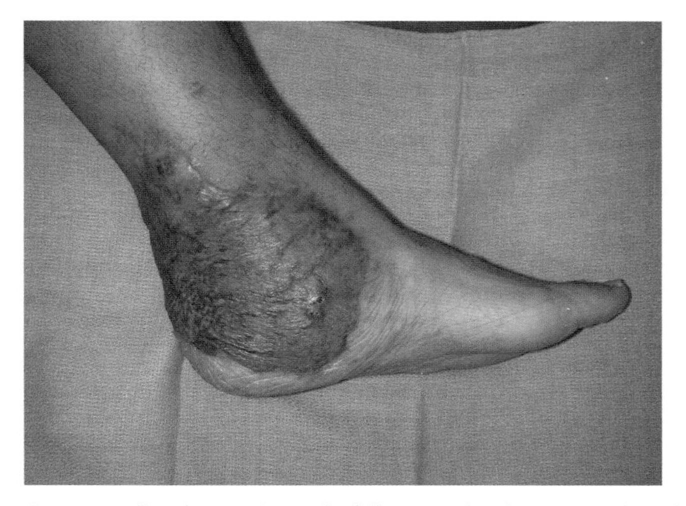

• **Fig. 49.25** Results at 9-month follow-up showing a good and acceptable contour of the left foot and ankle after the debulking procedure.

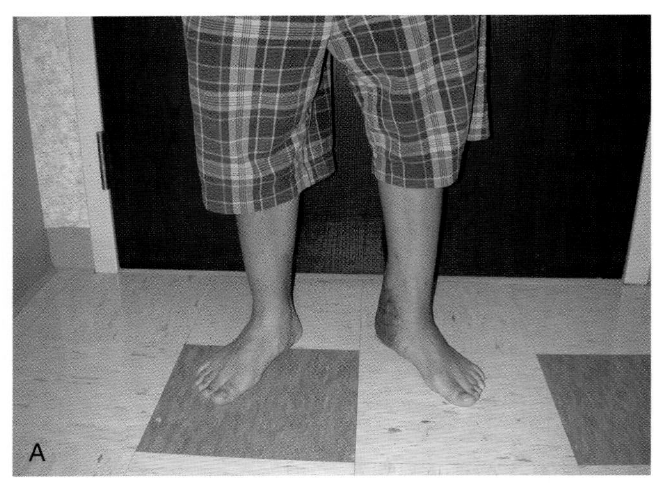

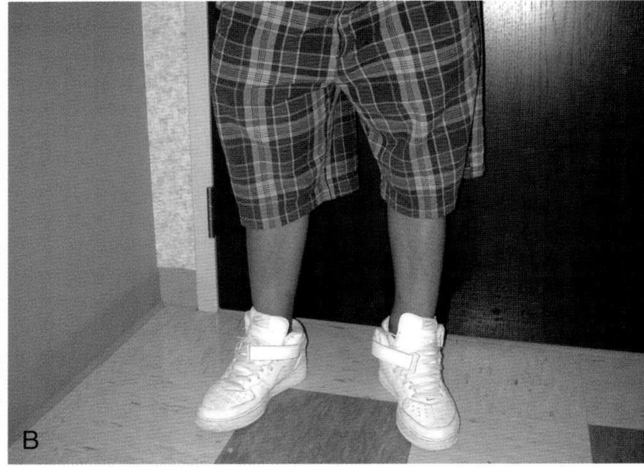

• **Fig. 49.26** Results at 9-month follow-up showing a good contour of the left foot and ankle in comparison with the contralateral normal site after the debulking procedure: (A) without a shoe; (B) with a shoe on.

foot and ankle wound reconstruction. He was discharged from hospital a week later after the second-stage procedure once he tolerated dangling protocol. All drains were removed during subsequent follow-up visits. The left foot and ankle wound and the skin graft over the muscle flap healed well (Fig. 49.20). He gradually began weight-bearing according to our standard protocols.

About 5 months after the initial resection and reconstruction, the patient underwent a debulking procedure of the healed free latissimus dorsi muscle flap over his left foot and ankle (Fig. 49.21). Under tourniquet control, a tangential excision was performed over the flap site in order to remove the bulky tissues of the flap (Fig. 49.22). An additional split-thickness skin graft was placed on the surface of the flap (Fig. 49.23). He had no postoperative complications and the flap site healed completely after debulking (Fig. 49.24).

Final Outcome

During an 18-month follow-up, the patient was symptom free and had good contour of his left foot and ankle with minimal scarring (Fig. 49.25). He had been able to wear shoes and was fully ambulating without difficulty (Figs. 49.26A and B). There has been no clinical evidence of local recurrence of the neurofibroma at the resection site.

Pearls for Success

Preoperative planning for complete resection of a large plexiform neurofibroma of the foot and ankle can be crucial. It is recommended to obtain complete imaging studies such as plain X-ray, MRI, and angiography in addition to a good physical examination of the affected areas. The neurovascular status of the foot and a possible bony invasion of the neurofibroma should also be evaluated. An MRI study, especially on postgadolinium T1-weighted images, can better define the extent of the tumor in the foot and ankle. An angiogram is useful to determine the vascular anatomy of the entire foot and ankle and the relationship between the major vessels and the plexiform neurofibroma and to facilitate operative planning for both tumor resection and subsequent microvascular anastomoses for free tissue transfer. A large plexiform neurofibroma of the foot and ankle can be managed by a complete resection of the tumor with preservation of major neurovascular structures, followed by a free tissue transfer for soft tissue reconstruction for a staged approach because after a lengthy resection of the tumor with significant blood loss, another possibly lengthy free tissue transfer for soft tissue coverage would not be optimal for either the patient or the surgeon. However, a good outcome can be achieved with the combination of good preoperative planning and a state-of-the-art reconstruction of the foot and ankle after complete resection of the tumor as two stage procedures, without local recurrence and/or wound healing complications.

Recommended Readings

Dorfman D, Pu LL. The value of color duplex imaging for planning and performing a free anterolateral thigh perforator flap. *Ann Plast Surg.* 2014;72(suppl 1):S6–S8.

Nazerali RS, Pu LL. Free tissue transfer to the lower extremity: a paradigm shift in flap selection for soft tissue reconstruction. *Ann Plast Surg.* 2013;70:419–422.

Pu LLQ. Free flaps in lower extremity reconstruction. *Clin Plast Surg.* 2021;48:201–214.

Pu LL, Vasconez HC. Large recurrent plexiform neurofibroma of the foot and ankle. *Microsurgery.* 2004;24:67–71.

Sakarya AH, Tsai KY, Hsu CC, et al. Free tissue transfers for reconstruction of weight-bearing heel defects: flap selection, ulceration management, and contour revisions. *J Plast Reconstr Aesthet Surg.* 2022;75:1557–1566.

50

Heel Reconstruction

CASE 1

Clinical Presentation

A 36-year-old White male developed a wound dehiscence following an open reduction and internal fixation of his calcaneus fracture by the orthopedic foot and ankle service (Fig. 50.1). He had sustained a right foot calcaneus fracture from a fall. He underwent soft tissue debridement by the orthopedic foot and ankle service, which left a complex heel wound with the exposed fracture site (Fig. 50.2). The plastic surgery service was asked by the primary service to provide soft tissue coverage to this complex posterior heel wound of the right foot.

Operative Plan and Special Considerations

For a complex heel wound, a medial plantar artery flap, a type B fasciocutaneous flap, can be selected as a valid reconstructive option. The flap receives a blood supply from the medial plantar artery, which is a continuation of the posterior tibial artery after bifurcation. The size of the flap's skin paddle can be up to 12 × 6 cm from the instep of the foot, which is in the non-weight-bearing area. The pedicle of the flap is under the fascia and the extent of the flap's arc of rotation depends on the level of bifurcation in the medial ankle (Fig. 50.3). The flap can be rotated posteriorly to cover a heel soft tissue defect. The donor site of the flap can be closed with a skin graft because it is in the non-weight-bearing area. A preoperative angiogram should be obtained to determine the blood supply to the foot and the level of bifurcation from the posterior tibial artery in the ankle.

Operative Procedures

Under general anesthesia, with the patient in the supine position, the right heel wound was debrided by the plastic surgery service. All unhealthy-looking skin or tissue was debrided and the wound was then irrigated with Pulsavac. After the definitive debridement, the heel wound, measuring 6 × 3.5 cm, looked fresh and clean (Fig. 50.4).

The medial plantar artery was mapped with a handheld Doppler and a 6 × 3.5 cm skin paddle of the flap was designed (Fig. 50.5). Under tourniquet control, the skin paddle was incised down to the fascia. The fascia around the skin paddle was incised and the pedicle was identified between the abductor and flexor digitorum brevis muscles. At the distal edge of the flap, the pedicle artery was divided with hemoclips and a subfascial dissection was performed. The medial plantar artery was included within the fasciocutaneous component of the flap and visualized all the time during the flap dissection. Additional pedicle dissection was performed through the extended proximal incision toward the heel wound (Fig. 50.6).

After the pedicle dissection had been completed and the tourniquet released, the flap appeared well perfused. It was rotated posteriorly to cover the heel wound (Fig. 50.7). The flap was then inset into the wound and approximated to the adjacent skin edges with several interrupted 3-0 nylon sutures in half-buried horizontal mattress fashion. A drain was placed under the flap before the final closure of the skin paddle. The medial ankle incision was closed with interrupted 3-0 nylon sutures and skin staples.

The flap donor site in the mid-plantar foot was closed with a split-thickness skin graft. It was harvested from the right lateral thigh with a dermatome. The skin graft was meshed to 1:1.5 ratio and then placed on the flap donor site and secured with multiple skin staples (Fig. 50.8). A bolster dressing was used to immobilize the skin graft.

Follow-Up Results

The patient did well postoperatively without any issues related to the medial plantar artery flap for soft tissue coverage of a posterior heel wound. He was discharged from hospital on postoperative day 5. The right heel wound healed without problems (Fig. 50.9) and the flap donor site skin graft took well. He was followed by the plastic surgery service for routine postoperative care and the orthopedic foot and ankle service for orthopedic care.

Final Outcome

During further follow-up, the right posterior heel wound after the flap reconstruction healed well with good contour and minimal scarring with no wound breakdown, recurrent infection, or contour issues. The flap donor site after skin grafting also healed well (Fig. 50.10), as did the calcaneus fracture. The patient has resumed his weight-bearing status and has returned to his normal activities as instructed.

Pearls for Success

A medial plantar artery flap can be elevated reliably to cover a posterior heel wound in the foot if only skin coverage is needed. A preoperative angiogram is necessary to evaluate the circulation in the foot and the level of bifurcation from the posterior tibial artery. The flap should be elevated as a fasciocutaneous flap and care

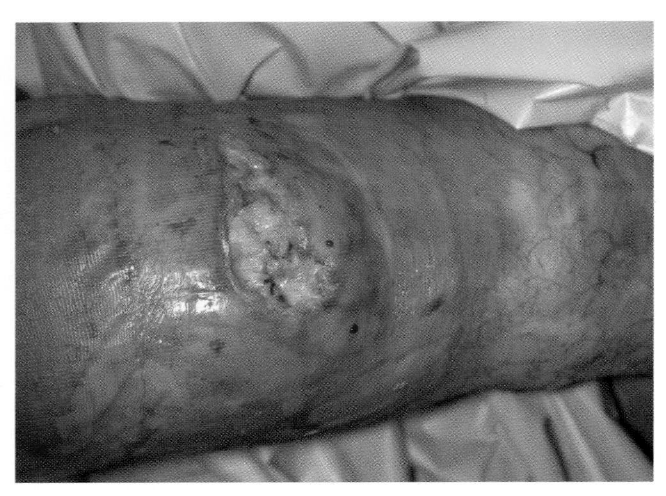

• **Fig. 50.1** A preoperative view showing a 6 × 3.5 cm open calcaneus wound of the right foot as a result of wound dehiscence from an orthopedic procedure.

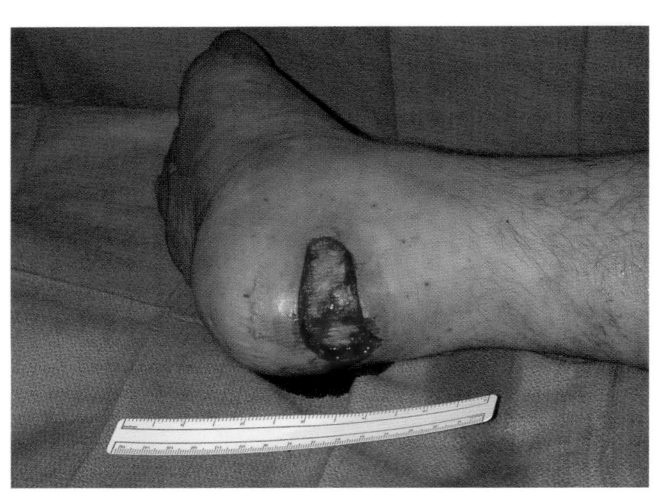

• **Fig. 50.4** An intraoperative view showing the calcaneus wound after definitive debridement by the plastic surgery service.

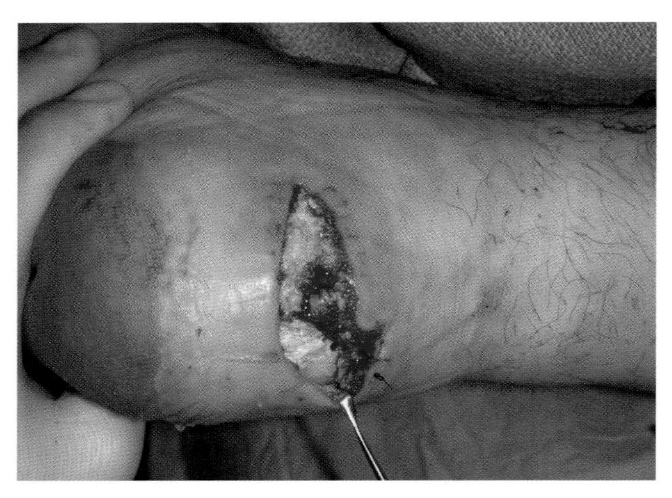

• **Fig. 50.2** An intraoperative view showing the calcaneus wound with the exposed fracture site after debridement by the orthopedic foot and ankle service.

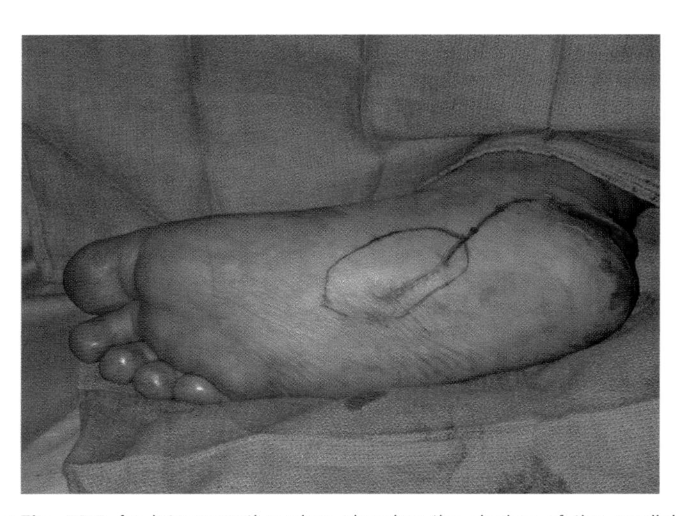

• **Fig. 50.5** An intraoperative view showing the design of the medial plantar artery flap. The pedicle should be incorporated within the flap.

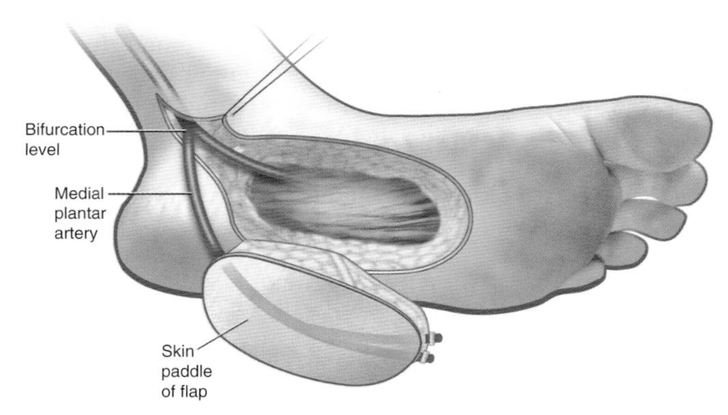

• **Fig. 50.3** A schematic diagram showing the level of bifurcation from the posterior tibial artery and the extent of the flap's arc rotation.

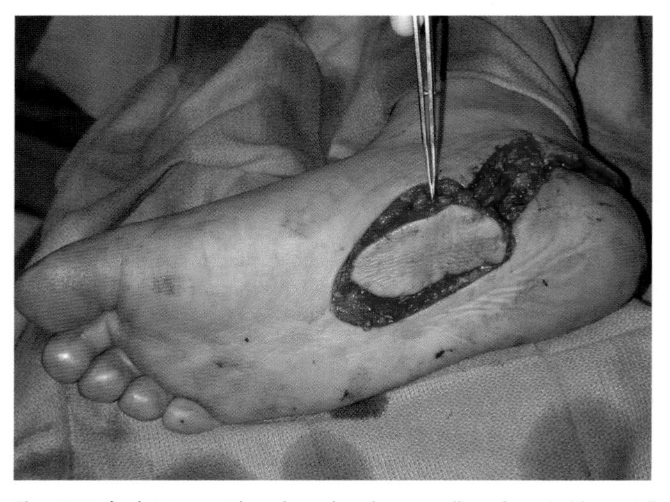

• **Fig. 50.6** An intraoperative view showing a well-perfused skin paddle of the flap after its dissection.

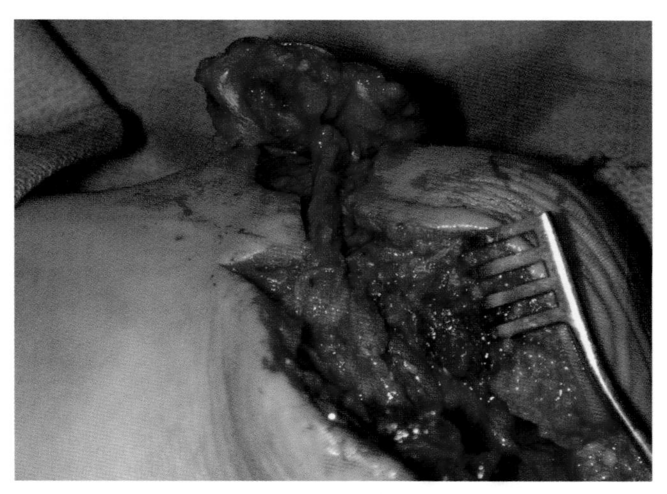

• **Fig. 50.7** An intraoperative view showing the completely elevated flap that was temporarily placed on the wound. The pedicle of the flap was through an opened subcutaneous tunnel.

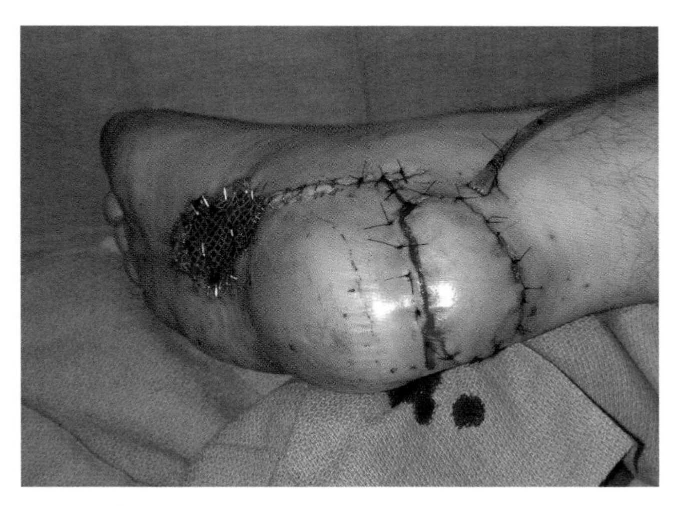

• **Fig. 50.8** An intraoperative view showing completion of the flap inset, closure of the opened subcutaneous tunnel, and the flap donor site closure with a skin graft.

should be taken to ensure that the medial plantar artery is included during the flap dissection. The pedicle artery is located under the fascia and can be visible. It can be located much deeper than the surgeon believes. The tourniquet is used for the skin paddle dissection, but additional pedicle dissection should be done after tourniquet release. The flap inset is relatively easy and the flap donor site can be closed with a skin graft. If the flap perfusion is not adequate after elevation because of vessel spasm, it can be placed back to the donor site and used later as a delayed flap for the same reconstruction. In general, arterial insufficiency of the flap is more common than venous congestion.

CASE 2

Clinical Presentation

A 53-year-old White male had a burn injury to his left heel about 20 years previously. He was treated in a foreign country with

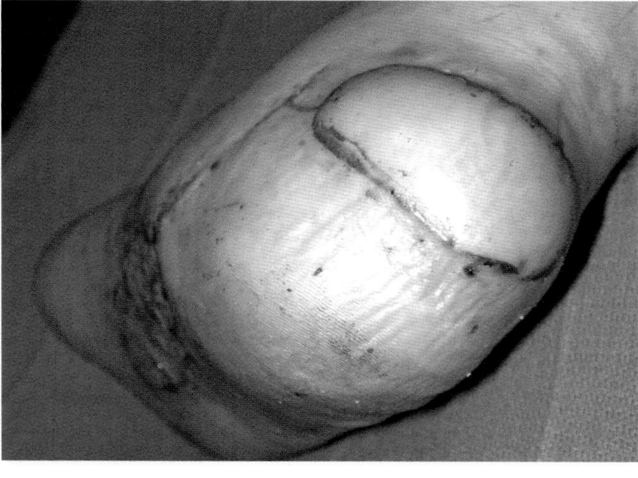

• **Fig. 50.9** Results at 5-week follow-up after the flap reconstruction showing well-healed calcareous wound with good contour.

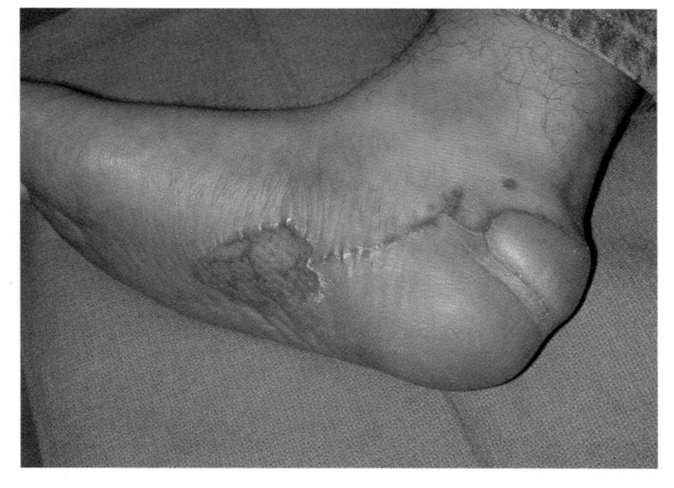

• **Fig. 50.10** Results at 7.5-month follow-up showing well-healed flap site and flap donor site with good contour and minimal scarring.

excision and skin grafting at that time. Unfortunately, for almost 10 years, the patient had a nonhealing ulcerative wound over his left heel. The wound was painful and never healed. He was referred by his primary care physician for definitive excision and subsequent wound coverage. On examination, there was 6 × 5 cm ulcerative wound over his left lateral heel and no scar was found over his lateral leg (Fig. 50.11).

Operative Plan and Special Considerations for Reconstruction

The distally based sural artery flap can be selected to cover a complex wound in the heel if the flap donor site is available and the pedicle of the flap in the lesser saphenous vein territory is not affected by previous trauma or surgery. The flap itself provides good skin coverage to the heel if it can be properly designed and dissected. The skin island over the gastrocnemius muscles can be harvested from the proximal two-thirds of the posterior leg. Once again, the flap receives blood supply primarily from three to six septocutaneous perforators arising from the peroneal artery in a

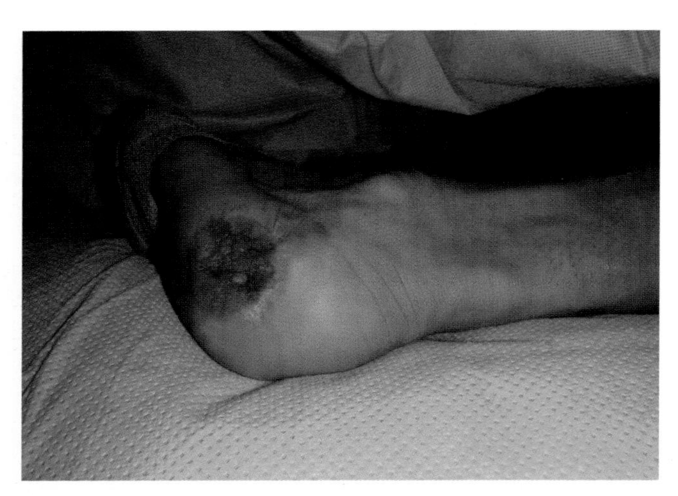

• **Fig. 50.11** A preoperative view showing a 6 × 5 cm ulcerative wound over the lateral heel of the left foot.

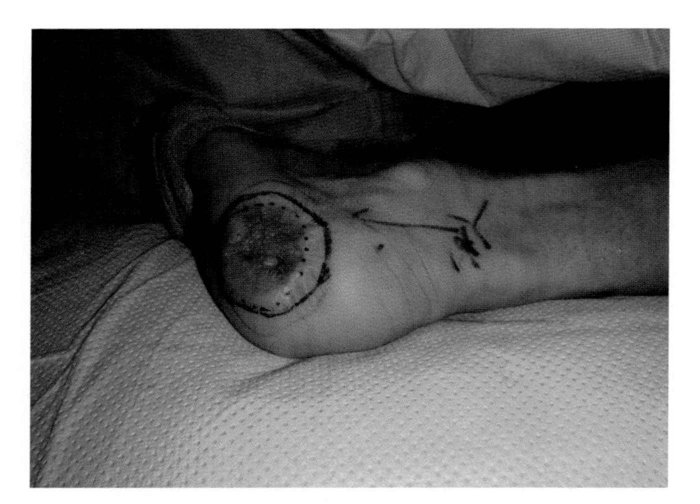

• **Fig. 50.12** An intraoperative view showing the plan for surgical excision of the ulcerative wound.

retrograde fashion. The peroneal artery should also be confirmed to be patent by a preoperative angiogram. The most proximal end of these perforators is located 4 to 7 cm proximal to the lateral malleolus. Its pedicle and skin paddle should include both the lesser saphenous vein and sural nerve systems within the adipofascial tissue once the flap is elevated. In general, the flap donor site can be closed primarily if its width is less than 4 cm.

Operative Procedures

Under general anesthesia, with the patient in the right lateral decubitus position, the left heel ulcerative lesion was marked with a 3 mm margin (Fig. 50.12). The skin and the entire ulcerative lesion were excised to the deep fascia. The ulcerative lesion was sent for a frozen section and the result was negative for Marjolin's ulcer.

A 6 × 5 cm skin paddle of the distally based sural artery flap was designed after the entire course of the lesser saphenous vein was mapped using a handheld Doppler between the Achilles tendon and the lateral malleolus. The pivot point of the flap turnover was marked at 6 cm above the lateral malleolus and a

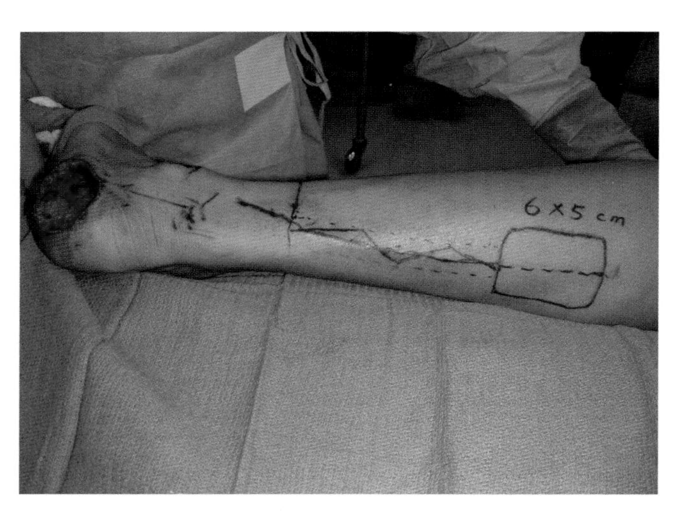

• **Fig. 50.13** An intraoperative view showing the design of the distally based sural artery flap as a turnover flap. The pivotal point of the flap turnover was 6 cm above the lateral malleolus. The pedicle would be elevated through a zigzag incision.

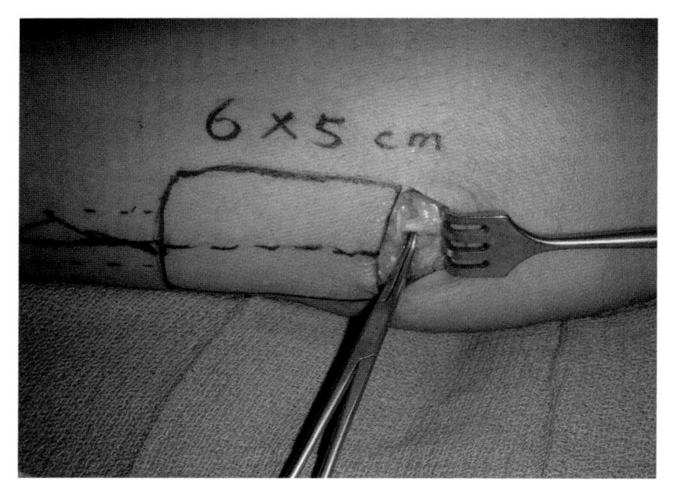

• **Fig. 50.14** An intraoperative view showing an exploration of the lesser saphenous vein (under the *forceps*) within the subcutaneous tissue plane. It would be divided during the flap elevation.

zigzag incision was marked for the pedicle dissection (Fig. 50.13). Under tourniquet control, the proximal incision of the flap was made to explore the lesser saphenous vein and its accompanying vessels, which were then divided (Fig. 50.14). The sural nerve and its accompanying vessels were then exposed through the fascia and also divided (Fig. 50.15). The skin island was elevated along the subfascial plane and completely elevated as a fasciocutaneous island flap. The adipofascial pedicle of the flap, about 2 cm wide, was identified through multiple zigzag incisions (Fig. 50.16). The flap was completely elevated based on the narrow pedicle and could be turned over, in a reverse fashion, to reach the heel wound (Fig. 50.17).

Once the tourniquet was released, the flap appeared well perfused. It was tunneled under the skin bridge between the pedicle and heel wound. An adequate size of tunnel had been created and the flap was tunneled through without direct compression to the pedicle. The flap was then placed into the

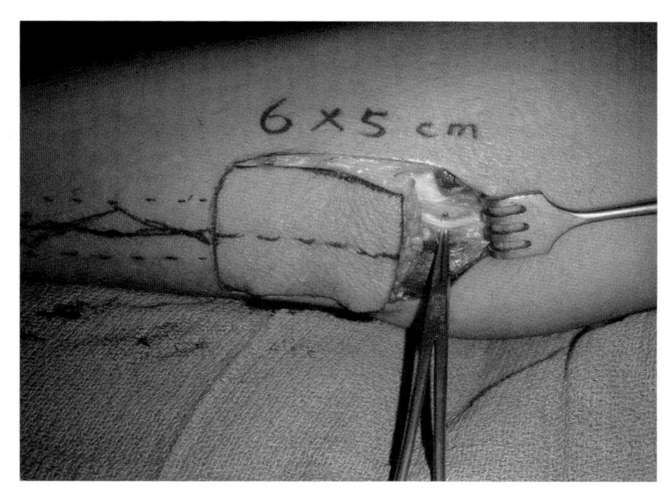

• **Fig. 50.15** An intraoperative view showing an exploration of the sural nerve (under the *forceps*) through the fascia. It would be divided during the flap elevation.

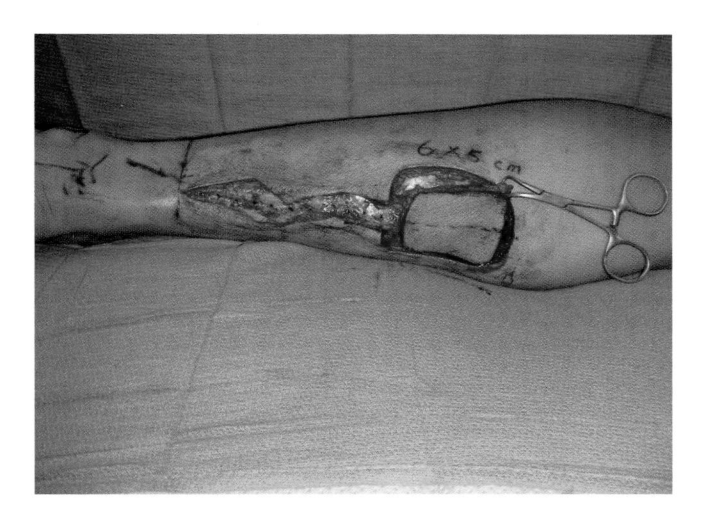

• **Fig. 50.16** An intraoperative view showing completion of the flap's skin paddle elevation but before the pedicle dissection. The pedicle was marked and could be made as narrow as 2 cm.

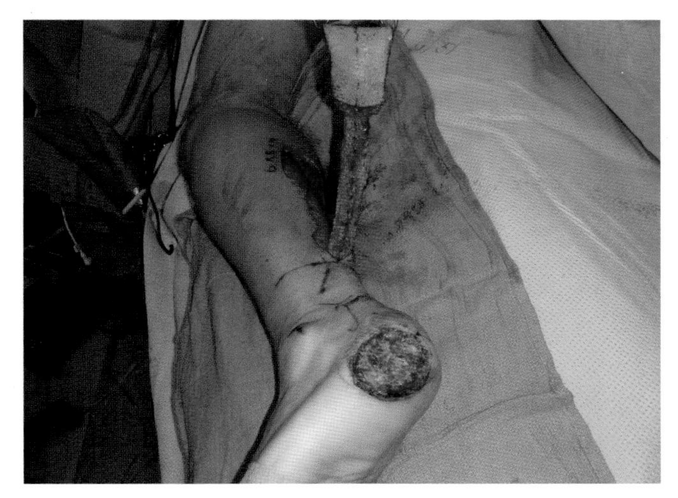

• **Fig. 50.17** An intraoperative view showing completion of the flap elevation. The flap could be turned over to cover this healed soft tissue defect.

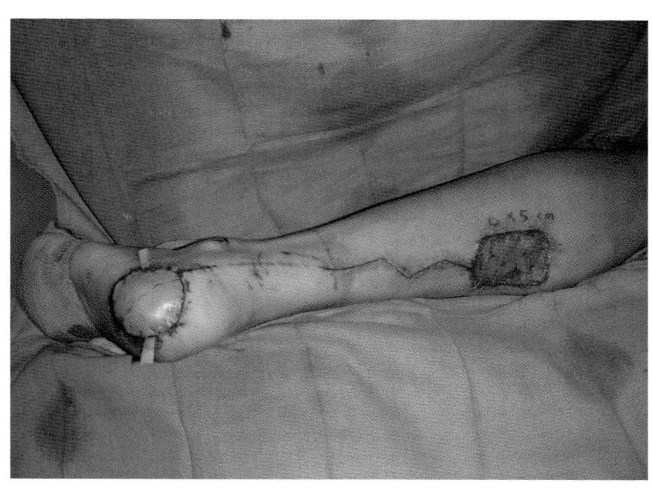

• **Fig. 50.18** An intraoperative view showing completion of the flap inset and closure of the flap's donor site and incision for the pedicle dissection.

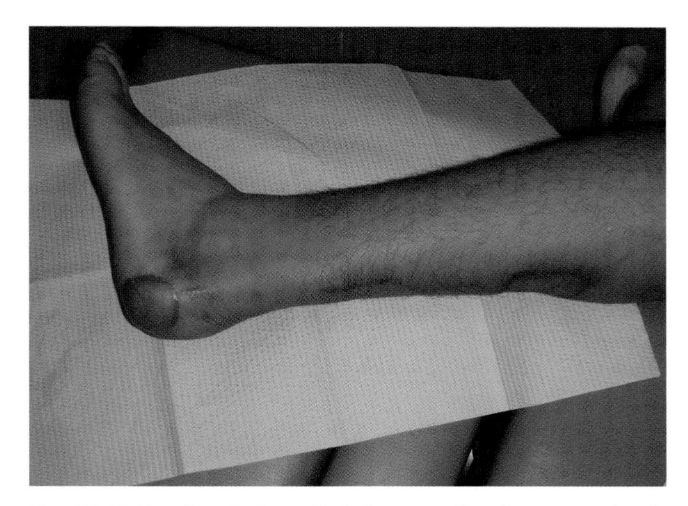

• **Fig. 50.19** Results at 3-month follow-up after flap reconstruction showing well-healed lateral heel wound of the left foot with good contour and minimal swelling. The flap donor site also healed well.

wound after trimming the excess flap tissue. A Penrose drain was placed under the flap and the flap was inset into the adjacent skin with several interrupted 3-0 Monocryl sutures in half-buried horizontal mattress fashion.

The zigzag skin incision was approximated in two layers. The deep dermal layer was approximated with several interrupted 3-0 Monocryl sutures. The skin was closed with Dermabond. The flap donor site was approximated as much as possible after undermining and the wound edge was tacked to the deep muscle layer with interrupted sutures. A split-thickness skin graft was harvested from the left thigh old skin graft donor site with a dermatome. The skin graft was left unmeshed, placed on the flap donor site, and secured with multiple skin staples (Fig. 50.18).

Follow-Up Results

The patient did well postoperatively without any issues related to the distally based sural artery flap for coverage of the heel wound in the

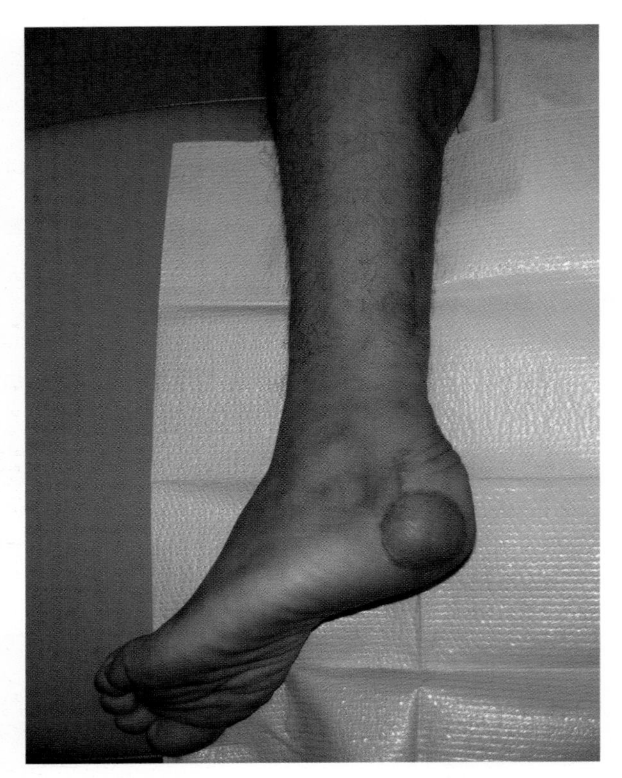

• **Fig. 50.20** Results at 7-month follow-up showing well-healed and stable lateral heel wound of the left foot with good contour and minimal scarring.

left foot. He was discharged from hospital on postoperative day 5. The left heel wound healed without problems (Fig. 50.19). He was followed by the plastic surgery service for routine postoperative care.

Final Outcome

During further follow-up, the left heel wound after the flap reconstruction had healed well with excellent contour and minimal scarring. There was no wound breakdown, recurrent infection, or contour issues related to the flap reconstruction (Fig. 50.20). The flap donor site after skin grafting also healed well. He has resumed his weight-bearing status and has returned to his normal activities as instructed.

Pearls for Success

A distally based sural artery flap can be used to cover a heel wound in the foot if only skin coverage is needed. It should be elevated as a fasciocutaneous flap that includes dual blood supply with both lesser saphenous vein and sural nerve systems. The adipofascial pedicle of the flap can be designed to be as narrow as 2 cm as long as both the lesser saphenous vein and sural nerve systems are included. This facilitates the pedicle turnover and tunneling through the skin bridge. In this way, the cosmetic outcome in the foot and ankle region can be optimal. However, if the skin tunnel is too tight, it can be opened and the pedicle can be covered with a skin graft. Postoperative venous congestion can be a problem and topical nitroglycerin paste or medicinal leech therapy may be used in addition to effective leg elevation. Inspection of the flap pedicle is warranted to ensure there is no direct compression. If venous congestion persists or worsens, the flap can be placed back into the donor site as the delay procedure. However, the flap may become too stiff for wound coverage. In addition, a supercharge to augment venous drainage between the proximal lesser saphenous vein and an adjacent vein in the foot can also be performed if the surgeon feels comfortable with the microsurgical technique.

Recommended Readings

Kececi Y, Sir E. Increasing versatility of the distally based sural flap. *J Foot Ankle Surg.* 2012;51:583−587.

Löfstrand JG, Lin CH. Reconstruction of defects in the weight-bearing plantar area using the innervated free medial plantar (instep) flap. *Ann Plast Surg.* 2018;80:245−251.

Mahmoud WH. Foot and ankle reconstruction using the distally based sural artery flap versus the medial plantar flap: a comparative study. *J Foot Ankle Surg.* 2017;56:514−518.

Pu LLQ. Locoregional flaps in lower extremity reconstruction. *Clin Plast Surg.* 2021;48:157−171.

Siddiqi MA, Hafeez K, Cheema TA, Rashid HU. The medial plantar artery flap: a series of cases over 14 years. *J Foot Ankle Surg.* 2012;51:790−794.

51

Foot Reconstruction

CASE 1

Clinical Presentation

A 54-year-old White male had a long history of complex congenital deformity of his right foot. He had several previous orthopedic procedures but unfortunately the hardware became infected. He underwent hardware removal by the orthopedic foot and ankle service, which left an open wound with scar tissue in the lateral foot, measuring 7 × 3.5 cm. The plastic surgery service was asked to provide soft tissue coverage for this open wound with the exposed underlying bone in his right lateral foot right after the orthopedic debridement (Fig. 51.1).

Operative Plan and Special Considerations for Reconstruction

A lateral foot wound can be reconstructed with a dorsalis pedis artery flap, elevated either as an island skin flap or as a rotation skin flap. The flap is a type B fasciocutaneous flap and receives blood supply primarily from the dorsalis pedis artery. It is thin, reliable, and mobile and can reach the lateral foot without difficulty. The usual size of the flap is 10 × 8 cm, but it can be designed larger. The sensate flap can also be made by incorporating a branch of the superficial peroneal nerve. A skin graft would be needed to close the flap's donor site. The posterior tibial artery should be evaluated for its patency in order to ensure the foot could still receive an adequate blood supply once the dorsalis pedis artery has been scarified.

Operative Procedures

Under general anesthesia, with the patient in the supine position, the plastic surgery part of the procedure started after the orthopedic part of the procedure had been completed by the orthopedic foot and ankle service. A large dorsalis pedis artery flap was designed as a rotation flap to cover the right lateral foot wound. Because of the medial foot incision made by the primary service, such an incision was incorporated in the flap design as a large rotational flap with a back cut if needed (Fig. 51.2).

The dorsalis pedis artery was mapped with a handheld Doppler and then marked (Fig. 51.3). Under tourniquet control, the skin incision was made through the subcutaneous tissue down to the fascia. The suprafascial dissection was performed and the flap was elevated sharply with a knife. The distal end of the dorsalis pedis artery was identified and divided with hemoclips near the distal skin edge of the flap. A large dorsal vein was also divided during the flap elevation. The flap dissection was done in a retrograde fashion. After completing the adequate flap dissection, the tourniquet was released. The flap appeared to be well perfused and the dorsalis pedis artery was included within the flap (Fig. 51.4). The flap was rotated into the right lateral foot wound and the excess flap tissue was excised (Fig. 51.5). A drain was inserted under the flap within the right lateral foot wound.

The flap inset was performed next. The flap closure was done with interrupted 3-0 Monocryl sutures in a half-buried horizontal mattress fashion. The flap donor area, measuring 15 × 5 cm, was closed with a skin graft. The split-thickness skin graft was harvested from the right lateral thigh with a dermatome, placed as a sheet graft over the dorsal foot donor site, and secured to the adjacent wound edge and flap with multiple skin staples (Fig. 51.6A and B). An occlusive dressing was applied to secure the skin graft. At the end of the procedure, a plantar splint was used to immobilize the ankle.

Follow-Up Results

The patient did well postoperatively without any issues related to the dorsalis pedis artery flap for the lateral foot wound coverage. He was discharged from hospital on postoperative day 5. The right lateral foot wound healed uneventfully (Fig. 51.7A and B). He was followed by the plastic surgery service for routine postoperative care and by the orthopedic foot and ankle service for orthopedic care.

Final Outcome

During further follow-up, the right lateral foot wound after the flap reconstruction healed well with good contour and minimal scarring and no wound breakdown, recurrent infection, or contour issues. The flap donor site after skin grafting also healed well (Fig. 51.8A and B). He has resumed his weight-bearing status and has returned to his normal activities as instructed.

Pearls for Success

The dorsalis pedis artery flap can be used to cover a dorsal foot wound either as an island flap or as a rotation flap. The flap is based on the dorsalis pedis artery and has relatively limited arc as a rotation flap. If a larger rotation flap is designed, it should include a back cut of the flap to increase the flap's arc of rotation. The donor site can be closed with a skin graft and its long-term outcome appears to be

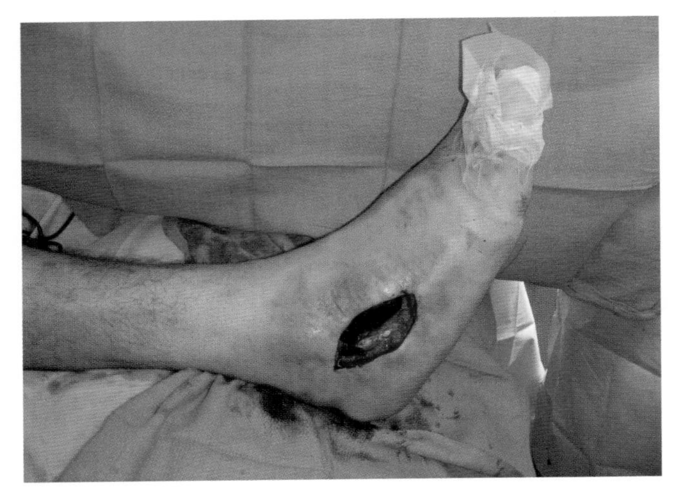

• **Fig. 51.1** A preoperative view showing a 7 × 3.5 cm lateral foot wound with exposed underlying bone.

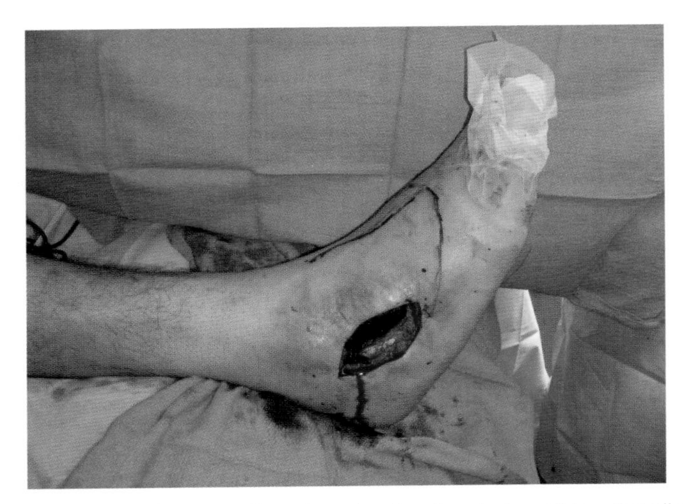

• **Fig. 51.2** An intraoperative view showing the design of the dorsalis pedis artery flap as a rotation flap. The pedicle was in the center of the flap and marked.

quite good. Care should be taken not to injure the pedicle vessel during the flap elevation. Suprafascial flap dissection can be performed so that a skin graft can be placed on the fascia for an optimal donor site wound closure. The flap is thin and reliable and can be considered as an excellent choice for a dorsal foot wound closure.

CASE 2

Clinical Presentation

A 46-year-old White male sustained a crushing injury to his right foot. He was initially operated on by the orthopedic foot and ankle service and multiple toe fractures were stabilized and the portion of the soft tissue wound was approximated. This had left a large dorsal foot wound, measuring 17 × 10 cm, with the exposed multiple extensor tendons. The plastic surgery service was consulted for soft tissue reconstruction of this large dorsal foot wound. His necrotic toes would be amputated during the definitive soft tissue wound coverage (Fig. 51.9).

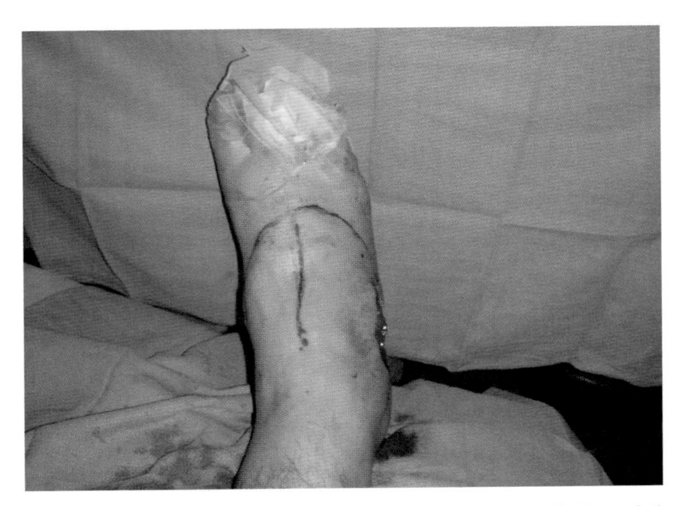

• **Fig. 51.3** A different intraoperative view showing the design of the dorsalis pedis artery flap as a rotation flap. The pedicle was in the center of the flap and marked.

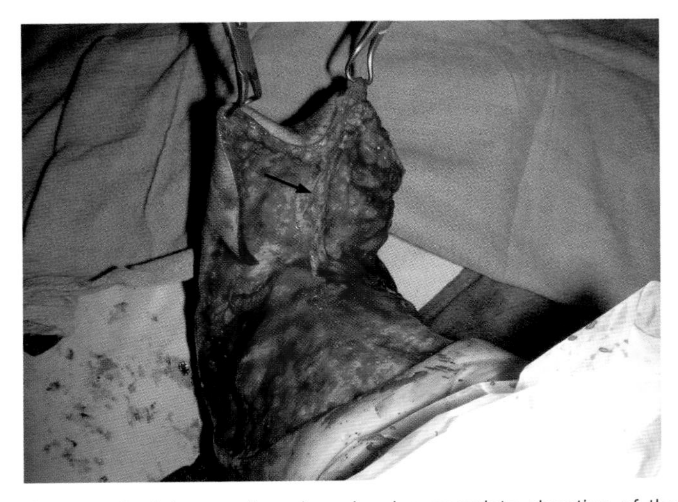

• **Fig. 51.4** An intraoperative view showing complete elevation of the flap. The pedicle (*arrow*) was included within the flap.

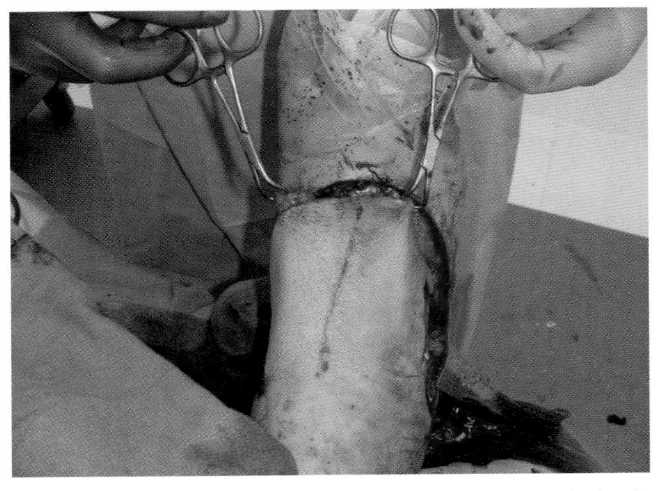

• **Fig. 51.5** An intraoperative view showing completion of the flap dissection. The flap could be rotated into the lateral foot wound without problem.

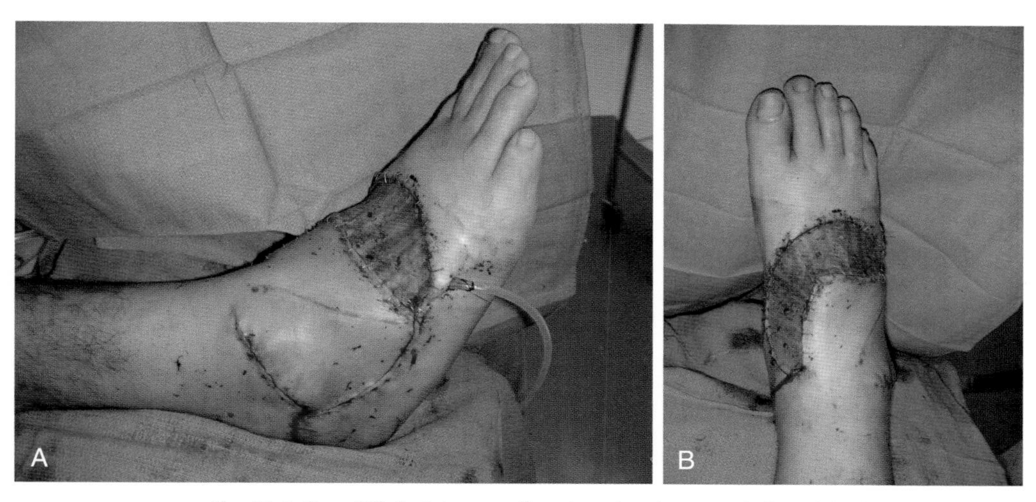

• **Fig. 51.6** (A and B) An intraoperative view showing completion of the flap inset. The flap's donor site was closed with a split-thickness skin graft.

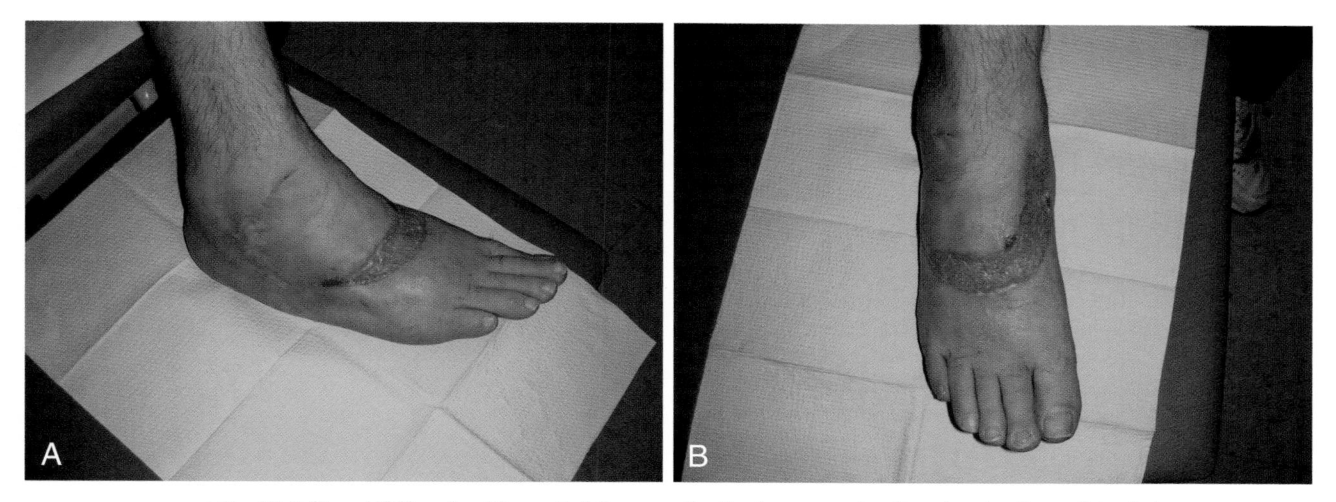

• **Fig. 51.7** (A and B) Results at 3-month follow-up after the flap reconstruction showing the well-healed lateral foot wound with good contour and minimal swelling.

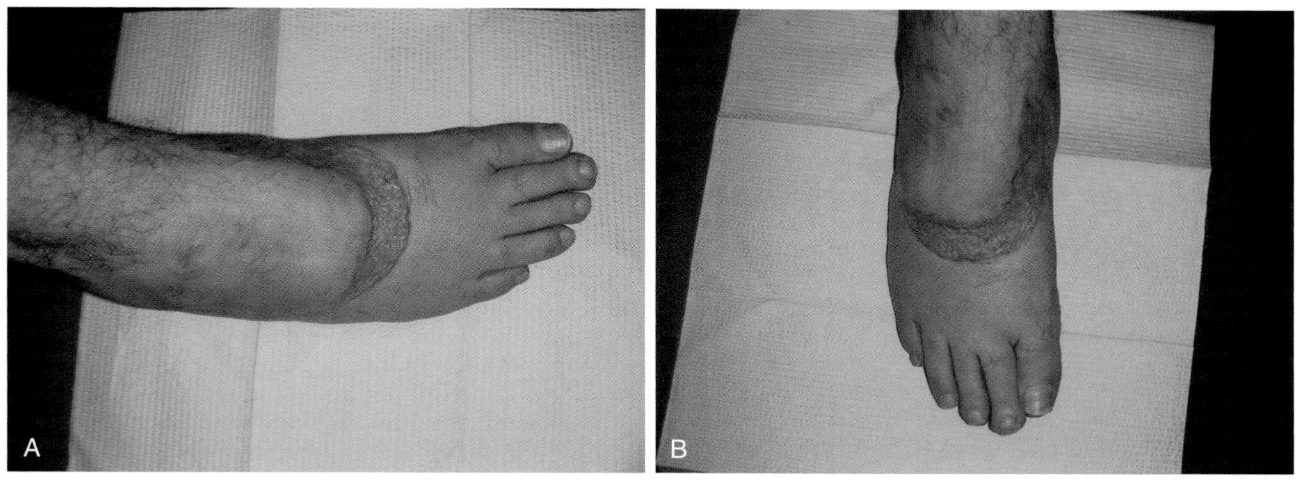

• **Fig. 51.8** (A and B) Results at 6-month follow-up showing the well-healed lateral foot wound with good contour and minimal scarring.

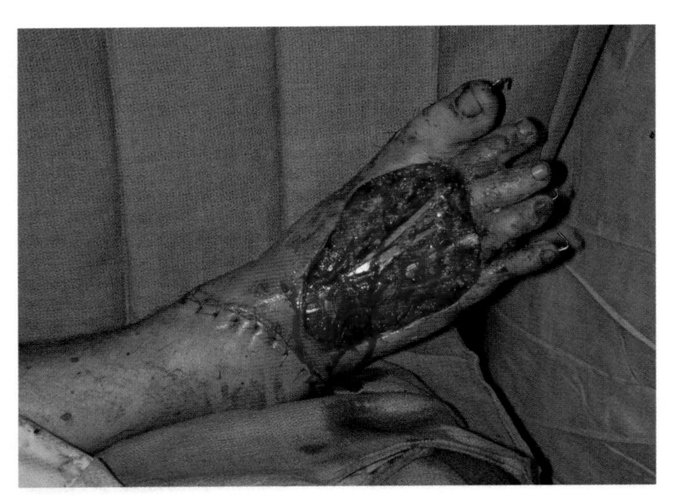

• **Fig. 51.9** A preoperative view showing a large right dorsal foot soft tissue defect, measuring 17 × 10 cm, as a result of a crushing injury. Three necrotic toes were also evidenced.

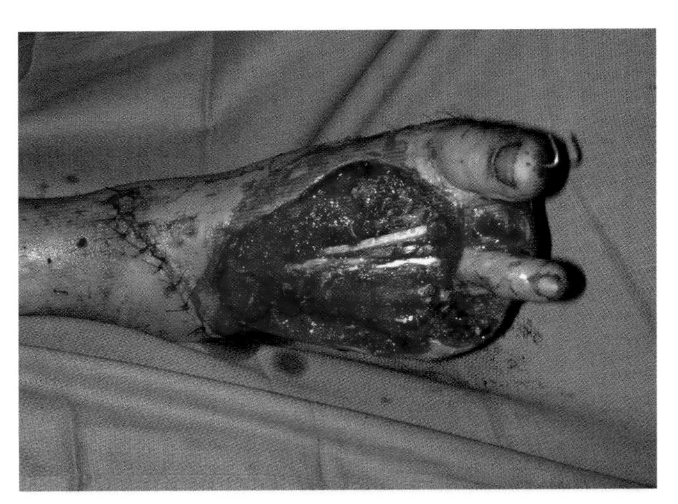

• **Fig. 51.10** An intraoperative view showing the appearance of the dorsal foot wound after a definitive wound debridement and amputation of three necrotic toes.

Operative Plan and Special Considerations

After assessing the soft tissue wound over the dorsum of the right foot, it appeared that the patient would need a large, thin, reliable skin coverage for this complex wound. Because his forearm was relatively large, a free radial forearm skin lap was considered a good option to provide adequate soft tissue reconstruction. The flap is reliable, thin, and versatile and can provide soft tissue coverage with an easy inset. The distal anterior tibial vessels or the dorsalis pedis vessels could serve as recipient vessels as long as they are outside the zone of injury. The foot had a normal vascular anatomy based on the preoperative angiogram. An Allen test was performed to confirm that the left nondominant hand would have adequate blood supply based only on the ulnar artery system.

Operative Procedures

Under general anesthesia, with the patient in the supine position, all unhealthy-looking skin or tissue in the right foot wound was debrided and the wound was irrigated with Pulsavac. Three necrotic toes were amputated by the orthopedic foot and ankle service (Fig. 51.10).

A free radial forearm skin flap was designed on the nondominant left forearm and a 17 × 10 cm skin paddle of the flap, oriented longitudinally, was designed (Fig. 51.11). Under tourniquet control, once the skin incision had been made through the fascia, subfascial dissection was performed for elevation of the skin paddle including the pedicle vessels that also contained the cephalic vein. With proximal zigzag incisions, the dissection of the pedicle in the forearm was made between the flexor carpi radialis muscle and brachioradialis muscle to the antecubital fossa. The radial artery and its venae comitantes as well as the cephalic vein were then divided with hemoclips after the recipient vessels had been dissected free, ready for microvascular anastomoses.

The distal anterior tibial vessels in the foot were explored. An incision was made by extending the dorsal wound proximally. After further dissection, both anterior tibial artery and vein were found to have good caliber and dissected out proximally beyond the foot for an adequate size of the vessels but also outside the zone of the injury. Under a microscope, the arterial microanastomosis was performed between the pedicle and the dorsalis pedis artery in an end-to-end fashion with interrupted 8-0 nylon sutures. The venous microanastomosis was also performed in an end-to-end fashion between the cephalic vein and the dorsalis pedis vein with interrupted 8-0 nylon sutures. After releasing all clamps, the flap appeared to be well perfused with a strong Doppler signal.

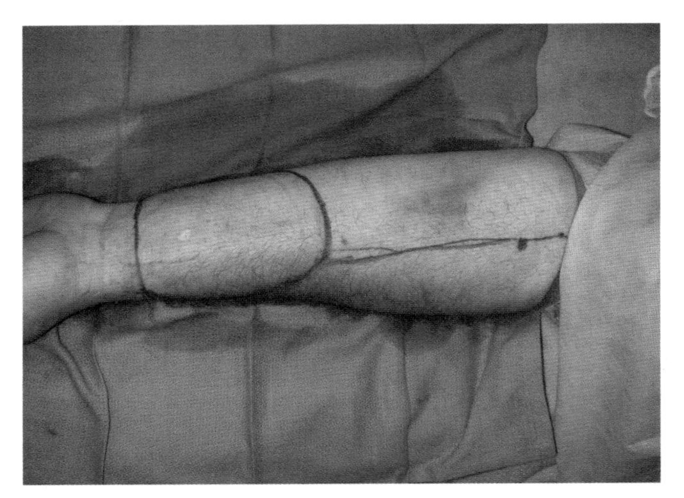

• **Fig. 51.11** An intraoperative view showing the design of the left free radial forearm flap. The radial artery in the forearm was also marked.

The flap inset was performed next. A drain was placed under the flap and the flap was then sutured to the adjacent skin edges of the wound with a 3-0 interrupted Vicryl suture in an interrupted half-buried horizontal mattress fashion. The incision over the pedicle appeared to be too tight and a skin graft was therefore placed over the pedicle for the wound closure (Fig. 51.12).

The forearm donor site skin incision was closed in two layers. A sheet split-thickness skin graft was harvested from the right lateral thigh with a dermatome and placed on the flap donor site and secured with a tie-over dressing.

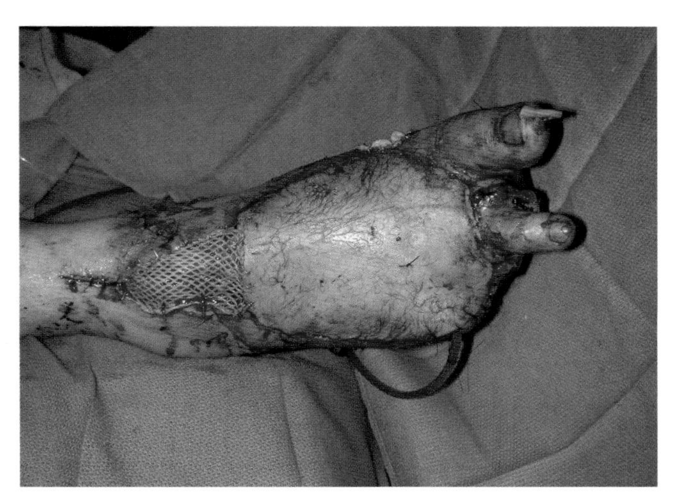

• **Fig. 51.12** An intraoperative view showing the completion of the free radial forearm flap inset and closure of the proximal incision including a skin graft over the pedicle of the flap.

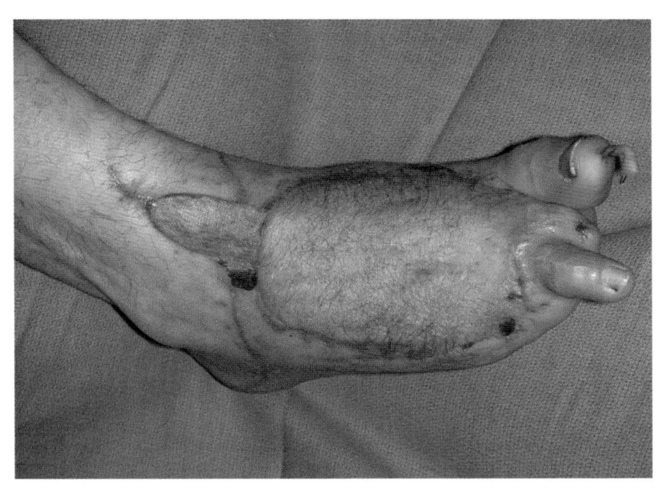

• **Fig. 51.13** Results at 7-week follow-up showing healed flap site and skin graft site.

Follow-Up Results

The patient did well postoperatively without complications related to the free radial forearm flap reconstruction. He was discharged from hospital on postoperative day 7 after tolerating dangling. The drain was removed during the first follow-up visit in 1 week. The right dorsal foot flap reconstruction site (Fig. 51.13) and the left forearm flap donor site healed well.

Final Outcome

During further follow-up, the right dorsal wound after the flap reconstruction continued to heal well (Fig. 51.14). The final contour after the flap reconstruction looked quite good (Fig. 51.15). The patient returned to weight-bearing activities and has been routinely followed by the orthopedic foot and ankle service for his orthopedic care.

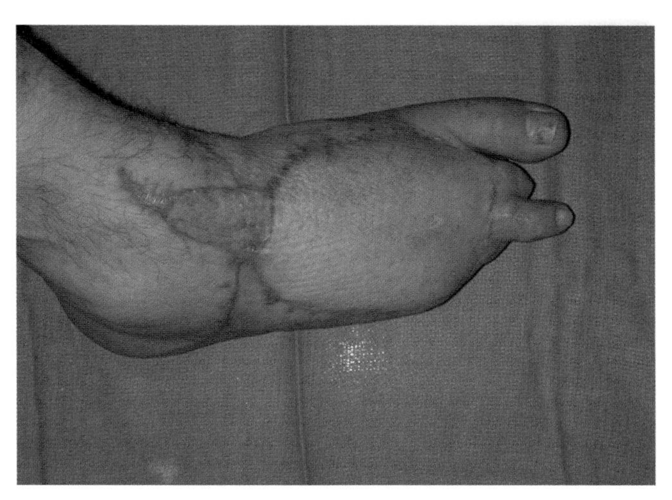

• **Fig. 51.14** Results at 4-month follow-up showing well-healed dorsal foot wound after the flap reconstruction with good contour and minimal scarring.

Pearls for Success

Although other free skin flaps can be an option for the same reconstruction, a free radial forearm skin flap can be an excellent choice for soft tissue reconstruction of a large dorsal foot wound. The flap can be harvested quickly from a nondormant forearm and provide a thin and malleable soft tissue coverage as a fast free tissue transfer. The cephalic vein should be considered a dormant vein and selected for a single venous anastomosis. A subfascial dissection of the flap can preferably be performed to provide a gliding surface over the underlying tendons. The distal anterior tibial vessels can be selected as recipient vessels for an easy end-to-end anastomosis as long as the recipient vessels are outside the zone of the injury. The pedicle of the flap can also be covered with a split-thickness skin graft if the closure of the incision is too tight.

CASE 3

Clinical Presentation

A 30-year-old African-American male sustained a left large dorsal foot wound after a previous orthopedic injury. He was operated on by the orthopedic foot and ankle service for wound debridement and internal fixation of a metatarsal fracture, which left a large open dorsal wound, measuring 15 × 9 cm, with exposed extensor tendons, fracture site, and hardware (Fig. 51.16). He was treated with vacuum-assisted closure therapy. The plastic surgery service was consulted for required soft tissue coverage, as a definitive reconstruction, to the left dorsal foot wound.

Operative Plan and Special Considerations

For this complex dorsal foot wound, a free skin flap, such as a free anterolateral thigh (ALT) perforator flap, was planned because the patient had a very thin layer of soft tissue in the thigh. The flap

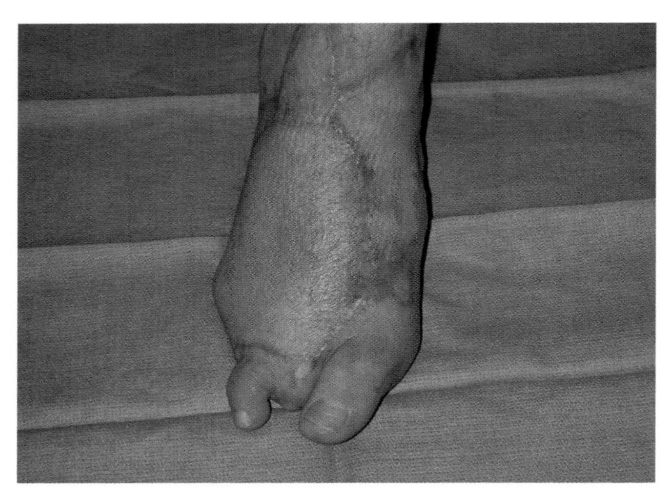

• **Fig. 51.15** Results at 10-month follow-up showing well-healed dorsal foot wound after flap reconstruction with good contour and minimal scarring.

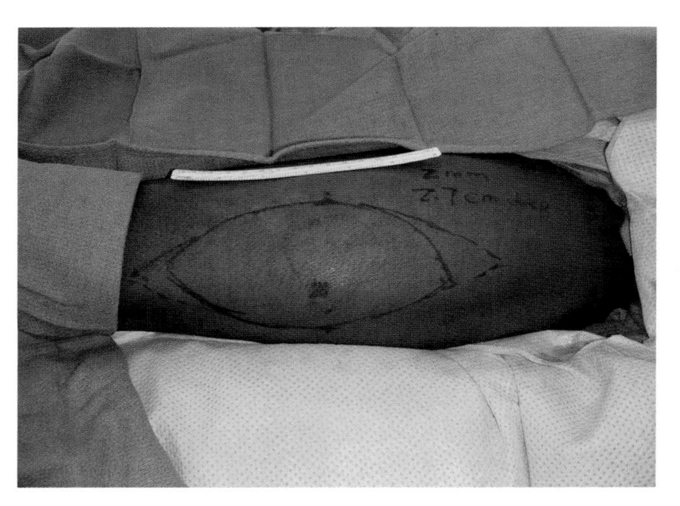

• **Fig. 51.17** An intraoperative view showing the design of the free ALT perforator flap with at least one good perforator that was confirmed by a preoperative duplex scan. The perforator was 2 mm in diameter with good blood flow and 2.7 cm deep from the skin level.

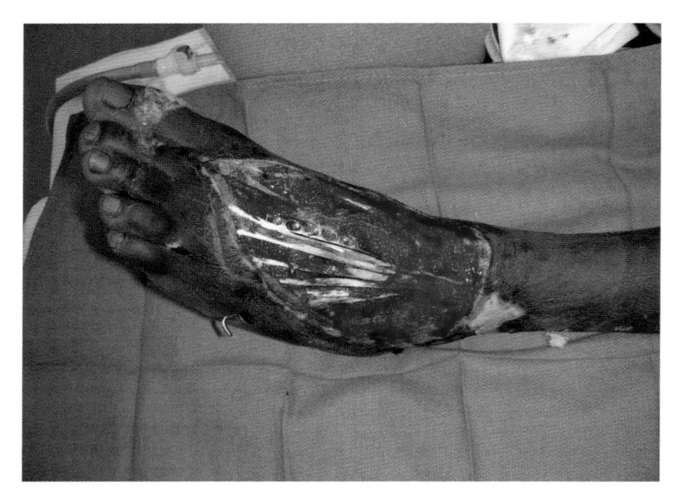

• **Fig. 51.16** A preoperative view showing a large (15 × 9 cm) and complex left dorsal foot wound with exposed extensor tendons, open fracture site, and hardware.

would provide adequate soft tissue reconstruction and good reconstructive outcome. Preoperative mapping of perforators with a duplex scan is performed routinely in the author's practice to determine which side should be selected as the ALT flap donor site. It helps the surgeon tremendously because the size and exact location of the perforator as well as its intramuscular course can be identified. This would make the perforator flap dissection no longer blind. A preoperative CT angiogram showed a normal vascular anatomy of the left leg and foot.

Operative Procedures

Prior to the procedure, a duplex scan identified a single large perforator 2 mm in diameter and about 2.7 cm intramuscular dissection would be anticipated. Under general anesthesia, with the patient in the supine position, the left dorsal foot wound was debrided, the skin edge was freshened, and all the colonized tissues were removed surgically. The wound was irrigated with Pulsavac and appeared to be clean and fresh after definitive debridement.

The left ALT perforator flap with a 15 × 9 cm skin paddle was designed (Fig. 51.17). The skin, subcutaneous tissue, and fascia were incised down to the muscle. The subfascial dissection of the flap was performed until close to the perforator. During dissection, several small perforators were divided because a large perforator had been identified preoperatively and the flap could be based on this single perforator. Once the perforator was clearly visualized, it was dissected free and the intramuscular dissection was performed. By exploring the intramuscular space between the rectus femoris and vastus lateralis muscles, the descending branch of the lateral circumflex femoral vessels (LCFV) was identified. After less than 3 cm intramuscular dissection, the perforator was found to join the descending branch of the LCFV. The descending branch was then divided distally with hemoclips. Further pedicle dissection was performed along with the descending branch in a retrograde fashion until it reached the profunda vessels (Fig. 51.18).

Before dividing the pedicle of the free ALT flap, the distal anterior tibial vessels were explored based on a normal preoperative angiogram. The skin incision was extended from the dorsal foot wound proximally and the anterior tibial vessels were identified in the space between the extensor pollicis longus and anterior tibialis muscle tendons. The anterior tibial artery and vein were dissected free. Both vessels appeared to be a good size and were prepared under loupe magnification for microvascular anastomosis.

The flap was temporarily inset into the defect and secured with small towel clips (Fig. 51.19). Under a microscope, the anterior tibial artery and vein were divided with hemoclips distally and their proximal ends were clamped temporarily with microvascular clamps. The arterial microanastomosis was performed in an end-to-end fashion with interrupted 8-0 nylon sutures. The venous

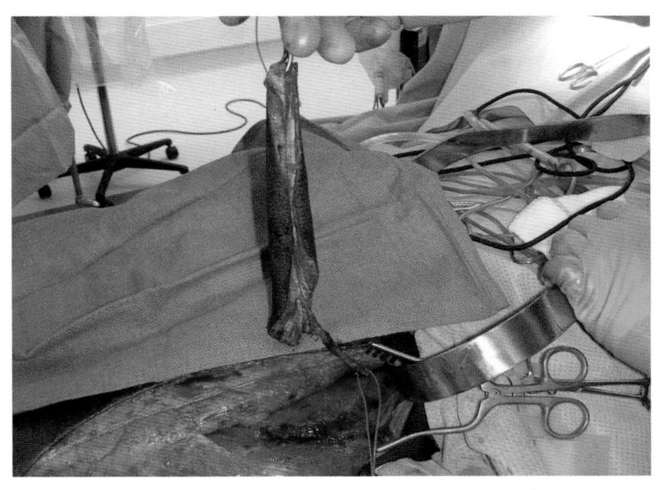

• **Fig. 51.18** An intraoperative view showing the elevated free ALT perforator flap prior to division of the pedicle.

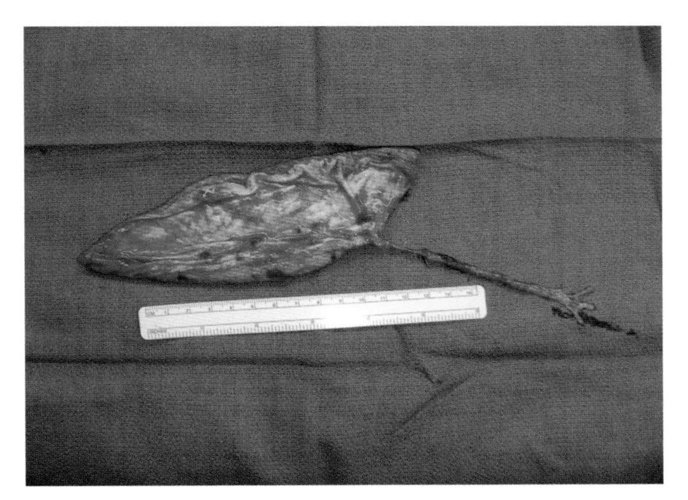

• **Fig. 51.19** An intraoperative view showing completion of the free ALT perforator flap dissection. The flap was elevated with the fascia making a fasciocutaneous flap.

microanastomosis was also performed in an end-to-end fashion but with a 2.5-mm coupler device. After all clamps had been released, the flap appeared to be well perfused with good Doppler signal. However, while placing a Cook Doppler probe, the arterial anastomosis appeared thrombosed. Therefore, the intraoperative decision was made to revise the arterial anastomosis.

The anterior wall of the arterial anastomosis was opened and a small white blood clot was removed manually. The artery was flushed with a heparinized saline solution. The anterior wall of the arterial anastomosis was repaired with two interrupted 8-0 nylon sutures. After the clamps had been released once more, the flap had a good profusion and a strong Doppler signal.

Once the arterial anastomosis appeared to be without problems, the flap inset was performed in two layers. A drain was

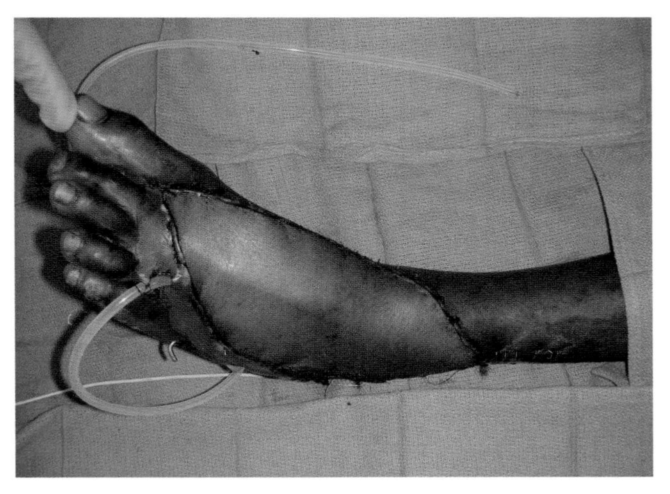

• **Fig. 51.20** An intraoperative view showing completion of the flap inset and closure of the incision used for exploration of the anterior tibial vessels.

inserted under the lateral aspect of the flap away from both anastomoses. The fascial layer was approximated to the adjacent deep tissue with 3-0 interrupted Monocryl sutures. The skin was closed with interrupted 3-0 Monocryl sutures in a half-buried horizontal mattress fashion. A small portion of the foot wound, measuring 6 × 5 cm, was covered with a split-thickness skin graft. The skin graft was harvested from the left anterior thigh with a dermatome, sutured to the skin edges of the wound with 5-0 chromic suture in a simple interrupted fashion. The skin graft was secured with an occlusive dressing. A posterior-based splint was applied at the end of procedure (Fig. 51.20).

The left thigh flap donor site was closed primarily after undermining. The fascial layer was approximated with several interrupted 2-0 PDS sutures. The deep dermal closure was done with interrupted 3-0 Monocryl sutures, followed by 3-0 V-Loc suture for the skin closure in a running subcuticular fashion.

Follow-Up Results

The patient did well postoperatively without any complications related to the free ALT perforator flap reconstruction for the coverage of the dorsal foot wound. He was discharged from hospital on postoperative day 10 after tolerating dangling. All drains were removed during subsequent follow-up visits. The dorsal foot wound flap reconstruction site healed well (Fig. 51.21), as did the left thigh ALT flap donor site (Fig. 51.22).

Final Outcome

The left dorsal foot wound after a free ALT flap reconstruction healed well with good contour and minimal scarring. The metatarsal fracture site also healed. The patient has resumed weight-bearing status and has returned to his normal activities. He has been followed by the orthopedic foot and ankle service for his care.

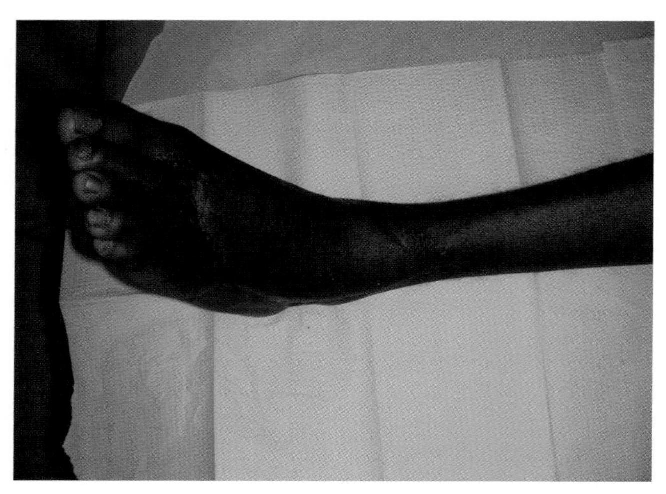

• **Fig. 51.21** Results at 10-week follow-up showing well-healed and stable left dorsal foot wound after free ALT flap reconstruction with good contour and minimal scarring.

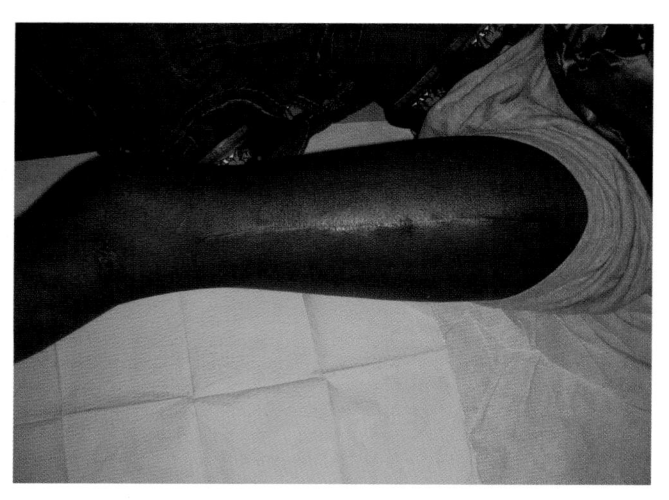

• **Fig. 51.22** Results at 10-week follow-up showing a well-healed flap's donor site in the left thigh.

Pearls for Success

For a large complex dorsal foot wound, a free ALT perforator flap can be a good reconstructive option in a thin patient with good to excellent contour. No flap debulking has been needed. The perforators can be mapped by a preoperative duplex scan and all necessary information including the size and blood flow of each perforator, the course of intramuscular dissection, and the location of the descending branch of the LCFV can be obtained. The flap can be based on either one or two perforators and their dissections would no longer be blind. The distal anterior tibial vessels can be selected as recipient vessels and both microvascular anastomoses, in end-to-end fashion, can be performed without difficulty. The fascial portion of the flap can provide a gliding surface over the extensor tendons and therefore a fasciocutaneous flap should be elevated.

Recommended Readings

Dorfman D, Pu LL. The value of color duplex imaging for planning and performing a free anterolateral thigh perforator flap. *Ann Plast Surg.* 2014;72(suppl 1):S6–S8.

Eubanks RD, Bowker HD, Al-Mufarrej F. Innervated dorsalis pedis advancement flap for burn foot contractures. *J Burn Care Res.* 2020;41:466–471.

Hsu CC, Loh CYY, Wei FC. The anterolateral thigh perforator flap: its expanding role in lower extremity reconstruction. *Clin Plast Surg.* 2021;48:235–248.

Nazerali RS, Pu LL. Free tissue transfer to the lower extremity: a paradigm shift in flap selection for soft tissue reconstruction. *Ann Plast Surg.* 2013;70:419–422.

Wong CH, Lin JY, Wei FC. The bottom-up approach to the suprafascial harvest of the radial forearm flap. *Am J Surg.* 2008;196:e60–e64.

Zeiderman MR, Pu LLQ. Free-style free perforator flaps in lower extremity reconstruction. *Clin Plast Surg.* 2021;48:215–223.

52 Complex Foot Reconstruction

Clinical Presentation

A 35-year-old White male sustained an accidental gunshot wound (GSW) to his left foot. The GSW (12 × 6 × 4 cm) was through-and-through to the medial aspect of the left midfoot with significant soft tissue loss. He also had a comminuted fracture of the first metatarsal with a 5-cm bony defect and complete destruction of the first metatarsophalangeal joint. The extensor hallucis longus tendon was completely destroyed. After initial wound debridement by the orthopedic trauma service, he was taken back to the operating room 2 days later for a second wound debridement by the orthopedic foot and ankle service. The bony stabilization of the first metatarsal was performed with K-wires at that time and the GSW of the left foot open fracture wound was filled with antibiotic beads. The plastic surgery service was consulted for soft tissue coverage of this complex foot wound with composite tissue loss (Fig. 52.1 A and B).

Operative Plan and Special Considerations

For this relatively small but through-and-through composite defect of the foot, a free gracilis muscle flap can be an excellent choice for soft tissue reconstruction. The gracilis muscle is a type II flap. It is a narrow strap-like muscle (24 × 5 × 1.5 cm) with a pedicle length averaging 6 cm. It has become the author's first choice to cover a small or medium-sized defect of the distal third tibial wound or foot. With many advances in surgical technique for flap dissection, the gracilis muscle can be used as a free muscle flap for various reconstructive needs. Its flap dissection can be relatively straightforward and pedicle length and size can be improved by dividing the branches of the medial circumflex femoral vessels to the adductor longus and brevis muscles. In this case, the proximal dorsalis pedis vessels could be dissected and used as recipient vessels for a comfortable and relatively easy end-to-end microvascular anastomosis. About 6 weeks after a free gracilis muscle flap transfer once the foot GSW healed, bone grafts could be performed to achieve fracture union of the first metatarsal.

Operative Procedures

Six days after the initial injury, the patient underwent a free gracilis muscle flap transfer to the left foot wound by the plastic surgery service. Under general anesthesia, with the patient in the supine position, the left foot open fracture wound was debrided. All colonized tissues were removed and the skin edge was freshened with a blade. The wound was irrigated with Pulsavac and looked clean and fresh after definitive wound debridement.

The proximal dorsalis pedis vessels were exposed through a zigzag incision. They were easily dissected free and would act as the recipient vessels. Both the artery and the vein were identified and dissected free under loupe magnification. Each vessel was then wrapped with a vessel loop.

A 20-cm longitudinal incision was made in the medial left thigh along a line between the pubic tubercle and the medial femoral condyle. The skin and subcutaneous tissue were incised and the fascia was opened. Once the anterior board of the gracilis muscle had been identified and dissected free, the adductor longus muscle was retracted laterally to expose the main pedicle vessels. After identifying the main pedicle of the gracilis muscle, all minor pedicles in the distal portion of the muscle were divided. The distal muscle was also divided near the origin. Proximally, the muscle insertion to the pubic tubercle was divided and the muscle dissection was completed. The pedicle dissection was performed under loupe magnification and during its dissection, all small branches were divided with microclips. The branches of the medial circumflex femoral vessels to the adductor longus and brevis were divided, which produced an additional 2 cm of pedicle length with a possible vessel diameter greater than 2.0 mm of the pedicle size. The pedicle vessels were divided with hemoclips from the profunda, ready for free tissue transfer.

The pedicle of the flap was prepared under loupe magnification. The artery and vein were then identified and separated. The artery was flushed with heparinized saline solution. One artery and two veins were prepared for microvascular anastomoses. After further preparation of the pedicle vessels under an operating microscope, the flap was temporarily inset into the through-and-through medial foot wound. Under an operating microscope, an end-to-end arterial microanastomosis was performed between the pedicle and the dorsalis pedis artery with an interrupted 8-0 nylon suture. The venous microanastomosis was performed with a 2.0-mm coupler device in an end-to-end fashion. Once all clamps had been released, the flap appeared to be well perfused with a strong Doppler signal.

The final inset of the flap was performed. A 10-mm flat JP was inserted into the wound under the flap. The muscle flap was placed inside the through-and-through wound and sutured to the adjacent skin edge with interrupted 3-0 Monocryl sutures in a half-buried horizontal mattress fashion. Both microvascular anastomoses were also covered with the flap. A split-thickness skin graft was harvested from the left lateral thigh. The skin graft was meshed to 1:1.5 ratio, placed over the muscle flap, and secured to the adjacent skin with skin staples (Fig. 52.2A and B).

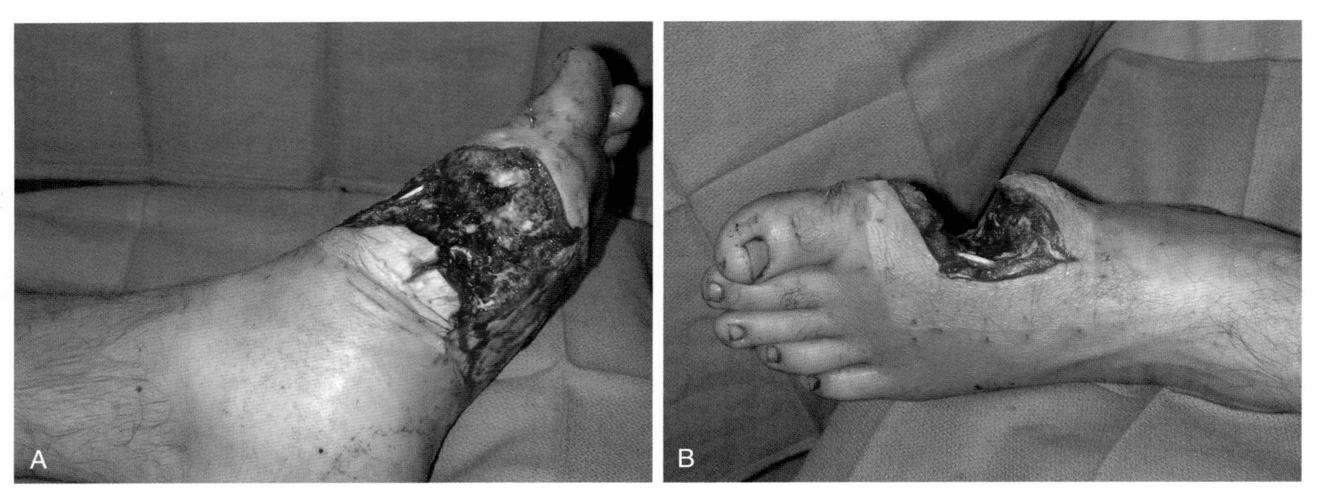

• **Fig. 52.1** (A and B) A preoperative view showing a 14 × 6 × 4 cm composite GSW in the left middle foot associated with a 5-cm gap of the first metatarsal.

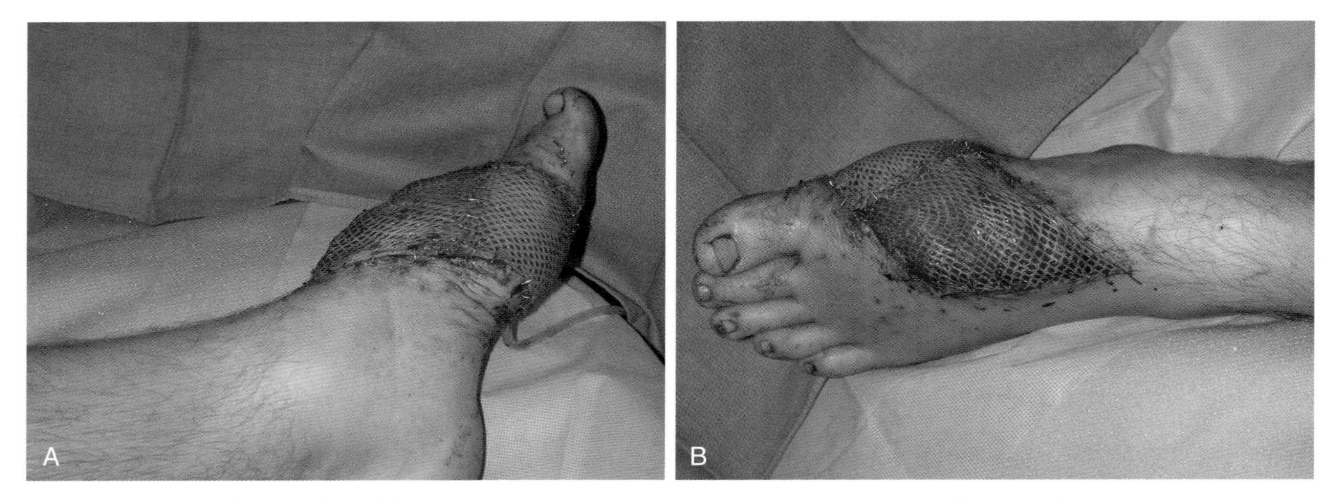

• **Fig. 52.2** (A and B) An intraoperative view showing completion of the free gracilis muscle flap transfer to the left middle foot after successful microvascular anastomoses.

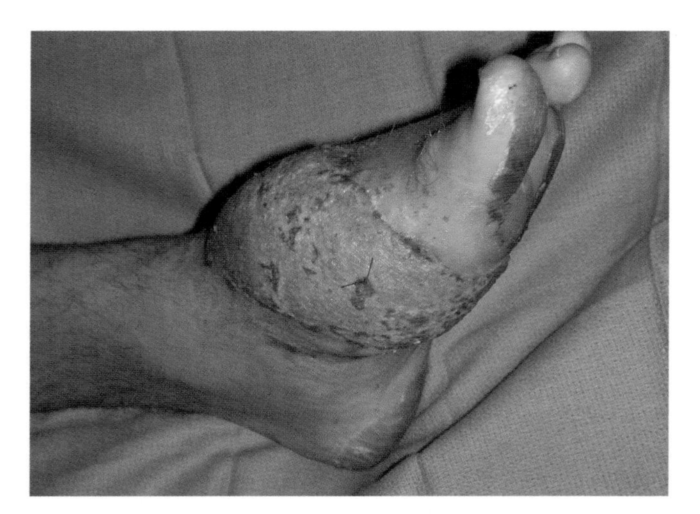

• **Fig. 52.3** The result at 4-week follow-up showing stable and well-healed left middle foot wound after the free gracilis muscle transfer.

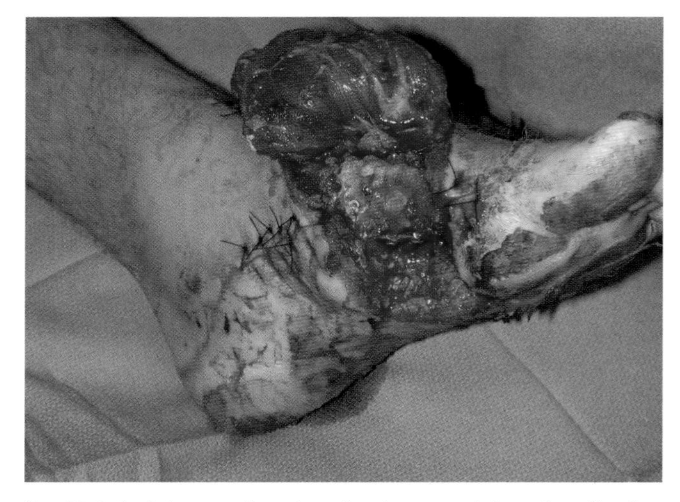

• **Fig. 52.4** An intraoperative view showing completion of an iliac bone graft 6 weeks after elevation of the free gracilis muscle flap.

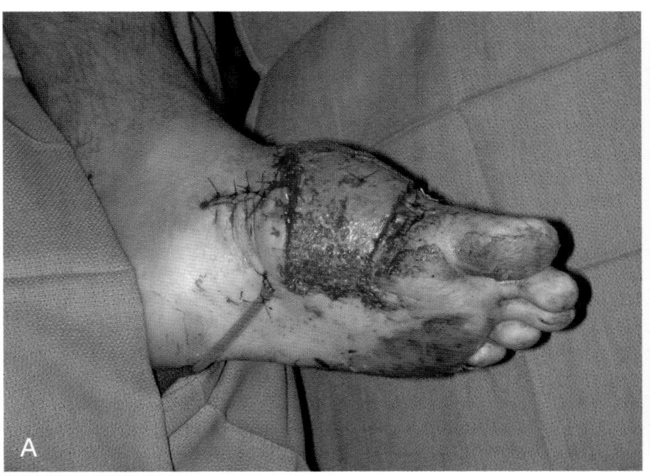

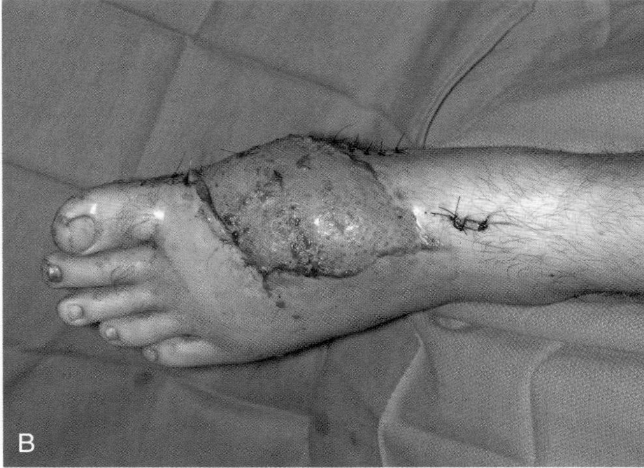

• **Fig. 52.5** (A and B) An intraoperative view showing complete coverage of the bone graft site with the previously elevated free gracilis muscle flap.

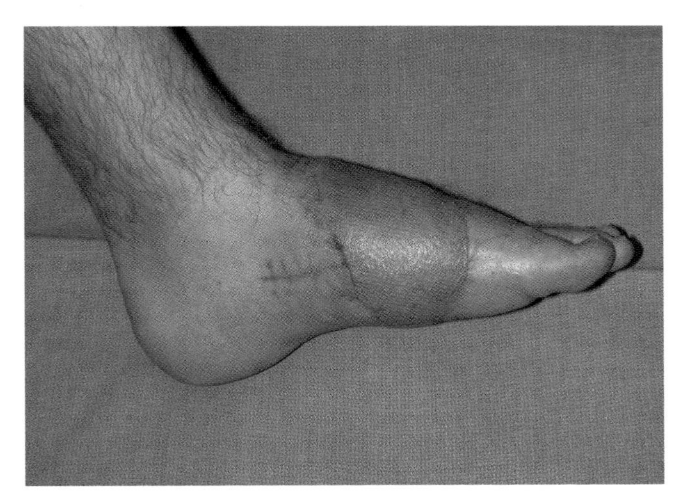

• **Fig. 52.6** The result at 2-month follow-up showing stable and well-healed left middle foot wound after elevation of the free gracilis muscle flap.

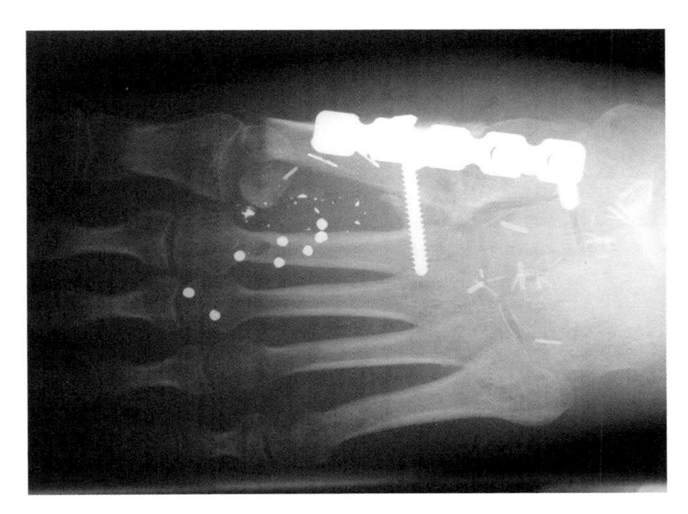

• **Fig. 52.7** An X-ray image at 4-month follow-up showing adequate bony union of the first metatarsal after the bone grafting procedure.

The left thigh gracilis muscle flap donor site was closed in two layers after placing a 10-mm flat JP drain. The deep dermal layer was approximated with interrupted 3-0 Monocryl sutures. The skin incision was closed with skin staples.

Follow-Up Results

The patient did well postoperatively without any complications related to the free gracilis muscle flap transfer for coverage of a through-and-though composite midfoot wound. He was discharged from hospital on postoperative day 6 after tolerating dangling protocol. All drains were removed during subsequent follow-up visits. The left foot GSW wound healed well after the free gracilis muscle flap transfer and the skin graft over the muscle flap also healed well (Fig. 52.3).

Final Outcome

Six weeks after the free gracilis muscle flap reconstruction for a through-and-through GSW of the left foot, the patient underwent an iliac bone graft to the first metatarsal bony gap by the orthopedic foot and ankle service once the flap was elevated by the plastic surgery service (Fig. 52.4). The flap was once again inset into the through-and-through foot wound without any problems (Fig. 52.5A and B). The flap site after elevation and inset healed well (Fig. 52.6). The first metatarsal fracture site achieved bony union after the bone graft procedure (Fig. 52.7). Eventually, the left foot through-and-through GSW wound healed well with good contour and minimal scarring (Fig. 52.8 A and B). The patient has resumed his normal activities and has been routinely followed by the orthopedic foot and ankle service (Fig. 52.9). The left thigh gracilis muscle flap donor also healed well with minimal scarring (Fig. 52.10).

Pearls for Success

A free gracilis muscle flap can be an excellent choice for a through-and-through GSW in the foot where soft tissue coverage should be performed first. The proximal two-thirds of the muscle is reliable based on the dominant pedicle vessels. The size of the flap

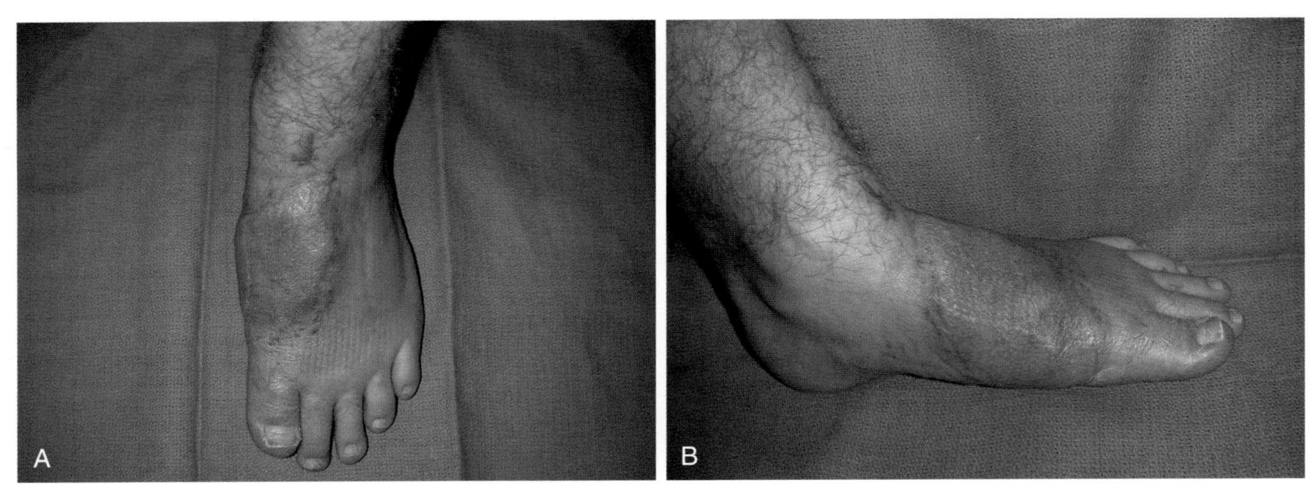

• **Fig. 52.8** (A and B) The result at 7-month follow-up showing stable and well-healed left middle foot wound after elevation of the free gracilis muscle flap.

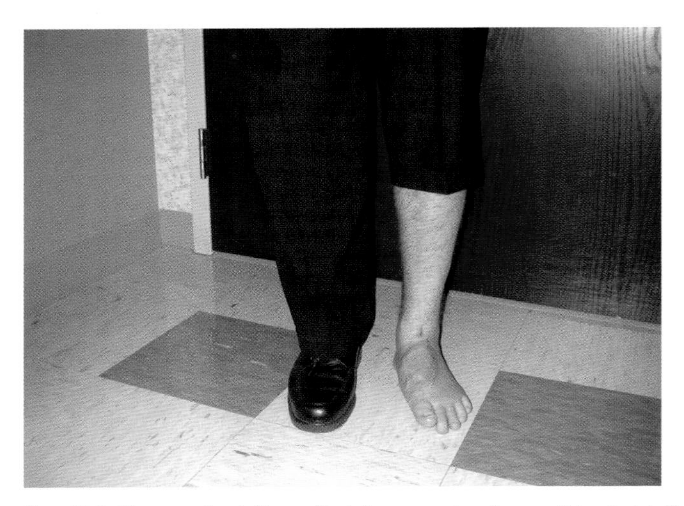

• **Fig. 52.9** The result at 7-month follow-up showing well-healed left middle foot wound after free gracilis muscle transfer with good contour and minimal scarring.

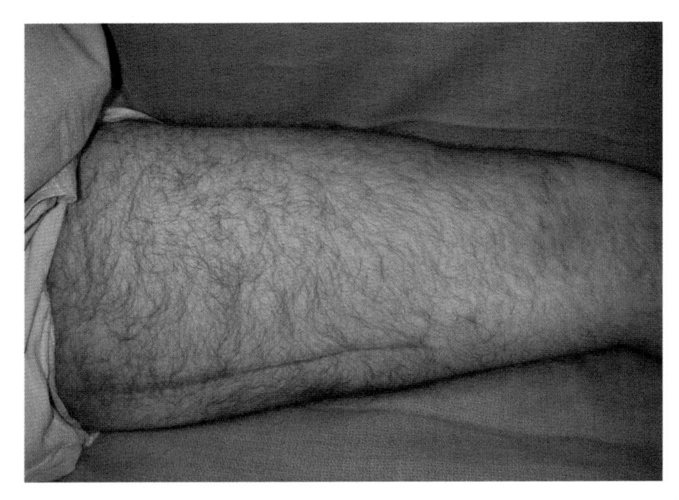

• **Fig. 52.10** The result at 7-month follow-up showing good contour and minimal scarring of the left thigh gracilis muscle flap donor site.

can make it an excellent option to cover the composite foot wound. The muscle can be harvested relatively quickly and has few donor site problems. Its pedicle length and size can be improved by dividing the branches of the medial circumflex femoral vessels to the adductor longus and brevis muscles. It is the author's preference to select the proximal dorsalis pedis vessels as the recipient vessels for the free tissue transfer to the middle foot. The proximity of the recipient vessels to the soft tissue defect and the size of the vessels make an end-to-end microvascular anastomosis less difficult to perform. If a subsequent bony reconstruction of the metatarsal is indicated, the healed free muscle flap can be elevated in 6 weeks and inset into the defect to cover a bone graft and a metal plate after an orthopedic procedure. The free gracilis muscle flap can shrink after 6 months so that the contour can be quite good after such a reconstruction in the foot.

Recommended Readings

Pu LL, Medalie DA, Lawrence SJ, Vasconez HC. Reconstruction of through-and-through gunshot wounds to the feet with free gracilis muscle flaps. *Ann Plast Surg*. 2003;50:286−291.

Pu LLQ. Free flaps in lower extremity reconstruction. *Clin Plast Surg*. 2021;48:201−214.

Redett RJ, Robertson BC, Chang B, Girotto J, Vaughan T. Limb salvage of lower-extremity wounds using free gracilis muscle reconstruction. *Plast Reconstr Surg*. 2000;106:1507−1513.

Wang CY, Han P, Chai YM, Lu SD, Zhong WR. Pedicled fibular flap for reconstruction of composite defects in foot. *Injury*. 2015;46: 405−410.

Index

Page number followed by "*f*" indicates figures.